D1458521

Human Genome
Epidemiology

HUMAN GENOME EPIDEMIOLOGY

Second Edition

Building the Evidence for Using Genetic Information to Improve Health and Prevent Disease

Edited by

MUIN J. KHOURY

SARA R. BEDROSIAN

MARTA GWINN

JULIAN P. T. HIGGINS

JOHN P. A. IOANNIDIS

JULIAN LITTLE

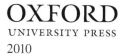

UNIVERSITY PRESS

2010

OXFORD
UNIVERSITY PRESS

Oxford University Press, Inc., publishes works that further
Oxford University's objective of excellence
in research, scholarship, and education.

Oxford New York
Auckland Cape Town Dar es Salaam Hong Kong Karachi
Kuala Lumpur Madrid Melbourne Mexico City Nairobi
New Delhi Shanghai Taipei Toronto

With offices in
Argentina Austria Brazil Chile Czech Republic France Greece
Guatemala Hungary Italy Japan Poland Portugal Singapore
South Korea Switzerland Thailand Turkey Ukraine Vietnam

Library of Congress Cataloging-in-Publication Data
Human genome epidemiology : building the evidence for using genetic information to improve health and prevent
disease / edited by Muin J. Khoury ... [et al.]. — 2nd ed.
p. ; cm.
Includes bibliographical references and index.
ISBN 978-0-19-539844-1
1. Genetic disorders—Epidemiology. 2. Medical genetics—Methodology. 3. Genomics. I. Khoury, Muin J.
[DNLM: 1. Genetics, Medical—methods. 2. Genetic Diseases, Inborn—epidemiology. 3. Genetic
Predisposition to Disease—epidemiology. 4. Genetic Screening. 5. Genome, Human. 6. Genomics.
QZ 50 H91674 2010]
RB155.5.H86 2010
616'.042—dc22
2009018899

Preface

In the first edition of *Human Genome Epidemiology* published in 2004, we discussed how the epidemiologic approach provides an important scientific foundation for studying the continuum from gene discovery to the development, applications, and evaluation of human genome information in improving health and preventing disease. Since 2004, advances in human genomics have continued to occur at a breathtaking pace. Although the concept of personalized healthcare and disease prevention often promised by enthusiastic scientists and the media is yet to be fulfilled, we are now seeing progress and rapid accumulation of data in many "omics" related research fields. New methods to measure genome variation on an unprecedented large scale have propelled a new generation of genome-wide association studies. Evaluation of rare variants and full sequencing at large-scale are rapidly becoming a reality. Also, we have seen the emergence of population-based biobanks in many countries with the objectives of quantifying longitudinally the joint influences of genetic and environmental factors on the occurrence of common diseases.

With all these ongoing developments, we have invited many authors who are leaders in the field to produce the second edition of *Human Genome Epidemiology*. Our aim is to inform readers of new developments in the genomics field and how epidemiologic methods are being used to make sense of this information. We do realize that the material presented in this book will be outdated even before it is published. However, the methodologic challenges and possible solutions to them will remain with us for quite some time. There is very little material remaining from the first edition of *Human Genome Epidemiology*.

This new edition is divided into five parts. In Part I, we revisit the fundamentals of human genome epidemiology. We first give an overview of the development and progress in applications of genomic technologies with a focus on genomic sequence variation (Chapter 2). We then give an overview of the multidisciplinary field of public health genomics that includes a fundamental role of epidemiologic methods and approaches (Chapter 3). We also present a brief overview of evolving methods for tracking and compiling information on genetic factors in disease (Chapter 4).

In Part II, we discuss methodologic developments in collection, analysis, and synthesis of data from human genome epidemiologic studies. We discuss the emergence of biobanks around the world (Chapter 5), the evolution of case-control studies and cohort studies in the era of GWAS (Chapter 6), and the emerging role of consortia and networks (Chapter 7). Next, we discuss methodologic analytic issues in GWAS (Chapter 8) and the analytic challenges of gene-gene and gene-environment interaction (Chapter 9). We then address issues of reporting of genetic associations

(Chapter 10), evolving methods for integrating the evidence (Chapter 11) as well as assessment of cumulative evidence and field synopses (Chapter 12).

In Part III, we provide several case studies that attempt to present an evolving knowledge base of the cumulative evidence on genetic variation in a variety of human diseases. As the information undoubtedly will change (even before the publication of the book), we stress here the importance of strong methodologic foundation for analysis and synthesis of information from various studies. The diseases shown in this section include three cancers: colorectal cancer (Chapter 13), childhood leukemia (Chapter 14), and bladder cancer (Chapter 15). We also present data from type 2 diabetes (Chapter 16), osteoporosis (Chapter 17), preterm birth (Chapter 18), coronary heart disease (Chapter 19), and schizophrenia (Chapter 20). Collectively, these chapters cover an impressive array of common complex human diseases and provide an epidemiologic approach to rapidly emerging data on gene-disease and gene-environment interactions.

In Part IV, we discuss methodologic issues surrounding specific applications of human genomic information for medicine and public health. We start in Chapter 21 with a review of the concept of Mendelian Randomization, an approach that allows us to assess the role of environmental factors and other biomarkers in the occurrence of human diseases using data on the association of genetic variation and disease endpoints. In Chapter 22, we discuss how clinical epidemiologic concepts and methods can be used to assess whether or not one or more genetic variants (e.g., genome profiles) can be used to predict risk for human diseases. Chapter 23 presents a major milestone for public health genomics, namely the publication of methods of systematic review and assessment of the clinical validity and utility of genomic applications in clinical practice. This chapter is a reprint of the published paper from the independent multidisciplinary panel, the EGAPP working group, supported by CDC and many partners. Chapter 24 briefly summarizes how reviews of the evidence on validity and utility of genomic information can be done systematically and rapidly, even in the face of incomplete information. Chapter 25 focuses on the crucial role of the behavioral and social sciences in assessing the impact and value of epidemiologic information on gene-disease associations. Chapter 26 addresses issues in evaluating developments in newborn screening. Chapter 27 provides an epidemiologic framework for the evaluation of pharmacogenomic applications in clinical and public health practice. Chapter 28 presents an overview of the relevance and impact of epigenomics in clinical practice and disease prevention. Finally, chapter 29 presents an epidemiologic framework for evaluating family health history as a tool for disease prevention and health promotion. Even in this genomics era, family history remains a strong foundation, not only for identifying single gene disorders, but also for stratifying individuals and populations by different levels of disease risk and implementing personalized interventions.

Finally, in Part V of the book, we present a few case studies of the application of epidemiologic methods of assessment of clinical validity and utility for several disease examples. These include two pharmacogenomic testing examples—initial treatment of depression with SSRIs (Chapter 30) and warfarin therapy (Chapter 31). We also present information on population screening for hereditary hemochromatosis (Chapter 32), a genetic disorder with incomplete penetrance that has attracted some attention over the past decade as a possible example of population screening in the genomics era.

The second edition of *Human Genome Epidemiology* is primarily targeted to basic, clinical, and population scientists involved in studying genetic factors in common diseases. In addition, the book focuses on practical applications of human genome variation in clinical practice and disease prevention. We hope that students, clinicians, public health professionals, and policy makers will find the book useful in learning about evolving epidemiologic methods for approaching the discovery and the use of genetic information in medicine and public health in the twenty-first century.

Atlanta	MJK, SB, MG
Cambridge	JH
Ioannina	JI
Ottawa	JL
2009	

Acknowledgments

We are grateful to the following individuals for reviewing drafts of selected book chapters:

Louise Acheson
Betsy Anagnostelis
Melissa Austin
Wylie Burke
Melinda Clyne
Rajvir Dahiya
W. David Dotson
Michael P. Douglas
Nicole Dowling
Jennifer L. Flome
Sara Giordano
Ridgely Fisk Green
Scott Grosse
Daurice A. Grossniklaus
Idris Guessous
Jennifer Harris
Steve Hawken
Terri Jackson
Candice Y. Johnson
Fontini Kavvoura
Katherine Kolor
Ruth Loos
Denise Lowe
Stephanie Melillo
Melanie Myers
Renée M. Ned
Nikolaos Patsopoulos
Paul Pharoah
Margaret Piper
Beth Potter
Jessica L. Rowell
Simon Sanderson
Linda Sharp
Camilla Stoltenberg

John Thompson
Rodolfo Valdez
Jan Vandenbroucke
David Veenstra
Bridget Wilcken
Lauren E. Williams
Quanhe Yang
Ajay Yesupriya
Wei Yu

Contents

PART III   Case Studies: Cumulative Assessment of the Role of Human Genome Variation in Specific Diseases

PART IV   Applications of Epidemiologic Methods for Using Genetic Information in Medicine and Public Health

PART V   Case Studies: Assessing the Use of Genetic Information in Practice for Specific Diseases

Contributors

SARA R. BEDROSIAN, BA, BFA
McKing Consulting Corporation
Office of Public Health Genomics
Centers for Disease Control and
    Prevention
Atlanta, GA

ALFRED O. BERG, MD, MPH
Department of Family Medicine
University of Washington
Seattle, WA

JONINE L. BERNSTEIN, PhD
Department of Epidemiology and
    Biostatistics
Memorial Sloan-Kettering Cancer Center
New York, NY

LARS BERTRAM, MD
Max-Planck Institute for Molecular Genetics
Berlin, Germany

NICK BIRKETT, MD, MSc
Department of Epidemiology and
    Community Medicine
University of Ottawa
Ottawa, ON, Canada

PAOLO BOFFETTA, MD
International Agency for Research on
    Cancer
Lyon, France

MELISSA L. BONDY, PhD
Department of Epidemiology
University of Texas
M.D. Anderson Cancer Center
Houston, TX

LINDA A. BRADLEY, PhD
Women & Infants Hospital
Department of Pathology and
    Laboratory Medicine
The Warren Alpert Medical School of
    Brown University
Providence, RI

MOLLY S. BRAY, PhD
Center for Human Genetics
Institute of Molecular Medicine and
    School of Public Health
University of Texas
Houston, TX

PAUL E. BRENCHLEY, PhD
Renal Research Laboratories
Manchester Institute of Nephrology and
    Transplantation
Royal Infirmary
Manchester, United Kingdom

PHILIPPA BRICE, PhD
Foundation for Genomics and
    Population Health (PHG Foundation)
Cambridge, United Kingdom

PATRICIA A. BUFFLER,
PhD, MPH
Division of Epidemiology
University of California
Berkeley School of Public Health
Berkeley, CA

PAUL R. BURTON, MD
Department of Health Sciences
University of Leicester
Leicester, United Kingdom

ADAM S. BUTTERWORTH,
MSc, PhD
*Department of Public Health and
    Primary Care
University of Cambridge
Cambridge, United Kingdom
and
UK HuGENet Coordinating Centre
Cambridge, United Kingdom*

NED CALONGE, MD, MPH
*Colorado Department of Public Health
    and Environment
Denver, CO*

HARRY CAMPBELL, MD, FRCP,
FFPH, FRSE
*Public Health Sciences
College of Medicine and Vet Medicine
University of Edinburgh
Edinburgh, United Kingdom*

JUAN PABLO CASAS, MD
*Department of Epidemiology and
    Population Health
London School of Hygiene and Tropical
    Medicine
London, United Kingdom*

STEPHEN J. CHANOCK, MD
*Laboratory of Translational Genomics
Division of Cancer Epidemiology and
    Genetics
National Cancer Institute, National
    Institutes of Health
Bethesda, MD*

ANAND P. CHOKKALINGAM,
PhD, MS
*Division of Epidemiology
School of Public Health
University of California at Berkeley
Berkeley, CA*

BARBARA COHEN, PhD
*Former Senior Editor
Public Library of Science
San Francisco, CA*

JOHN DANESH, MD, MBChB,
MSc, DPhil, FRCP
*Department of Public Health and
    Primary Care
University of Cambridge
Cambridge, United Kingdom*

GEORGE DAVEY SMITH, MD,
DSc, FRCP, F MED SCI
*MRC Centre for Causal Analyses in
    Translational Epidemiology
Department of Social Medicine
University of Bristol
Bristol, United Kingdom*

ALEX DEMARSH, MSc
*Department of Epidemiology and
    Community Medicine
University of Ottawa
Ottawa, ON, Canada*

SIOBHAN M. DOLAN, MD, MPH
*Albert Einstein College of Medicine
Montefiore Medical Center
Bronx, NY*

W. DAVID DOTSON, PhD
*Office of Public Health Genomics
Centers for Disease Control and
    Prevention
Atlanta, GA*

MICHAEL P. DOUGLAS, MS
*McKing Consulting Corporation
Office of Public Health Genomics
Centers for Disease Control and
    Prevention
Atlanta, GA*

CORNELIA M. VAN DUIJN, PhD
Department of Epidemiology
Erasmus University Medical Center
Rotterdam, The Netherlands

ROSS DUNCAN, PhD, MA
Department of Dermatology
Leiden University Medical Center
Leiden, The Netherlands

SHAH EBRAHIM, MSc, DM,
FRCP, FFPHM
London School of Hygiene and Tropical
  Medicine
London, United Kingdom

ERIK VON ELM, MD, MSc
Institute of Social and Preventive
  Medicine
University of Bern
Bern, Switzerland
and
German Cochrane Centre
Department of Medical Biometry and
  Medical Informatics
University Medical Centre
Freiburg, Germany

JONINE D. FIGUEROA, PhD,
MPH
Division of Cancer Epidemiology and
  Genetics
National Cancer Institute
Department of Health and Human
  Services
Bethesda, MD

ISABEL FORTIER, PhD
Public Population Project in Genomics
Montreal, QC, Canada
and
Department of Social and Preventive
  Medicine
University of Montreal
Montreal, QC, Canada

MATTHEW FREEDMAN, MD
Dana-Farber Cancer Institute
Boston, MA

HELENA FURBERG, PhD
University of North Carolina at Chapel
  Hill
Chapel Hill, NC

FRANCE GAGNON, MSc, PhD
University of Toronto
Dalla Lana School of Public Health
Toronto, ON, Canada

MONTSERRAT GARCIA-CLOSAS,
MD, MPH, DrPH
Division of Cancer Epidemiology and
  Genetics
National Cancer Institute
Bethesda, MD

JEAN GOLDING, PhD, DSc,
FMEDSCI
Paediatric and Perinatal Epidemiology
Bristol, United Kingdom

JESUS GONZALEZ-BOSQUET,
MD, PhD
Laboratory of Translational Genomics
Division of Cancer Epidemiology and
  Genetics
National Cancer Institute, National
  Institutes of Health
Bethesda, MD

JEREMY GRIMSHAW, MBChB,
PhD, FRCGP
Canada Research Chair in Health
  Knowledge Transfer and Uptake
Clinical Epidemiology Program
Ottawa Health Research Institute
Department of Medicine
University of Ottawa
Ottawa, ON, Canada

SCOTT D. GROSSE, PhD
National Center on Birth Defects and
  Developmental Disabilities
Centers for Disease Control and
  Prevention
Atlanta, GA

IRIS GROSSMAN, PhD
Pharmacogenetics Consulting
Cabernet Pharmaceuticals
Durham, NC

NELLEKE A. GRUIS, PhD
Harvard School of Public Health
Boston, MA

JAMES M. GUDGEON, MS, MBA
Intermountain Healthcare
Clinical Genetics Institute
Salt Lake City, UT

MARTA GWINN, MD, MPH
Office of Public Health Genomics
Centers for Disease Control and
  Prevention
Atlanta, GA

JAMES E. HADDOW, MD
Department of Pathology and
  Laboratory Medicine
Brown University, Alpert Medical School
Providence, RI

MIA HASHIBE, PhD
Gene–Environment Epidemiology Group
International Agency for Research on
  Cancer
Lyon, France

STEVEN HAWKEN, MSc
Department of Epidemiology and
  Community Medicine
University of Ottawa
Ottawa, ON, Canada

JULIAN P. T. HIGGINS, PhD
MRC Biostatistics Unit
Institute of Public Health
Cambridge, United Kingdom

DAVID J. HUNTER, MBBS, ScD
Program in Molecular and Genetic
  Epidemiology
Departments of Epidemiology and
  Nutrition
Harvard School of Public Health
Boston, MA

KIMBERLEY HUTCHINGS, MSc
Department of Epidemiology and
  Community Medicine
University of Ottawa
Ottawa, ON, Canada

CLAIRE INFANTE-RIVARD,
MD, PhD
Department of Epidemiology,
  Biostatistics, and Occupational Health
Faculty of Medicine
McGill University
Montreal, QC, Canada

JOHN P. A. IOANNIDIS, MD, PhD
Clinical and Molecular Epidemiology
  Unit
Department of Hygiene and
  Epidemiology
School of Medicine and Biomedical
  Research Institute
Foundation for Research and
  Technology-Hellas
University of Ioannina
Ioannina, Greece
and
Center for Genetic Epidemiology and
  Modeling
Department of Medicine
Tufts University School of Medicine
Boston, MA

A. CECILE J. W. JANSSENS, PhD
Department of Epidemiology
Erasmus University Medical Center
Rotterdam, The Netherlands

MARJO-RIITTA JARVELIN, MD, MSc, PhD
Department of Epidemiology and Public
*   Health*
Imperial College
London, United Kingdom
and
Department of Public Health Science and
*   General Practice*
University of Oulu
Oulu, Finland

CANDICE Y. JOHNSON, MSc
Department of Epidemiology and
*   Community Medicine*
University of Ottawa
Ottawa, ON, Canada

MUIN J. KHOURY, MD, PhD
Office of Public Health Genomics
*   Centers for Disease Control and*
*   Prevention*
Atlanta, GA
and
Division of Cancer Control and
*   Population Sciences*
National Cancer Institute
Bethesda, MD

RICHARD A. KING, MD
Genetics in Medicine
Minneapolis, MN

BARTHA M. KNOPPERS, PhD, O.C.
Centre of Genomics and Policy
Department of Human Genetics
McGill University
Montreal, QC

PETER KRAFT, PhD
Department of Epidemiology and
*   Biostatistics*
Program in Molecular and Genetic
*   Epidemiology*
Harvard School of Public Health
Boston, MA

JULIAN LITTLE, PhD
Canada Research Chair in Human
*   Genome Epidemiology*
Department of Epidemiology and
*   Community Medicine*
University of Ottawa
Ottawa, ON, Canada

BEATRICE MALMER, MD, PhD
Department of Radiation Sciences
Oncology
Umea University Hospital
Umea, Sweden

TERI MANOLIO, MD, PhD
Office of Population Genomics
National Human Genome Research
*   Institute*
Bethesda, MD

DEMETRIUS M. MARAGANORE, MD
Department of Neurology
Mayo Clinic
Rochester, MN

LINDSEY MASSON, PhD, MSc, BSc, RPHNUTR
Department of Public Health
University of Aberdeen
Aberdeen, Scotland, United Kingdom

DAVID B. MATCHAR, MD
Duke Center for Clinical Health Policy
  Research
Durham, NC
and
Department of Veterans Affairs Medical
  Center
Durham, NC
and
Duke-NUS Graduate Medical School
  Program in Health Services Research
Singapore

COLLEEN M. McBRIDE, PhD
Social and Behavioral Research Branch
National Human Genome Research
  Institute
Washington, DC

MARK I. McCARTHY, MD, FRCP, FMedSci
Oxford Centre for Diabetes,
  Endocrinology and Metabolism
University of Oxford
Oxford, United Kingdom
and
Wellcome Trust Centre for Human
  Genetics
University of Oxford
Oxford, United Kingdom
and
Oxford NIHR Biomedical Research
  Centre
Churchill Hospital
Oxford, United Kingdom

MONICA R. McCLAIN, PhD
Division of Medical Screening
Women & Infants Hospital
Providence, RI

JOHN McLAUGHLIN, PhD
Population Studies and Surveillance
Cancer Care Ontario
Toronto, ON, Canada
and
Prosserman Centre for Health Research
  at the Samuel Lunenfeld Research
  Institute
Toronto, ON, Canada

JOYCE B. J. VAN MEURS, PhD
Department of Internal Medicine
Erasmus MC
Rotterdam, The Netherlands

DAVID MOHER, PhD
Department of Epidemiology and
  Community Medicine
University of Ottawa
Ottawa, ON, Canada

JULIA A. NEWTON-BISHOP, PhD
Genetic Epidemiology Division
CR-UK Clinical Centre
Leeds, United Kingdom

THOMAS R. O'BRIEN, MD, MPH
Division of Cancer Epidemiology and
  Genetics
National Cancer Institute
Rockville, MD

JAMES M. OSTELL, PhD
Information Engineering Branch
National Center for Biotechnology
  Information
National Library of Medicine, NIH
Bethesda, MD

RYAN P. OWEN, PhD
PharmGKB
Genetics Department
Stanford University
Stanford, CA

ROBERTA A. PAGON, MD
*University of Washington
School of Medicine
Seattle, WA*

GLENN E. PALOMAKI, BS
*Department of Pathology and
    Laboratory Medicine
Brown University, Alpert
    Medical School
Providence, RI*

ANDREW PATERSON, MD
*Genetics of Complex Diseases
Hospital for Sick Children (SickKids)
Toronto, ON, Canada*

DIANA B. PETITTI,
MD, MPH
*Department of Biomedical
    Informatics
Arizona State University
Phoenix, AZ*

MARGARET PIPER, PhD
*Blue Cross Blue Shield Association
    Technology Evaluation Center
Chicago, IL*

TIMOTHY R. REBBECK, PhD
*Center for Clinical Epidemiology and
    Biostatistics
School of Medicine
University of Pennsylvania
Philadelphia, PA*

ELIO RIBOLI, PhD
*International Agency for
    Research on Cancer
Lyon, France
and
Imperial College
London, United Kingdom*

FERNANDO RIVADENEIRA, MD,
PhD
*Departments of Internal Medicine and
    Epidemiology
Erasmus MC
Rotterdam, The Netherlands*

NATHANIEL ROTHMAN, MD,
MPH, MHS
*Division of Cancer Epidemiology and
    Genetics
National Cancer Institute
Bethesda, MD*

GEORGIA SALANTI, PhD
*School of Medicine and Biomedical
    Research Institute
University of Ioannina
Ioannina, Greece*

NADEEM SARWAR, MPHIL, PhD
*Department of Public Health and
    Primary Care
University of Cambridge
Cambridge, United Kingdom*

SASKIA C. SANDERSON, PhD
*Genetics and Genomic Sciences
Mount Sinai School of Medicine
New York, NY*

PAUL SCHEET, PhD
*MD Anderson Cancer Center
Department of Epidemiology
University of Texas
Houston, TX*

DANIELA SEMINARA, PhD,
MPH
*Epidemiology and Genetics Research
    Program
Division of Cancer Control and
    Population Sciences
National Cancer Institute, NIH
Bethesda, MD*

LINDA SHARP, PhD
National Cancer Registry (NCR)
Cork, Ireland, United Kingdom

ALEXANDRE STEWART, PhD,
BScH, MSc
University of Ottawa Heart Institute
Ottawa, ON, Canada

EMANUELA TAIOLI, MD, PhD
University of Pittsburgh Cancer Institute
University of Pittsburgh Medical Center
Pittsburgh, PA

VALERIE TAIT, PhD
Department of Epidemiology and
   Community Medicine
University of Ottawa
Ottawa, ON, Canada

STEVEN M. TEUTSCH, MD,
MPH
Los Angeles County Department of
   Public Health
Los Angeles, CA

MUGDHA THAKUR, MD
Department of Psychiatry and
   Behavioral Sciences
Duke University Medical Center
Durham, NC

EVROPI THEODORATOU, PhD
Public Health Sciences
University of Edinburgh
Edinburgh, Scotland, United Kingdom

DUNCAN C. THOMAS, PhD
Biostatistics Division
Verna Richter Chair in Cancer Research
Department of Preventive Medicine
University of Southern California
Los Angeles, CA

NIC TIMPSON, PhD
Department of Social Medicine
University of Bristol
Bristol, United Kingdom

ANDRÉ G. UITTERLINDEN, PhD
Departments of Internal Medicine and
   Epidemiology
Erasmus MC
Rotterdam, The Netherlands

RODOLFO VALDEZ, PhD, MSc
Office of Public Health Genomics
Centers for Disease Control and
   Prevention
Atlanta, GA

DAVID L. VEENSTRA, PhD,
PharmD
Pharmaceutical Outcomes Research
   and Policy Program, and Institute for
   Public Health Genetics
University of Washington
Seattle, WA

MUKESH VERMA, PhD
Methods and Technologies Branch
Epidemiology and Genetics Research
   Program
Division of Cancer Control and
   Population Sciences
National Cancer Institute (NCI)
National Institutes of Health (NIH)
Bethesda, MD

PAOLO VINEIS, MD, MPH
Environmental Epidemiology
Imperial College
London, United Kingdom

CHRISTOPHER H. WADE, PhD, MPH
Social and Behavioral Research Branch
& Genome Technology Branch
National Human Genome Research
Institute
Washington, DC

NICK WAREHAM, PhD, MRC
Medical Research Council Epidemiology
Unit
Elsie Widdowson Laboratories
Cambridge, United Kingdom

GEORGE WELLS, MSc, PhD
Cardiovascular Research Methods
Centre
University of Ottawa Heart Institute
Ottawa, ON, Canada

MIRIAM WIENS, BSc MSc
Department of Epidemiology and
Community Medicine
University of Ottawa
Ottawa, ON, Canada

MARC S. WILLIAMS, MD
Intermountain Healthcare
Clinical Genetics Institute
Salt Lake City, UT

ROBIN E. WILLIAMSON, PhD
American Journal of Human Genetics
Boston, MA

DEBORAH M. WINN, PhD
Division of Cancer Control and
Population Sciences
National Cancer Institute
Bethesda, MD

PAULA W. YOON, ScD, MPH
Division for Heart Disease and Stroke
Prevention
Centers for Disease Control and
Prevention
Atlanta, GA

WEI YU, PhD, MS
Office of Public Health Genomics
Centers for Disease Control and
Prevention
Atlanta, GA

MAJA ZECEVIC, PhD, MPH
Lancet
New York, NY

RON ZIMMERN, MA, FRCP, FFPHM
Foundation for Genomics and
Population Health (PHG Foundation)
Cambridge, United Kingdom

GUANG YONG ZOU, PhD
Department of Epidemiology and
Biostatistics
University of Western Ontario
London, ON, Canada
and
Robarts Clinical Trials
Robarts Research Institute
London, ON, Canada

ELEFTHERIA ZEGGINI, PhD
Wellcome Trust Centre for Human
Genetics
University of Oxford
Oxford, United Kingdom
and
Wellcome Trust Sanger Institute
Wellcome Trust Genome Campus
Cambridge, United Kingdom

I

FUNDAMENTALS OF HUMAN GENOME EPIDEMIOLOGY REVISITED

1

Human genome epidemiology: the road map revisited

Muin J. Khoury, Sara R. Bedrosian, Marta Gwinn,
Julian Little, Julian P. T. Higgins, and John P. A. Ioannidis

In 2004, we published the book entitled *Human Genome Epidemiology: A Scientific Foundation for Using Genetic Information to Improve Health and Prevent Disease* (1). In it, we discussed how the epidemiologic approach provides an important scientific foundation for studying the continuum from gene discovery to the development, applications, and evaluation of human genome information in improving health and preventing disease. We called this continuum human genome epidemiology (or HuGE) to denote an evolving field of inquiry that uses epidemiologic applications to assess the population impact of human genetic variation on health and disease, and how the resulting information can be used to improve population health. We discussed and gave examples that illustrated that after the discovery of genetic variants associated with diseases, additional well-conducted epidemiologic studies are needed to characterize the population impact of gene variants on the risk for adverse health outcomes and to identify and measure the impact of modifiable risk factors that interact with gene variants. Epidemiologic studies are also required for evaluating clinical validity and utility of new genetic tests, to monitor population use of genetic tests and to determine the impact of genetic information on the health and well-being of different populations. The results of such studies will help medical and public health professionals integrate human genomics into practice.

The Rationale for a Second Edition of *Human Genome Epidemiology*

Since 2004, advances in human genomics have continued to occur at a breathtaking pace. Although the concept of personalized healthcare and disease prevention often promised by enthusiastic scientists and the media is yet to be fulfilled, we are now seeing rapid progress and accumulation of data in many "omics" related research fields such as transcriptomics, proteomics, and metabolomics (2). Results of the International HapMap project were published in 2005 (3), paving the way to more efficient methods to discover human genetic variations associated with a variety of common diseases of public health significance. New methods to measure genome variation on an unprecedented large scale (hundreds of thousands of genetic variants) have propelled a new generation of genome association studies (4). Evaluation of rare variants and full sequencing at large-scale are rapidly becoming a reality. Also, we have seen the emergence of population-based biobanks in many countries with the objectives of quantifying longitudinally the joint influences of genetic and environmental factors on the occurrence of common diseases (5).

Perhaps the single most important development in human genome epidemiology has been the emergence of genome-wide association studies (GWAS; 6). The continuous improvements in genome-wide analysis technologies, coupled with drastic reductions in price, have led to widespread applications of these technologies in large collaborative case-control, cross-sectional, and cohort studies. These studies have interrogated agnostically, without *a priori* hypotheses, variation in the whole genome, looking for differences in the distribution of genetic polymorphisms between individuals with and without disease. As of August 2009, more than 400 gene variants have been discovered and replicated as risk markers (but not necessarily true culprits) for a variety of common diseases of public health significance (7). As a result, we are seeing an unprecedented expansion in the number of publications of GWAS as well as studies of candidate genes with varying methodological quality. While the deposition of GWAS data in potentially accessible databases (8,9) could lead to avoidance of selective publication, protection from other biases (e.g., selection, confounding, misclassification) is still a real concern even with large GWA studies that are based on selected or noncomparable samples of cases and controls. In addition, new technology such as full genomic sequencing is likely to replace the current genome-wide SNP analysis platforms. Furthermore, we are seeing the emergence of the novel approaches of system biology, as well as the development of biomarkers based on gene expression profiles, epigenetic patterns, proteomic profiles, and so on. Each new development taxes our ability to make sense of the ever-increasing amount of data. We must continue to develop, apply, and sharpen our epidemiological approaches to study designs, analysis, interpretation, and knowledge synthesis.

From Gene Discovery to Clinical and Public Health Applications

The ongoing success of GWAS in uncovering genetic risk markers for many common diseases has renewed expectations of a new era of health care and public health practice (6,10,11). Already, we have a few examples of applications in clinical medicine and population health (see Table 1.1 for emerging examples). By and large, emerging applications are relatively rare in spite of the rapid advances in gene discovery, and for many of them, their benefits and cost-effectiveness are not well known. Therefore, there is an urgent need to understand the benefits and harms and to ensure high-quality implementation of new technologies (12). This includes improving the evidence base of outcomes of these technologies; the

Table 1.1 Examples of emerging applications of human genome discoveries for clinical practice and disease prevention

Type of Application	Examples of Proposed Applications
Therapeutic agents	Herceptin in treatment of breast cancer
Diagnostic tests	BRCA analysis in hereditary breast and ovarian cancer
Pharmacogenomic tests	Genetic testing for warfarin treatment
Prognostic tests	Tumor gene expression profiles in various cancers
Screening tests	Biomarkers for early detection of ovarian cancer
Risk assessment tests	Genome profiles in breast and prostate cancer

development of evidence-based guidelines for the use of genomic applications (13); the use of policy and legislation to prevent discrimination on the basis of genetic information (14); and the effective engagement of providers, researchers, and the general public. More recently, "direct to consumer" (DTC) offerings of genome-wide profiles have been developed and marketed by several companies, with the implicit, if not explicit, goal of providing information for improving individual health and preventing common diseases (15). The ready availability and complexity of these new DTC tests could strain the ability of consumers and the health care delivery system to determine the true value of applying extensive quantities of genomic data to health management. Proponents of DTC genome-wide profiles feel strongly that this approach can empower and educate individuals about disease prevention and health promotion. Others are concerned that the use of genome-wide profiles is based on an incomplete knowledge about the relationship between genetic variations and human diseases, and the lack of a full understanding of the optimal specific medical or lifestyle interventions that should be offered based on these test results (16). Questions also remain regarding the scope of individual genetic tests that should be included in genomic profiles, whether the underlying technologies are robust, and where the balance lies between potential benefits and harms (clinical utility) of these tests to individuals and populations (16,17). A 2007 report found several limitations in the existing US-based research and healthcare delivery infrastructure to create an evidence base of utilization and outcomes of gene-based applications (18). In addition, providers and the public have little understanding of genomics and genomics services (10). Overcoming these limitations would require coordinating efforts that span multiple disciplines of laboratory sciences, medicine and public health, including health services research, and outcomes research. The epidemiologic approach is at the intersection of all these disciplines.

The Emergence of Public Health Genomics

In the face of evolving technologies, we have witnessed in the past few years the emergence of "public health genomics," a multidisciplinary field concerned with the effective and responsible translation of genome-based knowledge and technologies to improve population health. This field is thriving in many countries and uses epidemiologic methods as a foundation for knowledge integration of genetic information in medicine and public health (19–21). Public health genomics uses population-based data on genetic variation and gene-environment interactions to develop, implement, and evaluate evidence-based tools for improving health and preventing disease. Public health genomics also applies systematic, evidence-based assessments of genomic applications in health practice and works to ensure the delivery of validated, useful genomic tools in practice.

Even with impressive advances in the basic sciences of gene discovery and characterization, reservations have been voiced about the potential benefits of medical applications of genomics; these reservations are based in part on the complex relationship between genetic variation and the environment with disease occurrence, as reflected in the modest associations between individual gene variants and disease outcomes, and the limited clinical validity and utility of using genetic information in the prediction of disease. Moreover, prematurely optimistic claims by researchers, the media, test developers, and commercial genomic enterprises may lead to unrealistic expectations among consumers and inappropriate use of genetic information. Also, an overemphasis on the genetics of human disease may divert attention from the importance of environmental exposures, social structure, and lifestyle factors (22). In public health practice, skepticism about genomics runs high among some practitioners whose traditional domains are the control of infectious diseases, environmental exposures, and health promotion for chronic disease prevention. To some, genomics research is perceived as a low-yield investment, as well as an opportunity cost, undercutting social efforts to address environmental causes of ill health. To others, public health applications of genomics are viewed only in terms of population screening, remaining limited to newborn screening programs (23). Still others reject genomics research as an unwarranted extension of the individual risk paradigm (24), citing the distinction between prevention in populations and in high-risk persons set out by Geoffrey Rose in 1985 (25). However, Rose was careful to present these approaches as complementary rather than mutually exclusive (25).

It can be argued that the integration of genomics into healthcare and disease prevention requires a strong medicine–public health partnership (26). Public health and health care often operate in different spheres, although medicine is part of the "public health system" (27). This "schism" can be overcome in genomics using a population approach to a joint translational agenda that includes (a) a focus on prevention, a traditional public health concern that is now a promise of genomics in the realm of personalized medicine; (b) a population perspective that requires a large amount of population level data to validate gene discoveries for clinical and population-level applications, especially given the modest associations between genetic factors and disease burden; (c) commitments to evidence-based knowledge synthesis and guideline development, especially with thousands of potential genomic applications emerging into practice; and (d) emphasis on health services research and the surveillance of population health to evaluate health outcomes, costs, and benefits in the "real world" (27).

Epidemiology and the Phases of Genomics Translation

As shown in Table 1.2, there are four phases of translation research in genomics, from gene discovery to population health impact (28). In addition to traditional genetic epidemiology, which has focused by and large on gene discovery, epidemiologic methods and approaches play a role in all four phases (see Table 1.2). Phase 1 (T1) research seeks to move a basic genome-based discovery into a candidate health application (e.g., genetic test/intervention). Phase 2 (T2) research assesses the value of a genomic application for health practice leading to the development of evidence-based guidelines. Phase 3 (T3) research attempts to move evidence-based guidelines into health practice, through delivery, dissemination, and diffusion research. Phase 4 (T4) research seeks to evaluate the "real world" health outcomes of a genomic application in practice. Because the development of evidence-based guidelines is a moving target, the types of translation research can overlap and provide feedback loops to allow integration of new knowledge. Although it is difficult to quantify how much of human genomics research is T1, we have estimated that no more than 3% of published research focuses on T2 and beyond (28). Indeed, evidence-based guidelines

Table 1.2 Human genome epidemiology and the phases of genomics translation: examples and application

Phase	*Notation*	*Types of Research*	*Examples*
T1	Discovery to candidate health application.	Phases 1 and 2 clinical trials; observational studies.	What is the magnitude of the association between genetic variants and disease risks? Is there gene-environment interaction?
T2	Health application to evidence-based practice guidelines.	Phase 3 clinical trials; observational studies; evidence synthesis and guidelines development.	What are the positive and negative predictive values of genetic factors in risk assessment?
T3	Practice guidelines to health practice.	Dissemination research; implementation research; diffusion research; Phase 4 clinical trials.	What proportion of individuals who meet guidelines criteria receive recommended care and what are the barriers to implementing practice guidelines?
T4	Practice to population health impact.	Outcomes research (includes many disciplines); population monitoring of morbidity, mortality, benefits and risks.	Does implementation of practice guidelines reduce disease incidence/improve outcomes?

Source: Adapted from Reference 28.
See Reference 28 for definition of terms.

and T3 and T4 research currently are rare (except in newborn screening, and selected testing for genetic disorders such as hereditary breast and ovarian cancer).

The Continued Need for Methodological Standards in Human Genome Epidemiology

Thus, the need for making sense of the avalanche of genetic and genomic data is more urgent than ever. This urgency is behind the continued growth of the Human Genome Epidemiology Network (HuGENet), a global collaboration of individuals and organizations who are interested in accelerating the development of the knowledge base on human genetic variation and population health and the use of this information in improving health and preventing disease (29). HuGENet has focused on developing methods and guidance to integrate and disseminate a global knowledge base on assessing the prevalence of genetic variants in different populations, genotype-disease associations, and gene-gene and gene-environment interactions, and evaluating genetic tests for screening and prevention. During the past three years, HuGENet has made many methodological and substantive contributions to the field. HuGENet has developed a Web-based searchable knowledge base (the HuGE Navigator) that captures ongoing publications in human genome epidemiology (30). The HuGE Navigator is searchable by disease, gene, and disease risk factors. Furthermore, in collaboration with several journals, HuGENet has sponsored the systematic reviews of the evidence on genotype-disease associations, using specific published guidelines and recommendations—the HuGENet handbook (31)—for carrying out this work, as well as for applying quantitative methods of synthesis. Since 2000, HuGENet collaborators have carried out more than 80 reviews on various diseases ranging from single gene conditions to common complex diseases. In 2005, HuGENet formed a network of investigator networks (32), which currently has 35 consortia, mostly disease-specific networks that are represented by hundreds of collaborators interested in sharing knowledge, experience, and resources in the conduct, analysis, and dissemination of results of human genome epidemiology investigations. In 2006, HuGENet conducted a workshop in collaboration with the global movement STROBE (STrengthening the Reporting of OBservational Epidemiology) to extend the now well-studied "STROBE reporting checklist" to include genetic associations, under the rubric of STREGA (STrengthening the REporting of Genetic Associations; 33). In addition, the HuGENet "network of networks" published a "road map" for using consortia-driven pooled meta-analyses to accelerate the knowledge base on gene-disease associations (34). With the publication of the HuGENet roadmap, the editors of *Nature Genetics* called for the development and online publication of peer reviewed, curated expert knowledge bases called "field synopses" that are regularly updated and freely accessible (35). HuGENet implemented the field synopsis concept in a meeting held in 2006 in Venice (36). The workshop participants generated interim guidelines for grading the cumulative evidence in genetic associations based on three criteria: (1) the amount of evidence;

(2) the extent of replication; and (3) protection from bias. The proposed scheme allows for three categories of descending credibility for each of these criteria and also for a composite assessment of "strong," "moderate," or "weak" credibility (36). In 2008, HuGENet collaborators conducted a workshop to discuss insights and experiences from several field synopses that represented the first efforts by multiple authors at grading the credibility of these associations on a massive scale. HuGENet participants emerged with a vision for collaboration that builds a reliable cumulative evidence for genetic associations and a transparent, distributed, and authoritative knowledge base on genetic variation and human health (37).

The HuGE Roadmap Revisited

With all these ongoing developments, we have invited many authors who are leaders in the field to produce the second edition of *Human Genome Epidemiology*. Our aim is to inform readers of new developments in the genomics field and how epidemiologic methods are being used to make sense of this information. We do realize that the material presented in this book will be outdated even before it is published. However, the methodological challenges and possible solutions to them will remain with us for quite some time. There is very little material remaining from the first edition of *Human Genome Epidemiology*.

This new edition is divided into five parts. In Part I, we give an overview of the development and progress in applications of genomic technologies, with a focus on genomic sequence variation (Chapter 2). We then give an overview of the multidisciplinary field of public health genomics that includes a fundamental role of epidemiologic methods and approaches (Chapter 3). We also present a brief overview of evolving methods for tracking and compiling information on genetic factors in disease (Chapter 4).

In Part II, we discuss methodological developments in collection, analysis, and synthesis of data from human genome epidemiologic studies. We discuss the emergence of biobanks around the world (Chapter 5), the evolution of case-control studies and cohort studies in the era of GWAS (Chapter 6), and the emerging role of consortia and networks (Chapter 7). Next, we discuss methodological analytic issues in GWAS (Chapter 8) and the analytic challenges of gene-gene and gene-environment interaction (Chapter 9). We then address issues of reporting of genetic associations (Chapter 10), evolving methods for integrating the evidence (Chapter 11), and assessment of cumulative evidence and field synopses (Chapter 12).

In Part III, we provide several case studies related to various diseases that attempt to present an evolving knowledge base of the cumulative evidence on genetic variation in a variety of human diseases. As the information undoubtedly will change (even before the publication of the book), we stress here the importance of strong methodological foundation for analysis and synthesis of information from various studies. The diseases shown in this section include three cancers: colorectal cancer (Chapter 13), childhood leukemia (Chapter 14), and bladder cancer (Chapter 15).

We also present data from type 2 diabetes (Chapter 16), osteoporosis (Chapter 17), preterm birth (Chapter 18), coronary heart disease (Chapter 19), and schizophrenia (Chapter 20). Collectively, these chapters cover an impressive array of common complex human diseases and provide an epidemiologic approach to rapidly emerging data on gene-disease and gene-environment interactions.

In Part IV, we discuss methodological issues surrounding specific applications of human genomic information for medicine and public health. We start in Chapter 21 with a review of the concept of Mendelian Randomization, an approach that allows us to assess the role of environmental factors and other biomarkers in the occurrence of human diseases using data on the association of genetic variation and disease endpoints. In Chapter 22, we discuss how clinical epidemiologic concepts and methods can be used to assess whether one or more genetic variants (e.g., genome profiles) can be used to predict risk for human diseases. Chapter 23 presents a major milestone for public health genomics, namely the publication of methods of systematic review and assessment of the clinical validity and utility of genomic applications in clinical practice. This chapter is a reprint of the published paper from the independent multidisciplinary panel, the EGAPP working group, sponsored by CDC and many partners. Chapter 24 briefly summarizes how reviews of the evidence on validity and utility of genomic information can be done systematically and rapidly, even in the face of incomplete information. Chapter 25 focuses on the crucial role of the behavioral and social sciences in assessing the impact and value of epidemiologic information on gene-disease associations. Chapter 26 addresses issues in evaluating developments in newborn screening. Chapter 27 provides an epidemiologic framework for the evaluation of pharmacogenomic applications in clinical and public health practice. Chapter 28 presents an overview of the relevance and impact of epigenomics in clinical practice and disease prevention. Finally, Chapter 29 presents an epidemiologic framework for evaluating family health history as a tool for disease prevention and health promotion. Even in this genomics era, family history remains a strong foundation, not only for identifying single gene disorders, but also for stratifying individuals and populations by different levels of disease risk and implementing personalized interventions.

Finally, in Part V of the book, we present a few case studies of the application of epidemiologic methods of assessment of clinical validity and utility for several disease examples. These include two pharmacogenomic testing examples—initial treatment of depression with SSRIs (Chapter 30) and warfarin therapy (Chapter 31). We also present information on population screening for hereditary hemochromatosis (Chapter 32), a genetic disorder with incomplete penetrance that has attracted some attention over the past decade as a possible example of population screening in the genomics era.

The second edition of *Human Genome Epidemiology* is primarily targeted at basic, clinical, and population scientists involved in studying genetic factors in common diseases. In addition, the book focuses on *practical* applications of human genome variation in clinical practice and disease prevention. We hope that students, clinicians, public health professionals, and policy makers will find the book useful in learning about evolving methods for approaching the discovery and the use of genetic information in medicine and public health in the twenty-first century.

References

1. Khoury MJ, Little J, Burke W, eds. *Human Genome Epidemiology: A Scientific Foundation for Using Genetic Information to Improve Health and Prevent Disease.* New York: Oxford University Press; 2004.
2. Nature Omics Gateway. Available at http://www.nature.com/omics/. Accessed May 28, 2009.
3. International HapMap Consortium. A haplotype map of the human genome. *Nature.* 2005;437:1299–1320.
4. Thomas DC. Are we ready for whole genome association studies? *CEBP.* 2006; 4:595–598.
5. Knoppers BM. Biobanking: international norms. *J Law Med Ethics.* 2005;33:7–14.
6. Manolio TA, Brooks LD, Collins FS. A Hapmap harvest of insights into the genetics of common disease. *J Clin Invest.* 2008;118:1590–1605.
7. National Human Genome Research Institute-Office of Population Genomics. A catalog of published genomewide association studies. Available at http://www.genome.gov/gwastudies/. Accessed May 28, 2009.
8. National Center for Biotechnology Information. Database on genotypes and phenotypes (dbGAP). Available at http://www.ncbi.nlm.nih.gov/gap. Accessed May 28, 2009.
9. National Cancer Institute. Cancer genetic markers of susceptibility (CGEMS). Available at http://cgems.cancer.gov/. Accessed May 28, 2009.
10. Feero WG, Guttmacher AE, Collis FS. The genome gets personal-almost. *JAMA.* 2008;299:1351–1352.
11. Department of Health and Human Services: personalized healthcare initiative. Available at http://www.hhs.gov/myhealthcare/. Accessed May 28, 2009.
12. Secretary's Advisory Committee on Genetics, Health and Society. US system of oversight of genetic testing. Available at http://www4.od.nih.gov/oba/SACGHS/reports/SACGHS_oversight_report.pdf. Accessed May 28, 2009.
13. Khoury MJ, Bradley L, Berg A, et al. The evidence dilemma in genomic medicine: the need for a roadmap for translating genomic discoveries into clinical practice. *Health Affairs.* 2008;27(6): 1600–1611. doi: 10.1377/hlthaff.27.6.1600
14. Hudson KL, Holohan MK, Collins FS. Keeping pace with the times—the Genetic Information Nondiscrimination Act of 2008. *N Engl J Med.* 2008;358:2661–2663.
15. Hogarth S, Javitt G, Melzer D. The Current Landscape for Direct-to-Consumer Genetic Testing: Legal, Ethical, and Policy Issues. *Ann Rev Genom Hum Genet.* 2008;9:161–182.
16. McGuire AL, Cho MK, McGuire SE, et al. The future of personal genomics. *Science.* 2007;317:1687.
17. Hunter DJ, Khoury MJ, Drazen JM. Letting the genome out of the bottle-will we get our wish. *N Engl J Med.* 2008;358:105–107.
18. Agency for Healthcare Research and Quality. Infrastructure to monitor utilization and outcomes of gene-based applications: an assessment. Available at http://effectivehealthcare.ahrq.gov/healthInfo.cfm?infotype=nr&ProcessID=63. Accessed May 28, 2009.
19. Burke W, Khoury MJ, Stewart A, et al. The path from genome-based research to population health: development of an international public health genomics network. *Genet Med.* 2006;8:451–458.

20. Khoury MJ, Bowen S, Bradley LK, et al. A decade of public health genomics in the United States, Centers for Disease Control and Prevention. *Public Health Genomics.* 2009;12:20–29.
21. Knoppers BM, Brand AM. From community genetics to public health genomics: what's in a name. *Public Health Genomics.* 2009;12:1–3.
22. Buchanan AV, Weiss KM, Fullerton SM. Dissecting complex disease: the quest for the philosopher's stone? *Int J Epidemiol.* 2006;35:562–571.
23. Rockhill B. Theorizing about causes at the individual level while estimating effects at the population level: implications for prevention. *Epidemiology.* 2005;16:124–129.
24. Holtzman NA. What role for public health in genetics and vice versa? *Community Genet.* 2006;9:8–20.
25. Rose G. Sick individuals and sick populations. *Int J Epidemiol.* 1985;14:32–38.
26. Khoury MJ, Gwinn M, Burke W, et al. Will genomics widen or help heal the schism between medicine and public health? *Am J Prev Med.* 2007;33:310–317.
27. Institute of Medicine. *Who Will Keep the Public Healthy? Educating Public Health Professionals for the 21st Century.* Washington, DC: National Academies Press; 2003.
28. Khoury MJ, Gwinn M, Yoon PW, et al. The continuum of translation research in genomic medicine: how can we accelerate the appropriate integration of human genome discoveries into healthcare and disease prevention. *Genet Med.* 2007;9:665–674.
29. Centers for Disease Control and Prevention. The Human Genome Epidemiology Network (HuGENet). Available at http://www.cdc.gov/genomics/hugenet/default.htm, Accessed May 28, 2009.
30. Yu W, Gwinn M, Clyne M, et al. A navigator for human genome epidemiology. *Nat Genet.* 2008;40:124–125. Also available online at http://www.hugenavigator.net/. Accessed May 28, 2009.
31. HuGENet handbook of HuGE reviews, edition 1.0 posted at http://www.genesens.net/_intranet/doc_nouvelles/HuGE%20Review%20Handbook%20v11.pdf. Accessed May 28, 2009.
32. Ioannidis JPA, Bernstein J, Boffetta P, et al. A network of investigator networks in human genome epidemiology. *Am J Epidemiol.* 2005;162:302–304.
33. STrengthening the REporting of Genetic Associations (STREGA). *Ann Intern Med.* February 3, 2009;150(3):206–215.
34. Ioannidis JPA, Gwinn M, Little J, et al. The Human Genome Epidemiology Network. A road map for efficient and reliable human genome epidemiology. *Nat Genet.* 2006;38:3–5.
35. Editorial. Embracing risk. *Nat Genet.* 2006;38:1.
36. Ioannidis JPA, Boffetta P, Little J, et al. Cumulative assessment of genetic associations: interim guidelines. *Int J Epidemiol.* 2008;37:120–132.
37. HuGENet workshop 2008: Networks, genomewide association studies and the knowledge base on genetic variation and human health. Available at http://www.cdc.gov/genomics/hugenet/hugewkshp_jan08.htm.. Accessed May 28, 2009.

2

Principles of analysis of germline genetics

Jesus Gonzalez-Bosquet and Stephen J. Chanock

Introduction

Armed with a comprehensive draft of the human genome, one of the first priorities was to develop a large-scale map of common genetic variation to investigate the role of genetics in human disease (1–3). Using the catalog of annotated common human variation, geneticists have begun to capitalize on the recent technical advances to investigate thoroughly the complexities of genetic variation and its contribution to complex human diseases and traits. Moreover, the age of the genomics revolution has spawned an opportunity to examine the interplay between environmental/lifestyle factors and genetic variation as well as the genetics of individual responses to medical intervention (e.g., pharmacogenomics) (4). A seminal step has been the characterization of common haplotypes in three continental populations, known as the International HapMap Project (http://www.hapmap.org); it has already reaped over 200 novel loci in the genome associated with human diseases/traits, primarily discovered by genome-wide association studies (GWAS) (5–8). Though these advances have focused on a component of genomic architecture, namely common genetic variants, parallel programs in comprehensive resequence analysis should yield a catalog of uncommon variants (1,000 genome project-HapMap3, http://www.hapmap.org/cgi-perl/gbrowse/hapmap3_B36) that will enable analysis of less common variants. In concert with the assessment of germline genetic variation, genomic characterization is underway using different platforms to integrate with gene expression data; these programs include the ENCODE (the ENCyclopedia Of DNA Elements) Project, which seeks to define functional elements (http://www.genome.gov/10005107) (9), and the Cancer Genome Atlas (TCGA), which is interrogating somatic and germline alterations in select cancers (10). Together, these new developments promise to accelerate the discovery and characterization of novel genomic mechanisms in human diseases and traits.

The age of genomics has ushered in a more ambitious approach toward scientific discovery, "team" science, in which resources and study populations are pooled to identify novel genetic markers (Figure 2.1). In this regard, GWAS survey thousands of the most common genetic variants across the genome, single nucleotide polymorphisms (SNPs) in an "agnostic manner" (in other words, unfettered by prior

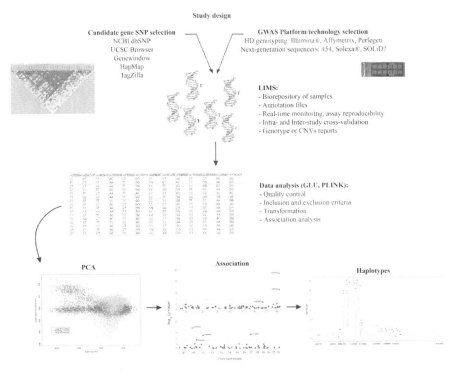

Figure 2.1 Workflow of a genotyping study: The panel depicts critical steps in the execution of a successful, high-quality, high-throughput genotyping study, starting from the design of the study with either a candidate approach or a genome-wide association study (GWAS) approach, and followed with an efficient Laboratory Information Management System (LIMS), required to track samples and processes, as well as with quality control capabilities. Powerful, specially designed and highly scalable software (PLINK, GLU) is needed for the increasingly complex data output analysis. These processes may include principal component analysis (PCA), association analysis, and haplotype reconstruction and association.

hypotheses) and require adequately powered follow-up studies for replication (11). It is this latter point that is central to the search for moderate- to high-frequency low-penetrance variants associated with human diseases and traits (12). Efforts to replicate are necessary to guard against the large number of apparent false positives, which can be due to chance or methodological biases in study design and execution (11,13,14). The emergence of high fidelity, highly parallel genotyping technologies make possible what was unimaginable a few years before. The generation of dense data sets with millions of genotypes creates new statistical challenges that are as daunting as are the issues of archiving and storage. Careful delineation of responsibilities among a team of scientists is necessary to ensure quality control and stable analytical results.

Until recently, the primary engine for gene discovery was the candidate approach, but it had yielded only a modicum of success (15). Usually, due to technical or budget constraints, a handful of genetic markers, either SNPs, microsatellites, or other markers, were chosen within one or several known genes (16). These genes were the "best bet," usually based on prior knowledge drawn from either laboratory or published association studies. The markers were chosen because they satisfied one or more conditions: (a) known or putative function either altering the coding region or the regulation of the gene or genomic region, (b) prior functional evidence emanating from the laboratory or a prior association study, or (c) exploration of regions flanking a locus based on patterns of linkage disequilibrium. Other approaches included studies of families with high penetrance of certain complex diseases.

Previously, family linkage studies have been utilized to identify rare genetic variants with high-penetrance susceptibility genes (17,18), but failed to be informative on more common genetic variants with low to moderate effect (16). The majority of linkage analysis studies also used genetic markers other than SNPs for mapping. In their seminal paper, Risch and Merikangas argued, "that the method that has been used successfully (linkage analysis) to find major genes has limited power to detect genes of modest effect, but that a different approach (association studies)...has far greater power, even if one needs to test every gene in the genome. Thus, the future of the genetics of complex diseases is likely to require large-scale testing by association analysis" (19).

Genetic Variation

Single Nucleotide Polymorphisms (SNPs)

The spectrum of human genetic variation is defined by both the frequency of polymorphisms, which can vary substantially between populations and the size of the variants. Interestingly, the difference between any two single human genomes is less than 0.5%. The most common sequence variation in the genome is the stable substitution of a single base, known as a single nucleotide polymorphism (SNP), which, by definition, is observed in at least 1% of a population. The minor allele frequency (MAF) is the lowest allele frequency observed at a locus in one particular population; and current estimates are that there are at least 8–10 million SNPs with a MAF greater than 1% (20–22), and 5 million SNPs with a MAF greater than 10% (2,20). As Figure 2.2 shows, there are a greater number of SNPs with lower MAFs. Interestingly, the majority of SNPs with a MAF greater than 15–20% are common to all human populations (7,23); for instance, nearly 85% of the more than 1.5 million SNPs are common to European American, Han Chinese, and African American populations. A small subset of high-frequency SNPs, less than 10%, appears to be private to a single population, again suggesting the common ancestry of all (23).

Human genetic variation is greatly influenced by geography, with genetic differentiation between populations increasing with geographic distance, and genetic diversity decreasing with distance from Africa; populations of African ancestry have the greatest diversity, resulting in shorter segments of linkage disequilibrium

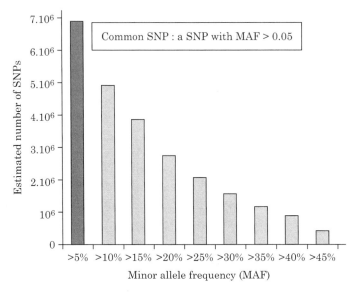

Figure 2.2   Estimated number of SNPs in the human genome as a function of their minor allele frequency (22).

(24–28). Alleles under positive selection increase in prevalence in a population and leave distinctive "signatures" or patterns of genetic variation in DNA sequence. These can be identified by comparison with the background distribution of genetic variation, primarily evolved under neutrality (15). In some cases, these "signatures," or differences in allele frequencies between populations, reflect major regional selective pressures, such as infectious diseases (e.g., malaria), environmental stresses (e.g., temperature), or diet (e.g., milk consumption) (29–31).

   In the age of candidate gene studies, SNPs were classified on the basis of a predicted effect in either the coding sequence or perhaps a region that could regulate transcription. A SNP situated in a translated genomic region, that is, exon, is known as a coding SNP, or cSNP. Furthermore, a subset of cSNPs change the translated amino acid sequence and are also known as nonsynonymous cSNPs; most coding SNPs do not alter the predicted amino acid and are known as synonymous SNPs. So far, a small subset of cSNPs have been conclusively associated with disease and even fewer have supporting laboratory evidence to provide plausibility (32,33). A proliferation of structural prediction software for proteins can assess the impact of amino acid variation *in silico* to predict conformational protein changes (Protein Data Bank, http://www.rcsb.org/pdb; Swiss-Model, http://swissmodel.expasy.org// SWISS-MODEL.html). New models and algorithms are regularly proposed that claim improved reliability for predicting deleterious changes in protein structure (34–36); without corroborative laboratory data, the predictions are merely *in silico* observations. Overall, between 50,000 and 250,000 SNPs could be functional, namely, nonsynonymous coding variants or regulators of gene expression or splicing (32,33). It is possible that some "functional" or causal SNPs contribute to regulatory differences in expression or genetic pathways (37–39), but most SNPs appear not to be functional and have been maintained on the backbone of an inherited block of DNA through generations.

The international public repository for SNPs is dbSNP (http://www.ncbi.nih.gov/SNP/), currently curating over 8 million human SNPs, nearly half of which have been validated with genotyping assay by the SNP Consortium and the International HapMap Project. A small percentage has been verified by sequencing (40,41). Roughly one-sixth may be not reliable, that is, are actually monoallelic, due to either genotyping or, more likely, sequencing errors (42,43). In general, the reported SNPs have been biased toward high-frequency variants in populations of European ancestry.

Despite their frequency, most SNPs are not inherited independently but in blocks, resulting in sets of SNPs transmitted together between generations (21,44,45). These blocks are defined by linkage disequilibrium (LD), which estimates the correlation between SNPs, and are often defined in chromosomal segments as haplotypes. The concept of LD permits investigators to look at a set of SNPs and determine proxies for other, untested SNPs (or tagSNPs) (46,47). This "indirect approach" is predicated on finding markers only, relegating the search for causal or functional variants to later work (Figure 2.3). Several tools have been developed to optimize the number of tagSNPs required to represent common haplotypes (Tagger, embedded in Haploview software, http://www.broad.mit.edu/mpg/haploview; TagZilla, http://tagzilla.nci.nih.gov) (48). Consequently, the indirect approach of using a limited set of tagSNP as a proxy of a LD block has emerged as the preferred approach utilized by GWAS to explore across the genome (49).

(a) Haplotype blocks: based on D' values for linkage disequilibrium (LD)

(b) Grouping of SNPs into bins based on r^2

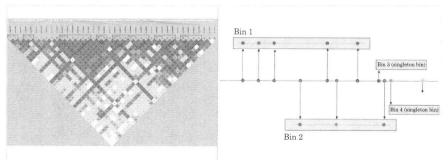

Figure 2.3 Strategy for SNP Selection: (a) SNP selection through haplotype blocks, based on the concept of linkage disequilibrium (LD). "TagSNPs" are proxies for other SNPs, (the so-called indirect approach) (50). (b) Selection of SNPs based on r^2, another measure of LD, which groups SNPs with high LD into "bins." TagSNPs are proxies for these loci included in each "bin" (51).

Currently, the catalog of uncommon variation, namely SNPs with MAF under 1%, is incomplete. The contribution of uncommon variants promises to unravel another portion of the genomic architecture, but it will require extensive rese-quencing analyses of large groups of subjects to identify the uncommon variants (4,9). These are rare variants, or mutations, with a strong familial component and a high penetrance, usually identified by classical Mendelian patterns of inheritance of a defined phenotype or disease within familial pedigrees. These variants are called disease mutations, and are widely cataloged in a public database, the Online Mendelian Inheritance in Man, or OMIM (http://www.ncbi.nlm.nih.gov/sites/entrez?db=OMIM/).

Structural Polymorphisms

Structural variations in the genome may be either cytologically visible or more commonly submicroscopic variants that have generated intense interest recently (52,53). These can include deletions, insertions, and duplications collectively known as copy number variations (CNVs), as well as less frequent inversions and transloca-tions (54,55) (Figure 2.4). Several of the inversions can be quite large, such as the 3.5 Mb on chromosome 17 seen in perhaps as much as 20% of the population (56). Although structural variants in some genomic regions have no obvious phenotypic consequence (57–59), CNVs have been shown to influence gene dosage, and there-fore might cause genetic disease, either alone or in combination with other factors (60). Some observations, either by the failure to assemble the draft genome sequence or by actual experimentation, estimate that segmental duplicated genomic sequence could involve between 5% and 10% of the genome (58,61,62).

Ongoing investigations and results so far suggest that common CNVs are less prevalent than previously reported (63). McCarroll et al. have recently shown that most common CNVs with high minor allele frequencies may be in linkage dis-equilbirum with common SNPs (64). Coordinated efforts are underway to estab-lish a comprehensive catalog of CNVs, such as the Database of Genomic Variants (http://projects.tcag.ca/variation/) (53,65), and the Human Structural Variation Database (http://humanparalogy.gs.washington.edu/structuralvariation/). The dif-ficulties in the assembly of genomic regions have underscored the complexity of structural variation, which was partly fueled by the recognition of a notable per-centage of SNPs that failed quality control in the International HapMap project; these were later determined to reside in regions now known to be enriched for CNVs (3,6,52,62,66).

Recent efforts have begun to establish standards for the identification, valida-tion, and reporting of CNVs (53). Despite the progress on CNV discovery due to the availability of several microarray platforms that can detect quantitative imbalances, there are still substantive technical challenges due to the breadth of polymorphic dif-ferences, for which analyses are particularly unstable. New algorithms have begun to emerge that should streamline moderate- to high-throughput, cost-effective meth-ods to "scan the genome" for inversions or translocations based on stable sequence

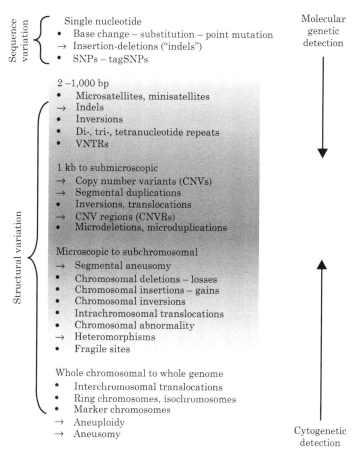

Sequence variation

Single nucleotide
- Base change – substitution – point mutation
→ Insertion-deletions ("indels")
- SNPs – tagSNPs

Molecular genetic detection

Structural variation

2 –1,000 bp
- Microsatellites, minisatellites
→ Indels
- Inversions
- Di-, tri-, tetranucleotide repeats
- VNTRs

1 kb to submicroscopic
→ Copy number variants (CNVs)
→ Segmental duplications
- Inversions, translocations
→ CNV regions (CNVRs)
- Microdeletions, microduplications

Microscopic to subchromosomal
→ Segmental aneusomy
- Chromosomal deletions – losses
- Chromosomal insertions – gains
- Chromosomal inversions
- Intrachromosomal translocations
- Chromosomal abnormality
→ Heteromorphisms
- Fragile sites

Whole chromosomal to whole genome
- Interchromosomal translocations
- Ring chromosomes, isochromosomes
- Marker chromosomes
→ Aneuploidy
→ Aneusomy

Cytogenetic detection

Figure 2.4   Challenges and standards in integrating surveys of structural variation: Range of genetic variation that have to be taken into account when designing and analyzing genotype studies (53).

assemblies (64,67–71). Improved determination of common CNV has been based on advances in techniques, such as tiling arrays, (which cover the genome through partial overlapping (tile-like) sets of fixed oligonucleotides), paired-end sequencing (sequence analysis of both ends of a larger fragment to improve alignment), and dense SNP genotyping platforms.

Short tandem repeats (STRs) represent a class of polymorphism, or microsatellite, that occurs when a pattern of two or more nucleotides are repeated in certain areas of the genome. STRs have been used for linkage analysis and forensic investigation. The patterns can range in length from 2 to 10 bp (usually tetra- or penta-nucleotide repeats) and they are typically located in noncoding regions. Four to five repeats are also robust, essentially error free and resistant to degradation in nonideal conditions. Shorter repeat sequences tend to suffer from artifacts such as stutter and preferential amplification (72,73). Longer repeat sequences are susceptible to environmental degradation and do not amplify by polymerase chain reaction (PCR) as well as shorter sequences. By genotyping enough STR loci and assessing their sequence repetitions at a given locus, it is possible to generate a unique genetic profile of an individual. Accordingly, STR genotype analysis has emerged as the industry standard for forensics (74).

Genotype Analysis

The standard for genotyping is to interrogate specific, unique loci in the genome after DNA amplification by PCR. One of the challenges of genotype analysis is that each allele in the genome must be assayed individually, unlike surveys of gene expression that can use a common signature, such as oligodT, to capture a high percentage of messenger RNA at once. An assay must be robust and reproducible in exceeding a sufficient threshold for detection, and even though amplification protocols are highly faithful, error can be introduced for SNP detection, particularly if there are neighboring SNPs that could alter allele-specific binding of probes or if local genomic sequence is enriched for GC content (Figure 2.5) (75,76). Moreover, the presence of genetic redundancy of part of the sequence (CNV) in the segment amplified or in neighboring SNPs, can undermine the fidelity of the assay, sometimes providing bias in allele calling (62). As observed in the HapMap project, CNVs can have implications for SNP assay design because the current method for assaying SNPs is based on amplification of local sequence surrounding the SNP of interest (52,66). With this method the presence of redundant sequences is amplified, either locally or elsewhere in the genome, and if there are polymorphisms between these different segments, the fidelity of the SNP assay is undermined.

Initially, restriction fragment length polymorphism (RFLP) assays were used to identify patterns of DNA broken into pieces by restriction enzymes and the size of the fragments were used to develop a footprint of the region of interest (77). RFLP analysis is laborious and error prone and has been largely abandoned for probe intensity and microchip technologies that can be easily scaled and reliably performed, such as differential hybridization, primer extension, ligation reactions, and allele-specific probe cleavage, all of which interrogate one SNP at a time.

The TaqMan® SNP genotyping assay (Applied Biosystems, Foster City, CA) is a PCR-based assay designed to interrogate a single SNP, using two locus-specific PCR primers and two allele-specific, labeled probes (78). The assay utilizes the inherent 5' exonuclease property of Taq polymerase. At the 5' end of each probe is an allele-specific reporter dye: the probe that hybridizes to one allele has one dye, while the other probe has a second, different dye. At the 3' end of both probes is a single universal quencher dye. These quencher dyes prevent the excitation and emission of the reporter dyes when in close proximity.

During PCR amplification, the two PCR primers anneal to the template DNA, and the detection probes anneal specifically to a complementary sequence, in the template DNA, between the forward and reverse primer sites. During the elongation

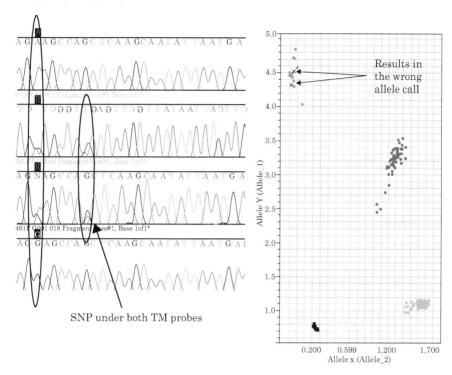

Figure 2.5 Fidelity of the genotyping assay: Error can be introduced in SNP detection, particularly if neighboring SNPs alter allele-specific binding of probes and bias allele calling. The presence of a neighboring SNP under both TaqMan (TM) probes (left panel) may bias the allele call (right panel).

step of each cycle, the Taq polymerase comes in contact, from the 5' end, with the reporter dye. Using Taq's exonuclease property, the reporter dye is released from the probe, and the fluorescence is released (i.e., no longer quenched by the quencher dye). In addition, the probe itself is also digested by the Taq polymerase. After 50 cycles of PCR, fluorescence from reporter dye #1 and/or reporter dye #2 accumulates, and this fluorescence is detected (post-PCR) on an ABI 7900ht Sequence Detection System.

Assays must be designed for unique flanking sequences and should not overlap any adjacent, neighboring SNPs or insertion/deletions. Throughput is moderate but can be increased with robotics or miniaturization of TaqMan assays, such as with Fluidigm or BioTrove (79,80).

The technical capacity to interrogate sets of SNPs in multiplex has improved greatly, mainly in predetermined fixed sets of SNPs. The capital cost of developing increasing densities of custom SNPs has presented a formidable barrier to follow-up large-scale analysis, necessitating selective attempted replication efforts. Technologies have been developed that are based on direct oligonucleotide hybridization with probe fluorescence detection, or by single base sequencing method, or chip-based mass spectrometry, that is, based on matrix-assisted laser desorption/ionization time-of-flight (MALDI-TOF) (81). MALDI is an ionization technique used in mass spectrometry that allows analysis of biomolecules by ionization, usually triggered by a laser beam. A matrix is used to protect the biomolecule from destruction. The mass spectrometer most used with the MALDI approach is the TOF (time-of-flight) mass spectrometer.

The custom bead-array technology by Illumina® (San Diego, CA) enables custom detection of more than 1,500 SNPs with excellent performance, and analysis of high-quality DNA generated by whole genome amplification assays (82,83). This system combines the high multiplexing of the genotype assays and the flexibility of Illumina's multisample array formats, and gives the opportunity to implement disease-related or pathway-specific custom panels.

The Illumina system is an Infinium® Assay protocol that features single-tube preparation of DNA followed by whole-genome amplification prior to genotyping thousands of unique SNPs. The target is hybridized to the bead-bound 50mer oligomer, and then the single-base extension is performed incorporating a labeled nucleotide for assay readout. This technology can be used to design custom sets of SNPs (between 7,600 and 60,000 bead types) with high efficiency (84). The successive platform designs include the HumanHap300, HumanHap500, and, lately, the Infinium HD (high-density) series with the Human1M-Duo BeadChips™, with over 1 million SNPs to be genotyped, primarily chosen as tagSNPs from HapMap II (7).

The Affymetrix microchip system uses the assay termed "whole-genome sampling analysis" (WGSA) for highly multiplexed SNP genotyping of complex DNA (85). This method amplifies a subset of the human genome through a single primer amplification reaction using restriction-enzyme-digested, adaptor-ligated human genomic DNA. After fragmentation, sequential labeling and hybridization to targets is required prior to scanning the microchip. The GeneChip® Human Mapping 500K Array, designed to space SNP markers across the genome, with higher density across genes, has been improved with the Genome-Wide Human SNP Array 6.0 that provides a dense set of SNPs (over 900,000 SNPs) and probes that monitor over 5,500 CNVs across the genome. The paucity of restriction enzyme sites in some areas of the genome limits the coverage of this platform technology within select genomic regions. The main difference between both platforms is coverage: the SNPs selected for the Illumina platform are primarily chosen according to the aggressive tag strategy, namely as proxy for untested SNPs, while the Affymetrix platform provides the coverage with spaced markers.

GWAS Genotyping Issues

In GWAS, the selection of SNPs for the initial scan is determined by the fixed content microchips, but the follow-up is defined by more expensive custom genotyping (86). In this regard, scalability presents a daunting challenge for follow-up studies (87).

The technical capacity to generate high-throughput genotypes may require sophisticated robotics for efficient laboratory flow as well as dedicated bioinformatics to handle both the size and complexity of the data. So despite the fact that the recent availability of new technologies and platforms has decreased the nominal price per genotype assayed and accelerated the whole process, all these variables have to be taken into consideration for execution of high-quality studies. An important part of the optimization process is the Laboratory Information Management System (LIMS) and robotic automation that accurately track samples for an efficient workflow management. Because of the elevated cost of these platforms, there is little flexibility in choosing individual SNPs to be included within the already designed, commercially available whole genome scans.

There are two high-density genotyping platforms that achieve calling capabilities of between 500,000 and 1 million SNPs, as well as probe content to interrogate CNVs: Affymetrix (Santa Clara, CA) and Illumina (San Diego, CA). Both platforms require between 300 and 700 ng of total high-quality DNA (usually at 50 ng/μl). An issue common to both platforms is the difficulty in assaying SNPs that reside close together (within 60 or fewer nucleotides). Denser sets of SNPs on commercial platforms have increased coverage, but not always for all populations.

Coverage, based on the HapMap II set of SNPs with minor allele frequencies greater than 5%, is also the main argument used in the scientific debate over the choice of platforms (7,48). Figure 2.6 illustrates the minimum linkage disequilibrium (LD) for any SNP assay assessed by the coefficient of correlation, r^2 for 2-SNP comparison. r^2 is a measure of LD, or how frequently two loci are transmitted together during meiosis, across generations. The closer r^2 is to 1.0, the closer it is to perfect LD; that is, both loci always segregate together. But as we learn more about LD, the complexity of LD patterns, and how these patterns are covered by SNPs, the common LD threshold of $r^2 > 0.8$ is being modified in some instances. Multimarker strategies have been proposed for analyzing more complicated loci.

Sequence Analysis

For nearly a quarter of a century, DNA sequence analysis by capillary electrophoresis has emerged as the primary technique for large and small-scale projects. Dideoxy-sequencing is based on the principle of terminating DNA synthesis, thus, generating fragments of varying length that can be assembled in order to read the specific DNA sequence; it is notable that the basic reaction is predicated on an amplification step by PCR and thus has an intrinsic error, albeit small but nonetheless predictable (88). The advent of the 96-capillary 3730/3730 xl DNA Analyzer (Applied Biosystems, Foster City, CA) was the central catalyst in the generation of the first draft sequence of the human genome (89). Efficient removal of unincorporated dye terminators and salts preceded capillary electrophoresis in which an electrical field is applied so that the negatively charged DNA fragments move

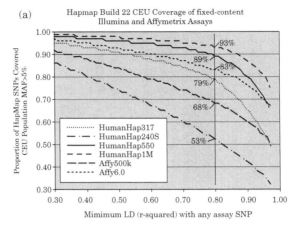

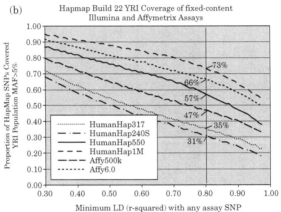

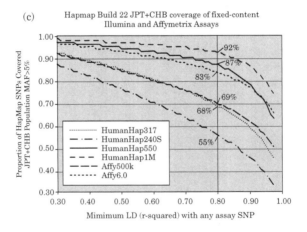

Figure 2.6   Genotyping platforms coverage of HapMap II SNPs: SNP coverage is plotted against linkage disequilibrium measured by the coefficient of correlation, r² for 2-SNP comparison. Panels: (a) HapMap CEU population: CEPH (Utah residents with ancestry from northern and western Europe USAB); (b) HapMap YRI population: Yoruba in Ibadan, Nigeria; (c) HapMap JPT population: Japanese in Tokyo, Japan, and CHB population: Han Chinese in Beijing, China.

through the polymer toward the positive electrode. Data collection software creates a raw data file, which needs further analysis with specialized software to translate the collected color-data images into the corresponding nucleotide bases. The technology has been widely used in genetics and comparative genomics (90) and it will continue to be used until the high-throughput sequencing technologies are commercially available.

Next-generation sequencers have been developed to process millions of sequence reads in parallel rather than in batches of 96 at a time, setting them apart from conventional capillary-based sequencing. Minimal input DNA for production of a library still yields read lengths shorter (35–250 bp, depending on the platform) than capillary sequencers (650–800 bp). Because of their novelty, sequencing reads accuracy and associated quality have to be validated, but the high number of reads provides increased coverage of each base position (9).

The Roche/454 GS-FLX sequencer works on the principle of "pyrosequencing," which uses the pyrophosphate molecule released on nucleotide incorporation by DNA polymerase to fuel a downstream set of reactions that ultimately produces light from the cleavage of oxyluciferin by luciferase (91). The DNA strands of the library are amplified *en masse* by emulsion PCR (92) on the surfaces of hundreds of thousands of agarose beads. Each agarose bead surface contains up to 1,000,000 copies of the original annealed DNA fragment to produce a detectable signal from the sequencing reaction. Imaging of the light flashes from luciferase activity records which templates are adding that particular nucleotide, and the light emitted is directly proportional to the amount of a particular nucleotide incorporated. The current 454 instrument, the GS-FLX, produces an average read length of 250 bp per sample (per bead), with a combined throughput of ~100 Mb of sequence data per 7-h run. By contrast, a single ABI 3730 programmed to sequence 24 × 96-well plates per day produces ~440 kb of sequence data in 7 h, with an average read length of 650° bp per sample (9).

The Illumina Genome Analyzer is based on the concept of "sequencing by synthesis" (Solexa® Sequencing technology) to produce sequence reads of ~32–40 bp from tens of millions of surface-amplified DNA fragments simultaneously. A mixture of single-stranded, adaptor oligo-ligated DNA fragments is incubated and amplified with four differentially labeled fluorescent nucleotides. Each base incorporation cycle is followed by an imaging step that identifies it, and by a chemical step that removes the fluorescent group. At the end of the sequencing run (~4 days), the sequence of each cluster is computed and subjected to quality control. A typical run yields ~40–50 million such sequences.

The Applied Biosystems SOLiD™ sequencer uses a unique sequencing process catalyzed by DNA ligase. Each SOLiD (Sequencing by Oligo Ligation and Detection) run requires ~5 days and produces 3–4 Gb of sequence data with an average read length of 25–35 bp. The specific process couples oligo adaptor-linked DNA fragments with 1-μm magnetic beads that are decorated with complementary oligos and amplifies each bead–DNA complex by emulsion PCR. AB SOLiD sequencing by ligation first anneals a universal sequencing primer, then goes through subsequent ligation of the appropriate labeled 8mer, followed by detection at each cycle by fluorescent readout. The unique attribute of this system is that an extra quality check of read accuracy is enabled that facilitates the discrimination of base calling errors from true polymorphisms or indel events, the so-called 2 base encoding (9).

Quality Control in the Laboratory

The success of genetic analysis of germline DNA by genotyping or sequence analysis is based on the efficient and meticulous handling of the samples from receipt through genetic analysis. Close coordination between the laboratory performing the extraction and the biorepository storing the DNA samples is optimal and protects against handling and biorepository errors, an under-appreciated problem. Standard operating procedures (SOPs) are mandatory for all steps and should be reviewed regularly for both improvements and quality control purposes. Genomic DNA of poor quality reduces completion rates and concordance, suggesting that DNA quality can alter accuracy of genotyping. In some cases, it can undermine the veracity of high-throughput genotyping platforms.

DNA quantification can be performed by spectrophotometric measurement of DNA optical density, by PicoGreen (Turner BioSystems, Sunnyvale, CA) analysis, NanoDrop™ spectrophotometer (NanoDrop Technologies, Wilmington, DE), or by real-time PCR analysis using a standardized TaqMan assay (93). Surprisingly, reproducibility in quantification is challenging and for this reason, quantification methods should be chosen for specific genotype/sequence platforms. Real-time PCR can provide a preliminary test for sample quality as it relates to robust analysis in a high-throughput laboratory, but performance still needs to be gauged with specific technologies. Spectrophotometry and the PicoGreen assay measure total DNA present, regardless of source or quality, whereas a real-time PCR assay measures the total "amplifiable" human DNA. Establishing DNA quantity by real-time PCR is critical for DNA from buccal swabs, cytobrush samples, or other nonblood sources, particularly as it relates to estimating the amount of competing nonhuman DNA. Even small differences between these techniques are important in assessing the amounts of single- and double-stranded DNA because accurate quantification is critical for optimizing the genotyping results.

In the high-throughput setting, there should be strong consideration for DNA fingerprinting of each sample with either a set of SNPs (probably more than 60 with high MAF SNPs) or a forensic panel of 15 small tandem repeats and amelogenin, also known as the AmpFLSTR Identifiler assay (Applied Biosystems). The former can be useful for assessing the sample quality for the specific technology used for "extreme genotyping," and is useful for determining contaminated samples as well as those likely to fail on a chip technology. Moreover, the individual profiles can be useful for verifying known duplicates and identifying unexpected duplicates. When the latter are observed, investigation should consider not only pre-genotyping laboratory or informatics errors but also laboratory errors with plates or reagents.

For some time, there has been intense interest in using whole-genome amplification (WGA) technology to revive molecular epidemiology studies with scant amounts of DNA. While the results have been encouraging, varying results reflect differences in fidelity of protocols and reagents. If performed optimally, WGA can generate large quantities of DNA for genotype assays, but with the caveat that approximately 5% of the genome is not faithfully represented. Regions with high GC content and telomeric regions are especially problematic, and data pertaining to these regions should be cautiously interpreted. With advances in genomic technologies that have evolved enough to permit the study of thousands of SNPs simultaneously from small quantities of DNA, the temptation to use WGA DNA in GWAS is great, but the performance does not reach the high standard observed with native DNA. Furthermore, efficiencies in whole-genome amplification have generated considerable enthusiasm, but have not yet reproducibly amplified the entire genome nor recaptured heavily degraded or damaged DNA. Two different approaches have been commercially optimized; the multiple displacement amplification approach utilizes a high-performance bacteriophage φ 29 DNA polymerase with degenerate hexamers or, alternatively, generation of libraries of 200–2,000 base-pair fragments created by random chemical cleavage of genomic DNA, followed by ligation of adaptor sequences to both ends and PCR amplification. Though there have been efforts to amplify a spectrum of DNA sources, including whole blood, dried blood, buccal cell swabs, cultured cells, and buffy coat cells, varying degrees of success have been reported. Under optimal conditions, the expected yield approaches 10,000-fold in genomic DNA overall. Many laboratories have observed that WGA of water control specimens generates a small, monoallelic signal, which can be called as a single allele (94). This underscores the care that must be given to both the quality control analysis and the software programs used for automating calls in high-throughput genotype analysis.

The design of all molecular epidemiology studies should include undisclosed duplicates taken from the same sample, and if possible replicates of different samples taken from the same individual. Duplicate testing is necessary to assess the quality of the DNA and the extraction process and its prior storage. For the new extreme genotyping technologies, the genotype concordance between duplicates usually exceeds 99.5%. Errors in genotyping, mainly due to loss of one of the heterozygous alleles, occur in well below 1% of samples for commercial and academic platforms and techniques of highest quality. If standard operating procedures are followed closely, completion rates should be greater than 95% for most studies, but may be slightly lower depending on the quality of genomic DNA. Completion rates below 90% should raise substantive concern about technical or analytical deficiencies, prompting repeat genotype analysis. In GWAS, because so many false positive results are observed, some of which could be due to genotype error, it is recommended that a second technology, such as TaqMan or sequencing, be performed to verify the accuracy and establish concordance (11). Though some have advocated using the fitness for Hardy–Weinberg proportion (Hardy–Weinberg equilibrium testing, or HWE), errors in HWE testing can catch major genotype errors but should probably not be used as a stringent threshold for excluding SNPs from analysis.

Bioinformatics

One of the daunting challenges of large-scale genotyping and sequence analysis is the bioinformatic workflow needed to archive, analyze, and access high-density data sets. Accordingly, the effectiveness of laboratory activities is predicated on the flow of information, from the choice of markers, choice of platforms and processes, and laboratory analysis including quality control and assessment through the management and presentation of data sets. Highly trained personnel are required to generate and manage both laboratory and analytical data in a high-throughput processing environment. A Laboratory Information Management System (LIMS) is required to track samples, assays, reagents, equipment, robotics, and processes through the entire workflow. The LIMS captures the movement of information, beginning in the biorepository of samples, and continuing through the delivery of final genotype or CNVs reports, and incorporates the results of experimental data, linked directly to *in silico* information via relational databases. Annotation files that include specific genomic coordinates and genotype assays are closely related to quality control in the sense that this information ensures the fidelity and accuracy of analyses; this is necessary because of the regular updates to the human genome sequence, HapMap and dbSNP databases. Rigorous quality-control and quality-assurance checks of the LIMS software by real-time monitoring should be implemented in order to maintain assay reproducibility and reliable data flow.

Storage of data and access to databases is necessary to enable the efficient analysis *in silico* of raw data generated by genotype and sequence platforms. Some have begun to advocate use of an Analytical Information Management System (AIMS) to receive and process high-density laboratory output. The purpose of the AIMS is to assess rigorously the quality of data and filter out suboptimal genotype or sequence data prior to conducting association or mutation testing. Table 2.1 outlines the major steps that should be considered in the "cleaning" of data prior to publication or data posting.

Standard operating procedures, defined in the laboratory, must be monitored *in silico* to achieve high quality data sets, especially because 10^6–10^9 data points can be generated per study. With continually increasing numbers of loci explored in newer systems, and study design including progressively more individuals in each study, data output is only going to increase, presenting by itself a logistical challenge. The use of scalable computational systems, with parallel computing and multiprocessor capabilities, is not optional any more. The software applications designed for the

Table 2.1 Issues for generation of final, publication-grade build of high-density genotype data

Filter out of samples with low completion rate (<90%)
Filter out SNP assays with low call rates (<90%)
Determination of fitness for Hardy–Weinberg proportion
Determine expected duplicates
Investigate unexpected duplicates
Assess concordance between duplicates
Search for cryptic relatedness between subjects
Assessment of population substructure (after filtering first-degree relatives)
Determine admixture with STRUCTURE analysis
Estimate population stratification (principal component analysis)
Recluster genotype calls
Validate significant genotype calls with second technology

data analysis have to be flexible enough to handle such a wide range of information, while still working in a multiprocessor environment.

There are two suites of tools that have been developed for archiving and management of dense data sets, such as those encountered in GWAS, that are publicly available, PLINK (http://pngu.mgh.harvard.edu/~purcell/plink/summary.shtml) (95), and Genetic Library Utilities, GLU (http://cgf.nci.nih.gov/glu/docs). PLINK, now in version 1.04, is a free, open-source whole-genome association analysis set, developed to conduct basic, large-scale analyses in a computationally efficient manner. PLINK enables investigators to perform analysis of genotype/phenotype data, and there is no support for the steps prior to the final analysis build, namely assistance with study design, generating genotype or CNV calls from raw data or quality control/quality assessment of genotype data sets. A new suite of tools, GLU (Genotype Library and Utilities) v. 1.0, is a Python-based suite created to manage, analyze, and report high-throughput SNP genotype data. It is also an open-source framework and a software package designed to effectively handle the amount of data created in high-density genotype assays. GLU is a powerful suite capable of performing quality-control analysis of datasets, identifying both duplicated samples and completion calling by samples or loci. It has a great flexibility in input format acceptance from almost all common formats and standards. Other data management features include merging and splitting of data sets, and transformation of any accepted file formats, including transforming to binary files, which do not require as much storage space as other file types. GLU has filter capacity based on powerful criteria for inclusion and exclusion as part of the quality-control/quality-assessment process. As a part of the workflow, GLU could perform call completion and duplication assessment. On the basis of these results, we may exclude samples/loci and build a curated data set (called "Build #") with only the genotypes to be analyzed.

The integration of TagZilla in the suite allows linkage disequilibrium estimation and a high-performance tagger-like application, as previously mentioned (see http://tagzilla.nci.nih.gov/).

Conclusion

In the last decade, there has been an unprecedented rate of discovery in human genetics, from the draft sequence of a human genome and its annotation to investigation of the genetic contribution to complex and Mendelian disorders. This has been the consequence of major advances in technical and informatics solutions that have shifted the paradigm of study toward genome-wide exploration. This paradigm shift could not have occurred without the foresight of establishing high-quality epidemiological studies that collected not only biospecimens but also detailed information on environmental exposures and lifestyle choices. The pursuit of applying human genomics to understanding the basis of human diseases and traits will advance as more efficient and effective techniques become available to sequence entire genomes, but it will be difficult to proceed without improving the measurements needed to assess environmental contributions to human disease.

So far, the technology has permitted the efficient scanning across the genome with common variants, but it is likely that in the future, we will be able to look at uncommon variants in the same manner. Eventually, we expect to conduct full genome sequencing, but the challenges will be substantial, both in parsing through the data and prioritizing what should be examined for biological relevance. Discovery of novel regions associated with disease is expected to continue at a rapid pace, but until a spectrum of large-scale screening tools for assessing functional elements in the genome is developed, the gap between discovery and understanding the biological basis of genetics will widen. In this regard, the interrogation of each region will require intense labor, which under present circumstances will be at a far slower pace than that of the discovery of novel regions in the genome associated with diseases or traits.

Once novel regions have been established, it will be possible to pursue the development of new preventive or therapeutic interventions, but again at a pace far slower than that of discovery. Similarly, the rush to introduce genetic markers into personal and public health decisions should be tempered by the commitment to conduct adequately powered, well-designed studies to address specific questions. Genetic testing of mutations or SNPs will require careful consideration of the context in which the information will be gathered, protected, and applied to a specific decision. Currently, community education of both the lay public and the genetics community will inevitably shift the ways in which we gather and apply the information now available using one or more of the new genetic platforms. As this occurs, it will be possible to comprehensively assess the contribution of different types of genetic variation to human disease. The daunting challenge lies in scripting the right sequence of studies that will take into account population genetics history, public health implications, and clinical paradigms that are designed to protect the confidentiality of individuals.

References

1. Human Genome Sequencing C. Finishing the euchromatic sequence of the human genome. *Nature.* 2004;431:931–945.
2. Lander ES, Linton LM, Birren B, et al. Initial sequencing and analysis of the human genome. *Nature.* 2001;409:860–921.
3. Venter JC, Adams MD, Myers EW, et al. The sequence of the human genome. *Science.* 2001;291:1304–1351.
4. Birney E, Stamatoyannopoulos JA, Dutta A, et al. Identification and analysis of functional elements in 1% of the human genome by the ENCODE pilot project. *Nature.* 2007;447:799–816.
5. The International HapMap Project. *Nature.* 2003;426:789–796.
6. The International HapMap C. A haplotype map of the human genome. *Nature.* 2005;437:1299–1320.
7. Frazer KA, Ballinger DG, Cox DR, et al. A second generation human haplotype map of over 3.1 million SNPs. *Nature.* 2007;449:851–861.
8. Manolio TA, Brooks LD, Collins FS. A HapMap harvest of insights into the genetics of common disease. *J Clin Invest.* 2008;118:1590–1605.
9. Mardis ER. The impact of next-generation sequencing technology on genetics. *Trends Genet.* 2008;24:133–141.
10. The Cancer Genome Atlas Research Network. Comprehensive genomic characterization defines human glioblastoma genes and core pathways. *Nature.* 2008;455:1061–1068.
11. Chanock SJ, Manolio T, Boehnke M, et al. Replicating genotype-phenotype associations. *Nature.* 2007;447:655–660.
12. Hunter DJ, Thomas G, Hoover RN, et al. Scanning the horizon: what is the future of genome-wide association studies in accelerating discoveries in cancer etiology and prevention? *Cancer Causes Control.* 2007;18:479–484.
13. Hirschhorn JN, Altshuler D. Once and again-issues surrounding replication in genetic association studies. *J Clin Endocrinol Metab.* 2002;87:4438–4441.
14. Skol AD, Scott LJ, Abecasis GR, et al. Joint analysis is more efficient than replication-based analysis for two-stage genome-wide association studies. *Nat Genet.* 2006;38:209–213.
15. Sabeti PC, Schaffner SF, Fry B, et al. Positive natural selection in the human lineage. *Science.* 2006;312:1614–1620.
16. Stratton MR, Rahman N. The emerging landscape of breast cancer susceptibility. *Nat Genet.* 2008;40:17–22.
17. Hall JM, Lee MK, Newman B, et al. Linkage of early-onset familial breast cancer to chromosome 17q21. *Science.* 1990;250:1684–1689.
18. Wooster R, Bignell G, Lancaster J, et al. Identification of the breast cancer susceptibility gene BRCA2. *Nature.* 1995;378:789–792.
19. Risch N, Merikangas K. The future of genetic studies of complex human diseases. *Science.* 1996;273:1516–1517.
20. Kruglyak L, Nickerson DA. Variation is the spice of life. *Nat Genet.* 2001;27:234–236.
21. Reich DE, Cargill M, Bolk S, et al. Linkage disequilibrium in the human genome. *Nature.* 2001;411:199–204.
22. Reich DE, Gabriel SB, Altshuler D. Quality and completeness of SNP databases. *Nat Genet.* 2003;33:457–458.

23. Hinds DA, Stuve LL, Nilsen GB, et al. Whole-genome patterns of common DNA variation in three human populations. *Science.* 2005;307:1072–1079.

24. Relethford JH. Global patterns of isolation by distance based on genetic and morphological data. *Hum Biol.* 2004;76:499–513.

25. Ramachandran S, Deshpande O, Roseman CC, et al. Support from the relationship of genetic and geographic distance in human populations for a serial founder effect originating in Africa. *Proc Natl Acad Sci USA.* 2005;102:15942–15947.

26. Li JZ, Absher DM, Tang H, et al. Worldwide human relationships inferred from genome-wide patterns of variation. *Science.* 2008;319:1100–1104.

27. Rosenberg NA, Pritchard JK, Weber JL, et al. Genetic structure of human populations. *Science.* 2002;298:2381–2385.

28. Romero IG, Manica A, Goudet J, et al. How accurate is the current picture of human genetic variation? *Heredity.* 2008;101:471–472.

29. Hughes AL, Packer B, Welch R, et al. Effects of natural selection on interpopulation divergence at polymorphic sites in human protein-coding loci. *Genetics.* 2005;170:1181–1187.

30. Sabeti PC, Varilly P, Fry B, et al. Genome-wide detection and characterization of positive selection in human populations. *Nature.* 2007;449:913–918.

31. Tishkoff SA, Reed FA, Ranciaro A, et al. Convergent adaptation of human lactase persistence in Africa and Europe. *Nat Genet.* 2007;39:31–40.

32. Chanock S. Candidate genes and single nucleotide polymorphisms (SNPs) in the study of human disease. *Dis Markers.* 2001;17:89–98.

33. Risch NJ. Searching for genetic determinants in the new millennium. *Nature.* 2000;405:847–856.

34. Miklos I, Novak A, Dombai B, et al. How reliably can we predict the reliability of protein structure predictions? *BMC Bioinformatics.* 2008;9:137.

35. Edwards YJ, Cottage A. Bioinformatics methods to predict protein structure and function. A practical approach. *Mol Biotechnol.* 2003;23:139–166.

36. Heringa J. Computational methods for protein secondary structure prediction using multiple sequence alignments. *Curr Protein Pept Sci.* 2000;1:273–301.

37. Erichsen HC, Chanock SJ. SNPs in cancer research and treatment. *Br J Cancer.* 2004;90:747–751.

38. Cargill M, Altshuler D, Ireland J, et al. Characterization of single-nucleotide polymorphisms in coding regions of human genes. *Nat Genet.* 1999;22:231–238.

39. Stephens JC, Schneider JA, Tanguay DA, et al. Haplotype variation and linkage disequilibrium in 313 human genes. *Science.* 2001;293:489–493.

40. Packer BR, Yeager M, Burdett L, et al. SNP500Cancer: a public resource for sequence validation, assay development, and frequency analysis for genetic variation in candidate genes. *Nucleic Acids Res.* 2006:D617–D621.

41. Stephens M, Sloan JS, Robertson PD, et al. Automating sequence-based detection and genotyping of SNPs from diploid samples. *Nat Genet.* 2006;38:375–381.

42. Marth G, Schuler G, Yeh R, et al. Sequence variations in the public human genome data reflect a bottlenecked population history. *Proc Natl Acad Sci USA.* 2003;100:376–381.

43. Marth GT, Korf I, Yandell MD, et al. A general approach to single-nucleotide polymorphism discovery. *Nat Genet.* 1999;23:452–456.

44. Bonnen PE, Wang PJ, Kimmel M, et al. Haplotype and linkage disequilibrium architecture for human cancer-associated genes. *Genome Res.* 2002;12:1846–1853.

45. Sabeti PC, Reich DE, Higgins JM, et al. Detecting recent positive selection in the human genome from haplotype structure. *Nature.* 2002;419:832–837.

46. Cardon LR, Abecasis GR. Using haplotype blocks to map human complex trait loci. *Trends Genet.* 2003;19:135–140.

47. Johnson GC, Esposito L, Barratt BJ, et al. Haplotype tagging for the identification of common disease genes. *Nat Genet.* 2001;29:233–237.
48. Barrett JC, Fry B, Maller J, et al. Haploview: analysis and visualization of LD and haplotype maps. *Bioinformatics.* 2005;21:263–265.
49. Stram DO, Haiman C, Hirschhorn JN, et al. Choosing Haplotype-Tagging SNP based on unphased genotype data using a preliminary sample of the unrelated subjects with AN example from the multiethnic cohort study. *Hum Hered.* 2003;55:27–36.
50. Gabriel SB, Schaffner SF, Nguyen H, et al. The structure of haplotype blocks in the human genome. *Science.* 2002;296:2225–2229.
51. Carlson CS, Eberle MA, Rieder MJ, et al. Selecting a maximally informative set of single-nucleotide polymorphisms for association analyses using linkage disequilibrium. *Am J Hum Genet.* 2004;74:106–120.
52. McCarroll SA, Altshuler DM. Copy-number variation and association studies of human disease. *Nat Genet.* 2007;39:S37–S42.
53. Scherer SW, Lee C, Birney E, et al. Challenges and standards in integrating surveys of structural variation. *Nat Genet.* 2007;39:S7–S15.
54. Kidd JM, Cooper GM, Donahue WF, et al. Mapping and sequencing of structural variation from eight human genomes. *Nature.* 2008;453:56–64.
55. Feuk L, Carson AR, Scherer SW. Structural variation in the human genome. *Nat Rev Genet.* 2006;7:85–97.
56. Stefansson H, Helgason A, Thorleifsson G, et al. A common inversion under selection in Europeans. *Nat Genet.* 2005;37:129–137.
57. Sharp AJ, Locke DP, McGrath SD, et al. Segmental duplications and copy-number variation in the human genome. *Am J Hum Genet.* 2005;77:78–88.
58. Sebat J, Lakshmi B, Troge J, et al. Large-scale copy number polymorphism in the human genome. *Science.* 2004;305:525–528.
59. Iafrate AJ, Feuk L, Rivera MN, et al. Detection of large-scale variation in the human genome. *Nat Genet.* 2004;36:949–951.
60. Inoue K, Lupski JR. Molecular mechanisms for genomic disorders. *Annu Rev Genomics Hum Genet.* 2002;3:199–242.
61. Bailey JA, Yavor AM, Massa HF, et al. Segmental duplications: organization and impact within the current human genome project assembly. *Genome Res.* 2001;11:1005–1017.
62. Bailey JA, Gu Z, Clark RA, et al. Recent segmental duplications in the human genome. *Science.* 2002;297:1003–1007.
63. Buckley PG, Mantripragada KK, Piotrowski A, et al. Copy-number polymorphisms: mining the tip of an iceberg. *Trends Genet.* 2005;21:315–317.
64. McCarroll SA, Kuruvilla FG, Korn JM, et al. Integrated detection and population-genetic analysis of SNPs and copy number variation. *Nat Genet.* 2008;40:1166–1174.
65. Khaja R, Zhang J, MacDonald JR, et al. Genome assembly comparison identifies structural variants in the human genome. *Nat Genet.* 2006;38:1413–1418.
66. Freeman JL, Perry GH, Feuk L, et al. Copy number variation: new insights in genome diversity. *Genome Res.* 2006;16:949–961.
67. Khaja R, Zhang J, MacDonald JR, et al. Genome assembly comparison identifies structural variants in the human genome. *Nat Genet.* 2006;38:1413–1418.
68. Istrail S, Sutton GG, Florea L, et al. Whole-genome shotgun assembly and comparison of human genome assemblies. *Proc Natl Acad Sci USA.* 2004;101:1916–1921.
69. Cooper GM, Zerr T, Kidd JM, et al. Systematic assessment of copy number variant detection via genome-wide SNP genotyping. *Nat Genet.* 2008;40:1199–1203.
70. Korn JM, Kuruvilla FG, McCarroll SA, et al. Integrated genotype calling and association analysis of SNPs, common copy number polymorphisms and rare CNVs. *Nat Genet.* 2008;40:1253–1260.

71. Barnes C, Plagnol V, Fitzgerald T, et al. A robust statistical method for case-control association testing with copy number variation. *Nat Genet.* 2008;40:1254–1252.

72. Goellner GM, Tester D, Thibodeau S, et al. Different mechanisms underlie DNA instability in Huntington disease and colorectal cancer. *Am J Hum Genet.* 1997;60:879–890.

73. Ballantyne KN, van Oorschot RAH, Mitchell RJ. Comparison of two whole genome amplification methods for STR genotyping of LCN and degraded DNA samples. *Forensic Sci Int.* 2007;166:35–41.

74. Roewer L, Krawczak M, Willuweit S, et al. Online reference database of European Y-chromosomal short tandem repeat (STR) haplotypes. *Forensic Sci Int.* 2001;118:106–113.

75. Pompanon F, Bonin A, Bellemain E, et al. Genotyping errors: causes, consequences and solutions. *Nat Rev Genet.* 2005;6:847–859.

76. Packer BR, Yeager M, Staats B, et al. SNP500Cancer: a public resource for sequence validation and assay development for genetic variation in candidate genes. *Nucleic Acids Res.* 2004;32:D528–D532.

77. Saiki RK, Scharf S, Faloona F, et al. Enzymatic amplification of beta-globin genomic sequences and restriction site analysis for diagnosis of sickle cell anemia. *Science.* 1985;230:1350–1354.

78. Livak KJ, Marmaro J, Todd JA. Towards fully automated genome-wide polymorphism screening. *Nat Genet.* 1995;9:341–342.

79. Brenan CJ. DNA-based molecular lithography for nanoscale fabrication. *IEEE Eng Med Biol Mag.* 2002;21:164.

80. Frederickson R. Fluidigm. *Chem Biol.* 2002;9:1161–1162.

81. Sun X, Ding H, Hung K, Guo B. A new MALDI-TOF based mini-sequencing assay for genotyping of SNPS. *Nucleic Acids Res.* 2000;28:E68.

82. Cunningham JM, Sellers TA, Schildkraut JM, et al. Performance of amplified DNA in an Illumina Golden Gate Bead Array assay. *Cancer Epidemiol Biomarkers Prev.* 2008;17:1781–1789.

83. Berthier-Schaad Y, Kao WH, Coresh J, et al. Reliability of high-throughput genotyping of whole genome amplified DNA in SNP genotyping studies. *Electrophoresis.* 2007;28:2812–2817.

84. Thomas G, Jacobs KB, Yeager M, et al. Multiple loci identified in a genome-wide association study of prostate cancer. *Nat Genet.* 2008;40:310–315.

85. Matsuzaki H, Loi H, Dong S, et al. Parallel genotyping of over 10,000 SNPs using a one-primer assay on a high-density oligonucleotide array. *Genome Res.* 2004;14:414–425.

86. Barrett JC, Cardon LR. Evaluating coverage of genome-wide association studies. *Nat Genet.* 2006;38:659–662.

87. McCarthy MI, Abecasis GR, Cardon LR, et al. Genome-wide association studies for complex traits: consensus, uncertainty and challenges. *Nat Rev Genet.* 2008;9:356–369.

88. Sanger F, Nicklen S, Coulson AR. DNA sequencing with chain-terminating inhibitors. *Proc Natl Acad Sci USA.* 1977;74:5463–5467.

89. Collins FS, Morgan M, Patrinos A. The Human Genome Project: lessons from large-scale biology. *Science.* 2003;300:286–290.

90. Shendure J, Mitra RD, Varma C, et al. Advanced sequencing technologies: methods and goals. *Nat Rev Genet.* 2004;5:335–344.

91. Margulies M, Egholm M, Altman WE, et al. Genome sequencing in microfabricated high-density picolitre reactors. *Nature.* 2005;437:376–380.

92. Dressman D, Yan H, Traverso G, et al. Transforming single DNA molecules into fluorescent magnetic particles for detection and enumeration of genetic variations. *Proc Natl Acad Sci USA.* 2003;100:8817–8822.

93. Haque KA, Pfeiffer RM, Beerman MB, et al. Performance of high-throughput DNA quantification methods. *BMC Biotechnol.* 2003;3:20.
94. Bergen AW, Haque KA, Qi Y, et al. Comparison of yield and genotyping performance of multiple displacement amplification and OmniPlex whole genome amplified DNA generated from multiple DNA sources. *Hum Mutat.* 2005;26:262–270.
95. Purcell S, Neale B, Todd-Brown K, et al. PLINK: a tool set for whole-genome association and population-based linkage analyses. *Am J Hum Genet.* 2007;81:559–575.

3

The public health genomics enterprise

Philippa Brice and Ron Zimmern

Introduction

The association between public health and genomics is relatively recent, emerging as a consequence of the prominence given to the human genome following the elucidation of the genetic code. Nevertheless, public health has for over a century shared a common history with human genetics through its links with the eugenics movement, and its quest to improve the health of future generations (1). It is likely that the original proponents of eugenics had altruistic intentions as they sought to apply emerging knowledge of Mendelian genetics to promote the fitness of populations; but modern society has now condemned their approaches to this goal as ethically repugnant, while modern science has demonstrated critical flaws in their understanding of hereditary (genetic) factors governing complex diseases and traits. Yet some continue to make the "complex connections" between public health and eugenics when they refer to the prenatal genetic screening programs of today (2).

The ideas behind eugenics were firmly based on *genetics*, the study of inherited variation in living organisms. *Genomics*, by contrast, is a wider term referring to the study of the structure and function of the genome and the role it plays in health and disease. The term *genomics* is now usually used in an even broader manner to encompass the entirety of genetic, cellular, and molecular biology, and in particular the explosion in knowledge and understanding that has resulted from the Human Genome Project. It is in this broadest sense, summarized later in the chapter as "genome-based knowledge," (3) that we employ the word *genomics*.

We refer to public health genomics as an *enterprise* to emphasize its importance, novelty, and difficulty, and its need for vision, boldness, and energy. It seems appropriate to do so because the potential benefits of genomic and postgenomic research for human health are both vast and desirable. The pace of change, although extremely fast when considered in relative terms, is nevertheless perceived by some as slow. This may be in part a reaction to the hype surrounding the "genomic revolution"; proponents of the Human Genome Project, in their enthusiasm to promote their endeavors, were somewhat overoptimistic in their estimation of the likely timescale for changes in health care due to emerging genomic understanding. They are not altogether to be blamed for this enthusiasm, because as the Human Genome Project has progressed, there has been an increasing realization that the complexity of the human body in health and disease, and the role of genetic factors in the regulation of these processes, are far greater than were originally imagined. While the prospects for genomic medicine are as bright as ever, the "revolution," as originally predicted by Francis Collins, former director of U.S. National Human Genome Research Institute (4), seems more likely to be a steady process of incremental change, and there are signs that some, at least, are gradually acknowledging this fact (5).

This chapter will consider first the origins and emergence of public health genomics as a subdiscipline of public health, moving on to a consideration of current practice with some specific examples, before finally looking at the future prospects for the field and its role within medicine and health care in the twenty-first century and beyond.

The Origins of Public Health Genomics

Scientific understanding of the fundamentals of genetics and molecular biology really took off in the latter half of the twentieth century, with a series of key discoveries such as the structure of DNA (6) and the elucidation of the genetic code (7). The 1980s and 1990s were a time of major progress for medical genetics, particularly chromosomal disorders and what are sometimes referred to as "genetic diseases"—monogenic, or single-gene, diseases, which typically show set patterns of inheritance and hence expression within affected families. In particular, it became possible to identify chromosomal regions involved in such diseases using family-based linkage studies and, more recently, genetic association studies. Though less than 100%, the association between the presence of variants in a given gene and the existence of a corresponding monogenic disease is very strong and amenable to genetic epidemiological analysis. Using rapidly developing techniques to isolate, amplify, and sequence specific regions of DNA, researchers were able to pinpoint the precise genes associated with major diseases, and to identify the mutations within these genes that led to disease. For example, the *DMD* gene was identified as the gene involved in Duchenne muscular dystrophy in 1986 (8), the *CFTR* gene as the gene involved in cystic fibrosis in 1989 (9), and the *HTT* gene as that involved in Huntington disease in 1993 (10). By 2008, the *Online Mendelian Inheritance in Man* (OMIM) database listed over 1,850 different rare, heritable diseases. These insights, combined with novel technologies and the development of genetic tests to identify the presence of key mutations, have greatly expanded the capacity of clinical geneticists to predict and diagnose monogenic diseases and to help affected families.

Understanding of the contribution of genetic factors to disease has grown enormously in the past 20 years, largely as a result of the sequencing of the human genome and related studies. The formal inception of the Human Genome Project (HGP) was in 1990, when an international consortium of centers in the United States, United Kingdom, France, Germany, Japan, and China, led and coordinated by the

U.S. National Institutes of Health (NIH) and the Department of Energy (DOE), set out to determine the complete sequence of the human genome. A first draft of the sequence was published in 2001 (11,12), and the HGP was formally completed in 2003, with the publication of 99% of the gene-containing regions to an accuracy of 99.99%; certain sections of the genome proved highly refractory to standard methods of sequencing (13). The twenty-first century is very much a "postgenomic" era; rather than simply putting into practice the fruits of the HGP (although this is certainly happening) many researchers are setting out to perform extraordinary feats of information collection and analysis, in order to make sense of the bewildering complexity that is the functional human genome. New landmark discoveries continue to emerge, notably within epigenomics (14), the study of the spatio-temporal regulation of gene expression via mechanisms *other* than DNA sequence; for example, the identification of RNA interference (15). Much remains to be determined. Yet, while a comprehensive understanding of the human organism remains a very distant goal (if indeed it will ever be entirely possible), the benefits to date have already been significant, not least in terms of disease genetics.

Unfortunately, the relationship between genetic variant and disease is frequently unclear, even for monogenic diseases. Relatively few show complete *penetrance*; penetrance refers to the probability that an individual with a specific genotype will develop the associated disease, over a defined period, that is, a lifetime. For example, while the lifetime penetrance of the dominant monogenic disorder Huntington disease can be as high as 100% for individuals with trinucleotide repeat expansions of 41 or more in the *HTT* gene (16), the lifetime clinical penetrance of the recessive monogenic disorder hereditary hemochromatosis (caused by inherited mutations in the *HFE* gene) is known to be low, with estimates ranging from less than 1% (17) to approaching 30% (18,19). The *expressivity* of a disease may also vary; that is, the degree and manner in which individuals with a given genotype show symptoms of disease. Cystic fibrosis is typically completely penetrant in childhood, but the nature and severity of disease varies; while most patients show multisymptomatic (multiorgan) forms of disease, some retain normal pancreatic function, and others show only mild respiratory symptoms (20). Nor is the identification of pathogenic mutations necessarily straightforward, even where the gene associated with the disease has been identified. In some cases, a specific mutation or small group of mutations causes a monogenic disease or chromosomal disorder, but in others, whole genes must be scanned for thousands of potential causative mutations, a phenomenon known as *allelic heterogeneity*. Clinical geneticists and specialist genetic counsellors must take into account all these complexities and more when discussing options and possibilities for genetic testing and reproductive strategies for families affected by monogenic diseases.

Determinants of Health

While public health genomics retains significant links to classical medical genetics, it is inevitably, as a discipline concerned with population health, intimately linked with the genetics of the more common, complex diseases that affect populations such as depression, cardiovascular disease, type 2 diabetes, cancer, Alzheimer disease, and asthma. The pathogenesis of such diseases is influenced by multiple contributory factors, and causation cannot be attributed primarily to any single genetic or environmental determinant, unlike monogenic or infectious diseases. In considering disease causation and progression, especially for complex diseases, internal or individual factors (genetic and behavioral) must be taken into account along with external (environmental, social, or political) factors (Figure 3.1). Early public health efforts were focused primarily on interventions against harmful environmental influences in order to improve the health of the population; for example, the provision of sanitation and clean water, unadulterated food, and decent living conditions. In the developed world during the latter half of the twentieth century, with the decreasing prevalence of infectious disease, emphasis moved toward prevention of the complex chronic diseases, particularly via behavioral interventions, such as promoting smoking cessation and weight loss. In the years leading up to the twenty-first century there has been increasing recognition that, from a public health perspective, understanding both the behavioral *and* genetic forms of "internal" factors (Figure 3.1), and the ways in which they interact in the pathogenesis of complex diseases, is important for disease prevention.

Knowledge of key gene–environment interactions can ideally permit a combined approach to disease prevention. This includes forms of genetic screening to identify high-risk population subgroups in whom an exaggerated response to a common environmental exposure may be predicted (21), with environmental risk assessment and interventions to prevent the onset, or minimize the impact, of disease. Currently, individuals' risk of disease is estimated based on a combination of clinical measures and environmental exposures, such as age, gender, family history, weight, smoking status, and alcohol consumption, with preventative measures directed against those at greatest risk of developing disease. Understanding the genetic factors that influence diseases may provide additional information that can refine and improve risk

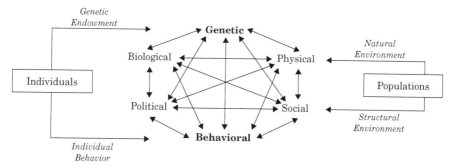

Figure 3.1   Determinants of health: interaction between internal or individual (genetic and behavioral) and external (environmental, social, or political) factors. Source: Adapted from Genetics, Health Care and Public Policy. Alison Stewart, Philippa Brice, Hilary Burton, Paul Pharoah, Simon Sanderson and Ron Zimmern, Cambridge University Press, 2007; Figure 1.1, page 3.

assessment, although the clinical utility of these refinements in risk estimation has yet to be determined.

Of note, the application of genetic knowledge in disease prevention as advocated by practitioners of public health genomics is primarily what has been referred to as "phenotypic prevention," that is, medical intervention to avert or delay the onset of disease in an at-risk patient (22). It is important to distinguish this from the alternative approach of "genotypic prevention," intervention to modify the genotype itself or to prevent the transmission of the genotype to the next generation, for example, via gene therapy or prenatal genetic diagnosis. Although such interventions may be offered to families affected by monogenic diseases via clinical geneticists, they are inappropriate for a population-based approach to disease prevention.

The Genetics of Complex Disease

Following on from work identifying the genes involved in monogenic diseases, the "second-wave" of genetic epidemiology proceeding from the HGP is the study of the genetics of common complex diseases. As has already been noted, the identification of genetic factors involved in the causation of such diseases is fraught with difficulty, since not only do multiple different factors influence most human diseases, they also interact with each other. However, this has not prevented researchers from attempting it, and in the past 10 years there have been numerous reports of significant links between a genetic variant and one form of disease or another. Unfortunately, the vast majority of these were not independently validated, and meta-analyses of multiple different studies often suggested that the true association was insignificant or extremely small. At the same time, each new publication was portrayed in the media in rather sweeping terms that are still employed today, such as *discovery of asthma gene offers new hope* (23), *depression gene discovered* (24), and *"fat" gene found by scientists* (25); communicating complex science of necessity requires simplistic explanations, and this combined with a natural journalistic tendency toward sensationalism meant that findings were often hyped.

It gradually became clear to the scientific community that searching for genetic variants involved in the pathogenesis of complex diseases in the same way that links had been made for Mendelian diseases was not effective enough; it proved more difficult than searching for a needle in a haystack, and small- to medium-scale genetic association studies (however well performed) were simply not highly powered enough to deliver the results. The contribution of any *one* genetic factor to a multigenic disease, even one conferring a relatively significant disease risk, is inevitably much smaller than a genetic factor that is effectively causative for a monogenic disease. Efforts therefore turned to the creation of huge disease cohorts large enough to yield meaningful and reliable results, such as the Wellcome Trust Case Control Consortium (26).

At the same time, Human Genome Project partners established new initiatives to generate data to support these efforts: the single nucleotide polymorphism (SNP) and Haplotype Mapping (HapMap) projects (27). These projects set out to create a map of common genetic variation in human populations, at the level of SNPs, and in particular, to identify and map key "tag" SNPs representative of groups of variants called haplotypes. The capacity to perform genome-wide scanning of SNPs for their possible association with disease has expanded steadily since the inception of the HapMap initiative; combined with new super-cohorts, results from the first large-scale genome-wide association studies (GWAS) began to emerge in 2006. By the end of 2007, more than 50 GWAS had been published in the major journals, reporting associations between selected genetic polymorphisms and diseases ranging from breast cancer (28) to Crohn's disease and type 2 diabetes (26,29,30). The results may be relatively modest, typically identifying variants that confer a relative risk of less than 2.0 for the disease in question (31), but they are robust. Such results represent the first steps in the mammoth task of trying to unravel the complex connections between genetics and disease. National and international collaboration continues to be the key to results, with new initiatives such as the Genetic Association Information Network (GAIN) (32) getting underway.

As human genome epidemiology expands, and understanding of the complex function of genes (and the environment) in health and disease gradually improves, the capacity for improved human health, thanks to novel methods of prevention, diagnosis, and treatment, increases (33). Although it is true that a comprehensive understanding remains a very distant prospect, the first examples of "genomic medicine" are already moving into clinical practice (34), and the vital bridging role of public health genomics in maximizing the potential health benefits becomes increasingly apparent.

The Emergence of Public Health Genomics

The specific discipline of public health genomics emerged in the 1990s, along with the major push to sequence the human genome (see Figure 3.2), as public health physicians began to realize the importance of genomics to different aspects of public health practice, particularly the potential applications of genetic testing (35). In the United States, the report of a Task Force on Genetics and Disease Prevention to the Centers for Disease Control and Prevention (CDC) led to the creation of a new Office of Genetics and Disease Prevention at CDC in 1997, later renamed the Office of Public Health Genomics (36). At around the same time, in the United Kingdom, expert advisory groups had similarly begun to recognize the potential new roles for genetics within the National Health Service (NHS), beyond the existing specialized genetics services. The Public Health Genetics Unit (PHGU) was established in Cambridge in 1997 (37), and was later succeeded by an independent charity, the Foundation for Genomics and Population Health (PHG Foundation). Over the past 10 years, public health genomics has gained increasing recognition as a discipline, with the establishment of academic centers (such as the Centers of Genomics and

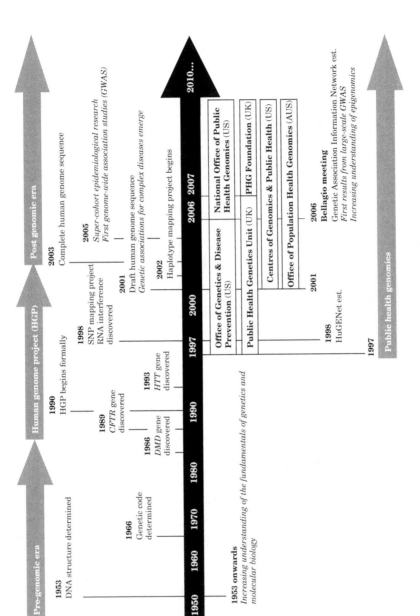

Figure 3.2   Timeline—the emergence of public health genomics.

Public Health at the Universities of Washington and Michigan in the United States, and the Center for Public Health Genetics at the University of Applied Sciences, Bielefeld, Germany) and various governmental and health care bodies in different countries (such as the Office of Population Health Genomics in the Department of Health of Western Australia).

The United Kingdom model for public health genetics was built around the Acheson definition of public health (38) and was originally defined as *the application of advances in genetics on the art and science of promoting health and preventing disease through the organised efforts of society* (39). This definition was intended to encompass "genetics" in the broadest sense, including both classical medical genetics and the new genetics and molecular biology of the genomic era. Disease prevention was similarly taken to include the whole spectrum of prevention, including interventions to arrest or delay disease progression and disability. Other proponents have similarly referred to public health genetics as the *challenge of interpreting the medical and public health significance of genetic variation within populations* (40) and the *intersection of genetics, public health, and preventive medicine* (41).

In 2005, 18 pioneers of public health genomics in the developed world came together to hold an expert workshop in Bellagio, Italy; funded by the Rockefeller Foundation, this group sought to agree on a formal definition for the discipline and take steps toward creating an effective international network of practitioners, to share and advance knowledge and practice. The experts in genome-based science, epidemiology, and public health, and law and ethics came from Canada, France, Germany, the United Kingdom, and the United States; together, they considered questions about the key concepts and aims that underlie public health genetics and the necessary inputs and outputs to achieve these goals. The first action was to agree on the use of "genomics" rather than "genetics," because it was felt to convey a more accurate impression of the breadth of the subject, incorporating not merely inheritance but also genomic knowledge and technologies proceeding beyond the scope of the original human genome project. Similarly, "population health" was considered to be a more useful term than "public health," since in some countries the latter has a more narrow definition that fails to include involvement in health service policy development and delivery. Finally, the enterprise of public health genomics was defined as *the responsible and effective translation of genome-based knowledge and technologies for the benefit of population health* (3).

This, then, is the overarching goal of public health genomics: the effective translation of novel biomedical understanding, tools, and techniques, into interventions that benefit human health. Translation is a key tenet, and another, which is interpreted in its broadest sense, encompassing not only the common concept of "bench to bedside" (primary translational research), but also what has been referred to as *the second gap in translation*, is the identification and evaluation of new and effective interventions (for example, novel tools for improved diagnosis, screening, or clinical management) and their implementation into clinical practice (42). This "second gap" in moving interventions into actual health care delivery, also dubbed "translation

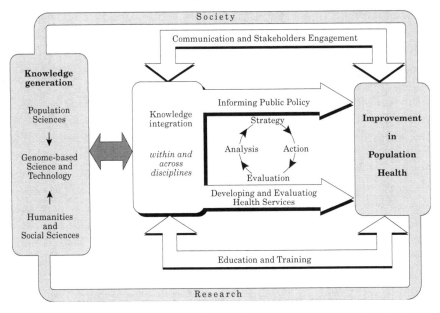

Figure 3.3   The Public Health Genomics Enterprise: moving interventions into health care delivery (translation to practice). Source: *Adapted from* Genome-based research and population health, 2006. *Report of an expert workshop held at the Rockefeller Foundation Study and Conference Center, Bellagio, Italy, April 14-20, 2005.*

to practice," (43) can seem minor relative to the challenges of moving from basic research to clinical trials ("translation to humans/patients"); but it is in many ways more complex, requiring the integration of multiple different sources and types of information to develop effective policies and strategies for improving the health of populations (Figure 3.3). Translation research in the context of genomic medicine has been further characterized as having four stages, or phases, moving from discovery to candidate health application (T1) and health application to evidence-based guidelines (T2), through to practice guidelines to health practice (T3), and practice to population health impact (T4) (44). Crucially, it requires more than research—even research with strictly translational focus—to achieve actual improvements in population health, which is why evaluation and development of health services and policy development are essential processes (Figure 3.3).

Obviously, since different countries have different health care systems, the exact process of policy development and movement into health practice will vary, but the guiding principles will be the same. In all cases, given the enormous investment of resources in basic and clinical biomedical research, unnecessary delay in the implementation of evidence-based strategies and interventions in health care is certainly undesirable, and yet the time lag remains. In recent years, proponents of public health genomics have played a key role in increasing awareness of this delay, and of strategies to combat it.

Central to the practice of public health genomics is interdisciplinarity, involving contributions from multiple areas of learning and expertise. From its inception, the field has brought together clinicians and scientists from a range of disciplines (notably public health, epidemiology, and the various forms of genetics, genomics, and molecular biology) with researchers from the social sciences, humanities, and other fields including law, philosophy, and ethics. Although linking together such disparate areas can be difficult, research and perspectives from all are essential, thanks to the aim of achieving "responsible" translation of biomedical advances into health benefits. This single word encompasses the manifold ethical, legal, and social implications (ELSI) arising from human genomics, the importance of which has been acknowledged from the beginning of the Human Genome Project itself, which devoted 3–5% of funding solely to work in this area.

The necessity for expert research and dialog in ELSI has been strengthened by public attitudes to genomic research and applications. Not only has the potential significance of genetic information been overemphasized, leading to the concept of *genetic exceptionalism*—the belief that genetic information is fundamentally distinct from any other forms of personal or medical information, and as such deserving of additional regulation (45)—but there is also a certain level of public distrust in the area of genetics and genomics. Some of this may be attributed to the legacy of eugenics; in the first half of the twentieth century, proponents of eugenics sought the improvement of human health, mental and physical capacity, for the benefit of populations. Although altruistic in origin, extreme supporters of the movement sought to impose unacceptable solutions, from selective sterilization to murder of those considered unfit. The concept that it was possible to distinguish simply between desirable and undesirable traits and select for or against them via selective breeding was, of course, completely flawed, since, as we now appreciate, even if it were possible to define such traits, they arise from multiple genetic and environmental influences and are therefore not amenable to manipulation via selective breeding.

Concerns about privacy and safety are important too; in insurance-based health care systems such as that of the United States, some fear that genetic information could be used as a bar against receiving treatment, if it were to reveal an increased risk of a certain disease or group of diseases. Fears of potential "genetic discrimination" also extend to other areas, notably employment. In the United Kingdom, research into the genetic modification of crops to increase resistance to disease suffered a public relations disaster in the 1990s, with a strong backlash against any form of "tampering with nature" that even now, for some, produces sinister overtones to the word "genetic" in almost any context. It is therefore essential that the development and implementation of health care tools and approaches should incorporate appropriate public and patient engagement and communication efforts. There are also issues that relate more specifically to population-based research and health programs and to genetic testing and screening, such as consent and confidentiality. Medical techniques in assisted reproduction raise moral issues for many, as do certain forms of research such as the derivation of human stem cells from embryos. The development and effective regulation of any such interventions, policies, and programs must therefore necessarily take into account expert input from many areas beyond that of biomedical science.

The incorporation of multiple different sources of data and expertise does, how-ever, pose a significant problem. Public health genomics therefore considers *knowledge integration* to be the key step in moving from genome-based knowledge and technologies into improved health of populations (46). In order to take into account all the relevant information, practitioners must analyze, synthesize, and com-prehend information and knowledge from many different disciplines, in order to properly inform the development and evaluation of health care policy and services (Figure 3.3). Although self-evident, this requirement for intelligent and well-in-formed knowledge brokers is contrary to the tradition of increasing specialization in both medicine and science; the structures of training are such that most individuals focus on an increasingly restricted area of practice and develop expertise primarily in this. While these experts are no less valuable today than in the past, there is an emerging need for a new generation of practitioners to support the experts; pub-lic health genomics embraces a groundbreaking attitude in requiring a "specialized generalist" approach to achieving its desired goals.

Of course, no single individual can amass sufficient expertise in enough fields to function alone; this is one reason why the practice of public health genomics has an essential requirement for interdisciplinarity. Suitable *knowledge management* support can facilitate this process and maximize the returns; for example, efficient systems and procedures for the identification and sharing of relevant information will aid timely interpretation, analysis, and action. However, since no one organi-zation can realistically employ all the experts it may ever need to cover the range of disciplines a given project in public health genomics might require, the second key aspect of knowledge integration comes into play: *knowledge brokering*. This is a process whereby practitioners of public health genomics can identify and bring together key individuals or bodies—for example, health service commissioners and managers; physicians, clinical geneticists, and other health care professionals; bio-medical scientists and health economists; patient and other stakeholder groups; and experts in law and regulation, ethics, philosophy, and sociology—and facilitate their interaction to produce suitable policy or service development. This may require input from the knowledge brokers, ranging from simple organization, informed network-ing, or literature review and synthesis, to commissioning or performing secondary research, auditing clinical practice across a whole region or country, or disseminat-ing findings, recommendations, or guidelines in an appropriate manner. An effec-tive knowledge brokering organization acts as a catalyst for change, by identifying needs, developing and streamlining work that addresses those needs, and moving it into health care practice.

There is increasing recognition of the overwhelming requirement for interdisci-plinary research and communication in order to achieve prompt transfer of inno-vations into clinical practice (47), and a movement toward creating groups and networks that will function in this manner. For example, the Canadian Health Services Research Foundation aims to address this gap between research and health care management and policy *by facilitating knowledge transfer and exchange;* new public-private partnerships such as the U.S. Biomarkers Consortium (48), which aims to support the development of *safe and effective medicines and treatments* from research right through to evaluation, regulatory approval, and suitable clinical practice guidance, are becoming more commonplace. In the same way, the need for expert knowledge brokers and intermediaries to "bridge the know-do gap for health services" (49) is also being acknowledged.

The Practice of Public Health Genomics

Genomics and Medicine

Genomics has the potential to transform medicine by generating new insights into the underlying genetic and biological basis of disease, including the genetic factors that may cause or significantly predispose individuals to develop specific disorders. This new knowledge provides previously unprecedented opportunities to prevent, detect, diagnose, and treat disease, and these are beginning to move into multiple areas of medicine to differing degrees (although genomic medicine is presently much more prominent in some services than others), as well as in public health practice. For example, the identification of mutations involved in monogenic disease and the development of specific genetic tests has permitted improved diagnosis; although there are relatively few therapeutic options for Mendelian diseases, in many cases there is scope to reduce or delay the morbidity associated with the condition. Diagnostic testing may be offered in the prenatal period to identify affected fetuses, and in some cases there is also an option for preimplantation genetic diagnosis (PGD), whereby early embryos generated via *in vitro* fertilization are screened for the presence of the disease-associated mutation, and only unaffected embryos are used to establish a pregnancy.

Genetic testing may also provide useful information with respect to potential therapeutic options. For example, Long QT Syndrome (LQTS), an inherited form of cardiac disease that involves defects in the ion channels of the heart, causes predisposition to arrhythmias and sudden cardiac death, especially in response to certain physiological triggers such as exercise. Mutations in several different genes can cause the syndrome, and knowing which form of LQTS is present can provide vital information for clinical management, both for patients and also for asymptomatic relatives who are found to possess the mutations. For example, different drugs are the therapeutic of choice for different subtypes of the syndrome, and different drugs may be contraindicated (50). Similarly, patients with different subtypes of the syndrome may be at increased risk of sudden cardiac death from different sorts of triggers that should be avoided; in LQTS1, exercise (especially swimming) involves the greatest risk, whereas for LQTS2, being woken by noise (such as an alarm clock) is the most common cause of death (51).

Moving beyond monogenic diseases, pharmacogenetic tests provide information about genetic factors that can influence interindividual variability in drug responses, and could potentially be used to direct the use of all sorts of medications for different indications, allowing clinicians to boost efficacy and reduce adverse reactions by selecting the most appropriate type and dose of drug for each individual patient. For example, responses to the widely prescribed anticoagulant drug warfarin are known to be influenced by the *CYP2C9* and *VKORC1* genotypes, and the drug has recently received an updated label from the U.S. Food and Drug Administration (FDA) to encourage the use of pharmacogenetic information in determining initial dose (52), although the clinical benefits of such testing have yet to be reliably confirmed (53).

In oncology, new tests that simultaneously analyze multiple genomic biomarkers such as gene expression or proteomic profiles have the potential to offer a more precise molecular diagnosis, prognosis, and in some cases also to predict or monitor responses to therapy. Tests that employ breast cancer gene expression profiles to predict likely outcome and direct the choice of treatment (with more aggressive therapy being used against tumors with profiles predictive of poor outcome) are already in development (54). Some high-profile new therapies can exploit the genetically determined molecular features of tumor cells for selectively targeted action. For example, Herceptin (trastuzumab) is used to treat HER2 positive breast tumors (55), while Glivec® (imatinib) uses molecular targeting directed against unique genetic features of chronic myeloid leukemia and gastrointestinal stromal tumor cells (56).

Public Health Genomics

How then do public health practitioners apply understanding of genetics and genomics to promote health and prevent disease in populations? The Bellagio group identified four key areas within public health genomics, proceeding from the interdisciplinary knowledge base (shown in Figure 3.3): the two broad categories of activity are informing public policy and developing and evaluating health services, which are critically underpinned by communication and stakeholder engagement and education and training (3). It is important to note that the diagram presents a conceptual framework for public health genomics, and the four areas of activity are not necessarily distinct in everyday practice. As set out in Figure 3.3, health service and policy development are the essential drivers for the translation of biomedical science and genomics into real changes in health care practice, which in turn will lead to genuine improvements in population health. The development of health services and health service policy, supported by efforts to ensure that relevant public policy and regulation are appropriate, are inherently pluralistic functions, involving many groups and activities, which is why the identification and engagement of appropriate stakeholders from the earliest stages is important, and effective communication is an ongoing requirement. Similarly, the delivery of changes to practice of necessity requires appropriate education and training. In this section, we focus on some selected examples of recent public health genomics work from the key categories of practice.

Informing Public Policy

It has been suggested that it will soon become critical for all forms of health care to employ evidence-based assessment of both new genetic tests and other forms of genomic technologies (57), as genomic medicine expands beyond medical genetics and oncology into other specialties. The evaluation and regulation of genetic tests have therefore been major themes in public health genomics in the last few years, and provide some good examples of recent work in national and international policy development. An Organisation for Economic Cooperation and Development (OECD) international expert meeting in 2006 developed policy recommendations on *The Evaluation of Clinical Validity and Clinical Utility of Genetic Tests (58)*. These included the need to establish international networks and develop an agreed-upon framework for genetic test evaluation, including consensus guidelines and quality standards for data and evidence, and suitable incentives and accountabilities to ensure compliance in different countries. The importance of developing processes and infrastructure for genetic test evaluation in individual countries was also emphasized. EuroGenTest, a European Union-funded network focused on all aspects of genetic testing, promotes harmonization of standards and good practice in member states and beyond, including consideration of quality management, information databases, public health, ethics and legal issues, new technologies, and education. Examples of recent work include the development of European Society of Human Genetics recommendations on *Patenting and licensing in genetic testing* (59) and new *Guidelines for Quality Assurance in Molecular Genetic Testing* (60).

United Kingdom-based work led by the PHG Foundation in this area includes a paper produced for the U.K. Genetic Testing Network, a body established to evaluate the effectiveness of new genetic tests and ensure the equitable provision of high standards of genetics services within the National Health Service (NHS), which provides a new framework for the evaluation of genetic tests (61) expanded from the original ACCE process (62). A later research report examines factors that influence how new genetic tests for common disease susceptibility enter routine clinical practice, emphasizing the need for appropriate clinical evaluation (63), while a meeting organized jointly with the Royal College of Pathologists produced a set of recommendations for the evaluation and regulation of clinical laboratory tests and complex biomarkers (64). In the United States, the Secretary's Advisory Committee on Genetics, Health, and Society (SACGHS), a multidisciplinary body that provides policy advice relating to genetic technologies for the U.S. Department of Health and Human Services, has released a report on the *U.S. System of Oversight of Genetic Testing* (65), which looks at systems to monitor information synthesis and interpretation, to determine standards for analytical and clinical validity and utility, and to ensure compliance. The Office of Public Health Genomics at CDC established the multidisciplinary Evaluation of Genomic Applications in Practice and Prevention (EGAPP) Working Group in 2005 with a specific brief to support a coordinated process for evaluating "genetic tests and other genomic applications" moving into clinical and public health practice; the group's first recommendations drew attention to the lack of evidence that the use of *CYP450* genotyping can improve clinical outcomes (66), despite the availability of a microarray-based test for this purpose that has received regulatory approval for marketing in both the United States (67) and Europe (68).

Another area of major policy development has been in biobanking. Biobanks, which are large-scale repositories of samples of blood, tissue, or other biological material linked with clinical and lifestyle data, are intended to facilitate population-level studies of the genetic and environmental determinants of disease, especially common forms of disease, with a view to improving prevention, diagnosis, and treatment.

Well known examples include the U.K. Biobank, CARTaGENE, Generation Scotland, the Western Australian Genome Health Project, the Estonian Genome Project, and LifeGene, but there are many others. Biobanks are governed in different ways: by specific legislation, or via internal systems. For example, the Estonian Genomic Database was created by an act of parliament and is governed by specific legislation, whereas the U.K. Biobank was established independently and has an independent Ethics and Governance Council, although it is subject to relevant existing legislation. Key issues that have arisen in policy development for the regulation and governance of biobanking initiatives have been focused mainly around ethical and legal issues of consent (69,70), confidentiality and identifiability (71), and property and benefit sharing (72); academic publications have reviewed these aspects of biobanks (73,74). Issues may vary depending on whether the biobank is a commercial or public body, or a public-private partnership. Public attitudes and opinions about biobanking are of particular significance, since most biobanks depend on recruiting volunteers to participate via programs of community engagement. Considerable scrutiny has therefore been devoted to this area, and there has been debate about public trust in such enterprises (75–79), as well as many programs of public engagement. Alternative approaches have been characterized as a "communication approach" to address public concerns, typified by the Estonian Genome Project, or a "partnership approach" to actively involve members of the public in decision-making processes (80). The Western Australia Office of Population Health Genomics is developing a deliberative engagement approach to biobanks, bringing together members of the public to discuss their concerns and priorities.

There are increasing moves toward collaborative genetic epidemiological research, in order to accumulate the very large samples needed to generate statistically highly powered epidemiological studies; for example, the Public Population Project in Genomics (P³G) is an international consortium established in 2007 for the development of a multidisciplinary infrastructure for combining and comparing large-scale population genomic studies (81). Similarly, the recently established European Biobank is intended to facilitate collaborative research projects by providing a central computerized system to link records on biological samples held in different research centers and biobanks across Europe; infrastructure and legal governance systems are scheduled to be in place by 2010. Increasing collaboration means that harmonization of national and international legislation, governance, and ethical guidelines for biobanks and other large-scale genetic research databases has become a significant issue. The P^{3}G initiative has multidisciplinary international working groups that provide leadership in key areas, including ethics, public engagement and governance. Attempts to draw together international guidelines have already been made; in 2002 the Human Genome Organisation (HUGO) Ethics Committee released a statement on human genomic databases (82,83), followed in 2003 by a World Health Organization (WHO) publication on the benefits and impact of genetic databases (84), and an *International Declaration on Human Genetic Data* from the United Nations Educational, Scientific and Cultural Organization (UNESCO) (85,86). A European Commission document reported on human biobanking legislation in different countries (87), while the Organisation for Economic Co-operation and Development (OECD) released *Creation and Governance of Human Genetic Research Databases* in 2006 (88). At the time of writing, a set of *Guidelines for Human Biobanks and Genetic Research Databases* was also in development (89), a process which included broad international consultation.

Developing and Evaluating Health Services

As previously mentioned, one of the key strategies in public health genomics is the application of genetic understanding and information to prevent disease, in particular by using information about genetic risk to allow more accurate risk assessment. For example, various genes have been identified that confer susceptibility to breast cancer. Rare high-penetrance allelic variants of the *BRCA1* (90,91) and *BRCA2* (92,93) genes cause hereditary breast-ovarian cancer syndrome, and confer a relative risk of 10–20-fold for breast cancer (94) with a lifetime penetrance of up to 91% (95). Prior to the identification of *BRCA1/2* and the development of genetic testing for mutations in these genes, risk of breast cancer could only be assessed based on family history, age, and other clinical factors, with women at greater risk being eligible for increased levels of surveillance (for example, by mammography and/or MRI). Now, however, women with a significant family history of breast and related cancers may be referred for genetic testing to identify *BRCA1/2* mutations. Not only does this provide a much more accurate estimate of risk for individuals in whom mutations are detected, but it also permits the testing of female relatives to determine whether or not they have inherited this genetic predisposition to disease, and hence whether or not increased surveillance or prophylactic interventions are warranted. Similarly, women in whom *BRCA1/2* mutations are identified are also known to be at a substantially increased risk of ovarian cancer (96), and clinical management needs to take this into account (97). However, mutations in the *BRCA* genes are present in only a minority of breast cancer cases, and much of the familial risk of the disease has yet to be explained. Recently, rare variants of other genes (such as *CHEK2, ATM, BRIP1,* and *PALB2)* have been found to confer moderate relative risks of 2–3-fold, and some common variants have also been shown to confer very low increases in relative risk, in the order of 1.07–1.26-fold (94), for example, the *FGFR2, TNRC9, MAP3K1,* and *LSP1* genes (28). Such discoveries have an immediate contribution to current understanding of the pathogenesis of breast cancer; in the future, if rapid and cost-effective methods of genotyping were to become available, it might eventually become feasible to include information on the presence of such variants in the assessment of breast cancer risk for individuals. A recent analysis of the prospects for using risk information based on more common, lower susceptibility alleles for breast cancer concluded that although such risk profiles did not provide enough discrimination to be useful for individualized disease prevention, they could potentially inform risk stratification to direct population screening measures (98).

Similarly, new forms of genetic screening and testing are also being used in the management of other common forms of cancer such as colorectal cancer. As with breast cancer, a small proportion of colorectal cancer cases are attributable to rare high-penetrance mutations in susceptibility genes; for example, mutations in certain mismatch repair genes (notably *MLH1, MSH2, MSH6,* and *PMS2*) can cause Lynch syndrome/hereditary nonpolyposis colorectal cancer (HNPCC), which accounts for 2–3% of colorectal cancer cases (99,100). Individuals with Lynch syndrome are at an increased risk not only of colorectal tumors, but also of other tumors, including ovarian and endothelial cancer in women (101). Referral criteria based on clinical and pathological findings combined with family history can identify those patients at greatest risk of having Lynch syndrome, who may then be referred for direct mutation analysis. As with *BRCA1/2* mutation analysis, this is a lengthy and expensive procedure, but a form of molecular screening for tumor-related features such as immunohistochemistry (IHC) or microsatellite instability (MSI) testing of tumor tissue can further stratify the referred "high risk" population into categories to identify those in whom full mutation analysis is warranted (101,102), although there is debate over the optimal strategy for combining different measures of HNPCC risk (103). However, a much larger proportion of colorectal cancer cases (15–30%) are estimated to include a genetic component than those accounted for by Lynch syndrome and other cancer syndromes (102), and there are also prospects for increasing understanding of the genetics of colorectal cancer finding application in risk stratification in the future; population screening for multiple common, low-penetrance variants associated with increased disease risk could identify individuals with above-population risk who could then receive increased levels of surveillance (104).

Newborn screening of infants is one of the most well-established examples of public health genomics in practice, and up to 40 million newborns receive such testing each year (105). The aim is to identify specific genetic diseases, typically those where prompt diagnosis allows effective therapeutic intervention. For example, diagnosis of the rare inborn error of metabolism phenylketonuria (PKU) and careful control of phenylalanine in the diet during infancy and childhood prevents severe mental retardation; screening for PKU was introduced in the 1960s, and screening for other conditions have followed. The capacity to identify serious genetic disorders has been significantly boosted in recent years by the advent of new molecular genetic tests, coupled with tandem mass spectrometry, which allows high-throughput testing for multiple conditions. In fact, it has made possible the identification of infants affected by diseases for which there is no cure, raising ethical debate about whether or not it is appropriate to offer screening for conditions in the absence of a highly effective intervention (106). Practice varies in different countries; for example, in Finland, only congenital hypothyroidism is screened for (105), while the United Kingdom newborn screening program tests for phenylketonuria, congenital hypothyroidism, sickle-cell disorders (hemoglobinopathies), and cystic fibrosis, with medium-chain acyl-CoA dehydrogenase deficiency (MCADD) scheduled to join the panel of conditions by 2009. The American College of Medical Genetics (ACMG) has produced recommendations for the uniform screening of a much larger uniform panel of 29 conditions across the United States, including other forms of metabolic disorder (107), while in Germany the Federal Ministry for Health and Social Security opted to restrict the screening panel to ten disorders (108).

Rapid developments in forms of genetic testing and treatments for inherited diseases have made it necessary to reassess the structure and delivery of various specialist health services. In the United Kingdom, the PHG Foundation has completed several projects around the evaluation and review of specialist services within the National Health Service (NHS). The basic model for the evaluation of health services is built around a stakeholder group of relevant medical and scientific specialists, health service commissioners and service providers, representatives of patients and support organizations, and experts in relevant disciplines such as law, ethics, health economics, and education. Public health genomics practitioners provide expertise in public health and epidemiology, along with wider skills in policy development, facilitation, and knowledge brokering, in order to unite and lead the gathered experts in their analysis and interpretation efforts. Typically, it is found that genetics services need to work in close cooperation with many different specialities to provide optimal care for patients with forms of genetic disorder. A needs assessment and service review focused on inherited forms of metabolic disease, where patients need access to a very wide range of biochemical and molecular tests for diagnosis and monitoring, as well as access to various forms of specialist support services, including dietetics and enzyme replacement therapies (109). The ways in which health services would need to adapt in order to take full advantage of emerging scientific knowledge and clinical tools, and policy issues that would be important in the development of future services were considered in the production of strategic recommendations with respect to service commissioning and provision, and health professional training and guidance.

Communication and Stakeholder Engagement

Appropriate engagement with relevant stakeholders is important not only as part of specific projects, but also much more broadly across the many issues and applications relevant to public health genomics, including primary and secondary research efforts. Given the multidisciplinary basis of the field, it may be necessary to facilitate dialog between professionals from very disparate backgrounds, along with representatives of patients and the wider public. In response to this need, public health genomics has traditionally focused very much on network-based working, and is supported by an international collaborative network, established by the Bellagio group (35). The Genome-based Research and Population Health Network (GRaPH-*Int*) was formally launched at the fourth International DNA Sampling Conference in Montreal in June 2006; the administrative hub is funded by the Public Health Agency of Canada. GRaPH-*Int* is a network of organizations and individuals who share an interest in public health genomics, and seek to transform knowledge and technologies into public policies, programs, and services for the benefit of public health. Crucially, the network integrates knowledge arising from a range of different disciplines, and hence the appellation *Int* may be taken to represent not only "international" but also "interdisciplinary" and "integrated." Besides supporting dialog between members and developing an integrated knowledge base for public health genomics, the network also has more specific goals to encourage communication and stakeholder engagement, promote education and training, and inform public policy in relevant areas. The "founder organizations" of GRaPH-*Int* are the U.S. Office of Public Health Genomics at CDC; the U.K. Foundation for Genomics and Population Health (PHG Foundation); and HumGen, a Canadian-based international collaborative database on the legal, ethical, and social aspects of human genetics. Other participating organizations include other international networks such as the Human Genome Epidemiology Network (HuGENet), the Network of Investigator Networks in Human Genome Epidemiology, the Public Population Project in Genomics (P³G Consortium), and the Public Health Genomics European Network (PHGEN). GRaPH-*Int* is therefore a "network of networks," a complicated structure but one that is necessary to effectively coordinate input from multiple different clinical and academic disciplines, in different organizations throughout different countries.

Education and Training

Public health genomics is intimately associated with education and training, largely due to a general lack of understanding of genetics among health professionals. In addition to a growing need for basic awareness of genetics and disease across health services, there is also a requirement for public health professionals in particular to understand the implications of genome-based knowledge and technologies for public health practice in the twenty-first century, including the importance of genomic variation as a determinant of health and the opportunities for application of genetic understanding and tools for improved risk estimation. Incorporation of public health genomics into mainstream public health training remains poorly advanced. However, various efforts have been and will continue to be made to provide opportunities for specialist training in the discipline, and availability of training is likely to rise in the near future, as this is an area of increasing focus. Examples include dedicated graduate degree courses available from different centers, such as the Masters and PhD programs in *Public Health Genetics* at the University of Washington Institute for Public Health Genetics in the United States, or the new Masters course in *Public Health Genomics* offered by Cranfield University in the United Kingdom. Where full degree courses are not yet available, some centers may offer short modules specifically on public health genomics within public health training, such as Masters Degrees in public health or epidemiology via association with centers of excellence. The PHG Foundation in the United Kingdom has provided specialist input to courses run by the University of Cambridge and the University of Hong Kong. The German Center for Public Health Genetics in Bielefeld has plans to introduce a public health genomics module centered on governance and policy, ethics, law, and economics, while the Michigan Center for Genomics and Public Health and Michigan Public Health Training Center (MPHTC) in the United States offer an Internet-based training module on genomic awareness (110) suitable for introducing public health professionals to the relevance of genomic advances, in addition to a cross-disciplinary module on *Public Health Genetics* for graduate students. International participants in both the PHGEN and GraPH-*Int* networks are working toward increased provision of relevant education and training.

It is important to note that although formal courses are valuable, public health specialists and other interested professionals may move into public health genomics by research and practice in relevant areas. A suitable knowledge base in public health genomics can be built effectively by training or experience in different key components of the discipline, such as genetic epidemiology, genomic medicine, and the ethical, legal, and social aspects of genomics, and these are available from many different international centers. Just as the public health community needs to learn about genomics in health and the wider issues (including awareness of relevant areas of law, the social sciences, and humanities) nonpublic health practitioners (such as those with backgrounds in genetics, general medicine, or the social sciences) should ideally have some understanding of the principles of public health and epidemiology. For example, in the United Kingdom, *Genetics and Health Policy* (GHP) courses provided by the then Public Health Genetics Unit between 2000 and 2006 sought to train a core of health service-related professionals (including physicians, nurses, genetic counselors, commissioners, managers, and policy makers) in order to establish a knowledge base within the National Health Service. Of course, no single person can ever become truly expert in all of the subdisciplines that contribute to public health genomics, but an awareness and appreciation of the key issues is essential; combined with appropriate participation in multidisciplinary networks to allow access to the relevant expertise as required, this allows a broad range of individuals to work effectively within the field.

Educational requirements in developing nations are rather different; the role of public health genomics at the present time is crucially focused on provision of training and resources for basic genetics services. For example, the *Capability* project, a collaborative venture between experts from Europe and centers of excellence in Argentina, Egypt, and South Africa, is attempting to build capacity for the transfer of genetic knowledge into primary health care practice and disease prevention (111), and is linked with the international Partnerships for Perinatal Health network, which seeks to build global expertise in the prevention of morbidity and mortality associated with birth defects and preterm birth. Working with less well-developed nations and, where possible, offering opportunities for collaboration and training is generally considered to be an important component of public health genomics; although major financial constraints may prevent the application of the most advanced tools and approaches for improved health arising from genomic knowledge, there is plenty of scope for the application of basic principles of public health and genetics.

The Prospects for Public Health Genomics

As knowledge of human genome epidemiology, human genomics, and related technologies continues to emerge, what will the role of public health genomics become in the future? A longstanding schism between public health and the rest of medicine has been noted to exist (46,112); although both seek to improve human health, the former is based upon population-level approaches to prevent disease, focused on environmental determinants of health, while the latter concentrates on biological mechanisms of pathology and prevention and treatment at the individual level. The role of genomics, as the effective basis of all molecular medicine, is more obviously inherent (and has been more readily acknowledged) within medicine than public health, where perceptions of the impact and potential of genomics are frequently low. And yet these divisions—of medicine from public health, of genomics from population health—inevitably hinder progress toward the shared goal of better health. Public health genomics, in recognizing the merits of both genomics *and* evidence-based interventions to improve population health, could act as a bridge to join the two.

If the vision of public health genomics—to see genomic medicine embedded throughout human health services as the utility of genomic information and advanced biomedical techniques and interventions grows—is realized, we expect that the term itself will, within a relatively short time, become redundant. In addition, the key principles of driving the realization of health benefits from new knowledge and applications will, we hope, be adopted across the board. Not only are the public and health service professionals hungry for these benefits, but also a responsive health service must combine evidence-based assessment of the merits of each intervention with a swift and flexible response to the results of such assessment, facilitating the incorporation into clinical practice, albeit within the inevitable economic restrictions. Just as the Bellagio meeting identified the key drivers and outputs of the public health genomics enterprise, practitioners are now seeking to set out ways in which both public health and medicine may move toward timely translation from research into clinical practice, from traditional to genomic medicine. A proposed framework emerging from public health genomics rests on four key areas: an increasing focus on disease prevention, a population perspective, commitment to evidence-based knowledge integration, and emphasis on health services research (44).

Certainly, the twenty-first century provides the perfect opportunity for all areas of medicine to move forward in partnership toward better health. Of course, some fields are likely to see the impact of genomics much sooner than others; current applications are still largely confined to clinical genetics and monogenic diseases, with oncology following behind, but broader applications are coming into health care practice; novel "omics" such as the use of proteomic, transcriptomic, and metabolomic biomarkers are moving toward application in both oncology and infectious disease, while understanding of genomic mechanisms in the development of complex diseases such as obesity, diabetes, cardiovascular and respiratory disease is driving the development both of new population approaches to prevention and novel therapeutic interventions. However, virtually all forms of medicine can benefit from the principles of public health genomics now by embracing both multidisciplinary and translational research. In this instance, we refer to translational research in its broadest sense, encompassing not only primary but also secondary translation into tangible health benefits.

Conclusions

The public health genomics enterprise has a clear purpose, one that merits the necessary efforts to direct and uphold the process, and to deliver the desired endpoints. The ultimate goals of medicine are the subject of considerable debate, but in recent years there has been a shift toward a more comprehensive approach that embraces not only the relief of pain, the provision of care, and (where possible) a cure, but also the prevention of disease and premature death, the promotion of health, and the pursuit of a peaceful death (113). Public health genomics is built around the prevention of morbidity and mortality and the promotion of health, and seeks these benefits at the population level in addition to that of individual patients. This is a paradigm that should, we believe, not only unite genomics and epidemiology, medicine and public health, but also underpin all health services and biomedical research in the modern world.

References

1. Pernick MS. Taking better baby contests seriously. *Am J Public Health*. May 2002;92(5):707–708.
2. Lippman A. Eugenics and public health. *Am J Public Health*. Januray 2003;93(1):11.
3. Genome-based research and population health. Report of an expert workshop held at the Rockefeller Foundation Study and Conference Center, Bellagio, Italy. Available at http://www.phgfoundation.org/file/2205. Accessed April 14–20, 2005.

4. Collins FS. Shattuck lecture—medical and societal consequences of the Human Genome Project. *N Engl J Med*. July 1, 1999;341(1):28–37.
5. Kamerow D. Waiting for the genetic revolution. *BMJ*. January 5, 2008;336(7634):22.
6. Watson JD, Crick FH. Molecular structure of nucleic acids; a structure for deoxyribose nucleic acid. *Nature*. April 25, 1953;171(4356):737–738.
7. Nobel Prizes for Medicine, 1968. *Nature*. October 26, 1968;220(5165):324–325.
8. van Ommen GJ, Verkerk JM, Hofker MH, et al. A physical map of 4 million bp around the Duchenne muscular dystrophy gene on the human X-chromosome. *Cell*. November 21, 1986;47(4):499–504.
9. Rommens JM, Iannuzzi MC, Kerem B, et al. Identification of the cystic fibrosis gene: chromosome walking and jumping. *Science*. September 8, 1989;245(4922):1059–1065.
10. A novel gene containing a trinucleotide repeat that is expanded and unstable on Huntington's disease chromosomes. The Huntington's Disease Collaborative Research Group. *Cell*. March 26, 1993;72(6):971–983.
11. Lander ES, Linton LM, Birren B, et al. Initial sequencing and analysis of the human genome. *Nature*. February 15, 2001;409(6822):860–921.
12. McPherson JD, Marra M, Hillier L, et al. A physical map of the human genome. *Nature*. February 15, 2001;409(6822):934–941.
13. Finishing the euchromatic sequence of the human genome. *Nature*. October 21, 2004;431(7011):931–945.
14. Callinan PA, Feinberg AP. The emerging science of epigenomics. *Hum Mol Genet*. April 15, 2006;15 Spec No 1:R95–R101.
15. Fire A, Xu S, Montgomery MK, et al. Potent and specific genetic interference by double-stranded RNA in Caenorhabditis elegans. *Nature*. February 19, 1998;391(6669):806–811.
16. Walker FO. Huntington's disease. Lancet. January 20, 2007;369(9557):218–228.
17. Beutler E, Felitti VJ, Koziol JA, et al. Penetrance of 845G--> A (C282Y) HFE hereditary haemochromatosis mutation in the USA. *Lancet*. January 19, 2002;359(9302):211–218.
18. Bacon BR, Britton RS. Clinical penetrance of hereditary hemochromatosis. *N Engl J Med*. January 17, 2008;358(3):291–292.
19. Allen KJ, Gurrin LC, Constantine CC, et al. Iron-overload-related disease in HFE hereditary hemochromatosis. *N Engl J Med*. January 17, 2008;358(3):221–230.
20. Kulczycki LL, Kostuch M, Bellanti JA. A clinical perspective of cystic fibrosis and new genetic findings: relationship of CFTR mutations to genotype-phenotype manifestations. *Am J Med Genet A*. January 30, 2003;116(3):262–267.
21. Cooper RS. Gene-environment interactions and the etiology of common complex disease. *Ann Intern Med*. September 2, 2003;139(5 Pt 2):437–440.
22. Juengst ET. "Prevention" and the goals of genetic medicine. *Hum Gene Ther*. December 1995;6(12):1595–1605.
23. Highfield, R. Discovery of asthma gene offers new hope. *The Telegraph*. July 11, 2002.
24. Depression gene discovered. *Daily Mail*. November 18, 2005.
25. "Fat" gene found by scientists. Available at http://www.timesonline.co.uk/tol/news/uk/health/article1647517.ece. Accessed April 13, 2007.
26. The Wellcome Trust Case Control Consortium. Genome-wide association study of 14,000 cases of seven common diseases and 3,000 shared controls. *Nature*. June 7, 2007;447(7145):661–678.
27. Guttmacher AE, Collins FS. Realizing the promise of genomics in biomedical research. *JAMA*. September 21, 2005;294(11):1399–1402.
28. Easton DF, Pooley KA, Dunning AM, et al. Genome-wide association study identifies novel breast cancer susceptibility loci. *Nature*. June 28, 2007;447(7148):1087–1093.
29. Sladek R, Rocheleau G, Rung J, et al. A genome-wide association study identifies novel risk loci for type 2 diabetes. *Nature*. February 22, 2007;445(7130):881–885.

30. Rioux JD, Xavier RJ, Taylor KD, et al. Genome-wide association study identifies new susceptibility loci for Crohn disease and implicates autophagy in disease pathogenesis. *Nat Genet*. May 2007;39(5):596–604.

31. Khoury MJ, Little J, Gwinn M, et al. On the synthesis and interpretation of consistent but weak gene-disease associations in the era of genome-wide association studies. *Int J Epidemiol*. April 2007;36(2):439–445.

32. Manolio TA, Rodriguez LL, Brooks L, et al. New models of collaboration in genome-wide association studies: the Genetic Association Information Network. *Nat Genet*. September 2007 ;39(9):1045–1051.

33. Khoury MJ, Davis R, Gwinn M, et al. Do we need genomic research for the prevention of common diseases with environmental causes? *Am J Epidemiol*. May 1, 2005;161(9):799–805.

34. Willard HF, Angrist M, Ginsburg GS. Genomic medicine: genetic variation and its impact on the future of health care. *Philos Trans R Soc Lond B Biol Sci*. August 29, 2005;360(1460):1543–1550.

35. Khoury MJ. From genes to public health: the applications of genetic technology in disease prevention. Genetics Working Group. *Am J Public Health*. December 1996;86(12):1717–1722.

36. 10 Years of Public Health Genomics at CDC 1997–2007. Available at http://www.cdc. gov/genomics/activities/file/print/2007-12_10yr_web.pdf. Accessed December 1, 2007.

37. Zimmern R. Genetics services. Briefing encounters. *Health Serv J*. April 29, 1999; 109(5652):24–25.

38. Acheson D. *Committee of Inquiry into the Future Development of the Public Health Function*. London: HMSO; 1988.

39. Stewart A, Brice P, Burton H, et al. *Genetics, Health Care and Public Policy*. Cambridge: Cambridge University Press; 2007.

40. Omenn GS. Public health genetics: an emerging interdisciplinary field for the post-genomic era. *Annu Rev Public Health*. 2000;21:1–13.

41. Coughlin SS. The intersection of genetics, public health, and preventive medicine. *Am J Prev Med*. February 1999;16(2):89–90.

42. Cooksey D. *A Review of UK Health Research Funding*. London: HMSO; 2006.

43. Westfall JM, Mold J, Fagnan L. Practice-based research—"Blue Highways" on the NIH roadmap. *JAMA*. January 24, 2007;297(4):403–406.

44. Khoury MJ, Gwinn M, Yoon PW, et al. The continuum of translation research in genomic medicine: how can we accelerate the appropriate integration of human genome discoveries into health care and disease prevention? *Genet Med*. October 2007;9(10):665–674.

45. Murray TH. Genetic exceptionalism and future diaries: is genetic information different from other medical information? In: Rothstein MA, ed. *Genetic Secrets:Pprotecting Privacy and Confidentiality in the Genetic Era*. New Haven: Yale University Press; 1997:60–73.

46. Khoury MJ, Gwinn M, Burke W, et al. Will genomics widen or help heal the schism between medicine and public health? *Am J Prev Med*. October 2007;33(4):310–317.

47. Sussman S, Valente TW, Rohrbach LA, et al. Translation in the health professions: converting science into action. *Eval Health Prof*. March 2006;29(1):7–32.

48. Zerhouni EA. Translational research: moving discovery to practice. *Clin Pharmacol Ther*. January 2007;81(1):126–128.

49. Lomas J. The in-between world of knowledge brokering. *BMJ*. January 20, 2007;334(7585):129–132.

50. Chung WK. Implementation of genetics to personalize medicine. *Gend Med*. September 2007;4(3):248–265.

51. Schwartz PJ. The congenital long QT syndromes from genotype to phenotype: clinical implications. *J Intern Med*. January 2006;259(1):39–47.

52. Gage BF, Lesko LJ. Pharmacogenetics of warfarin: regulatory, scientific, and clinical issues. *J Thromb Thrombolysis*. February 2008;25(1):45–51.

53. Anderson JL, Horne BD, Stevens SM, et al. Randomized trial of genotype-guided versus standard warfarin dosing in patients initiating oral anticoagulation. *Circulation*. November 27, 2007;116(22):2563–2570.

54. Sotiriou C, Piccart MJ. Taking gene-expression profiling to the clinic: when will molecular signatures become relevant to patient care? *Nat Rev Cancer*. July 2007; 7(7):545–553.

55. Chan A. A review of the use of trastuzumab (Herceptin) plus vinorelbine in metastatic breast cancer. *Ann Oncol*. July 2007;18(7):1152–1158.

56. Collins I, Workman P. New approaches to molecular cancer therapeutics. *Nat Chem Biol*. December 2006;2(12):689–700.

57. Evans J, Khoury MJ. Evidence based medicine meets genomic medicine. *Genet Med*. December 2007;9(12):799–800.

58. Kroese M, Elles R, Zimmern R. *The Evaluation of Clinical Validity and Clinical Utility of Genetic Tests*. Cambridge: PHG Foundation, Cambridge; 2007.

59. Ayme S, Matthijs G, Soini S. Patenting and licensing in genetic testing. *Eur J Hum Genet*. April 2008;16(4):405–411.

60. OECD Guidelines for Quality Assurance in Molecular Genetic Testing, 2007. Available at http://www.oecd.org/document/24/0,3343,en_2649_34537_1885208_1_1_1_1,00&&en-USS_01DBC.html. Accessed 2007.

61. Burke W, Zimmern R. *Moving Beyond ACCE: An Expanded Framework for Genetic Test Evaluation*. Cambridge, UK: PHG Foundation; 2007.

62. ACCE: a model process for evaluating data on emerging genetic tests. In: Khoury M, Little J, Burke W, eds. *Human Genome Epidemiology*. Oxford: Oxford University Press; 2004:217–233.

63. Melzer D, Hogarth S, Liddell K, et al. *Evidence and Evaluation: Building Public Trust in Genetic Tests for Common Diseases*. Cambridge, UK: PHG Foundation; 2008.

64. Furness P, Zimmern R, Wright C, et al. The *Evaluation of Diagnostic Laboratory Tests and Complex Biomarkers*. Cambridge, UK: PHG Foundation/Royal College of Pathologists; 2008.

65. Secretary's Advisory Committee on Genetics Health and Society. U.S. System of Oversight of Genetic Testing: A Response to the Charge of the Secretary of Health and Human Services. Available at http://oba.od.nih.gov/oba/SACGHS/reports/SACGHS_oversight_report.pdf. Accessed April 2008.

66. Evaluation of Genomic Applications in Practice and Prevention (EGAPP) Working Group. Recommendations from the EGAPP Working Group: testing for cytochrome P450 polymorphisms in adults with nonpsychotic depression treated with selective serotonin reuptake inhibitors. *Genet Med*. December 2007;9(12):819–825.

67. AmpliChip CYP450 test. *Med Lett Drugs Ther*. August 2005;47(1215–1216):71–72.

68. News in Brief. *Pharmacogenomics*. December 2004;5(7):763–765.

69. Hansson MG, Dillner J, Bartram CR, et al. Should donors be allowed to give broad consent to future biobank research? *Lancet Oncol*. March 2006;7(3):266–269.

70. Maschke KJ. Alternative consent approaches for biobank research. *Lancet Oncol*. March 2006;7(3):193–194.

71. Lowrance WW, Collins FS. Ethics. Identifiability in genomic research. *Science*. August 3, 2007;317(5838):600–602.

72. Winickoff DE. Partnership in U.K. Biobank: a third way for genomic property? *J Law Med Ethics*. 2007;35(3):440–456.

73. Greely HT. The uneasy ethical and legal underpinnings of large-scale genomic biobanks. *Annu Rev Genomics Hum Genet*. 2007;8:343–364.

74. Cambon-Thomsen A. The social and ethical issues of post-genomic human biobanks. *Nat Rev Genet.* 2004;5(11):866–873.

75. Tutton R, Kaye J, Hoeyer K. Governing UK Biobank: the importance of ensuring public trust. *Trends Biotechnol.* June 2004; 22(6):284–285.

76. Neidich AB, Joseph JW, Ober C, et al. Empirical data about women's attitudes towards a hypothetical pediatric biobank. *Am J Med Genet A.* February 1, 2008;146(3):297–304.

77. Kettis-Lindblad A, Ring L, Viberth E, et al. Genetic research and donation of tissue samples to biobanks. What do potential sample donors in the Swedish general public think? *Eur J Public Health.* August 2006;16(4):433–440.

78. Hansson MG. Building on relationships of trust in biobank research. *J Med Ethics.* July 2005;31(7):415–418.

79. Petersen A. Securing our genetic health: engendering trust in UK Biobank. *Sociol Health Illn.* March 2005;27(2):271–292.

80. Godard B, Marshall J, Laberge C, et al. Strategies for consulting with the community: the cases of four large-scale genetic databases. *Sci Eng Ethics.* July 2004;10(3):457–477.

81. Knoppers BM, Fortier I, Legault D, et al. The Public Population Project in Genomics (P3G): a proof of concept? Eur J Hum Genet. June 2008;16(6):664–665.

82. Statement on human genomic databases, December 2002. *J Int Bioethique.* September 2003;14(3–4):207–210.

83. Human Genome Organisation Ethics Committee. Statement on Human Genomic Databases. 2002. Available at http://www.hugo-international.org/img/genomic_2002.pdf.

84. Laurie G. Genetic databases: assessing the benefits and the impact on human and patient rights—a WHO report. *Eur J Health Law.* March 2004;11(1):87–92.

85. Abbing HD. International declaration on human genetic data. *Eur J Health Law.* March 2004;11(1):93–107.

86. UNESCO BC. International Declaration on Human Genetic Data. 2003. Available at http://unesdoc.unesco.org/images/0013/001312/131204e.pdf#page=27.

87. European Commission DEBAaF. Survey on opinions from National Ethics Committees or similar bodies, public debate and national legislation in relation to human biobank. December 2004. Available at http://ec.europa.eu/research/biosociety/bioethics/documents_en.htm.

88. Organisation for Economic Co-operation and Development. Creation and Governance of Human Genetic Research Databases. October 2006, ISBN 92-64-02852-8. Available at http://www.oecd.org/document/50/0,3343,en_2649_34537_37646258_1_1_1_1,00.html

89. Organisation for Economic Co-operation and Development. Guidelines for Human Biobanks and Genetic Research Databases. Available at www.oecd.org/sti/biotechnology/hbgrd. Accessed April 2008.

90. Hall JM, Lee MK, Newman B, et al. Linkage of early-onset familial breast cancer to chromosome 17q21. *Science.* December 21, 1990;250(4988):1684–1689.

91. Miki Y, Swensen J, Shattuck-Eidens D, et al. A strong candidate for the breast and ovarian cancer susceptibility gene BRCA1. *Science.* October 7, 1994;266(5182):66–71.

92. Wooster R, Bignell G, Lancaster J, et al. Identification of the breast cancer susceptibility gene BRCA2. *Nature.* December 21, 1995;378(6559):789–792.

93. Tavtigian SV, Simard J, Rommens J, et al. The complete BRCA2 gene and mutations in chromosome 13q-linked kindreds. *Nat Genet.* March 1996;12(3):333–337.

94. Stratton MR, Rahman N. The emerging landscape of breast cancer susceptibility. *Nat Genet.* January 2008;40(1):17–22.

95. Robson M, Offit K. Clinical practice. Management of an inherited predisposition to breast cancer. *N Engl J Med.* July 12, 2007;357(2):154–162.

96. Antoniou A, Pharoah PD, Narod S, et al. Average risks of breast and ovarian cancer associated with BRCA1 or BRCA2 mutations detected in case series unselected for family history: a combined analysis of 22 studies. *Am J Hum Genet.* May
2003;72(5):1117–1130.
97. Roukos DH, Briasoulis E. Individualized preventive and therapeutic management
of hereditary breast ovarian cancer syndrome. *Nat Clin Pract Oncol.* October 2007;
4(10):578–590.
98. Pharoah PD, Antoniou AC, Easton DF, et al. Polygenes, risk prediction, and targeted
prevention of breast cancer. *N Engl J Med.* June 26, 2008;358(26):2796–2803.
99. Lynch HT, de la Chapelle A. Hereditary colorectal cancer. *N Engl J Med.* March 6,
2003;348(10):919–932.
100. de la Chapelle A. Genetic predisposition to colorectal cancer. *Nat Rev Cancer.* October
2004;4(10):769–780.
101. Ponz dL, Bertario L, Genuardi M, et al. Identification and classification of hereditary
nonpolyposis colorectal cancer (Lynch syndrome): adapting old concepts to recent
advancements. Report from the Italian Association for the study of Hereditary Colorectal
Tumors Consensus Group. *Dis Colon Rectum.* December 2007;50(12):2126–2134.
102. Vasen HF, Moslein G, Alonso A, et al. Guidelines for the clinical management of Lynch
syndrome (hereditary non-polyposis cancer). *J Med Genet.* June 2007;44(6):353–362.
103. Bonis PA, Trikalinos TA, Chung M, et al. Hereditary nonpolyposis colorectal cancer:
diagnostic strategies and their implications. *Evid Rep Technol Assess (Full Rep).* May
2007; 150:1–180.
104. Sengupta N, Gill KA, Macfie TS, et al. Management of colorectal cancer: A role for
genetics in prevention and treatment? *Pathol Res Pract.* 2008;204(7):469–477.
105. McCabe LL, McCabe ER. Expanded newborn screening: implications for genomic
medicine. *Annu Rev Med.* 2008;59:163–175.
106. Bailey DB, Jr, Skinner D, Davis AM, et al. Ethical, legal, and social concerns about
expanded newborn screening: fragile X syndrome as a prototype for emerging issues.
Pediatrics. March 2008;121(3):e693–e704.
107. Newborn screening: toward a uniform screening panel and system. *Genet Med.* May
2006;8(Suppl 1):1S–252S.
108. Pollitt RJ. International perspectives on newborn screening. *J Inherit Metab Dis.* April
2006;29(2–3):390–396.
109. Burton H. Metabolic pathways: networks of care. PHG Foundation, November 2005.
Available at http://www.phgfoundation.org/pages/serviceprojects.htm#metabolic.
110. Michigan Public Health Training Center. Six Weeks to Genomic Awareness. Available
at https://practice.sph.umich.edu/mphtc/site.php?module=courses_one_online_course&
id=108. Accessed April 2008.
111. Capability. Available at http://www.capabilitynet.eu/.
112. White KL. *Healing the Schism. Epidemiology, Medicine, and the Public's Health.* New
York: Springer-Verlag; 1991.
113. Callahan D. Remembering the goals of medicine. *J Eval Clin Pract.* May 1999;5(2):
103–106.

4

Navigating the evolving knowledge of human genetic variation in health and disease

Marta Gwinn and Wei Yu

Genomics

Twentieth-century developments in biology and statistics established genetics as a science and led to the discovery of causal loci for many single-gene disorders. In the 1960s, Dr. Victor A. McKusick began compiling a continuously updated catalog of genes and diseases; first published in book form, the catalog went online in 1987 as Online Mendelian Inheritance in Man, or OMIM (http://www.ncbi.nlm. nih.gov/omim/). By the 1990s, OMIM was adding more than 150 disease-related genetic variants per year, nearly all of them rare mutations discovered in families (1). Since then, the declining costs and increasing efficiency of new technologies (especially automation and microarrays) have prompted an unprecedented outpouring of genomic data that has been compared with a "tsunami" for its potential to overwhelm capacity for data management and analysis (2,3).

Bioinformatics

The development of computational technology and methods to organize, archive, visualize, and share genomic data gave rise to the field of bioinformatics (4). In 1988, the National Library of Medicine (a component of the National Institutes of Health) created the National Center for Biotechnology Information (NCBI, http:// www.ncbi.nlm.nih.gov/) to provide "an integrated, one-stop, genomic information infrastructure for biomedical researchers from around the world." NCBI has become a central repository for genomic sequence data in humans and other species and has developed many other public databases, such as dbSNP (http://www.ncbi. nlm.nih.gov/SNP/, for single nucleotide polymorphisms, or SNPs) and Entrez Gene (http://www.ncbi.nlm.nih.gov/sites/entrez?db=gene, for genes) (5,6). Perhaps the most prominent and widely used NCBI database is PubMed (http://www.ncbi.nlm. nih.gov/pubmed/), a continuously updated, public database of more than 18 million citations for biomedical literature. Entrez (http://www.ncbi.nlm.nih.gov/Entrez/) is the search engine that allows searching across all NCBI databases.

The international Human Genome Project's early commitment to data sharing helped stimulate the construction of other, online genomic data repositories and tools for use by researchers and the public. For example, the UCSC Human Genome Browser (http://genome.ucsc.edu/), launched in 2002, created a framework for displaying multiply annotated sequence data at any scale throughout the genome (7). The UCSC Genome Browser Database has continued to evolve, adding many web-based applications for viewing, manipulating, and analyzing the data (8).

The Human Genome Organization (HUGO, http://www.hugo-international.org) was founded in 1988 to foster coordination among large-scale human genome mapping and sequencing projects around the world. The HUGO Gene Nomenclature Committee maintains a database of approved, unique gene names and symbols, which currently includes more than 28,000 genes (http://www.genenames.org) (9). The Human Genome Variation Society (HGVS) has begun a grass-roots effort to compile a list of locus-specific databases (LSDBs), which are curated collections of mutations, often reported with associated phenotypic information (10). Recently, NCBI embraced these efforts by allowing users to search, annotate, and submit human genome sequence variants to the dbSNP database by using HGVS standard nomenclature (http://www.ncbi.nlm.nih.gov/projects/SNP/tranSNP/tranSNP.cgi) (11).

Human Genome Epidemiology

Genomic data are relevant to public health to the extent that they can be translated into knowledge useful for prevention, prediction, diagnosis, and treatment of disease. Human genome epidemiology is the basic science for translating genomic research, relating genetic variation with variability in health status among well-defined groups of people. Analyzing these data in terms of measured individual and group characteristics is a complex, multidimensional problem.

During the past several years, the Human Genome Epidemiology Network (HuGENet™) has laid out a process for knowledge synthesis and evaluation in human genome epidemiology. The underlying framework for this process is a "network of networks": a collection of formal and informal collaborations organized according to location, funding source, or research interests (12) (see Chapter 7). The HuGENet "road map" for knowledge synthesis and evaluation defines a cycle that begins with reporting of research results and continues through systematic review and synthesis, grading of evidence, and feedback to research investigators and sponsors (13).

HuGE Navigator

Since 2001, HuGENet has maintained an online knowledge base in human genome epidemiology known as HuGE Navigator (http://www.hugenavigator.net) (14). The core data are extracted from PubMed weekly by a combination of automated and manual processes. A single curator selects relevant abstracts and indexes them by gene, study type (observational, meta-analysis, pooled analysis, clinical trial, genome-wide association), and category (of genotype prevalence, gene–disease association, gene–environment interaction, pharmacogenomics, and evaluation of genetic tests).

Human genome epidemiology accounts for only a small fraction of the published scientific literature in human genetics or genomics. Identifying relevant articles is a "needle in a haystack" problem that requires maximizing both sensitivity and specificity. In 2001, about 2,500 (5%) of nearly 50,000 PubMed citations on human genetics or genomics were included in the HuGE Navigator database. In 2007, PubMed added more than 67,000 new articles on human genetics or genomics and more than 5,000 (8%) met HuGE Navigator inclusion criteria (Figure 4.1). The rapid growth of this literature threatened to overwhelm the sole database curator; furthermore, an evaluation of sensitivity found that as many as 20% of relevant articles were being missed (15).

In 2006, HuGE Navigator introduced a new search strategy based on data and text mining algorithms; this approach reduced by 90% the number of citations reviewed by the curator each week, while increasing recall (sensitivity) to 97.5% (16). To make the database more accessible and useful to interdisciplinary researchers, HuGE Navigator added a user interface and an integrated set of new applications for exploring genetic associations, candidate gene selection, and investigator networks (17). Some of these applications are described in the following text.

HuGE Literature Finder (http://www.hugenavigator.net/HuGENavigator/startPagePubLit.do) is the core application of HuGE Navigator (18). The use of nonstandard terminology in published literature is a major obstacle to efficient

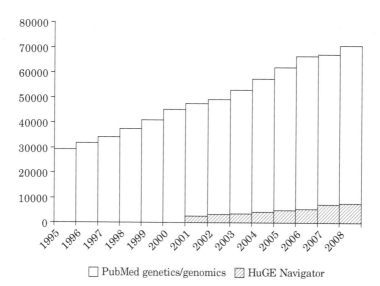

☐ PubMed genetics/genomics ▨ HuGE Navigator

Figure 4.1   PubMed articles on human genetics and genomics, 1995–2008, ** and articles included in HuGE Navigator, 2001–2008 *.

* database queries August 2009.
** PubMed query: gene OR genetic OR genome OR genomic.

searching and synthesis of information in human genome epidemiology. To address this problem, HuGE Navigator uses Unified Medical Language System (UMLS, http://www.nlm.nih.gov/research/umls/) concept unique identifiers (CUIs) to index PubMed abstracts in the database. Medical subject headings (MeSH) constitute one of the controlled vocabularies in UMLS; HuGE Navigator converts MeSH terms assigned by PubMed staff to UMLS CUIs. To index genes, HuGE Navigator uses HUGO gene symbols as well as Entrez Gene identifiers and gene aliases to supplement the content-rich UMLS metathesaurus. HuGE Navigator thus allows users to perform free-text queries, which enhances search sensitivity and makes more information available to the user. A filtering feature allows users to stratify query results by indexing terms (disease, gene, study type, category), as well as by author, journal, year, and country of publication. Genome-wide association studies (GWAS) are flagged and linked to the National Human Genome Research Institute's (NHGRI) Catalog of Published Genome-Wide Association Studies (http://www.genome. gov/26525384).

Phenopedia and Genopedia provide summary views of the HuGE Literature database by disease (MeSH term) and gene (HUGO gene symbol). Disease term definitions and gene-centered data are accessible from either view. Phenopedia (http://www.hugenavigator.net/HuGENavigator/startPagePhenoPedia.do) is disease-centered, displaying a frequency table of association studies, meta-analyses, and GWAS by gene. Phenopedia is a springboard for an important goal of the HuGENet roadmap: to develop an online encyclopedia containing disease-specific summaries of existing knowledge about genetic factors (see Chapter 20). Phenopedia also provides links to Web sites for disease-specific research consortia, databases, and other resources.

Genopedia *(http://www.hugenavigator.net/HuGENavigator/startPagePedia.do)* is gene-centered, displaying a frequency table of association studies, meta-analyses, and GWAS by gene. Genopedia links at the gene level to other databases containing detailed sequence data, as well as relevant information on molecular pathways, genetic variation, and genotype prevalence, genetic associations, gene expression, and genetic testing.

HuGE Investigator Browser *(http://www.hugenavigator.net/HuGENavigator/ investigatorStartPage.do)* creates domain-specific investigator networks by automatically parsing author affiliation data in PubMed records (17). This example of data mining provides a new way to explore and build investigator networks that are crucial to the HuGENet strategy. Nevertheless, it is only a starting point because the information available from PubMed is limited to first authors and ambiguity in author names and affiliations cannot be completely resolved.

GeneProspector(http://www.hugenavigator.net/HuGENavigator/geneProspector StartPage.do) ranks genes in order of available evidence for association with diseases or potential interactions with environmental risk factors. Published GWAS findings and meta-analyses are weighted more than individual association studies and availability of animal data is used to break ties (19).

Variant Name Mapper *(http://www.hugenavigator.net/HuGENavigator/ startPageMapper.do)* is an example of HuGE Navigator applications that assist users in conducting analyses, such as systematic reviews of genetic associations (20). Variant Name Mapper maps common names for genetic variants to their corresponding rs numbers (assigned by dbSNP). In the absence of a universal nomenclature for genetic variants, rs numbers provide a key for comparison, especially with results of commercial chips for GWAS

HuGE Watch *(http://www.hugenavigator.net/HuGENavigator/startPageWatch. do)* offers a general overview of publication trends in human genome epidemiology by year, by country, and by journal. Even these minimal data can offer useful information (21). For example, results of HuGE Watch queries show that although the number of published gene–disease association studies more than tripled from 2001 through 2008, the number examining gene–environment interactions remained small (Figure 4.2).

HuGE Navigator can be used to generate summary impressions of research activity in human genome epidemiology, as well as in such specialized subdomains as meta-analyses, clinical trials, and evaluations of genetic tests. HuGE Navigator can also serve as a starting point for systematic reviews and meta-analyses of gene– disease associations, providing a quick orientation to the literature captured by PubMed. For example, examining frequently studied gene–disease associations can suggest which ones lack a recent meta-analysis (22). Although PubMed is the largest single database of biomedical publications, it does not include all journals. As outlined in the HuGE Review Handbook (available online at: http://www.genesens. net/_intranet/doc_nouvelles/HuGE%20Review%20Handbook%20v11.pdf), a comprehensive review requires searching other publication databases (such as Science

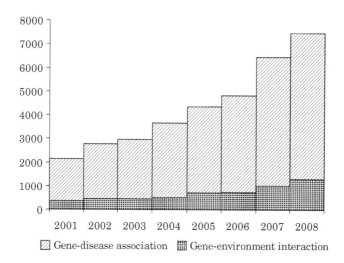

Figure 4.2 PubMed articles included in HuGE Navigator, 2001–2008.* gene–disease associations and gene–environment interactions.

* database queries August 2009.

Citation Index, EMBASE, and BIOSIS) and other data sources (23). Inevitably, the reviewer must do the work to collect the articles, conduct hand searches, and abstract and analyze the data.

Networking Knowledge

Accelerated production of genomic data has prompted the proliferation of databases. Since 1996, the *Nucleic Acids Research* journal has published an annual genomic database issue and compiled an online directory (http://www.oxfordjournals.org/ nar/database/a/); in 2008, the cumulative number of databases topped 1,000 for the first time (24). Reporting on the "annual stamp collecting edition," science blogger Duncan Hull (http://www.nodalpoint.org) asked, "As we pass the one thousand databases mark... I wonder what proportion of these databases will never be used?" (25). Simply capturing and storing data online—without the capacity to process or analyze it—does little to transform it into useful information. In a special issue dedicated to "big data," *Nature* magazine editorialized, "Researchers need to adapt their institutions and practices in response to torrents of new data—and need to complement smart science with smart searching" (26).

Although vastly challenging, assembly of the first human genome sequence was essentially a linear puzzle. Through annotation, analysis, and knowledge synthesis, the genome sequence is now just one dimension in a complex, multidimensional system of relationships at many levels. Understanding these relationships requires an interconnected data system, as well as tools for navigation. For example, NCBI's Entrez search engine connects NCBI databases that extend from the level of SNPs to phenotypes. The network of links among NCBI databases can be explored visually online at http://www.ncbi.nlm.nih.gov/Database/datamodel/.

The HuGE Navigator exploits existing knowledge infrastructures, including HUGO, UMLS, and especially NCBI databases. The HuGE Literature database is compiled from PubMed abstracts; HuGE Navigator's controlled vocabulary includes MeSH terms (as part of UMLS); and HuGE Navigator further mines PubMed data for author and journal information. In turn, Entrez Gene links to the HuGE Navigator, which also supplies citations for Entrez Gene's GeneRIFs (References Into Function) annotated bibliography (27).

Standardization of gene names and identifiers is now widely accepted, allowing HuGE Navigator to link to many other gene-centered databases. For epidemiology and downstream translation, however, disease-centered data are more important. Unfortunately, existing disease ontologies are far more intricate and less precise than those for genes, and no single, best system prevails. To define phenotypes, the HuGE Navigator employs MeSH terms, which are assigned by expert coders when publication abstracts are entered in PubMed; however, many other controlled vocabularies in the Unified Medical Language System (UMLS) have been developed for medical and biomedical research purposes. For example, the Systematized Nomenclature of Medicine—Clinical Terms (SNOMED CT, http://www.snomed.org) was designed to capture clinical care and research data; its use requires a license, which in the United States is provided by the National Library of Medicine (http://www.nlm.nih.gov/research/umls/Snomed/snomed_ main.html). The International Classification of Diseases (ICD, http://www.who. int/classifications/icd/en/index.html) developed by the World Health Organization is used worldwide for reporting morbidity and mortality statistics. Each of these vocabularies has advantages and disadvantages and the mapping from one to another (e.g., via UMLS) is not always straightforward.

Currently, various disease-specific summaries of genetic associations can be found scattered throughout the published literature and across many domain-specific Web sites, such as the PDQ Cancer Information Summaries: Genetics (http:// www.cancer.gov/cancertopics/pdq/genetics). Two well-recognized, online resources for disease-oriented summaries are OMIM and GeneReviews (http://www.geneclinics.org/profiles/all.html); both of these focus largely on uncommon, single-gene disorders.

The HuGENet collaboration aspires to develop an updated, online encyclopedia containing disease-specific summaries of existing knowledge about genetic factors— including genotype–phenotype associations, gene–gene and gene–environment interactions, and available genetic tests. This ambition faces many fundamental obstacles that are intrinsic to the way that research in this area is currently funded, conducted, published, and evaluated; nevertheless, some possible prototypes exist.

An instructive example is the AlzGene knowledge base (http://www.alzforum. org/res/com/gen/alzgene/), which is a component of the Alzheimer Research Forum Web site (http://www.alzforum.org/). AlzGene was the basis for a comprehensive systematic review and meta-analysis of Alzheimer disease genetic association studies published in 2007 (28). The database is continuously updated with primary research data abstracted from articles captured in PubMed. Users can search the database by gene and polymorphism, as well as by study, to obtain tables that summarize studied populations and results. An alternative view of the data includes allele and genotype frequencies stratified by race and ethnicity, along with meta-analysis results displayed as a forest plot. Other components of the Alzheimer Research Forum Web site include a bibliography, a research news digest, a conference calendar, and information on disease management and drug development. Now 10 years old, the Alzheimer Research Forum calls itself a "thriving scientific web community," which promises to evolve further via informatics as a resource for sharing "richly contextualized information" among researchers, practitioners, and affected families (29).

Challenges

Building the knowledge base in human genome epidemiology involves organizing, sharing, mining, interpreting, and evaluating the results of genomic research from a population perspective. This effort faces many technical, scientific, and social challenges, which can be met only by unprecedented levels of interaction across multiple levels of the research enterprise and cooperation among individual scientists, research groups, institutions, and agencies.

Controlled vocabularies and ontologies (which specify terms, concepts, and relationships) have become fundamental devices for organizing and sharing information within specific domains (30), and are particularly important for human genome epidemiology, which is concerned with integrating heterogeneous types of information (e.g., on genetic variants, individual traits, population characteristics) and the quantitative relationships among them. Naming all the elements in these domains and consistently modeling the relationships between them is a challenge of daunting scale and complexity. Human genome epidemiology should encourage the consistent use of interoperable ontologies for human phenotypes to permit collection, sharing, analysis, and synthesis of information by humans and computers (31).

Describing human genetic variation presents technical challenges. The HUGO system of unique gene names and symbols has become a widely accepted standard; however, development of a nomenclature for genetic variants is still evolving (32). Systematic review and synthesis of gene–disease associations require specific data at the level of genetic variants. As a central repository for SNPs and other genetic variants, dbSNP assigns each variant a unique accession number (rs number). Consistent use of rs numbers in abstracts that report genetic associations would substantially enhance capacity for data mining and knowledge synthesis in this field.

During the last decade, the Internet has become the preeminent infrastructure for building scientific knowledge through dissemination, annotation, and synthesis. Technical innovations such as XML (Extensible Markup Language) have enhanced the basis for data mining, and open access scientific journals have helped create a rich substrate (33). Overall, the trend in biomedical research is toward development of a "cyberinfrastructure" that integrates databases, network protocols, and computational tools together across research domains (34,35). The Cancer Biomedical Informatics Grid (caBIG, https://cabig.nci.nih.gov/) is a well-established model, dedicated to managing knowledge and supporting collaboration in cancer research.

Only recently have advances in genotyping technology permitted large-scale epidemiologic studies of gene–disease association and gene–environment interaction. NHGRI has sponsored a number of such studies through two large initiatives, the Genetic Association Information Network (GAIN, http://www.genome.gov/19518664) and the Genes, Environment, and Health Initiative (GEI, http://www.genome.gov/19518663). An integral component of these initiatives is an online data repository, dbGaP, (the database of Genotypes and Phenotypes, http://www.ncbi.nlm.nih.gov/sites/entrez?Db=gap), developed in collaboration with NCBI. In addition, NHGRI maintains a summary online "catalog" of published novel and statistically significant results of these studies (http://www.genome.gov/26525384), which are also indexed by HuGE Navigator. None of these resources, however, can capture all of the measured genetic associations (regardless of prior probability, size, or statistical significance) in a format amenable to knowledge synthesis.

In principle, online data repositories could be equipped with tools for summary analysis and meta-analysis of gene–disease associations. Recently, however, concern that even simple prevalence data for a sufficient number of SNPs could be matched with other genotype data to identify individual persons led several large data repositories to modify their public data access policies and to remove summary genotype prevalence data from public view (36,37). Together, current developments in genomics and informatics technologies are challenging traditional approaches to maintaining confidentiality of research data (38). Reliance on routine electronic data safeguards (such as removing personally identifying information) is clearly inadequate (39). Because privacy and confidentiality are socially defined concepts, their meaning and value must be considered from humanistic as well as scientific perspectives.

Genetics and epidemiology have grown from "cottage industries" to "big science," built on large-scale research collaborations and consortia (40,41). Although technology makes big science possible, it is still a thoroughly human enterprise shaped by social priorities, incentives, and expectations. Appropriate policies and norms for collecting, curating, publishing, and sharing data will have major implications for the developing knowledge base in genomics, including human genome epidemiology (42). In *the* "big data" issue of *Nature*, a group of authors from diverse fields, fifteen different institutions, and four countries wrote of the need to organize research output and recognize the role of knowledge management in the biological sciences:

> Biocuration, the activity of organizing, representing and making biological information accessible to both humans and computers, has become an essential part of biological discovery and biomedical research. But curation increasingly lags behind data generation in funding, development and recognition. (43)

They further observed that "As publication has become a mainly digital endeavor…, publications and biological databases are becoming increasingly similar" and recommended the use of reporting-structure standards to improve cross-referencing and indexing, and thus to increase the visibility and value of scientific research findings. For human genome epidemiology, an initial step in this direction is an extension of the *STrengthening the Reporting of OBservational studies in Epidemiology* (STROBE) statement to genetic association studies (44) (see Chapter 10). As an interdisciplinary effort to integrate information from many domains across many dimensions, human genome epidemiology can take a leading role in coordinated efforts to improve knowledge synthesis.

References

1. Peltonen L, McKusick V. Genomics and medicine. Dissecting human disease in the post-genomic era. *Science.* 2001;291(5507):1224–1229.
2. *Bioinformatics.* Available at http://www.businessweek.com/bw50/content/mar2001/bf20010323_198.htm. Accessed October 14, 2008.

3. National Cancer Institute. caBIG: the launch of a bioinformatics community. *NCI Cancer Bulletin.* 2004;1(9):5–6.
4. Attwood, TK. The quest to deduce protein function from sequence: the role of pattern databases. *Int J Biochem Cell Biol.* 2000;32(2):139–155.
5. Sherry ST, Ward MH, Kholodov M, et al. dbSNP: the NCBI database of genetic variation. *Nucleic Acids Res.* January 1, 2001;29(1):308–311.
6. Maglott D, Ostell J, Pruitt KD, et al. Entrez Gene: gene-centered information at NCBI. *Nucleic Acids Res.* 2005;33:D54–D58.
7. Kent WJ, Sugnet CW, Furey TS, et al. The human genome browser at UCSC. *Genome Res.* 2002;12(6):996–1006.
8. Karolchik D, Kuhn RM, Baertsch R, et al. The UCSC Genome Browser Database: 2008 update. *Nucleic Acids Res.* 2008;36:D773–D779.
9. Bruford EA, Lush MJ, Wright MW, et al. The HGNC Database in 2008: a resource for the human genome. *Nucleic Acids Res.* 2008;36:D445–D448.
10. Horaitis O, Talbot CC, Jr, Phommarinh M, et al. A database of locus-specific databases. *Nat Genet.* 2007;39(4):425.
11. den Dunnen JT and Antonarakis SE. Mutation nomenclature extensions and suggestions to describe complex mutations: a discussion. *Hum Mutat.* 2000;15(1):7–12.
12. Seminara D, Khoury MJ, O'Brien TR, et al. The emergence of networks in human genome epidemiology: challenges and opportunities. *Epidemiology.* 2007;18(1):1–8.
13. Ioannidis JP, Gwinn M, Little J, et al. A road map for efficient and reliable human genome epidemiology. *Nat Genet.* 2006;38(1):3–5.
14. Yu W, Gwinn M, Clyne M, et al. A navigator for human genome epidemiology. *Nat Genet.* 2008;40(2):124–125.
15. Lin BK, Clyne M, Walsh M, et al. Tracking the epidemiology of human genes in the literature: the HuGE Published Literature database. *Am J Epidemiol.* 2006;164(1):1–4.
16. Yu W, Clyne M, Dolan SM, et al. GAPscreener: an automatic tool for screening human genetic association literature in PubMed using the support vector machine technique. *BMC Bioinformatics.* 2008;9:205.
17. Yu W, Yesupriya A, Wulf A, et al. An automatic method to generate domain-specific investigator networks using PubMed abstracts. *BMC Med Inform Decis Mak.* 2007;20;7:17.
18. Yu W, Yesupriya A, Wulf A, et al. An open source infrastructure for managing knowledge and finding potential collaborators in a domain-specific subset of PubMed, with an example from human genome epidemiology. *BMC Bioinformatics.* 2007;8:436.
19. Yu W, Wulf A, Liu T, et al. Gene Prospector: An evidence gateway for evaluating potential susceptibility genes and interacting risk factors for human diseases. *BMC Bioinformatics.* December 8, 2008;9:528.
20. Yu W, Ned R, Wulf A, et al. The need for genetic variant naming standards in published abstracts of human genetic association studies.. *BMC Research Notes* 2009;2:56.
21. Yu W, Wulf A, Yesupriya A, et al. HuGE Watch: tracking trends and patterns of published studies of genetic association and human genome epidemiology in near-real time. *Eur J Hum Genet.* 2008;16:1155–1158.
22. Yesupriya A, W Yu, Clyne M, et al. The continued need to synthesize the results of genetic associations across multiple studies. *Genet Med.* 2008;10:633–635.
23. Frodsham AJ, Higgins JP. Online genetic databases informing human genome epidemiology. *BMC Med Res Methodol.* 2007;7:31.
24. Galperin MY. The Molecular Biology Database Collection: 2008 update. *Nucleic Acids Res.* January 2008; 36(Database issue):D2–D4. Epub November 19, 2007.
25. One thousand databases high and rising. Available at http://www.nodalpoint.org/2008/01/18/one_thousand_databases_high_and_rising. Accessed October 14, 2008.

26. Anonymous. Community cleverness required. *Nature.* 2008;455(7209):1.
27. Mitchell JA, Aronson AR, Mork JG, et al. Gene indexing: characterization and analysis of NLM's GeneRIFs. *AMIA Annu Symp Proc.* 2003;2003:460–464.
28. Bertram L, McQueen MB, Mullin K, et al. Systematic meta-analyses of Alzheimer disease genetic association studies: the AlzGene database. *Nat Genet.* 2007;39(1):17–23.
29. Clark T, Kinoshita J. Alzforum and SWAN: the present and future of scientific web communities. *Brief Bioinform.* 2007;8(3):163–171.
30. Bodenreider O, Stevens R. Bio-ontologies: current trends and future directions. *Brief Bioinform.* 2006;7(3):256–274.
31. Smith B, Ashburner M, Rosse C, et al. The OBO Foundry: coordinated evolution of ontologies to support biomedical data integration. *Nat Biotechnol.* 2007;25:1251–1255
32. den Dunnen JT, Antonarakis SE. Mutation nomenclature extensions and suggestions to describe complex mutations: a discussion. *Hum Mutat.* 2000;15(1):7–12.
33. Brown PO, Eisen MB, Varmus HE, et al. Why PLoS became a publisher. *PLoS Biol.* 2003;1(1): E36.
34. Stein LD. Towards a cyberinfrastructure for the biological sciences: progress, visions and challenges. *Nat Rev Genet.* 2008;9(9): 678–688.
35. Buetow KH. Cyberinfrastructure: empowering a "third way" in biomedical research. *Science.* 2005;308(5723):821–824.
36. Homer N, Szelinger S, Redman M, et al. Resolving individuals contributing trace amounts of DNA to highly complex mixtures using high-density SNP genotyping microarrays. *PLoS Genet.* 2008;4(8):e1000167.
37. Zerhouni EA, Nabel EG. Protecting Aggregate Genomic Data. *Science.* October 3, 2008;322(5898):44. Epub September 4, 2008.
38. Lunshof JE, Chadwick R, Vorhaus DB, et al. From genetic privacy to open consent. *Nat Rev Genet.* 2008;9(5):406–411.
39. McGuire AL, Gibbs RA. Genetics. No longer de-identified. *Science.* 2006;312(5772):370–371.
40. Hoover RN. The evolution of epidemiologic research: from cottage industry to "big" science. *Epidemiology.* January 2007;18(1):13–17.
41. Kreeger K. Consortia, "big science" part of a paradigm shift for genetic epidemiology. *J Natl Cancer Inst.* 2003;95(9):640–641.
42. Foster MW, Sharp RR. Share and share alike: deciding how to distribute the scientific and social benefits of genomic data. *Nat Rev Genet.* 2007;8(8):633–639.
43. Howe D, Costanzo M, Fey P, et al. Big data: The future of biocuration. *Nature.* 2008;455(7209):47–50.
44. von Elm E, Altman DG, Egger M, et al. The Strengthening the Reporting of Observational Studies in Epidemiology (STROBE) statement: guidelines for reporting observational studies. *PLoS Med.* 2007;4(10):e296.

II

METHODS AND APPROACHES FOR DATA COLLECTION, ANALYSIS, AND INTEGRATION

5

The global emergence of epidemiological biobanks: opportunities and challenges

Paul R. Burton, Isabel Fortier, and Bartha M. Knoppers

Introduction

A biobank may be defined as "An organized collection of human biological material (e.g., blood, urine, or extracted DNA) and associated information stored for one or more research purposes" (1). Many biobanks are "disease specific" (2). That is, they include samples and data from (usually) a large number of cases of a specific disease, or pathology specimens of a particular type (e.g., a tumor or a brain bank). Disease-specific biobanks may be combined with appropriate sets of controls (3) to provide a foundation for powerful case-control studies (4). Moreover, some case-control studies can legitimately be viewed as biobanks in their own right (5). Another major class of biobanks is designated "population-based." Recruits into these studies are sampled from a defined target population with no explicit attempt to over- or under-sample subjects based on current disease status. Most population-based biobanks are cohort studies, although some have a simple cross-sectional design (2,6). Given the study design parallels with traditional epidemiology, it is clear that, from the perspective of the population science, there is nothing particularly new about the modern concept of "biobanking" (2). The only real departures from long-standing tradition are the sheer size of the largest initiatives now being proposed, the particular emphasis that is placed on obtaining biological material, and the greatly enhanced biotechnological capability that now exists to store, process, and analyze biological samples.

That said, there *has* been a crucial change in the philosophy of the underlying science. Many contemporary biobanks, particularly *population-based* biobanks, are being set up as general purpose research infrastructures with little emphasis being placed on testing specific scientific hypotheses. Rather, they are being designed, as far as is practicable, to optimize future scientific opportunity and to enable sharing of the resource across the biomedical research community as a whole. At the same time, by actively harmonizing study design and conduct, it is hoped to facilitate the sharing of data and samples between biobanks so as to promote powerful pooled analyses and rigorous replication studies. This change in philosophy has important implications for the opportunities and challenges of contemporary biobanking that are the focus of this chapter.

Opportunities: The Scientific Role of Biobanks

The last decade has seen a fundamental shift in genetic epidemiology, from studies of genetic linkage to studies of genetic association (7). This is based on assumptions about the validity of the common disease common variant hypothesis (8–12), which implies that genetic determinants of common complex diseases will typically exhibit weak etiological effects (13) and will be identified more powerfully using association studies (14). Some association studies are based on family designs (15,16) but most involve unrelated individuals (13,16,17) and are either stand-alone case-control studies (16–18) or case-control comparisons nested within cohort studies (19–22). A genetic association study addresses the question: "is genetic variant G systematically associated with disease D across a population?" This may be viewed as *traditional epidemiology applied to genotypes or alleles* (7), and so the association paradigm supports the integration of environmental and lifestyle determinants (as in conventional epidemiology) with genomic determinants to explore direct and interactive effects on disease-related traits.

Until recently, this approach was open to serious question (11–13,17,23–32). But, a series of recent publications has demonstrated that, not only in theory but also *in practice*, it is possible—given an adequate sample size—to reliably detect and replicate genetic associations with complex diseases in general population samples (33). For example, this has now been shown in: type 1 diabetes (4,34); type 2 diabetes (4,35–38); coronary heart disease (4,39–41); breast cancer (42,43); colorectal cancer (44–46); prostate cancer (47,48); age-related macular degeneration (49–51); and Crohn's disease (4,52). These successes are crucial, because the rationality of an extensive international investment in biobanks, each enrolling large numbers of unrelated individuals, is critically dependent on the assumption that etiological effects—both genetic and lifestyle—*can* be detected by association studies. But if these successes *do* provide a justification for further investment in biobanking, how may these biobanks be used, and how, if at all, will their role differ from that of conventional epidemiological studies?

A Foundation for Association Analyses Based on Case-control Comparisons

The outcome variable in most association studies in human genomic epidemiology is either a binary disease phenotype (disease present [yes/no]) or a quantitative trait related directly to the disease of interest, or to a component of a putative causal pathway leading to that disease. The etiological determinants of primary interest may be genetic variants, environmental/lifestyle exposures, or gene–environment or gene–gene interactions. When the outcome is binary, such an analysis is typically based on a case-control comparison (outcome-dependent sampling). Such a comparison may be undertaken in the context either of a stand-alone case-control study or of a nested case-control analysis in a cohort. When the outcome is quantitative, direct analysis involving that outcome may be based on data from a cross-sectional or a cohort study.

A Foundation for Exposure-based Analyses

Unlike case-control comparisons, exposure-based analyses select subjects from a biobank on the basis of *exposure*. The most important class of exposure-based analyses will probably be "genotype-based studies," which are poised to become a common and important use of biobanks. For example, 100 subjects may be sampled because they exhibit a particular genetic variant, while a further 100 may be selected—as a comparison group—that do not have that variant. With appropriate consents, the selected participants may be invited to attend for follow-up investigation. If they agree, potentially intensive bioclinical exploration can be undertaken of intermediate causal pathways leading to the disease of interest. Here, biobanks with a population-based cohort design are ideal. Not only do they include prospectively collected lifestyle/environmental information, but unlike disease-specific biobanks, the initial ascertainment mechanism places no probabilistic constraints on the distribution of intermediate phenotypes. Furthermore, when genotyping costs fall and entire cohorts can comprehensively be genotyped or sequenced, the vast size of an adequately powered cohort means that even relatively uncommon genetic variants or environmental exposures will be present in sufficient numbers for meaningful analysis.

Investigation of the Determinants of Disease Progression

Both disease-based and population-based biobanks provide a good framework for studying determinants that modulate disease progression. In both settings, subjects that have a disease of interest can be followed longitudinally (by face-to-face or remote review, or by tracking in electronic health information systems) and phenotypic changes can be related to genetic and environmental/lifestyle factors.

A Foundation for Family-based Studies Including Linkage Studies

If familial relationships can be defined within a biobank, then the potential for undertaking family-based studies exists. Assuming appropriate consideration is given to relevant ethico-legal issues, this is possible in several situations: (i) if the study recruits families rather than individuals (e.g., Generation Scotland) (53); (ii) if the data in the study can be record linked to population-based genealogies (e.g., deCODE) (40); (iii) if demographic information can be collected enabling relatives to be identified via record linkage (54); and (iv) if extensive genotyping can be undertaken and relatives identified using DNA-based approaches (55,56).

Perhaps the most important form of family-based analysis that might be undertaken is genetic linkage analysis (57), particularly for disease-related traits that are quantitative or are very common binary disease states. But, the potential value of a biobank as a foundation for many types of family-based analyses can be enhanced by downstream extension studies: additional members of "informative" families can be approached, recruited, and investigated in detail.

A Source of "Common" Controls

The principles underpinning Mendelian Randomization (18,20,58) ensure that environmental and lifestyle determinants and genetic variants are unlikely to confound a genetic effect of interest and that inferences should not be distorted by reverse causality. As an additional and important corollary, case-control studies of the direct association between a genetic variant and a complex disease are relatively robust to the manner in which the controls are selected (18). One set of controls that is reasonably representative of the general population as a whole may therefore be used as a *common control series* and compared to more than one set of cases. This was the basis of the successful Wellcome Trust Case Control Consortium (WTCCC) (4) project. Here, a national population-based biobank (the 1958 Birth Cohort) (3) provided a cost-effective way to generate one set of common controls. A large national biobank may also be used to generate a common control series for a scientifically important subpopulation, for example, as a source of common controls for case-series deriving from a relatively large ethnic-minority subpopulation.

From a scientific perspective, the roles of contemporary biobanks are really no different than those of traditional epidemiological studies. The spectrum of uses to which biobanks will be put is precisely the same as that of more traditional studies, and the design challenges are equivalent. But, this perspective misses the point that it is not the science itself that is changing (except in its technological sophistication) but, rather, the *philosophy* of how that science is implemented. Unlike many traditional epidemiological projects, most biobanks are, quite explicitly, infrastructural resources. They are not set up to answer specific scientific questions, but rather to provide powerful platforms for biomedical and epidemiological science that will enable future research to be undertaken more effectively and at lower cost. Thus, from a strategic perspective, most individual biobanks are deliberately designed so as to fulfil a number of different roles, and much of the thinking that goes into study design focuses on two things: (i) the management of data and samples is aimed at optimizing future utility in terms of a wide range of potential uses, including those that are yet to be invented; (ii) very careful account must be taken of the need to collect, process, store, and release data and samples in ways that optimize information quality, minimize information loss, and promote the prospect for future use by other researchers and of pooling with other biobanks. Thus, the difference between biobanks and traditional epidemiological studies is not so much in their science, but rather in the strategic thinking that must go into their conception, design, set up, and use.

Challenges

There is no doubt that biobanks offer many exciting scientific opportunities. But their design, construction, management, and maintenance all present important scientific and ethico-legal challenges. This section explores some of the important challenges that must be faced. This is not intended as a comprehensive review of *all* challenges faced by biobanks—that would take a whole book—rather it is aimed at addressing some of the most critical challenges that are influencing the design and set up of biobanks right now.

Scientific Challenges

Small effect sizes. Although alternative strategies might have been adopted (23), an informal collective decision has been taken to base preliminary exploration of the etiological architecture of the complex diseases on the assumption that at least some important causal determinants will satisfy the Common Disease Common Variant (CDCV) hypothesis (8–12). This is the principal logic underpinning the extensive international investment in biobanks enrolling large numbers of unrelated individuals. But the decision to invest in this way has "self-fulfilling" consequences. For example, if common complex diseases are caused by a mixture of common variants with small effects and rare family-specific variants with large effects, the current generation of biobanks will only identify the former with adequate power. This means that, in designing biobanks that recruit unrelated individuals, it is essential to ensure that they *are* capable of detecting the small effect sizes that are plausible under the CDCV hypothesis.

But, what is *plausible*? To date, the majority of associations between chronic diseases and genetic variants that have reliably been identified and replicated are characterized by allelic or genotypic relative risks of 1.5 or less (4,13,34–52). Many fall in the range of 1.1–1.3, and although effect sizes may be greater for causal variants than for markers in linkage disequilibrium, it would be unwise to assume that the gain will be substantial. Furthermore, it is likely that it is the genuinely larger effects that have been identified first and that the "average" effect sizes that are currently observed are positively biased by the "winners" curse (59,60). In consequence, if the aim is to properly explore causal architecture under the CDCV hypothesis, it must be accepted (42) that many important effects will probably be more difficult to detect than those typically found to date and that research infrastructures are required that will enable the detection of main effects corresponding to relative risks smaller than 1.3.

However, this raises an important question: is there any scientific value in identifying relative risks of such a size? From the perspective of traditional epidemiology and public health, this depends on the prevalence and severity of the disease and on the prevalence of the at-risk determinant. Even relative risks in the range of 1.1–1.3 might theoretically generate many thousands of potentially avoidable cases of a common disease caused by a common exposure. More often, however, small relative risks will be associated with small attributable risks and, despite understandable optimism (61), it seems unlikely that they will play a major role in, for example, identifying high-risk population subgroups—or high-risk individuals—to target prevention or early diagnosis (20). But this misses the central point, which is that the primary aim of contemporary genomic epidemiology is to inform us about the causal architecture of the complex diseases. Each additional quantum of knowledge has the potential to provide an important insight that might ultimately have a dramatic impact on disease prevention or management. This implies that scientific interest may logically focus on *any* causal association that can convincingly be identified and replicated—it need not be "strong" by any statistical criterion. We therefore agree (2,20) with Khoury and Gwinn who argue that "each investigation that increases our understanding of gene–environment interaction, etiological heterogeneity, pathogenesis, and natural history of common diseases adds to a knowledge base for estimating risks and guiding interventions to improve population health" (62).

But can small relative risks be interpreted anyway? In 1995, Taubes argued that: "[observational epidemiological studies]... are so plagued with biases, uncertainties, and methodological weaknesses that they may be inherently incapable of accurately discerning... weak associations" (63). In other words, if entirely realistic levels of confounding and reverse causality can generate an artefactual odds ratio of, say, 1.3, can any useful conclusion, whatsoever, be drawn from an observed odds ratio of 1.25? Fortunately, many of the arguments underlying this bleak, but compelling, assessment are greatly mitigated in human genome epidemiology (18). Randomization (segregation and assortment) at gamete formation renders simple phenotype–genotype associations robust to lifestyle confounding and to uncertainty in the direction of causality (20). In other words, enhanced inferential rigor is a direct, but wholly fortuitous, consequence of what is sometimes called Mendelian Randomization (20,58,64). Despite important caveats (20,58,65), small effects reflecting the direct impact (main effects) of genetic determinants or the differential impact of genetic variants in diverse environmental backgrounds (gene–environment interactions) are therefore rendered more meaningful than their counterparts in traditional environmental epidemiology.

Analytic complexity. The fundamental challenges presented by the need to detect small effect sizes are further compounded by the complexity of the background noise from which they must be discriminated. Analytic complexity arises from at least three sources: first, complexity in the underlying biology (e.g., etiological heterogeneity and sequential causal pathways with multiple components); second, errors in assessment of both outcomes and exposure that are fundamental to even the best measurement technology that is available; third, complexity arising from decisions about study design and analysis (e.g., complex correlation structures are fundamental to both family and longitudinal designs). This subsection will consider some of the key issues in more detail.

a) Many studies test a plethora of hypotheses simultaneously. Methods that appropriately adjust for this (66–69) make the inferential process more conservative and true effects harder to find. The impact can be substantial. For example, a simple Bonferroni correction controlling the genome-wide type 1 error rate to 5% for a genome-wide association study (GWAS) testing 500,000 SNPs requires that individual SNPs are tested at $p < 10^{-7}$ (70). Similarly, for testing SNPs in a vague candidate gene where the prior odds against an association might often exceed 1,000:1 (68), the approach based on the False Positive Report Probability (69) demands the equivalent of testing at approximately $p < 10^{-4}$ to keep the proportion of "significant" findings that are "false positives" to $\approx 10\%$.

b) The underlying focus of contemporary bioscience is not on investigating the effect of a single SNP or a single lifestyle determinant, but rather on exploring a "'web of causation' involving multiple and complex pathways, perhaps involving many genes and environmental substrates" (68). Teasing out the component associations that together form a causal chain is technically difficult (71), and typically of lower power than studying a single association in isolation (65).

c) Complex causal structures are commonly associated with nonindependence of observational units. Under many designs in genetic epidemiology, a correlation structure is generated that must be addressed appropriately. Such correlation may be informative in its own right (72,73), but it can be difficult to deal with technically (74,75), and often leads to a loss of statistical power.

d) Errors in the assessment of either exposures or outcomes can seriously impair statistical power (33,76) (see below) and can bias parameter estimates (75,77).

e) Etiological determinants that are unknown, or have not been measured, can also impact on the identification of an etiological factor of scientific interest (33).

f) Mendelian randomization provides no protection against the confounding/over-dispersion caused by latent differences in population ancestry between populations being compared (78,79).

How big is big? The striking inconsistency (11–13,17,24–32) of genetic association studies until very recently (4,13,34–52) can reasonably be blamed on a wide variety of different scientific and technical issues (24,26,28,30,80–85). However, the fundamental difficulty underpinning almost all specific explanations has been the difficulty of distinguishing small biological effects from the underlying analytic complexity. Even the most cursory review of study design makes it clear that the common route to failure has been a consistent, and serious, lack of statistical power (24,26,28,30,80–85). However, this presents a major challenge: how large should stand-alone and nested case-control studies really be, if they *are* to power contemporary gene discovery? And, crucially, will the current generation of "large" initiatives (2,4,86) (http://www.p3gobservatory.org; http://www.genome.gov/17516722) generate enough power to study the *joint* effects of genes and environment (87)? These challenges are absolutely fundamental. Governments and funding agencies worldwide are considering investment in population genomics. Difficult strategic decisions, with imposing price tags and important opportunity costs, are being taken. Accurate power calculations are therefore needed to determine realistic sample size requirements.

Conventional power calculations (88) indicate that having 400 cases and 400 controls provides less than 1% power to detect (at $p < 0.0001$) an odds ratio of 1.4 for a binary "at-risk" genotype with a general population frequency of 9.75% (this corresponds to the prevalence of an "at-risk" genotype arising from a dominant risk-determining allele with a minor allele frequency [MAF] of 5%). There is no doubt that a study involving several hundred cases and controls demands extensive hard work. It is also true that such studies are "large" by historical standards. But the reality is that to generate a power of 80%, such a study would actually require 4,000 cases and 4,000 controls.

But even these figures substantially understate the challenge that really faces us. Conventional power calculations ignore many important aspects of analytic complexity (see above). For example, in a study of type 2 diabetes diagnosed on the basis of "*GP diagnosis or HbA1C ≥ 2 SD (standard deviations) above the population mean*" (89), account should be taken of the sensitivity (89.1%) and specificity (97.4%) of the diagnostic test (89). Equally, appropriate consideration should be given to the impact of genotyping error, and of unmeasured risk factors causing heterogeneity in baseline disease risk. Using an R-based (90) simulation-based power-calculation engine (ESPRESSO) jointly developed by P³G and UK Biobank (33,91) (see http://www.p3gobservatory.org/powercalculator.htm), these complexities can be taken into full account. This approach may be used to mimic the conventional power calculation undertaken above, by assuming that disease and genotype are assessed without error and that there is no heterogeneity in disease risk. This confirms a requirement for ≈4,000 cases and 4,000 controls. But, if the sensitivity and specificity of disease assessment is taken into account, if the genotyping error is assumed to equate to incomplete linkage disequilibrium with an R^2 of 0.8 (92), and if heterogeneity in disease risk is reflected in an assumed 10-fold ratio in the risk between subjects on high (95%) and low (5%) centiles of population risk, the estimated sample size requirement more than *doubles* to 8,500 cases and 8,500 controls.

It is clear that sample size requirement has many important determinants. The ESPRESSO power calculator was therefore used to generate sample size profiles, for main effects and for gene–environment interactions, across a range of different bioclinical scenarios (Figures 5.1 and 5.2). Two things are clear.

First, the power to detect genetic effects (both main effects and interactions) is strongly influenced by assessment error (33,76). In reality, genotyping errors are consequent upon a mixture of true errors in genotyping, inefficiencies in the calling algorithm, and incomplete linkage disequilibrium (LD) (4,92). Although they are modelled here as if they are caused solely by incomplete LD, this merely provides a convenient way to describe the magnitude of the error in a manner that can readily be understood. Thus, $R^2 = 1.0$ equates to no genotyping error, and $R^2 = 0.8$ corresponds to an error equivalent to the minimum LD between markers on the Affymetrix 500k chip and SNPs on HapMap 2 (92). In relation to errors in the assessment of lifestyle

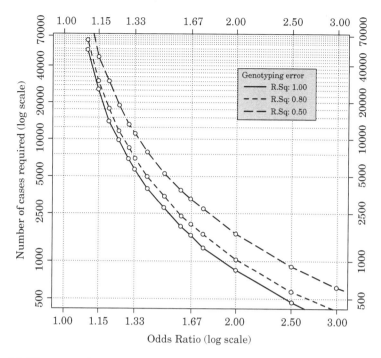

Figure 5.1 The required number of cases (vertical axis) required in an unmatched case-control study with four times as many controls as cases to provide 80% power to detect (at p < 0.0001) a true odds ratio (horizontal axis) associated with a genetic main effect. The genetic variant is a dominantly acting allele with a population prevalence of 5%—this generates a binary "at-risk" genotype with a prevalence of 9.75%. Error in the assessment of genotype is assumed to be equivalent to incomplete linkage disequilibrium with $R^2 = 1.0$, 0.8, or 0.5. There is assumed to be a 10-fold difference in baseline risk of disease between a subject on the 5% and 95% centiles of population risk. The disease is assumed to be type 2 diabetes assessed using a test with 89.1% sensitivity and 97.4% specificity.

determinants, it is assumed that the binary exposure arises from dichotomization of an underlying quantitative latent variable measured with the reliability specified. For the purposes of illustration, Table 5.1 lists lifestyle measures with reliabilities corresponding approximately to those presented in Figure 5.2.

Second, it is clear (33) that sample size requirements are *very large*. Even in a relatively well-powered setting, for example, a main effect reflecting the impact of a genotype assessed without error in a vague candidate gene (taking statistical significance at $p = 10^{-4}$), Figure 5.1 indicates that ≥2,500 cases are needed for 80% power to detect an odds ratio of 1.5 under the conditions detailed in the figure legend. An odds ratio of 1.2 demands more than 10,000 cases and for a GWA study testing at $p < 10^{-7}$ the required sample sizes all increase by a further 70%. The study sizes needed for gene–environment interactions are yet more demanding (Figure 5.2). Even in the absence of measurement error, an interaction odds ratio of 2.0 demands nearly 5,000

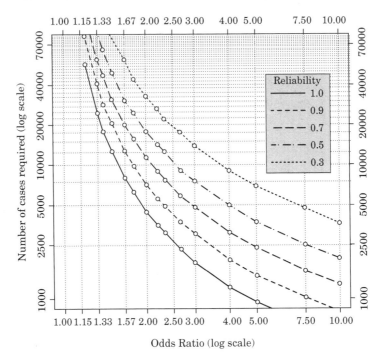

Figure 5.2   The required number of cases (vertical axis) required in an unmatched case-control study with four times as many controls as cases to provide 80% power to detect (at p < 0.0001) a true odds ratio (horizontal axis) associated with a gene–environment interaction. The interaction is between a binary "at-risk" genotype with a prevalence of 9.75% (as Figure 5.1), and a binary environmental determinant with a prevalence of 50%. The "at-risk" status of the environmental determinant is assumed to have been generated by dichotomization of a latent normally distributed variable measured with the range of reliabilities indicated. Error in the assessment of genotype is assumed to be equivalent to incomplete linkage disequilibrium with $R^2 = 0.8$. There is assumed to be a 10-fold difference in baseline risk of disease between a subject on the 5% and 95% centiles of population risk. The disease is assumed to be type 2 diabetes assessed using a test with 89.1% sensitivity and 97.4% specificity.

cases to provide 80% power, and in a more realistic setting—a moderate odds ratio (1.67) and an environmental factor measured with reliability 0.7 (93)—the required number of cases increases to 20,000. Many entirely realistic situations can be envisaged in which the sample size requirement will be larger still.

However, do these calculations overstate the problem by focusing on genes with binary (e.g., dominant) effects, rather than genes with ordered effects across the three genotypes generated by two alleles (e.g., a multiplicative model that is *additive on the scale of log odds*) (4)? Empirical evidence (data not shown) indicates that if an additive genetic model is valid and is fitted, sample size requirements typically fall between 5% and 50% relative to the binary model. However, the largest reduction

Table 5.1 Formal estimates of test–retest reliability for a number of exemplar lifestyle/environmental determinants that are widely studied

Reliability of Measurement	Lifestyle/Environmental Factor
≥0.95	Body mass index (BMI) calculated from measured height and weight in various studies (94)
≈0.9	Measured hip or waist circumference (94,95)
≈0.7	Blood pressure measurement in the Intersalt Study (93)
≈0.5	Many nutritional components in a dietary recall study, mean of four 24-hour assessments (84)
≈0.3	Many nutritional components in a dietary recall study, a single 24-hour assessment (84)

in sample size requirement is exhibited by SNPs with common minor alleles, and for them, a gain in power is often unimportant. Rather, it is SNPs with *rare* minor alleles that are subject to severe limitations in their statistical power (Figure 5.1), but in that setting there are very few subjects that are homozygous for the minor allele, and an additive variant therefore acts almost as if it were binary. In the case of a MAF of 5%, the sample size requirement for the additive model is typically 95% of that used for the binary model. Furthermore, variants with dominant or recessive effects on the risk of disease are not esoteric rarities, and if the additive model is *invalid*, power will actually be lost by assuming it to be true.

In the light of all of these considerations, it would appear that if general purpose research platforms (e.g., biobanks) based on unrelated individuals are to be set up, they must be capable of supporting analyses as large as the very largest that are currently going to press (4,34–52). But if this number of cases is to be recruited, from where can they be obtained? In particular, if some are to be generated as incident cases in cohort studies, how large must such cohorts be, and how long might one reasonably have to wait to generate five, ten, or twenty thousand cases? As a rough guide (33,91), Table 5.2 presents the estimated times to generate incident cases of 16 selected chronic diseases in U.K. Biobank: a cohort study recruiting 500,000 subjects (50% male, aged 40–69 years) from across Great Britain. The estimates are based on simulations using national age–sex specific rates of death and disease incidence. They are appropriately adjusted for migration, anticipated withdrawal from the study, and the fact that healthy cohorts are typically healthier, on average, than the general populations from which they are drawn (33,91).

Ethico-legal Challenges

The human genome project and its ethico-legal implications attracted the close attention of policy makers starting in the early 1990s. This has not held true for epidemiological biobanks. The planning, funding, and public participation in the building of such infrastructures constantly face both systemic and policy barriers: systemic,

Table 5.2 The expected time after the commencement of recruitment by which
U.K. Biobank will have generated 1,000, 2,500, 5,000, 10,000, and 20,000 cases
of 16 important complex diseases

	Time to Achieve 1,000 Cases (in Years)	Time to Achieve 2,500 Cases (in Years)	Time to Achieve 5,000 Cases (in Years)	Time to Achieve 10,000 Cases (in Years)	Time to Achieve 20,000 Cases (in Years)
Bladder cancer	11	19	31	—	—
Breast cancer (F)	4	6	10	17	40
Colorectal cancer	5	9	14	22	42
Prostate cancer (M)	6	9	14	22	41
Lung cancer	7	12	19	34	—
Non-Hodgkins lymphoma	11	22	—	—	—
Ovarian cancer (F)	12	26	—	—	—
Stomach cancer	16	29	—	—	—
Stroke	5	8	12	18	28
MI and coronary death	2	4	5	8	13
Diabetes mellitus	2	3	4	6	10
COPD	4	6	8	13	23
Hip fracture	7	11	15	21	31
Rheumatoid arthritis	7	14	27	—	—
Alzheimer disease	7	10	13	18	23
Parkinson disease	6	10	15	23	37

due to their sheer size, cost, and duration; policy, due to conflation with gene-hunting
studies and their societal implications (97). Furthermore, once a biobank has successfully overcome the systemic and policy barriers (98), it is then faced with a range of
additional ethico-legal issues associated with the fundamental scientific research that
is its primary aim (99). Key topics covered in this subsection include: public understanding of biobanks; rational approaches to ethical review; maintenance of privacy
and security; effective consent; and international interoperability.

Public understanding. The daily bombardment of scientific "breakthroughs,"
(100) including the "map" of the human genome (101), and now the role of genetic
and environmental determinants in causing common diseases (4), has left the public
both perplexed and sceptical about the arrival of yet another "genomic" enterprise. Policy makers and the general public alike find it difficult to comprehend
that a biobank is not a scientific "experiment" in itself but is a resource providing
a platform for future research. In agreeing to participate in a biobank, there are

no personal benefits to be anticipated; no drugs, medical devices, or interventions will be used (except in an initial cursory clinical assessment); any exciting scientific discoveries will typically take decades to emerge; and—bizarrely, from the perspective of many participants—the scientists would prefer to recruit healthy subjects than those with preexisting disease. These characteristics all place the construction of such infrastructures outside the traditional perception of biomedical research. Fortunately, much has been learned about strategies for public engagement (not just "education") (102), but the resources required are enormous and beyond the budgets of many biobanks.

Ethics review. The metaphorical "Thermopylae" of many biomedical research projects is the ethics review. Most contemporary ethics committees have not previously encountered epidemiological biobanks and have limited experience and understanding of many of the relevant issues. Although this creates a perfect opportunity for education, it also leads to serious misunderstandings and delays, particularly when norms are applied that are simply not suited to the real nature of biobanks. For example, to be completely transparent, biobanks must downplay any personal biomedical benefits while highlighting the potential for unpredictable (exciting) future research. But, ethics committees expect to see neutral, "scientific" descriptions that avoid inducement and speculation. The fundamental problem is that participants in the creation of such infrastructure are not really acting as research participants at all; or not, at least, in the widely recognized sense. Rather, they are volunteering as "global citizens" in offering long-term access to their DNA and personal data with no expectation of a personal return. It is true that the preliminary clinical assessment is an important drawing card, but this merely highlights the increasing absence of a personal, general practitioner in the lives of many citizens; in an ideal world, this preliminary clinical assessment would not be seen as a personal benefit at all. From the perspective of an experienced member of a typical ethics committee, these characteristics of a biobank project fall entirely outside the norms of clinical research, usually undertaken in sick patients, and often based on clinical trials. It is true that an equivalent situation does arise in Phase 1 clinical trials, but precisely because this is so, volunteers are usually paid, which is not the case for biobanks. To compound the problem, ethics committees rarely include epidemiologists, population geneticists, or anyone else with experience in building sample and data infrastructure open to third-party researchers.

Privacy and security. There is widespread cynicism about the efficacy of the security of modern biobanks. This arises for several reasons. The first is the recognized impossibility of guaranteeing that an individual can never be identified. The very provision of a DNA sample defies an absolute guarantee, even though such identification may be exceedingly unlikely. Second, as concerns the notion of identifiability, personal data legislation only applies when an individual is identifiable. Only recently has this been confirmed to mean that for all practical and reasonable intents and purposes, a person is not to be considered identifiable if coding mechanisms have been put in place (103). Third, the sophistication of modern encryption and informatics privacy tools are widely misunderstood and underestimated. Fourth, the rigor of the formal mechanisms overseeing data and sample access is often not recognized. Without necessarily excluding the private sector or eventual commercialization, access to both data and samples is strictly controlled and often involves a separate, independent access committee (104). Fifth, the public has become all too accustomed to hearing of major data security blunders arising from deliberate malpractice or from managerial incompetence. No security system can ever guarantee against deliberate criminal intent, but the comprehensive protocols, checks and counterchecks applied by a typical biobank should provide reliable protection against security lapses (105). The same checks and governance hold for data sharing activities. This heightened security serves to balance the broad consent provided for future research and international access and ensures that the trust of participants in proper stewardship of the samples and data is maintained.

Consent. A fundamental characteristic of—particularly large population-based—epidemiological biobanks is that they must necessarily seek broad consent to use banked data and samples for scientific projects that may take place far in the future and may entail technology and methods that are yet to be conceived. Furthermore, in order for the vast national and international investment in biobanks to optimally meet the expectations and needs of the populations that fund them, it is crucial that consent covers broad access to third party researchers. This constellation of characteristics distinguishes large-scale epidemiological biobanks from almost all forms of traditional biomedical science, including clinical trials, traditional projects in epidemiology and genetic epidemiology, and research based on pathology collections linked to clinical records (106). When a study has enrolled hundreds of thousands of recruits, it is no simple matter (indeed it may be impossible) to reconsent everybody years later. It is therefore crucial that the consent is correctly phrased the first time. Qualitative evidence suggests that consent forms are read and understood by participants in ways that may differ very markedly from the understanding of those writing them (107)—often less rigidly—and it is crucial that biobanks recognize that investment in a well-worded consent form may not only increase recruitment rates, but can also enhance future scientific opportunity.

International interoperability. The ultimate challenge lies in ensuring that epidemiological biobanks can exchange data and materials across boundaries dividing legal and ethical jurisdictions. This is important not only for technical reasons (e.g., increased statistical power and access to a richer array of environmental and cultural exposures, etc.) but also because science of such a fundamental nature must be *international* in its scope, funding, and benefit to society. It is essential that scientists from around the world, including those from developing countries, are able to construct and access biobanking resources, and to validate, compare, replicate, and refine data, samples, and analyses that are central to the needs of their populations. To that end, it is not only broad consent with a long-term time horizon that is essential, but the need for national and international, public and possibly commercial access is paramount as well, and careful thought at the outset needs to be put into material and data transfer agreements.

Responding to the challenges

It should be clear that the science of biobanking faces a number of important challenges. However, two in particular would appear to be fundamental. From the perspective of the science, the primary challenge is to increase the quantity, quality, and utility of the information that will ultimately be stored as data and samples in the biobanks being set up today. On the ethico-legal side, the challenge is to ensure that everybody (governments, nongovernmental organizations, policy makers, funders, researchers, the general public, and study participants) understands what modern biobanking is *really* about, and that legal systems and ethical review mechanisms as applied to biobanks are therefore enabling and fit-for-purpose. Regulatory and governance systems must promote good practices—that facilitate effective science—without imposing risk or unnecessary cost on willing and consenting participants, and must enhance the prospect of legitimate information flow around the world.

Optimizing Information Content

There is little doubt that many scientific questions of fundamental importance will only be answerable given access to very large amounts of high-quality data in a format that promotes integration between biobanks. These considerations are particularly critical if we wish to set up multipurpose research platforms to provide a robust infrastructure for future studies of the joint effect of genes and environment.

If we do, then in designing these platforms, a number of key issues must be kept in mind. First, sample size calculations must be realistic. If the scientific goal is to reach the moon, a "moon-rocket" is required, not a commercial airliner—even if the latter flies perfectly well and is much cheaper. Second, optimal use must be made of alternative, and complementary, study designs. Cohort studies, case-control, cross-sectional, and family-based studies *all* have appropriate roles and consideration must also be given to recruiting subjects in all age groups: at birth, in childhood, in middle age, and in the elderly. Furthermore, once a platform has been built, it must be used in a manner that maximizes its utility, for example, it should be considered as a basis for disease-based sampling (case-control analyses), exposure-based sampling (e.g., genotype-based studies), and intensive laboratory-based studies of causal pathways. Third, appropriate emphasis must be placed on the *quality* of information and samples, whether they are collected at recruitment or longitudinally. Data and sample handling and storage protocols must also be optimized to ensure flexibility for future technological and scientific developments that are as yet unpredictable.

Fourth, the capacity to track large numbers of healthy subjects longitudinally must be enhanced, ideally using electronic methods, and appropriate investment must be made in deep phenotyping of consenting subjects once a disease event has been identified. Fifth, the mathematical models used to analyze data in genomic and genetic epidemiology must be efficient as well as valid. When sample sizes are in the tens or hundreds of thousands, an analysis that is 90% efficient may nevertheless waste millions of dollars. Investment should therefore be made in developing optimized approaches. Furthermore, there must be a willingness to accept that a definitive analysis may take a week, because the approach that takes 10 minutes is only 95% efficient. Sixth, we must develop standardized procedures for data and sample collection, processing, storage, and sharing so that compatible information can easily be integrated between biobanks (2,20). *Harmonization* defines a philosophy of standardizing those aspects that *can* be the same between studies while acknowledging that there is strength in diversity and developing sharing mechanisms that also deal optimally with the *unavoidable difference* between studies (2). Harmonization comes in two basic flavors: *retrospective*, which aims to optimize the mapping of preexisting information from one study onto the equivalent information from other studies, and *prospective*, where questionnaires and standard operating procedures for emerging studies are rendered as similar as possible ahead of time. The two approaches are complementary and both are important. Seventh, we must develop tools and information systems enabling researchers to identify where data and samples of potential value may be sited and indicating how to obtain permission to access them, and instructions on how to abstract, interpret, and use them (http://www.p3gobservatory.org). Finally, we must develop internationally agreed quality criteria by which biobanks may be judged in order that we may flag those data sources that are of high enough quality to make it worthwhile for researchers to invest their time in trying to find them.

Optimizing Understanding and Ethico-legal Structures

Biobanking presents individual nations and the global community with new ethico-legal challenges that we must work through together. There is a pressing need for effective dialog between governments, nongovernmental organizations, funding agencies, scientists and technologists, experts in ethico-legal and social issues, health interest groups, and the general public. A broad and shared understanding of what biobanking is about must be achieved. This provides the best way to ensure that it is the issues that *really* concern participants, scientists, and the general public that are given the greatest weight when new biobanks are set up.

Such a dialog will necessarily take time, but it is also critical to recognize that things must move forward without unwarranted delay. New biobanks are being designed and constructed right now. Every contemporary biobank that is set up under an unnecessary ethical or legal constraint that prohibits national or international sharing is an opportunity lost: for the scientists involved; for the governments and populations that funded it; and, most importantly, for the participants who agreed to give up time and biosamples on the assumption that they would be used in an optimal way to further future developments in bioscience and thereby the health of generations to come. Rather, we should, where possible, aim for consent to be as broad as possible, and for access and material transfer agreements to be secure but not unnecessarily restrictive. Legalistic or protectionist ethics cannot and should not prevent or block the opportunity of individuals to participate in large-scale population research if they are willing to do so and freely provide informed consent. Participants *must* be afforded appropriate protection against unscrupulous activity, but if what is entailed is properly and fully explained and if participants are willing to act as "citizens of the world" through their ongoing contribution to a biobank, why should they be prevented from doing so? It is only by optimizing the potential for national and international sharing of data and samples that we can ensure a maximum return on the altruistic investment made by these global citizens.

We must also try to move away from the "safe" thinking that is built into some regulatory mechanisms. Some of this thinking echoes earlier times, before the information revolution made international data sharing a reality. It reflects understandable, but often inappropriate, concerns that arise from media-based exposure to deliberate malpractice or large-scale "informatic" incompetence (105) in other walks of life. Some ethico-legal commentators appear to believe that it is their primary role, and the role of the "system," to guard against scientists that wish to behave like crooked financiers or incompetent public officials. A perhaps more moderate perspective might acknowledge that the natural position of a biobank scientist is to act like a medical or a legal practitioner. Many are medical and/or legal professionals in their own right, and they more than willingly embrace the sanctity of the doctor–patient and attorney–client relationship in other settings without the need to repeatedly justify this *a priori* in front of a regulatory committee.

Getting It Together

Substantial work has already been completed, but we are currently taking the first few steps of a long journey. The imperative to undertake this route and to travel it together has been recognized by a number of major international bodies and organizations. These include, but are not limited to: P³G and PHOEBE (particularly population-based biobanks); ISBER (particularly tissue-based biobanks); HuGENet™ (particularly case-control studies); NCI and OECD (particularly developing baseline working standards for biobanks); and BBMRI (particularly infrastructural development). It is to be hoped that the enabling philosophy and international spirit of collaboration that characterized the Human Genome Project (108,109) and the HapMap Project (110,111) will be equally effective in ensuring the ultimate success of what can reasonably be viewed as a direct descendant of these initiatives. That is, an international network of harmonized biobanks that will allow us to explore, understand, and ultimately control how genes and lifestyle/environment act together to determine health and disease in human society.

Acknowledgments
The work underpinning this chapter has been supported by the core research programs of P³G (the Public Population Project in Genomics) and CARTaGENE funded by Genome Canada and Genome Quebec, and of PHOEBE (Promoting Harmonization of Epidemiological Biobanks in Europe) funded by the European Union under the Framework 6 program. The program of research in genetic epidemiology in Leicester is also funded in part by MRC Cooperative Grant #G9806740 and Wellcome Trust Grant #086160/Z/08/A. The power calculations reported in the chapter were generated using simulation-based methods that were initially developed with the support of UK Biobank and its joint funders: Wellcome Trust, Medical Research Council, Department of Health, Scottish Executive, and Northwest Regional Development Agency. We gratefully acknowledge the hard work of Anna Hansell, Imperial College, who undertook the original calculations that generated the figures in Table 5.2.

References

1. P3G and PHOEBE Consortia. The Biobank Lexicon http://www.p3gobservatory.org/lexicon/list.htm. Accessed 25 May, 2009.
2. Burton P, Fortier I, Deschenes M, Hansell A, Palmer L. Biobanks and biobank harmonization. In: Davey SG, Burton P, Palmer L, eds. An Introduction to Genetic Epidemiology. Bristol: Policy Press; In press 2009.
3. Power C, Elliott J. Cohort profile: 1958 British birth cohort (National Child Development Study). *Int J Epidemiol*. 2006;35(1):34–41.
4. Wellcome_Trust_Case_Control_Consortium. Genome-wide association study of 14,000 cases of seven common diseases and 3,000 shared controls. *Nature*. 2007;447:661–678.
5. Clarke R, Xu P, Bennett D, et al. Lymphotoxin-alpha gene and risk of myocardial infarction in 6,928 cases and 2,712 controls in the ISIS case-control study. *PLoS Genet*. 2006;2(7):e107.
6. Husebekk A, Iversen O-J, Langmark F, Laerum OD, Ottersen OP, Stoltenberg C. *Biobanks for Health—Report and Recommendations from an EU Workshop*. Oslo: Technical report to EU Commission; 2003.
7. Burton PR, Tobin MD, Hopper JL. Key concepts in genetic epidemiology. *Lancet*. 2005;366(9489):941–951.
8. Lander ES. The new genomics: global views of biology. *Science*. 1996;274(5287):536–539.
9. Reich DE, Lander ES. On the allelic spectrum of human disease. *Trends Genet*. 2001;17(9):502–510.
10. Pritchard JK, Cox NJ. The allelic architecture of human disease genes: common disease-common variant or not? *Hum Mol Genet*. 2002;11(20):2417–2423.
11. Hirschhorn JN, Lohmueller K, Byrne E, Hirschhorn K. A comprehensive review of genetic association studies. *Genet Med*. 2002;4(2):45–61.
12. Lohmueller KE, Pearce CL, Pike M, Lander ES, Hirschhorn JN. Meta-analysis of genetic association studies supports a contribution of common variants to susceptibility to common disease. *Nat Genet*. 2003;33(2):177–182.
13. Hattersley AT, McCarthy MI. What makes a good genetic association study? *Lancet*. 2005;366(9493):1315–1323.
14. Risch N, Merikangas K. The future of genetic studies of complex human diseases. *Science*. 1996;273:1516–1517.
15. Hopper JL, Bishop DT, Easton DF. Population-based family studies in genetic epidemiology. *Lancet*. 2005;366(9494):1397–1406.
16. Cordell HJ, Clayton DG. Genetic association studies. *Lancet*. 2005;366(9491):1121–1131.

17. Palmer LJ, Cardon LR. Shaking the tree: mapping complex disease genes with linkage disequilibrium. *Lancet.* 2005;366(9492):1223–1234.

18. Clayton D, McKeigue PM. Epidemiological methods for studying genes and environmental factors in complex diseases. *Lancet.* 2001;358(9290):1356–1360.

19. Breslow NEDNE. *Statistical Methods in Cancer Research.* Volume 2—The design and analysis of cohort studies. Lyon: International Agency for Research on Cancer; 1987.

20. Davey Smith G, Ebrahim S, Lewis S, Hansell AL, Palmer LJ, Burton PR. Genetic epidemiology and public health: hope, hype, and future prospects. *Lancet.* 2005;366(9495):1484–1498.

21. Manolio TA, Bailey-Wilson JE, Collins FS. Genes, environment and the value of prospective cohort studies. *Nat Rev Genet.* 2006;7(10):812–820.

22. Collins FS. The case for a US prospective cohort study of genes and environment. *Nature.* 2004;429(6990):475–477.

23. Terwilliger JD, Weiss KM. Confounding, ascertainment bias, and the blind quest for a genetic "fountain of youth." *Ann Med.* 2003;35(7):532–544.

24. Ioannidis JP, Ntzani EE, Trikalinos TA, Contopoulos-Ioannidis DG. Replication validity of genetic association studies. *Nat Genet.* 2001;29(3):306–309.

25. Tabor HK, Risch NJ, Myers RM. Opinion: candidate-gene approaches for studying complex genetic traits: practical considerations. *Nat Rev Genet.* 2002;3(5):391–397.

26. Weiss KM, Terwilliger JD. How many diseases does it take to map a gene with SNPs? *Nat Genet.* 2000;26(2):151–157.

27. Goldstein DB, Ahmadi KR, Weale ME, Wood NW. Genome scans and candidate gene approaches in the study of common diseases and variable drug responses. *Trends Genet.* 2003;19(11):615–622.

28. Cardon LR, Bell JI. Association study designs for complex diseases. *Nat Rev Genet.* 2001;2(2):91–99.

29. Terwilliger JD, Goring HH. Gene mapping in the 20th and 21st centuries: statistical methods, data analysis, and experimental design. *Hum Biol.* 2000;72(1):63–132.

30. Buchanan AV, Weiss KM, Fullerton SM. Dissecting complex disease: the quest for the Philosopher's Stone? *Int J Epidemiol.* 2006;35(3):562–571.

31. Moonesinghe R, Khoury MJ, Janssens AC. Most published research findings are false-but a little replication goes a long way. *PLoS Med.* 2007;4(2):e28.

32. Chanock SJ, Manolio T, Boehnke M, et al. Replicating genotype-phenotype associations. *Nature.* 2007;447(7145):655–660.

33. Burton PR, Hansell AL, Fortier I, et al. Size matters: just how big is BIG?: Quantifying realistic sample size requirements for human genome epidemiology. *Int J Epidemiol.* 2009;38(1):263–273.

34. Todd JA, Walker NM, Cooper JD, et al. Robust associations of four new chromosome regions from genome-wide analyses of type 1 diabetes. *Nat Genet.* 2007;39(7):857–864.

35. Grant SF, Thorleifsson G, Reynisdottir I, et al. Variant of transcription factor 7-like 2 (TCF7L2) gene confers risk of type 2 diabetes. *Nat Genet.* 2006;38(3):320–323.

36. Zeggini E, Weedon MN, Lindgren CM, et al. Replication of genome-wide association signals in U.K. samples reveals risk loci for type 2 diabetes. *Science.* 2007;316:1336–1339.

37. Saxena R, Voight BF, Lyssenko V, et al. Genome-wide association analysis identifies loci for type 2 diabetes and triglyceride levels. *Science.* 2007;316(5829):1331–1336.

38. Scott LJ, Mohlke KL, Bonnycastle LL, et al. A genome-wide association study of type 2 diabetes in Finns detects multiple susceptibility variants. *Science.* 2007;316(5829):1341–1345.

39. Samani NJ, Erdmann J, Hall AS, et al. Genomewide association analysis of coronary artery disease. *N Engl J Med.* 2007;357(5):443–453.

40. Helgadottir A, Thorleifsson G, Manolescu A, et al. A common variant on chromosome 9p21 affects the risk of myocardial infarction. *Science.* 2007;316(5830):1491–1493.
41. McPherson R, Pertsemlidis A, Kavaslar N, et al. A common allele on chromosome 9 associated with coronary heart disease. *Science.* 2007;316(5830):1488–1491.
42. Easton DF, Pooley KA, Dunning AM, et al. Genome-wide association study identifies novel breast cancer susceptibility loci. *Nature.* 2007;447(7148):1087–1093.
43. Stacey SN, Manolescu A, Sulem P, et al. Common variants on chromosomes 2q35 and 16q12 confer susceptibility to estrogen receptor-positive breast cancer. *Nat Genet.* 2007;39(7):865–869.
44. Haiman CA, Le Marchand L, Yamamato J, et al. A common genetic risk factor for colorectal and prostate cancer. *Nat Genet.* 2007;39(8):954–956.
45. Tomlinson I, Webb E, Carvajal-Carmona L, et al. A genome-wide association scan of tag SNPs identifies a susceptibility variant for colorectal cancer at 8q24.21. *Nat Genet.* 2007;39(8):984–988.
46. Zanke BW, Greenwood CM, Rangrej J, et al. Genome-wide association scan identifies a colorectal cancer susceptibility locus on chromosome 8q24. *Nat Genet.* 2007;39(8):989–994.
47. Gudmundsson J, Sulem P, Steinthorsdottir V, et al. Two variants on chromosome 17 confer prostate cancer risk, and the one in TCF2 protects against type 2 diabetes. *Nat Genet.* 2007;39(8):977–983.
48. Gudmundsson J, Sulem P, Manolescu A, et al. Genome-wide association study identifies a second prostate cancer susceptibility variant at 8q24. *Nat Genet.* 2007;39(5):631–637.
49. Klein RJ, Zeiss C, Chew EY, et al. Complement factor H polymorphism in age-related macular degeneration. *Science.* 2005;308(5720):385–389.
50. Haines JL, Hauser MA, Schmidt S, et al. Complement factor H variant increases the risk of age-related macular degeneration. *Science.* 2005;308(5720):419–421.
51. Edwards AO, Ritter R, 3rd, Abel KJ, Manning A, Panhuysen C, Farrer LA. Complement factor H polymorphism and age-related macular degeneration. *Science.* 2005;308(5720):421–424.
52. Rioux JD, Xavier RJ, Taylor KD, et al. Genome-wide association study identifies new susceptibility loci for Crohn disease and implicates autophagy in disease pathogenesis. *Nat Genet.* 2007;39(5):596–604.
53. Smith BH, Campbell H, Blackwood D, et al. Generation Scotland: the Scottish Family Health Study; a new resource for researching genes and heritability. *BMC Med Genet.* 2006;7:74.
54. Hansen J, Alessandri PT, Croft ML, Burton PR, de Klerk NH. The Western Australian Register of Childhood Multiples: effects of questionnaire design and follow-up protocol on response rates and representativeness. *Twin Res.* 2004;7(2):149–161.
55. Sheehan NA, Egeland T. Structured incorporation of prior information in relationship identification problems. *Ann Hum Genet.* 2007;71(Pt 4):501–518.
56. Sheehan N, Egeland T. Adjusting for founder relatedness in a linkage analysis using prior information. *Hum Hered.* 2008;65(4):221–231.
57. Teare DM, Barrett JH. Genetic linkage studies. *Lancet.* 2005;366(9490):1036–1044.
58. Davey Smith G, Ebrahim S. "Mendelian randomization": can genetic epidemiology contribute to understanding environmental determinants of disease? *Int J Epidemiol.* 2003;32(1):1–22.
59. Beavis WD. The power and deceit of QTL experiments: lessons from comparitive QTL studies. *Proceedings of the Forty-Ninth Annual Corn & Sorghum Industry Research Conference.* Washington, DC: American Trade Association; 1994:250–266.
60. Zondervan KT, Cardon LR. Designing candidate gene and genome-wide case-control association studies. *Nat Protoc.* 2007;2(10):2492–2501.

61. Collins FS. Shattuck lecture—medical and societal consequences of the Human Genome Project. *N Engl J Med*. 1999;341(1):28–37.
62. Khoury MJ, Gwinn M. Genomics, epidemiology, and common complex diseases: let's not throw out the baby with the bathwater! *Int J Epidemiol*. 2006;35(5):1363–1364; author reply 1364–1365.
63. Taubes G. Epidemiology faces its limits. *Science*. 1995;269(5221):164–169.
64. Tobin MD, Minelli C, Burton PR, Thompson JR. Commentary: development of Mendelian randomization: from hypothesis test to "Mendelian deconfounding." *Int J Epidemiol*. 2004;33(1):26–29.
65. Didelez V, Sheehan N. Mendelian randomization as an instrumental variable approach to causal inference. *Stat Methods Med Res*. 2007;16(4):309–330.
66. Benjamini Y, Hochberg Y. Controlling the false discovery rate: a practical and powerful approach to multiple testing. *J R Stat Soc Series B*. 1995;57:289–300.
67. Weller JI, Song JZ, Heyen DW, Lewin HA, Ron M. A new approach to the problem of multiple comparisons in the genetic dissection of complex traits. *Genetics*. 1998;150:1699–1706.
68. Thomas DC, Clayton DG. Betting odds and genetic associations. *J Natl Cancer Inst*. 2004;96(6):421–423.
69. Wacholder S, Chanock S, Garcia-Closas M, El Ghormli L, Rothman N. Assessing the probability that a positive report is false: an approach for molecular epidemiology studies. *J Natl Cancer Inst*. 2004;96(6):434–442.
70. Thomas DC. Are we ready for genome-wide association studies? *Cancer Epidemiol Biomarkers Prev*. 2006;15(4):595–598.
71. Lauritzen S, Sheehan N. Graphical models for genetic analyses. *Stat Sc*. 2003;18(4):489–514.
72. Khoury M, Beaty T, Cohen B. *Fundamentals of Genetic Epidemiology*. Oxford: Oxford University Press; 1993.
73. Burton P, Tiller K, Gurrin L, Cookson W, Musk A, Palmer L. Genetic variance components analysis for binary phenotypes using generalized linear mixed models (GLMMs) and Gibbs sampling. *Genet Epidemiol*. 1999;17(2):118–140.
74. Burton PR, Scurrah KJ, Tobin MD, Palmer LJ. Covariance components models for longitudinal family data. *Int J Epidemiol*. 2005;34:1063–1067.
75. Zeger SL, Liang KY. An overview of methods for the analysis of longitudinal data. *Stat Med*. 1992;11(14–15):1825–1839.
76. Wong MY, Day NE, Luan JA, Chan KP, Wareham NJ. The detection of gene-environment interaction for continuous traits: should we deal with measurement error by bigger studies or better measurement? *Int J Epidemiol*. 2003;32(1):51–57.
77. Burton P, Gurrin L, Sly P. Extending the simple linear regression model to account for correlated responses: an introduction to generalized estimating equations and multi-level mixed modelling. *Stat Med*. 1998;17(11):1261–1291.
78. Schaid DJ, Elston R, Olsen J, Palmer L. *Disease Marker Association*. Chichester: Wiley; 2002:206–217.
79. Marchini J, Cardon LR, Phillips MS, Donnelly P. The effects of human population structure on large genetic association studies. *Nat Genet*. 2004;36(5):512–517.
80. Risch NJ. Searching for genetic determinants in the new millennium. *Nature*. 2000;405(6788):847–856.
81. Little J, Khoury MJ, Bradley L, et al. The human genome project is complete. How do we develop a handle for the pump? *Am J Epidemiol*. 2003;157(8):667–673.
82. Ioannidis JP, Gwinn M, Little J, et al. A road map for efficient and reliable human genome epidemiology. *Nat Genet*. 2006;38(1):3–5.

83. Khoury MJ, Millikan R, Little J, Gwinn M. The emergence of epidemiology in the genomics age. *Int J Epidemiol.* 2004;33:936–944.
84. Khoury MJ, Little J, Gwinn M, Ioannidis JP. On the synthesis and interpretation of consistent but weak gene-disease associations in the era of genome-wide association studies. *Int J Epidemiol.* 2007;36(2):439–445.
85. Little J, Bradley L, Bray MS, et al. Reporting, appraising, and integrating data on genotype prevalence and gene-disease associations. *Am J Epidemiol.* 2002;156(4):300–310.
86. Collins R, UK Biobank Steering Committee. *UK Biobank: Protocol for a Large-scale Prospective Epidemiological Resource.* Manchester: UK Biobank Coordinating Centre; 2007.
87. Hunter DJ. Gene-environment interactions in human diseases. *Nat Rev Genet.* 2005;6(4):287–298.
88. Armitage P, Berry G. *Statistical Methods in Medical Research,* 3rd ed. Oxford: Blackwell Scientific Publications; 1994.
89. Rohlfing CL, Little RR, Wiedmeyer HM, et al. Use of GHb (HbA1c) in screening for undiagnosed diabetes in the U.S. population. *Diabetes Care.* 2000;23(2):187–191.
90. R Development Core Team. *A Language and Environment for Statistical Computing.* Vienna, Austria: R Foundation for Statistical Computing; 2008.
91. Burton PR, Hansell A. UK *Biobank: the Expected Distribution of Incident and Prevalent Cases of Chronic Disease and the Statistical Power of Nested Casecontrol Studies.* Manchester, UK: UK Biobank Technical Reports; 2005.
92. Barrett JC, Cardon LR. Evaluating coverage of genome-wide association studies. *Nat Genet.* 2006;38(6):659–662.
93. Dyer AR, Shipley M, Elliott P, for the Intersalt Cooperative Research Group. Urinary electrolyte excretion in 24 hours and blood pressure in the INTERSALT study: I. estimates of reliability. *Am J Epidemiol.* 1994;139(9):927–939.
94. Klipstein-Grobusch K, Georg T, Boeing H. Interviewer variability in anthropometric measurements and estimates of body composition. *Int J Epidemiol.* 1997;26(Suppl 1):S174–S180.
95. Rimm EB, Stampfer MJ, Colditz GA, Chute CG, Litin LB, Willett WC. Validity of self-reported waist and hip circumferences in men and women. *Epidemiology.* 1990;1(6):466–473.
96. Grandits GA, Bartsch GE, Stamler J. Method issues in dietary data analyses in the Multiple Risk Factor Intervention Trial. *Am J Clin Nutr.* 1997;65(suppl):211S–227S.
97. Knoppers BM, Kent A. Policy barriers in coherent population-based research. *Nat Rev Genet.* 2006;7(1):8.
98. Knoppers BM, Kent A. Tool-sharing issues in coherent population-based research. *Nat Rev Genet.* 2006;7(2):84.
99. P3G_Consortium. See P3G Observatory—Ethics, Governance and Public Engagement: http://www.p3gobservatory.org/repository/ethics.htm. Accessed 25 May, 2009.
100. Condit CM. How geneticists can help reporters to get their story right. *Nat Rev Genet.* 2007;8(10):815–820.
101. Lander ES, Linton LM, Birren B, et al. Initial sequencing and analysis of the human genome. *Nature.* 2001;409(6822):860–921.
102. Godard B, Marshall J, Laberge C. Community engagement in genetic research: results of the first public consultation for the Quebec CARTaGENE project. *Community Genet.* 2007;10(3):147–158.
103. Working Party Document No. WP 136: Opinion N° 4/2007 on the concept of personal data. Available at http://ec.europa.eu/justice_home/fsj/privacy/docs/wpdocs/2007/wp136_en.pdf.

104. Knoppers BM, Abdul-Rahman MH, Bedard K. Genomic databases and international collaboration. *King's Law J.* 2007;18(2):291–312.

105. Wintour P. Lost in the post—25 million at risk after data discs go missing. *Guardian.* November 21, 2007;1.

106. Helgesson G, Dillner J, Carlson J, Bartram CR, Hansson MG. Ethical framework for previously collected biobank samples. *Nat Biotech.* 2007;25(9):973–976.

107. Dixon-Woods M, Ashcroft RE, Jackson CJ, et al. Beyond "misunderstanding": written information and decisions about taking part in a genetic epidemiology study. *Soc Sci Med.* 2007;65(11):2212–2222.

108. International Human Genome Sequencing Consortium. Finishing the euchromatic sequence of the human genome. *Nature.* 2005;431:931–945.

109. Venter JC, Levy S, Stockwell T, Remington K, Halpern A. Massive parallelism, randomness and genomic advances. *Nat Genet.* 2003;33(Suppl):219–227.

110. The International HapMap Project. The International HapMap Project. *Nature.* 2003;426(6968):789–796.

111. Altshuler D, Brooks L, Chakravarti A, Collins F, Daly M, Donnelly P. A haplotype map of the human genome. *Nature.* 2005;437(7063):1299–1320.

6

Case-control and cohort studies in the age of genome-wide associations

Teri Manolio

Introduction

The advent of genome-wide association studies (GWAS) has revolutionized research on the genomics of complex diseases and traits (1). In what has been called one of the greatest bursts of discovery in the history of medical research (2), this technique has identified over 400 loci for nearly 100 common diseases and traits in the past 4 years (Table 6.1). GWAS use dense maps of single nucleotide polymorphisms (SNPs) to capture the vast majority of common variation, that is, variant alleles with a frequency of at least 5% in the population. Much of the success of these studies has been attributed to their assaying, in thousands of unrelated subjects, hundreds of thousands of SNPs selected primarily for their ability to capture common genomic variation rather than for their location in known genes or regulatory regions. GWAS thus assess genetic variation genome wide in an almost "agnostic" fashion, unconstrained by current imperfect understanding of genome structure and function (3). The GWA approach is revolutionary because it permits interrogation of the entire human genome at hitherto unattainable levels of resolution, unconstrained by prior hypotheses regarding genetic associations with disease. It can also be problematic because the massive number of statistical tests performed presents an unprecedented potential for false positive results, leading to new stringency in acceptable levels of statistical significance and requirements for replication of findings (2).

This novel approach has led to one of the major surprises in recent gene discovery—most of the SNPs newly identified as being associated with common diseases and traits are not in genes previously suspected of being related to specific diseases, and some are in regions containing no known genes at all (1). For example, only 33 (9.5%) of the first 348 GWA-identified SNPs are in coding regions or in 5' or 3' untranslated regions of genes, while roughly 45% are intronic and the remaining 45% are not near any known genes (4). New insights into potential pathogenic mechanisms and possible preventive or therapeutic strategies provided by these findings have included implication of the inflammation pathway in age-related macular degeneration (5), the bacterial-engulfment and processing pathway in inflammatory bowel disease (6), and the nicotine receptor pathway in lung cancer (7).

Table 6.1 Diseases and traits studied using genome-wide association testing assaying 100,000 variants or more, March 2005–August 2009

Eye diseases
- Macular degeneration
- Glaucoma

Cancer
- Lung cancer
- Prostate cancer
- Breast cancer
- Colorectal cancer
- Bladder cancer
- Neuroblastoma
- Melanoma
- Basal cell cancer
- *TP53* cancer predilection
- Acute and chronic lymphocytic leukemia
- Follicular lymphoma
- Thyroid cancer
- Myeloproliferative syndrome
- Testicular germ cell cancer
- Glioma
- Ovarian cancer
- Pancreatic cancer

Gastrointestinal diseases
- Cleft palate
- Inflammatory bowel disease
- Celiac disease
- Hirschsprung disease
- Gallstones
- Cirrhosis
- Drug-induced liver injury

Cardiovascular conditions
- ECG intervals
- Coronary disease
- Coronary spasm
- Atrial fibrillation/flutter
- Stroke
- Intracranial aneurysm
- Hypertension
- Hypertension diuretic response
- Aortic aneurysm/peripheral arterial disease

(Continued)

Table 6.1 Continued

- Lipids/lipoproteins
- Warfarin dosing
- Ximelegatran adverse response

Neuropsychiatric conditions

- Parkinson disease
- Amyotrophic lateral sclerosis
- Multiple sclerosis
- Multiple sclerosis interferon-β response
- Progressive supranuclear palsy
- Tauopathies
- Alzheimer disease
- Variant Creutzfeldt–Jakob disease
- Cognitive ability
- Memory
- Hearing, otosclerosis
- Restless legs syndrome
- Essential tremor
- Nicotine dependence
- Alcohol dependence
- Methamphetamine dependence
- Pain
- Panic disorder
- Neuroticism
- Schizophrenia
- Schizophrenia iloperidone response
- Bipolar disorder
- Bipolar disorder lithium response
- Family chaos
- Narcolepsy
- ADHD
- Personality traits

Autoimmune and infectious diseases

- Rheumatoid arthritis
- Rheumatoid arthritis anti-TNF response
- Systemic lupus erythematosus
- Juvenile idiopathic arthritis
- Behçet's disease
- Osteoarthritis
- Psoriasis
- Kawasaki disease

Table 6.1 Continued

- Sarcoidosis
- Pulmonary fibrosis
- Chronic obstructive pulmonary disease/lung function
- Cystic fibrosis severity
- Asthma
- Chronic rhinosinusitis
- Atopic dermatitis
- HIV setpoint/progression
- Chronic hepatitis B
- Severe malaria

Diabetes, renal disease, and anthropometry
- Type 1 diabetes
- Type 2 diabetes
- Diabetic nephropathy
- End-stage renal disease
- Kidney stones
- Obesity, body mass index, waist
- Insulin resistance, metabolic traits
- Height
- Osteoporosis
- Menarche
- Menopause/ovarian failure
- Male pattern baldness
- Male infertility

Laboratory/other traits
- Fetal hemoglobin
- Platelet mass/volume
- Transferrin levels
- C-reactive protein
- ICAM-1 levels
- Eosinophil numbers
- Total IgE levels
- Urate levels, gout
- Protein levels
- Folate pathway, vitamins
- β-Carotene levels
- Recombination rate
- Telomere length
- Pigmentation

Table 6.2 Proportion of familial risk of complex diseases
explained by genome-wide studies to date

Disease	Number of Loci	Genetic Risk Explained
Breast cancer (8)	7	5%
Crohn's disease (9)	32	10% overall variance, 20% of genetic risk
Diabetes (10)	18	6%
Systemic lupus erythematosus (11)	6	15%

Another major surprise stemming from these findings has been the predominantly modest increases in risk associated with these variants (1). Of the first 200 variants related to discrete diseases or dichotomized traits, for example, 50% were associated with odds ratios less than 1.3 or less, and only 15% carried odds ratios greater than 2.0 (4). Despite very large sample sizes and extensive collaborative efforts, often involving tens of thousands of patients and hundreds of investigators, GWA findings to date have explained only a small portion of the heritability of complex diseases such as breast cancer, diabetes, Crohn's disease, and systemic lupus erythematosus (Table 6.2). The failure to find many variants of large effect has been attributed to natural selection working to eliminate such variants from the population; tag SNPs assayed by current genotyping platforms having varying degrees of linkage disequilibrium with the true causative variants, leading to underestimation of effect; structural variants (insertions, deletions, duplications, inversions) or rare variants poorly assayed by current methods; and unaccounted-for effects of regulatory, epigenetic, or environmental modifiers of genetic variants.

Environmental modifiers of the effects of genetic variants, or gene–environment interactions, have received increased attention in recent years due to the recognition that genetic variants alone are unlikely to explain most of the recent increases in chronic diseases (12). Such increases are more likely due to environmental and behavioral changes interacting with a genetic predisposition, suggesting that failing to identify and control environmental modifiers of disease risk could mask important associations with genetic variants or misestimate the magnitude of their effects (13). Identifying environmental modifiers of these variants may also be essential in mitigating the risk conferred by these variants. Population-based genetic association studies with detailed characterization of environmental exposures are critical and underused resources for identifying potential interacting factors (14,15). This chapter explores the substantial and complementary strengths offered by the two main approaches to these studies, case-control and cohort designs, in the search for the genetic and environmental influences on common diseases.

Case-control Studies in the Era of Genome-wide Association

The great majority of GWAS conducted to date have used the case-control design, in which allele frequencies in persons with the trait or disease of interest are compared to those in a disease-free comparison group. These studies are often easier and cheaper to conduct than prospective cohort studies, in which participants are identified and characterized prior to disease onset and then followed forward in time to the occurrence of disease (Figure 6.1). Speed and efficiency may be maximized if sufficient numbers of cases and controls can be assembled rapidly, as is often the case in clinical series of patients presenting for medical care. Cases and controls are typically investigated retrospectively for evidence of genetic and other risk factors and environmental exposures that existed prior to disease onset, and thus likely contributed to disease development.

Although the case-control design is often selected for its ease and low cost during initial efforts to identify risk factors for common diseases, for the study of rare diseases it actually has important advantages over the prospective cohort design. These include facilitating the identification and recruitment of study subjects, since the design starts with diagnosed cases of disease, often from specialized referral centers. The prospective cohort design, in contrast, requires the follow-up of large numbers of people who will never develop a rare disease to identify the few cases who do. Schlesselman provides a salient illustration, estimating that a cohort study of a condition occurring at a rate of 8 cases per 1,000 persons would require observation

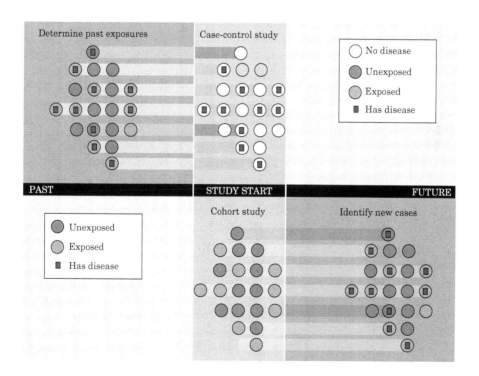

Figure 6.1 Assessing associations in case-control and cohort studies. Source: *Reprinted with permission from (16). Copyright © 2008 Massachusetts Medical Society. All rights reserved.*

of 3,889 exposed and 3,889 unexposed subjects to detect a two-fold increase in risk (17). A case-control study, in contrast, would require only 188 cases and 188 controls. If the prevalence of disease were lower, at 2 cases per 1,000, cohorts of approximately 15,700 exposed and 15,700 unexposed subjects would be needed to detect a two-fold increased risk, but a case-control study would still require only 188 cases and 188 controls.

The case-control design also permits assessment of multiple exposures in relation to disease outcome, provided those exposures can be measured after disease has occurred. This may be especially relevant if biological specimens have been collected and stored prior to disease onset, permitting targeted measurement of specific analytes in cases of interest and suitable controls. It may also permit more detailed assessment of a particular exposure (such as occupational or dietary history), collected retrospectively in small, selected numbers of cases and controls.

Despite these advantages, case-control studies are particularly prone to several of the sources of bias described in Table 6.3. A key requirement for a bias-free case-control study is that cases be representative of all persons who develop the disease under study. Because cases are often identified in the clinical setting, typically through review of medical records, mild cases or those that lead to early mortality are likely to be missed, leading to prevalence-incidence or survival bias. This is a particular problem if a sizeable subset of cases suffers a rapid and fatal course (as in coronary disease or some cancers), so that "etiologic" factors identified among the subset of survivors are actually more related to survival or a benign prognosis (18).

Another requirement is that controls be representative of all persons at risk for the disease. In this respect, potential threats to the representativeness of cases are also important among controls, especially nonresponse bias. Differential response rates related to genetic background may arise between cases and controls due to differences between these groups in prevalence of a family history of disease. The tendency for persons with a positive family history to be more likely to participate can be an important type of respondent bias in genetic studies (19). Findings from a biased group of cases or controls may not be generalizable to the population at large or may be frankly invalid, although these biases can often be identified and compensated for, particularly by selecting a control group that is matched on many of the potential confounding factors. Matching has its pitfalls, however, since once a factor is matched upon, so that it is evenly distributed between cases and controls, it can no longer be examined for association with disease. In addition, the difficulty in finding matching controls rapidly escalates with the number of factors matched upon. In general, unless one is certain that a given factor is related to disease etiology, it is probably better not to match on it so that it can be examined in analysis.

One solution to the lack of a "perfect" control group is to utilize more than one type of control group. One group of controls might be selected from the same hospital as the cases; another control group might use neighborhood controls,

Table 6.3 Biases in case-control and cohort designs

Type of Bias	Description
Biases that relate to subject selection (17,18)	
Prevalence–incidence or survival bias	Selection of existing cases that are currently available for study will miss fatal and short episodes, and might miss mild or silent cases.
Nonresponse (or respondent) bias	Differential rates of refusal or nonresponse to inquiries between cases and disease-free comparison subjects.
Diagnosis (or diagnostic suspicion) bias	Knowledge of a subject's exposure to a putative cause of disease can influence both the intensity and outcome of the diagnostic process.
Referral (or admission-rate) bias	Cases who are more likely to receive advanced care or to be hospitalized—such as those with greater access to health care or with coexisting illnesses—can distort associations with other risk factors in clinic-based studies, unless the same referral or admission biases are operative in disease-free comparison subjects.
Surveillance bias	If a condition is mild or likely to escape routine medical attention, cases are more likely to be detected in people who are under frequent medical surveillance.
Biases that relate to measuring exposures and outcomes (18)	
Recall bias	Questions about specific exposures might be asked more frequently of cases, or cases might search their memories more intensively for potential causative exposures.
Family information bias	The flow of family information about exposures or illnesses can be stimulated by, or directed to, a new case in its midst.
Exposure suspicion bias	Knowledge of a patient's disease status can influence the intensity and outcome of the search for exposure to a putative cause.

Source: Adapted from Reference 15.

where each control is matched by neighborhood to a case, or family controls, who share much of the case's genetic background but are unaffected by disease. Use of multiple control groups is often considered to be methodologically superior because the biases in one group may be minimized in the other and vice versa. Associations can be assessed in the two groups separately: if few differences are found, one may have greater confidence in the conclusions drawn. If more than one control group is used, one group might be selected to be matched and another unmatched.

Use of a common comparison group for multiple groups of disease cases has been employed successfully, primarily as a cost-saving measure, in GWAS by the Wellcome Trust Case Control Consortium (20). Despite initial skepticism that a single control group would permit detection of association signals in multiple disparate diseases, nearly all the findings from that study have been replicated in studies using more traditional control groups. This suggests that initial identification of SNPs associated with disease may be robust to these potential biases, although this approach may not provide unbiased measures of association (21). Selection of controls is among the most difficult, and most heavily criticized, aspect of case-control studies; indeed, it has been suggested that the ideal control group probably does not exist (22).

A third requirement for a bias-free case-control study is that collection of risk factor and exposure information should be the same for cases and controls. This can be difficult to ensure, especially for information collected in the course of clinical care, since invasive diagnostic approaches to rule out disease cannot be justified in healthy controls. Data collection methods should thus be developed that can be applied equally to both groups. Even this approach, however, cannot control for potential recall bias among the cases, which can substantially influence estimation of self-reported environmental exposures. This occurs when disease status influences the reporting of exposures, for example, when questions about exposure to a putative cause may be asked many times of known cases (or they may repeatedly search their memories) but only once of those without disease.

The presence of any of these forms of bias can severely affect the validity and generalizability of any observational study of disease etiology. Although concerns about recall bias tend to be dismissed in genetic studies because determination of the key exposure (a genetic variant) does not rely on recall, and the temporal nature of the genetic association is also clear, the potential for bias remains in selection of cases and controls and in assessment of other exposures that may act to modify any genotype-phenotype associations found. Limiting the collection of risk factor or biomarker information to the period prior to disease onset, if time of onset can be clearly defined, will reduce biases in risk factor ascertainment related to clinical care or awareness of disease status. Such use of premorbid risk factor information will also strengthen inferences regarding the temporal nature of risk relationships, a key element in determining causality. Unless extensive records exist prior to disease diagnosis, however, many key exposures such as dietary patterns or medication use cannot be collected retrospectively and premorbid risk factor information is often not available.

Another requirement for a valid case-control study, particularly in the genomic era, is that ancestral geographic origins and predominant environmental exposures of cases not differ dramatically from those of controls. Fortunately, the collection of ancestry informative markers and potential environmental confounders permits adjustment for differences in genetic background and environmental exposures, as long as there is some commonality between cases and controls. These adjustments must be applied carefully, however, to avoid overadjusting for variants or exposures that may actually be causal (15).

Finally, case-control studies typically permit investigation of only one primary outcome, the condition by which cases are defined. Since complex diseases rarely occur in isolation, and often share risk factors, the ability to examine genetic and environmental risk factors for a number of conditions once costly genomic assays have been performed is a major advantage of cohort studies that measure many outcomes in the same study subjects. Both study designs, however, often include measures of continuous traits such as height, lipids, or blood pressure that can then be used in secondary or combined analyses with other studies. Particularly successful examples of this approach in GWAS include the identification of the *FTO* variant related to obesity in what was initially a diabetes case-control study (23) and of 20 loci related to height in a combined analysis of cohort and case-control studies focused on a variety of diseases (24).

The case-control design also carries more assumptions, as detailed above, than the cohort design (Table 6.4). If these are not met, spurious associations and faulty

Table 6.4 Study designs used in genome-wide association studies

Design	Assumptions	Advantages	Disadvantages
Case-control	Cases and controls are drawn from the same population	Short time frame	Prone to a number of biases, including population stratification
	Cases are representative of all cases of the disease, or limitations on diagnostic specificity and representativeness are clearly specified	Large numbers of cases and controls can be assembled	Cases are usually prevalent cases, may miss fatal or short episodes, or mild or silent cases
	Genomic and epidemiologic data are collected similarly in cases and controls	Optimal epidemiologic design for studying rare diseases	Overestimate relative risk for common diseases
	Differences in allele frequencies relate to the outcome of interest rather than differences in background population between cases and controls		
Cohort	Subjects under study are more representative of the population from which they are drawn	Cases are incident (developing during observation) and free of survival bias	Large sample size needed for genotyping if incidence is low
	Diseases and traits are ascertained similarly in persons with and without the gene variant	Direct measure of risk	Expensive and lengthy follow-up
		Fewer biases than case-control studies	Existing consent may be insufficient for GWA genotyping or data sharing
		Continuum of health-related measures available in population samples not selected for presence of disease	Requires variation in trait being studied
			Poorly suited for studying rare diseases

Source: Adapted from Reference 21.

inferences may result. If well-established principles of epidemiologic design are adhered to, however, case-control studies can produce valid results that, especially for rare diseases, may not be obtainable in any other way. Unfortunately, genetic association studies using case-control methodologies have often not adhered to these principles. The often sharply abbreviated descriptions of cases and controls and lack of comparison of key characteristics in GWA reports can make evaluation of potential biases and replication of findings quite difficult (15,25).

Cohort Studies in the Era of Genome-wide Association

Fewer GWAS have utilized the cohort design, for many of the reasons of cost and efficiency noted above, but there are notable exceptions. The National Heart, Lung, and Blood Institute (NHLBI) has supported genome-wide genotyping of 500,000 SNPs in three generations of participants in the landmark Framingham Heart Study, and has made these data available through a controlled access process managed by the National Institutes of Health (http://www.ncbi.nlm.nih.gov/sites/entrez?db=gap). The richness of such a research resource is demonstrated by an earlier scan of 100,000 SNPs in the first two Framingham generations, which resulted in a burst of 17 concurrent publications reporting initial genome-wide associations with a vast array of conditions and traits (26). Genome-wide genotyping has also been applied to 25,000 women participating in the Women's Genome Health Study (27), and will be added to several other NHLBI cohorts in the near future. Notable GWAS that have utilized prospective cohort designs include breast and prostate cancer studies from the National Cancer Institute's Cancer Genetic Markers of Susceptibility (CGEMS) project (28,29). Additional studies of pancreatic, lung, and bladder cancer are also underway in this program.

Cohort studies involve collecting extensive baseline information in a large number of persons who are then followed to assess the incidence of disease in subgroups defined by genetic variants. Although cohort studies are typically more expensive and take longer to conduct than case-control studies, they often include subjects who are more representative of the population from which they are drawn than are clinical series. They also typically include a vast array of health-related characteristics and exposures for which genetic associations can be sought.

A major advantage of the prospective cohort design is that it permits standardized and detailed collection of premorbid exposure information tailored to meet the goals of the study. Assessment of environmental risk factors, and thus of potential gene–environment interactions, is typically more extensive and less prone to bias in prospective cohort studies than in case-control studies, making the former much more suitable for studying environmental influences on disease risk. Recall bias in particular is avoided by collecting information prior to disease onset.

Another key aspect of the prospective cohort design is that all participants are followed in a systematic way so that all cases of disease have an equal likelihood of being detected. This feature is important as it minimizes biases in case identification—particularly prevalence-incidence bias—that are typically encountered in clinical series. Time of disease onset can also be defined more clearly in prospective cohort studies than in case-control studies, and multiple disease outcomes can be studied.

Requirements for a generalizable prospective cohort study are that people recruited into the cohort have similar genetic and environmental exposures and disease risk to those who are not recruited, and that cohort members who are "lost" to follow-up have similar exposures and disease risk to those remaining. A third requirement is that likelihood of detection of disease is independent of the exposure of interest and of potential confounding factors such as age, access to medical care, and other exposures. This ensures similarity of data collection (and avoidance of bias) between exposed and unexposed persons. Although at present there is little concern that a participant's genetic make-up might directly influence the intensity or outcome of clinical diagnosis or treatment efforts, this may change as findings from GWAS become incorporated into clinical screening and diagnostic algorithms.

Ascertainment methods and outcome definitions should be the same in all cohort members and should not differ in relation to genetic or environmental exposures. Changes in exposure history should be assessed by repeated collection of exposure information and analyzed by appropriate longitudinal statistical techniques. Cohort studies that rely on outcomes identified in the course of clinical care are prone to many of the biases discussed above for case-control studies, so most prospective cohort studies implement a regular schedule of follow-up in which all participants are systematically investigated for occurrence of disease and changes in exposure. The need for such ongoing follow-up has been one of the major criticisms of prospective cohort studies, as it is time intensive and costly.

Other important limitations of the prospective cohort design include the large sample size needed to produce sufficient numbers of incident disease cases, and the typically long duration needed for these cases to accrue. In addition, the need to identify and collect information on risk factors of interest before disease cases have accrued adds to complexity and cost, but is often the only way to obtain valid, unbiased exposure information for prediction of disease.

The Problem of False Positive Findings

Analysis of GWA data is relatively straightforward, typically comparing the frequency of each allele or biallelic genotype in persons with and without disease. Complexity in analysis emerges due to the multiple testing carried out in GWAS, in that these same association tests are repeated for each of the 100,000 to over 1 million SNPs assayed. At the usual $p < 0.05$ level of significance, an association study of 1 million SNPs will show 50,000 SNPs to be "associated" with disease, almost all falsely positive and due to chance alone. The most common manner of dealing with this problem is to reduce the false positive rate by applying the Bonferroni correction, in which the conventional p-value is divided by the number of tests performed (21). A 1 million SNP survey would thus use a threshold of $p < 0.05/10^6$, or 5×10^{-8}, to identify associations unlikely to have occurred by chance. This correction has been criticized as overly conservative because it assumes independent associations of each SNP with disease while they are known to be correlated to some degree due to linkage disequilibrium (LD), or the tendency of SNPs located near each other on a chromosome to be inherited together. Other approaches have been proposed, including estimation of the false discovery rate, or proportion of significant associations that are actually false positives; false positive report probability, or probability that the null hypothesis is true given a statistically significant finding; and estimation of Bayes factors that incorporate the prior probability of association based on characteristics of the disease or the specific SNP (21). The Bonferroni correction has been the most commonly employed correction for multiple comparisons in GWA reports to date (1).

The threat of false positives has been widely recognized in the candidate gene literature—indeed, it may seem that nearly as much has been written about failure to replicate candidate gene associations as about the initial associations themselves (30). Potential reasons for failure to replicate are legion but include differences between study populations in the allele frequency of interest, in genetic background or environmental exposures, or in the host of potential biases that can afflict both case-control and cohort studies as described above. Many initial reports, especially in small studies prone to sampling bias, may simply have been spurious (i.e., due to chance alone). A comprehensive review of 600 candidate genes associated with common diseases reported that only six of those studied three or more times had been consistently replicated (31); similar comprehensive reviews have produced similar outcomes, and have generated a lively debate on what constitutes sufficient evidence for association.

This debate was largely resolved in a consensus development meeting conducted by the National Cancer Institute and the National Human Genome Research Institute, which produced a series of recommendations on what constitutes replication in GWAS (25). Key criteria for replication include study of the same or very similar phenotype and population, demonstration of a similar magnitude of effect and significance, in the same genetic model and same direction, for the same SNP and the same allele, as the initial report. Once replication became accepted as the *sine qua non* for reporting genetic associations (32), lack of reproducibility of genetic associations dropped sharply. Lack of replication may be varyingly attributed to differences in ancestral background between cases and controls or differences in phenotype definition, as well as selection biases, genotyping errors, and so on. At present, the best way of resolving these inconsistencies appears to be additional replication studies with ever larger sample sizes, though this may not be feasible for rare conditions or for associations identified in unique populations.

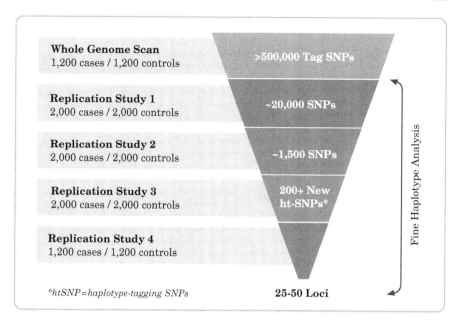

Figure 6.2 Replication strategy for a genome-wide analysis study of prostate cancer.
Source: *Reprinted from http://cgems.cancer.gov.*

Many GWAS use multistage designs to reduce the number of false positives while minimizing the number of costly genome-wide scans performed and retaining statistical power. Genome-wide scans are typically performed on an initial group of cases and controls and then a smaller number of associated SNPs is replicated in a second or third group of cases and controls of varying sizes (Figure 6.2). Some studies start with small numbers of subjects in the initial scan but carry forward large numbers of SNPs to minimize false negatives, while others start with more subjects but carry forward a smaller proportion of associated SNPs. Optimal proportions of subjects and SNPs in each phase have yet to be determined, but carrying forward a small proportion (<5%) of stage 1 SNPs will often mean limiting the associations ultimately identified to those of relatively large effect (21).

Importance of Genotyping Quality Control and Population Stratification

Genotyping errors, especially if occurring differentially between cases and controls, are an important cause of spurious associations and must be carefully sought and corrected. A number of quality control assessments should be applied both on a per-sample and a per-SNP basis. Checks on sample identity to avoid sample mix-ups should be described, and a minimum rate of successfully genotyped

SNPs per sample (usually 80–90% of SNPs attempted) should be reported. Once samples failing these thresholds are removed, individual SNPs across the remaining samples are subjected to further checks or "filters" for probable genotyping errors, including (i) the proportion of samples for which a SNP can be measured (the SNP call rate, typically >95%); (ii) the minor allele frequency (often >1%), as rarer SNPs are difficult to measure reliably; (iii) severe violations of Hardy-Weinberg equilibrium (often $p < 10^{-4}$); (iv) Mendelian inheritance errors in family studies; and (v) concordance rates in duplicate samples (typically >99.5%). Additional checks on genotyping quality should include careful visual inspection of genotype "cluster plots," or intensity values generated by the genotyping assay to ensure that the strongest associations do not merely reflect genotyping artifact (20,25). Genotype assignments of the most strongly associated SNPs should also be confirmed using a different method. Associations with any known "positive controls," such as the repeatedly replicated association of *TCF7L2* with type 2 diabetes (25), should be reported to increase confidence in the consistency of findings with prior reports.

Assessment of genotyping quality may be particularly important in case-control studies where case and control samples are collected or handled differently (33). This may be more of a problem with samples from disease cases, which may have been collected over an extended period of case accrual or in varied circumstances, or which have very small amounts of DNA requiring whole genome amplification prior to genotyping. Differences in DNA or genotype quality between cases and controls can be often quantified and adjusted for, or assignment of genotypes ("genotype calling") may need to be performed separately in cases and controls. Such differences must be systematically assessed, however, if they are to be identified and controlled for, and this step is easily overlooked.

Confounding due to "population stratification" has been cited as a major threat to the validity of genetic association studies, but its true importance is a matter of debate (34). It arises from variations in allele frequency between population subgroups, such as those defined by ethnicity or geographic origin, who in turn differ in their risk for disease. GWAS may then falsely identify the subgroup-associated genes as related to disease. Population stratification should be assessed and reported in GWAS, typically by examining the distribution of test statistics generated from the thousands of association tests performed (as by, for example, the chi-squared test) and assessing their deviation from the distribution expected under the null hypothesis of no SNP associated with the trait. Deviations from the null distribution suggest that either the assumed distribution is incorrect, or that the sample contains values arising in some other manner, as by a true association (25). Since the underlying assumption in GWAS is that the vast majority of assayed SNPs are not associated with the trait, strong deviations from the null may suggest important differences in population genetic structure. Several effective statistical methods are now available to correct for population stratification and are a standard component of rigorous GWA analyses (20).

Limitations of GWAS

Identification of a robustly replicating SNP-disease association is a crucial first step in identifying disease-causing genetic variants and developing suitable treatments, but it is only a first step (21). Association studies essentially identify a genomic location related to disease but provide little information on gene function, unless one has happened to identify a SNP with a predictable effect on gene expression or the transcribed product. Examination of known SNPs in high LD with the associated SNP may identify variants with plausible biologic effects, or sequencing of a suitable surrounding interval may be undertaken to identify rarer variants with more obvious functional implications. Tissue samples or cell lines can be examined for expression of the gene variant. Other functional studies may include genetic manipulations in cell or animal models, such as knockouts or knockins (35).

The potential for false positive results, lack of information on gene function, insensitivity to rare variants and structural variants, large sample sizes needed, and possible biases due to case and control selection and genotyping errors are important limitations of GWAS that have been detailed above. The often limited information available on environmental exposures and other nongenetic risk factors in early GWAS will make it difficult to assess gene–environment interactions.

Many of the design and analysis features of GWAS deal with minimizing the false positive rates while maintaining power to identify true positive associations. These same efforts to reduce false positives, however, may result in overlooking a true association, especially if only a small number of SNPs is carried over from the initial scan into replication studies. It is important to note that the most robust findings, those that "survive" multiple rounds of replication, are often not the most statistically significant associations in the initial scan, and may not even be in the top few hundred or few thousand associations. For example, the microseminoprotein-beta (*MSMB*) gene variant identified as the strongest association ($p < 7 \times 10^{-13}$) with prostate cancer in a combined stage 1 plus stage 2 study of 5,000 cases and 5,000 controls, was ranked 24,233th of 527,869 SNPs in the stage 1 scan (29). Had the investigators not carried forward the top 5% of associated SNPs into their second stage, this very plausible candidate gene, which produces a primary constituent of semen and is a proposed prostate cancer biomarker, would have been missed. Another cause of false negative results is the lack of the genetic variant of relevance on the genotyping platform, or lack of variation in that SNP in the population under study. As the number of SNPs and diversity of populations represented on genotyping platforms increase, this should become less of a problem.

An important question generated by these early GWAS relates to the small proportion of heritability, or familial clustering, explained by the genetic variants identified to date, as noted in Table 6.1. Debate continues as to whether the rest of the genetic influence might reside in a long "tail" of common SNPs with very small odds ratios, or in structural variants poorly assayed by current platforms, or in rarer variants of larger effect, or in interactions among common variants or with the environment. It is also possible that familial clustering due to genetic factors has been overestimated, and that important but overlooked or poorly measured environmental influences shared among family members may account for more familial clustering than previously appreciated. This remains to be determined, but it is important to keep in mind that even small odds ratios or rare variants can point the way toward valuable therapeutic strategies, such as the development of HMG-CoA reductase inhibitors arising from identification of LDL-receptor mutations in familial hypercholesterolemia (1).

Emerging Role of Population-based Studies in the GWA Era

The flood of GWA findings from case-control and cohort studies has led to follow-up replication, fine-mapping, sequencing, and functional studies in experimental systems to determine the biologic mechanisms of the associations, but much remains to be learned from well-characterized human population samples in which potentially causative variants have been, or could be, assayed. Important clues to gene function can be identified by examining associations with related or intermediate phenotypes such as hormone levels or bone density. More importantly, the potential population impact of variants of interest may be poorly described by the often highly selected or otherwise nonrepresentative group of cases in whom they were initially identified. Just as geneticists explore the "genetic architecture" of complex traits, defining the number and type of alleles associated with a trait and the mechanisms of their effects, so epidemiologists can explore the "epidemiologic architecture" of putative causal variants identified in GWAS—their population prevalence; prevalence in race/ethnic subgroups; relative risk of rigorously defined, incident disease; consistency of association across subgroups defined by age, sex, race/ethnicity, or exposures; and potential modifiability of associated risk. Such information is critical to determining the health implications of a given variant and the priority it should receive for identifying and testing interventions to reduce its associated risk. This information may also be quite valuable in exploring gene function, since the epidemiologic approach of genetic investigation, starting from observed phenotypic characteristics and moving more proximally to gene pathways and sequence variants, complements well the laboratory approach of moving from DNA sequence to function to phenotype.

More importantly, defining the risk associated with a specific genotype is essentially an epidemiologic problem, similar to characterizing any other risk factor, and requiring a detailed understanding of bias, confounding, and interaction. Such investigations may best be undertaken by experienced epidemiologists using data from the large-scale, prospective, population-based studies they have designed and carried out, because of the complexity of these datasets and the potential biases involved in exposure assessment and follow-up. Clinical trials, particularly primary prevention trials, may provide similarly representative and well-characterized population samples, with the added value of randomized interventions that may suggest potential avenues for modifying genotype-phenotype associations.

Population-based studies thus have a key role to play in the genomic era, in which addition of genome-wide genotyping often represents a comparatively small additional investment to the painstaking identification, recruitment, examination, and follow-up efforts already devoted to these cohorts. Case-control and cohort studies are both critical to genomic discovery, with case-control studies being especially useful for rare diseases and cohort studies for unbiased assessment of nongenetic exposures. The need for very large sample sizes to detect genetic variants of small effect has promoted formation of large collaborative consortia, often involving tens of thousands of samples (8,23,24). Such collaborations also provide intriguing opportunities for targeted studies of risk factors (both genetic and environmental) of comparatively unusual phenotypes such as sudden coronary death at young age or subarachnoid hemorrhage that might not be possible in any single cohort alone. Widespread data sharing, as through databases such as the Database of Genotype and Phenotype (dbGaP) of the National Center for Biotechnology Information (36), will facilitate the availability and responsible use of these valuable research resources. The value of population-based studies for finding initial associations, and for characterizing their importance on a population basis and among key subgroups, should not be underestimated. The best is yet to come for these studies as they embrace the genomic era.

References

1. Manolio TA, Brooks LD, Collins FS. A HapMap harvest of insights into the genetics of common disease. *J Clin Invest.* 2008;118:1590–1625.
2. Hunter DJ, Kraft P. Drinking from the fire hose—statistical issues in genome wide association studies. *N Engl J Med.* 2007;357:436–439.
3. Carlson CS. Agnosticism and equity in genome-wide association studies. *Nat Genet.* 2006;38:605–606.
4. Hindorff LA, Junkins HA, Manolio TA. A Catalog of Published Genome-Wide Association Studies. Available at: www.genome.gov/26525384. Accessed August 9, 2008.
5. Klein RJ, Zeiss C, Chew EY, et al. Complement factor H polymorphism in age-related macular degeneration. *Science.* 2005;308:385–389.
6. Rioux JD, Xavier RJ, Taylor KD, et al. Genome-wide association study identifies new susceptibility loci for Crohn's disease and implicates autophagy in disease pathogenesis. *Nat Genet.* 2007;39:596–604.
7. Amos CI, Wu X, Broderick P, et al. Genome-wide association scan of tag SNPs identifies a susceptibility locus for lung cancer at 15q25.1. *Nat Genet.* 2008;40:616–622.
8. Easton DF, Pooley KA, Dunning AM, et al. Genome-wide association study identifies novel breast cancer susceptibility loci. *Nature.* 2007;447:1087–1093.
9. Barrett JC, Hansoul S, Nicolae DL, et al. Genome-wide association defines more than 30 distinct susceptibility loci for Crohn's disease. *Nat Genet.* 2008;40:955–962.

10. Lango H, The UK Type 2 Diabetes Genetics Consortium, Palmer CN, et al. Assessing the combined impact of 18 common genetic variants of modest effect sizes on type 2 diabetes risk. *Diabetes*. November 2008;57(11):3129–3135. Epub June 30, 2008.

11. International Consortium for Systemic Lupus Erythematosus Genetics (SLEGEN), Harley JB, Alarcón-Riquelme ME, et al. Genome-wide association scan in women with systemic lupus erythematosus identifies susceptibility variants in ITGAM, PXK, KIAA1542 and other loci. *Nat Genet*. 2008;40:204–210.

12. Chakravarti A, Little P. Nature, nurture, and human disease. *Nature*. 2003;421:412–414.

13. Ordovas JM, Corella D, Demissie S, et al. Dietary fat intake determines the effect of a common polymorphism in the hepatic lipase gene promoter on high-density lipoprotein metabolism: evidence of a strong dose effect in this gene-nutrient interaction in the Framingham Study. *Circulation*. 2002;106:2315–2321.

14. Collins FS. The case for a US prospective cohort study of genes and environment. *Nature*. 2004;429:475–477.

15. Manolio TA, Bailey-Wilson JE, Collins FS. Genes, environment and the value of prospective cohort studies. *Nat Rev Genet*. 2006;7:812–820.

16. Manolio T. Novel risk markers and clinical pratice. N Engl J Med. October 23, 2003;349(17):1587–1589.

17. Schlesselman JJ. *Case-Control Studies: Design, Conduct, and Analysis*. New York: Oxford University Press; 1982.

18. Sackett DL. Bias in analytic research. *J Chron Dis*. 1979;32:51–63.

19. Wang SS, Fridinger F, Sheedy KM, et al. Public attitudes regarding the donation and storage of blood specimens for genetic research. *Community Genet*. 2001;4:18–26.

20. Wellcome Trust Case Control Consortium. Genome-wide association study of 14,000 cases of seven common diseases and 3,000 shared controls. *Nature*. 2007;447:661–678.

21. Pearson TA, Manolio TA. How to interpret a genome-wide association study. *JAMA*. 2008;299:1335–1344.

22. Wacholder S, Silverman DT, McLaughlin JK, et al. Selection of controls in case-control studies. III. Design options. *Am J Epidemiol*. 1992;135:1042–1050.

23. Frayling TM, Timpson NJ, Weedon MN, et al. A common variant in the FTO gene is associated with body mass index and predisposes to childhood and adult obesity. *Science*. May 11, 2007;316(5826):889–894.

24. Weedon MN, Lango H, Lindgren CM, et al. Genome-wide association analysis identifies 20 loci that influence adult height. *Nat Genet*. May 2008;40(5):575–583.

25. Chanock SJ, Manolio T, Boehnke M, et al. Replicating genotype-phenotype associations. *Nature*. 2007;447(7145):655–660.

26. Cupples LA, Arruda HT, Benjamin EJ, et al. The Framingham Heart Study 100K SNP genome-wide association study resources: overview of 17 phenotype working group reports. *BMC Med Genet*. 2007;8(Suppl 1):S1.

27. Ridker PM, Chasman DI, Zee RY, et al. Rationale, design, and methodology of the Women's Genome Health Study: A genome-wide association study of more than 25,000 initially healthy American women. *Clin Chem*. February 2008;54(2):249–255.

28. Hunter DJ, Kraft P, Jacobs KB, et al. A genome-wide association study identifies alleles in FGFR2 associated with risk of sporadic postmenopausal breast cancer. *Nat Genet*. July 2007;39(7):870–874.

29. Thomas G, Jacobs KB, Yeager M, et al. Multiple loci identified in a genome-wide association study of prostate cancer. *Nat Genet*. March 2008;40(3):310–315.

30. Hattersley AT, McCarthy MI. What makes a good genetic association study? *Lancet*. October 8, 2005;366(9493):1315–1323.

31. Hirschhorn JN, Lohmueller K, Byrne E, et al. A comprehensive review of genetic association studies. *Genet Med.* March-April 2002;4(2):45–61.

32. Todd JA. Statistical false positive or true disease pathway? *Nat Genet.* 2006;38(7):731–733.

33. Clayton DG, Walker NM, Smyth DJ, et al. Population structure, differential bias and genomic control in a large-scale, case-control association study. *Nat Genet.* November 2005;37(11):1243–1246.

34. Wacholder S, Rothman, N, Caporaso N. Counterpoint: bias from population stratification is not a major threat to the validity of conclusions from epidemiological studies of common polymorphisms and cancer. *Cancer Epidemiol Biomarkers Prev.* 2002;11:513–520.

35. Frayling TM, McCarthy MI. Genetic studies of diabetes following the advent of the genome-wide association study: where do we go from here? *Diabetologia.* 2007;50:2229–2233.

36. Mailman MD, Feolo M, Jin Y, et al. The NCBI dbGaP database of genotypes and phenotypes. *Nat Genet.* 2007;39:1181–1186.

7

The emergence of networks in human genome epidemiology: challenges and opportunities

Daniela Seminara, Muin J. Khoury, Thomas R. O'Brien,
Teri Manolio, Marta Gwinn, Julian Little,
Julian P. T. Higgins, Jonine L. Bernstein, Paolo Boffetta,
Melissa L. Bondy, Molly S. Bray, Paul E. Brenchley,
Patricia A. Buffler, Juan Pablo Casas,
Anand P. Chokkalingam, John Danesh, George Davey Smith,
Siobhan M. Dolan, Ross Duncan, Nelleke A. Gruis,
Mia Hashibe, David J. Hunter, Marjo-Riitta Jarvelin,
Beatrice Malmer, Demetrius M. Maraganore,
Julia A. Newton-Bishop, Elio Riboli, Georgia Salanti,
Emanuela Taioli, Nic Timpson, André G. Uitterlinden,
Paolo Vineis, Nick Wareham, Deborah M. Winn,
Ron Zimmern, and John P. A. Ioannidis

Introduction

Large-scale "big science" is advocated as an approach to complex research problems in many scientific areas (1). Epidemiologists have long recognized the value of large collaborative studies to address important questions that are beyond the scope of a study conducted at a single institution (2). We define networks (or, interchangeably, consortia) as groups of scientists from multiple institutions who cooperate in research efforts involving, but not limited to, the conduct, analysis, and synthesis of information from multiple population studies. Networks, by virtue of their greater scope, resources, population size, and opportunities for interdisciplinary collaboration, can address complex scientific questions that a single team alone cannot (3).

There is a strong rationale for using networks in human genome epidemiology particularly. Genetic epidemiology benefits from a large-scale population-based approach to identify genes underlying complex common diseases, to assess associations between genetic variants and disease susceptibility, and to examine potential gene–environment interactions (4–6). Because the epidemiologic risk for an

Reprinted with permission from *Epidemiology.* 2007 Jan;18(1):1–8.

individual genetic variant is likely to be small, a large sample size is needed for adequate statistical power (7). Power issues are even more pressing for less common disease outcomes. Replication in different populations and exposure settings is also required to confirm and validate results. The adoption of common guidelines for the conduct, analysis, reporting, and integration of studies across different teams is essential for credible replication. Transparency in acknowledging and incorporating both "positive" and "negative" results is necessary to direct subsequent research. Furthermore, newer and more efficient genotyping technologies must be integrated rapidly into current and planned population studies (8,9). Networks can support studies with sample sizes large enough to achieve "definitive" results, promote spin-off research projects, and yield faster "translation" of results into clinical and public health applications. Networks can also foster interdisciplinary and international collaboration (10). Lastly, networks can assemble databases that are useful for developing and applying new statistical methods for large data sets (11).

The experience of established networks provides an important knowledge base on which to develop recommendations for improving future efforts (12). The Human Genome Epidemiology Network (HuGENet) recently launched a global network of consortia working on human genome epidemiology (13). This Network of Investigator Networks aims to create a resource to share information, to offer methodologic support, to generate inclusive overviews of studies conducted in specific fields, and to facilitate rapid confirmation of findings. In October 2005, HuGENet brought together representatives from established and emerging networks to share their experiences at a workshop in Cambridge, United Kingdom (14). In advance of the meeting, a qualitative questionnaire was distributed to workshop participants. The questionnaire elicited information on experiences and practices in building and maintaining consortia. This chapter reports on the numerous challenges and their possible solutions as identified by the workshop participants (summarized in Table 7.1) as well as new opportunities offered by the network approach to genetic and genomic epidemiology.

Scientific Approach

Selection of Scientific Questions

To date, most networks have targeted projects originating from preliminary evidence of specific associations or for the purpose of genetic linkage. In most consortia, projects are selected through group discussion and informal or semiformal (e.g., voting) prioritization of candidate gene targets. Most networks try to focus on the best possible candidates to generate definitive evidence, but, given the large proportion of false positives in genetic epidemiology (15), there is considerable uncertainty about the criteria for selecting such targets. Possible criteria include the number and consistency of published reports for a specific gene, the presence of a high-profile controversy in the literature, strong *a priori* biologic plausibility, potentially high population-attributable risk (e.g., a common polymorphism) supporting linkage evidence from genome-wide data, and candidates derived from genome-wide association screens (16,17).

Table 7.1 Challenges faced by networks of investigators in human genome epidemiology and possible solutions

Major Challenges	Possible Solutions
Resources for establishing the initial infrastructure, supporting consortia implementation, and adding new partners	New and more flexible funding mechanisms: planning grants, collaborative research grants Coordination among national and international funding agencies and foundations Appropriate evaluation criteria for continuation of funding
Coordination: minimize administration to maximize scientific progress and avoid conflicts	Clear leadership structure: steering committee and working groups Early development of policies and processes Cutting-edge communication technology
Selection of target projects	Questions that can be uniquely addressed by collaborative groups Preliminary supportive evidence High-profile controversial hypothesis Biologic plausibility Genomewide evidence
Variable data and biospecimen quality from participating teams	Eligibility criteria based on sample size Sound and appropriate study design Accurate phenotype outcome and genotype assessments State-of-the-art biospecimen repositories
Handling of information from nonparticipating teams and of negative results	Integration of evidence across all teams and networks in a field Comprehensive reporting to maintain transparency Curated updated encyclopedia of knowledge base
Collection, management, and analysis of complex and heterogeneous data sets	Central informatics unit or coordinating center "Think tank" for analytic challenges of retrospective and prospective data sets Centralization of genotyping Standardization or harmonization of phenotypic and genotypic data Standardization of quality control protocols across participating teams
Anticipating future needs	Rapid integration of evolving high throughput genomic technologies Consideration of centralized platforms Maximizing use of bioresources Public–private partnerships Development of analytic approaches for large and complex data sets
Communication and coordination	Web-based communication: web sites and portals Teleconferences and meeting support
Scientific credits and career development	Upfront definition of publication policies Mentorship of young investigators Change in tenure and authorship criteria

(Continued)

122

Table 7.1 Continued

Major Challenges	Possible Solutions
Access to the scientific community at large and transparency	Data-sharing plans and policies Support for release of public data sets Availability and dissemination of both "positive" and "negative" results Encyclopedia of knowledge
Peer review	Review criteria appropriate for interdisciplinary large science Education of peer scientists to consortia issues Inclusion of interdisciplinary expertise in initial review groups
Informed consent	Anticipation of data and biospecimen sharing requirements and careful phrasing of informed consent Sensitivity to local and national legislations

Networks are often focused on candidate genes involved in pathogenesis of the disease outcome or in biologic pathways involving environmental exposures such as metabolism of carcinogens (18). For example, the WECARE consortium on genetics of cancer and radiation exposure (19) has addressed individual genes that lie within pathways related to double-strand breaks caused by radiation damage. Consortia are increasingly used to replicate findings from hypothesis-free genome-wide approaches. For example, consortia are attempting to replicate findings from two-stage genome-wide association studies of Parkinson disease (20) and breast cancer (21). With decreasing genotyping cost and the expressed interest of funding agencies in genome-wide association studies (22), some consortia are coordinating large-scale genotyping and replication of whole genome association designs (23).

Prospective and Retrospective Components

Networks use information and biologic specimens from ongoing or established cohort and case-control studies with data on phenotypes. Phenotype information may have been accumulated either retrospectively or prospectively depending on the study design. Participating teams with prospective designs usually continue collecting phenotype information.

Regarding genotyping, several consortia perform meta-analyses of individual-level data using studies in which all genotyping has already been done and data have been published. Some consortia include additional genotyping from teams that have not yet done or published such genotyping; for other consortia, prospective genotyping represents the majority of the data. Increasingly, prospective genotyping is coordinated to test novel candidate gene variants or variants identified by genome-wide approaches.

Handling of Information from Nonparticipating Teams

Many networks do not encompass all teams working on the disease or subject matter of interest. For some common diseases (e.g., breast cancer), there are two or more organized multiteam consortia in addition to nonorganized teams (24–26). Some consortia attempt analyses that include outside data to examine the robustness of their findings. Integration of evidence across networks and across participating and nonparticipating teams remains a challenge in developing all-encompassing synopses of the evidence on specific gene–disease associations (27).

Launching a Network

Network Characteristics
Consortia in the Network of Investigator Networks comprise between 5 and 521 teams. Subject numbers range from 3,000 to over half a million. Elements deemed essential for launching a network are a strong scientific rationale, the agreement of all teams to work together and combine data on overarching research questions, and the ability to support initial communication, coordination, identification, and recruitment of partners. True integration of disciplines can be challenging because different disciplines are typically housed in discrete departments and have different scientific cultures. Interdisciplinary training is important for bridging these gaps.

Established networks have coalesced through different processes. Frequently, the initiation of a network includes the gathering of information on available resources from several groups of investigators actively involved in research in the same field. Dissemination of information on integrated research aims, resources, and possible contributors ultimately leads to the identification of specific projects to be pursued. This process creates a forum for scientific exchange and more targeted collaborations (28). Networks tend to expand their membership over time and loss of partner teams is uncommon (29,30).

Although network membership tends to be inclusive, there is concern that inclusion of flawed data jeopardizes the validity of the collaborative results. For this reason, some consortia have eligibility criteria based on appropriateness of study design and phenotypic accuracy.

Organization and Coordinating Centers

Networks use different models of steering and coordination. Working groups focused on specific topics are common within the largest networks. For example, the International Head and Neck Cancer Epidemiology (INHANCE) network (31) requires all members to participate in at least one of seven working groups that focus on scientific issues or projects such as age at cancer onset, nonsmokers and nondrinkers, tobacco and alcohol, genetics and DNA repair, human papilloma virus prognosis and survival, and occupational factors. The Genetics of Melanoma (GenoMEL) network (32) has a Steering Committee, a Scientific Advisory Board, a Patient Advocacy Group, and an Ethics Committee as well as several topic-specific working groups. Some networks have separate statistical, genetic, and clinical coordinating centers, whereas others centralize these functions. A primary coordinator or chair and a small steering group are usually essential for the network to operate efficiently. Sometimes it is difficult to trace in detail what happens at the local level of participating sites. Minimizing and streamlining administration to maximize the conduct of science is essential.

Funding

Funding sources include governmental and public health agencies as well as private foundations. Funding from for-profit companies and full partnership with industry-sponsored teams has been rare, although some consortia have partnered with private companies for specific projects. For example, the Colon Cancer Family Registry worked with specific companies to perform a systematic mutational analysis of the participants enrolled (33). Funding, especially for infrastructure, is a key limiting factor. Difficulties also exist occasionally for obtaining funding to support activities beyond the originally proposed specific projects despite demonstrated productivity of the network. Some consortia have a single source for primary funding (typically National Institutes of Health or European Commission grants), but most networks have diverse, sometime project-specific, sources of funding. For example, the Birth Cohorts Consortium had a total of 64 funders over the past 8 years. In some countries, participation in a consortium can constitute a strong leverage to obtain national funds.

Standardization Within the Network

Data Management
Efficient and accurate data management is very important because poor-quality data from one or more teams may undermine an otherwise excellent collaboration. Data typically flow to one coordinating center, but some consortia have multiple data coordinating centers with complementary functions.

Networks use various data quality assurance practices and checks for logical errors and inconsistencies. Networks that have invested heavily in quality assurance believe that the effort was worthwhile, because errors may occur even under the best circumstances (34). Logical errors (inconsistencies in the contributed data) are usually easy to identify and readily solved through communication with the team investigators. Examples include out-of-range values, inversion of coding of phenotypes, improper or inconsistent allele calling, and inconsistent cross-coding in databases. Logical errors may reveal deeper problems with contributed data. Queries regarding missing data may yield additional information with some additional effort from the team. Some consortia have instituted in-person training for collecting genotype and phenotype data in addition to ongoing quality control checks. Some networks have developed and published explicit policies of quality assurance for phenotype or genotype data (25).

Standardization or Harmonization of Phenotypes and Other Measurements

Data standardization is best implemented at the beginning of a *de novo* collaborative study, when tools for data collection and definition of data items are developed. Data standardization achieves agreement on common data definitions to which all data layers must conform. Each data item is given a common name, definition, and value set or format. When standardization is not possible (e.g., different questionnaires or criteria have been used historically by different teams), harmonization of data items is suggested—and sometimes required by the funding agencies. Data harmonization is useful when data sets are already collected from originally independent studies focusing on similar questions or field of inquiry. The harmonization process seeks to maximize the comparability of data from two or more information systems with the goal of reducing data redundancy and inconsistencies as well as improving the quality and format of data.

Standardization or harmonization is crucial for a network to perform better than single studies, and these processes increase the credibility of the derived evidence. Phenotypes and other nongenetic measurements may be difficult to standardize across teams. For example, Parkinson disease has several sets of accepted diagnostic criteria and teams may use different criteria that have high concordance. It is often challenging to reassess phenotype using alternative criteria. In some diseases, there may be no consensus regarding the most important phenotypes to study. For example, 21 pharmacogenetic studies in asthma analyzed 483 different end points (35).

Conversely, the assembled data of some networks have been used to define subphenotypes of disease that would not have been evident with lower statistical power (36). Networks may help achieve harmonization, even when single-team studies have been inconsistent in preferred definitions and outcomes. For example, in the HIV consortium, access to primary data allowed for harmonized definitions of seroconverter and seroprevalent subjects and for the outcome (clinical AIDS) (37), although these variables had been defined inconsistently by the teams. In contrast, the InterLymph consortium standardizes the diagnosis of lymphoma subtypes through a coordinated review of a subset of slides from each numbered study (38). One criterion of the importance and success of a network may be its ability to adopt standards for phenotypes and covariates to prevent the use of inconsistent definitions in subsequent studies.

In some networks, phenotypes are assessed in prospectively ascertained cases or through an extensive reexamination of phenotypes of existing cases. Consortia also use training sessions on phenotyping, photographs (e.g., for moles in melanoma family members), and central review to enhance consistency of data.

Standardization of Genotypes

Most networks have not performed central genotyping of all samples, but exceptions exist (31,39). Shipping specimens is sometimes challenging in collaborations among geographically dispersed teams and regulatory considerations may also prohibit centralized genotyping. For example, some teams are prohibited from shipping specimens by their protocol, local legislation, or their funding agency. Several networks use a semicentralized approach in which some teams ship their samples to a central laboratory, whereas others perform onsite genotyping.

Quality control of genotype results is usually straightforward, but additional checks are required in a multiteam collaboration. Some networks use published genotype data without quality checks beyond what each individual team implemented in their laboratory (e.g., repeat genotyping of a random sample of specimens). In the absence of centralized quality control, consortia must depend on *post hoc* analyses such as deviation from Hardy-Weinberg equilibrium proportions in the controls (40), to identify possible genotyping (or other) errors. Large between-study heterogeneity in the final analyses may also reflect measurement errors. However, sizeable errors may still be missed with these methods.

Several networks, including the Public Population Project in Genomics (P^3G), check genotype results through exchange of blinded samples between groups. Another approach is to ship samples of known (ideally sequence-verified) genotypes to all participating laboratories. Alternatively, a sample of specimens that were genotyped locally may be shipped to a central laboratory for confirmation. Experience suggests that the reliability of each laboratory should not be taken for granted. Serious errors have occurred (e.g., inverse reporting of genotype results that produces an inverse association) that could only be detected by rigorous quality control mechanisms. Error rates may be considerable even for single nucleotide polymorphisms (SNPs) and can depend on a laboratory's methodology and expertise. This is particularly relevant because most gene–disease associations have modest effect sizes that could be obscured by small laboratory errors.

Other Organizational Issues

Communication and Web Site Development

Networks use face-to-face meetings, e-mail, teleconferences, and password-protected web sites to communicate with an increasing preference for electronic communication (for details, see web sites cited in Reference 14). Web sites promote visibility and diffuse basic information on the network, activities, and products (e.g., publications). Portals provide password-protected access for more sensitive information, which is essential to communication within and between teams as well as venues for private scientific interaction with fellow members. Some networks have developed principally as registers of data from multiple groups and their data management is entirely web-based, such as the meta-analysis on DNA repair and cancer risk (41).

Publication and Authorship

Explicit review and publication policies are best established early in the life of a network to avoid later dissent. For each manuscript, a core writing team is essential for developing an initial draft and incorporating comments from coauthors. Most consortia use individual-name authorships, which result in a long list of authors. The first author is typically the leader of the specific project. Some networks use tiered authorship (authors and separate lists of additional contributors and separate acknowledgments). Group authorship may also be used, but errors in tracking publications in PubMed and the Science Citation Index may occur (42). Intellectual property rights may also be an issue in consortia. A carefully crafted agreement involving all partners should be formulated at the outset.

Authorship position and principal investigator status on funded grants are critical for promotion of junior investigators. In the long run, networks will likely produce fertile ground for career development by assuring expert interdisciplinary mentorship and providing opportunities for developing productive scientific collaborations, but in emerging consortia, more senior investigators tend to assume major responsibilities and receive the corresponding authorship credit and grant funding. Some consortia have developed explicit policies of ensuring opportunities for young investigators. Changes in funding mechanisms, tenure criteria, and publication credit are needed to support consortia as a tool for both the rapid advancement of scientific knowledge and the development of new independent investigators (43).

Access to Data and Nonselective Availability of Data

Network-developed data and resources should be accessible to the larger scientific community and networks should develop data-sharing policies that support this requirement. Standardization of data-sharing policies is needed and could be facilitated by regulations and policies formulated by funding agencies (44).

It is important that both "positive" and "negative" results be reported to avoid publication bias (45). By their very nature, networks may be the last line of defense against selective reporting and resulting publication biases and should strive to identify and include high-quality, but previously unpublished, data.

Peer Review Process

Interdisciplinary science requires interdisciplinary peer review. Education of peer scientists and establishment of initial review groups with appropriate interdisciplinary expertise are vital to evaluate accurately the merit of consortia proposals.

Interdisciplinary research teams take time to assemble and require unique resources (46–48). Targeted funding mechanisms may be needed, especially to build infrastructures for emerging consortia. Criteria for evaluation of productivity by funding agencies should take into account the planning and time to establish the necessary infrastructure.

Informed Consent

Networks need flexibility to address emerging scientific questions. Informed consent should allow data sharing and support broad areas of research conducted by multiple investigators at different institutions in different countries. Examples of elements to be included in such informed consent have been published and adopted by some existing consortia (49). However, the variable requirements of Institutional Review Boards at different institutions in considering the incorporation of these elements and the great heterogeneity of privacy legislation at the state, national, and international level may complicate data and biospecimen sharing in large consortia (50).

Other Challenges and Opportunities

The meeting participants identified a number of additional challenges. For example, inclusiveness criteria are challenging and should be balanced against proper quality assurance. Single teams should be free to pursue their research priorities, and their promising results may then be replicated by the consortium at large. All "negative" results should be fully recorded, preferably in an open access environment, to avoid wasted duplication of effort and confusion in the field. Plurality may also reflect the existence of multiple networks in the same field with similar or very different designs. Accurate registration of membership may mitigate overlap and maximize comparison and replication of results. Upfront study registration has been adopted for clinical trials: ClinicalTrials.gov accepts nonrandomized studies and already has 4,000 or more in its database. Central tracking of genome-wide association studies is being planned by the National Institutes of Health as a means to minimize publication and reporting biases, maximize transparency and data access rapidly advance research, and maximize funding allocation (22). Rapid and continuous integration of cutting-edge genomic and other technologies is a challenge. This may require the adoption of centralized technology platforms, which may be supported by public–private partnerships such as the GAIN initiative (46). Long-term planning should take into account the fact that laboratory techniques are rapidly becoming cheaper and easier to apply on a large-scale basis. The development, maintenance, and standardization across teams of high-quality biologic repositories (or "biobanks") are a further challenge. The ultimate goal is to maximize bioresources through various valid strategies such as immortalized cell lines, whole genome amplification, pooling, tissue microdissection, or multiplex microarrays as deemed appropriate.

Table 7.2 Potential for networks to contribute to research progress in human genome epidemiology

Improve the quality of primary studies
Improve the standards of clinical, laboratory, and statistical methods
Strengthen the quality of international collaborative studies, and thereby reduce language and publication biases (50)
Provide empirical evidence for developing the optimal criteria for grading the credibility of evidence for genetic association studies (51)
Facilitate testing of between-studies heterogeneity in both allele frequencies and size of genetic effects across participating groups studying different populations
Facilitate replication of complex associations involving entire loci or pathways in large-scale data sets
Support methodologic development

Many of the challenges facing networks, if properly addressed, may yield opportunities, as summarized in Table 7.2.

Conclusions

The HuGENet Network of Investigators Networks seeks to provide an open forum for communication and sharing of expertise in statistical and laboratory methods, policies, and procedures among consortia. Consortia are encouraged to create a core registry that would include basic information on their participating teams and on the characteristics of their studies and target populations. This wider knowledge base would improve efficiency in planning further studies and allow for faster replication of results needing validation. Another HuGENet Network of Investigator Networks effort aims at developing an online encyclopedia of genomic epidemiology, maintaining updated information on results from ongoing studies. Such "synopses" of evidence are underway for several diseases, experimenting with various formats that would be comprehensive and flexible enough to cover the needs of a rapidly developing field (52–54). Ultimately, if interdisciplinary "large science" human genome epidemiology is to succeed, academic institutions, funding agencies, and scientific journals must incorporate policies, processes, and rewards that support team science while respecting individual creativity. This will require a fundamental change, which is already afoot, from a research culture of "rugged individualism" to one of teamwork.

References

1. Large Scale Biomedical Science: Exploring Strategies for Future Research; Committee on Large Scale Science and Cancer Research. IOM Report; 2003.
2. Seminara D, Obrams GI. Genetic epidemiology of cancer: a multidisciplinary approach. *Genet Epidemiol.* 1994;11:235–254.
3. Relationship of blood pressure, serum cholesterol, smoking habit, relative weight and ECG abnormalities to incidence of major coronary events: final report of the pooling project. The Pooling Project Research Group. *J Chronic Dis.* 1978;4:201–306.

4. Kreeger K. Consortia "big science": part of a paradigm shift for genetic epidemiology. *J Natl Cancer Inst.* 2003;95:640–641.

5. Khoury MJ. The case for a global human genome epidemiology initiative. *Nat Genet.* 2004;36:1027–1028.

6. Collins FS. The case for a US prospective cohort study of genes and environment. *Nature.* 2004;429:475–477.

7. Ioannidis JPA, Trikalinos TA, Khoury MJ. Implications of small effect sizes of individual genetic variants on the design and interpretation of genetic association studies of complex diseases. *Am J Epidemiol.* October 1, 2006;164(7):609–614. Epub August 7, 2006.

8. Hirschhorn JN, Daly MJ. Genome-wide association studies for common diseases and complex traits. *Nat Rev Genet.* 2005;6:95–108.

9. Thomas DC, Haile RW, Duggan D. Recent developments in genome-wide association scans: a workshop summary and review. *Am J Hum Genet.* 2005;77:337–345.

10. Caporaso NE. Why have we failed to find the low penetrance genetic constituents of common cancers? *Cancer Epidemiol Biomarkers Prev.* 2002;11:1544–1549.

11. Timpson NJ, Lawlor DA, Harbord RM, et al. C-reactive protein and its role in metabolic syndrome: mendelian randomisation study. *Lancet.* 2005;366:1954–1959.

12. Rogers S, Dowling E, Valle C, et al. The Trends and Development in Consortia as a Tool for Genetic Research in Epidemiology. *Proceedings of AACR Frontiers in Cancer Prevention and Research*; 2005;C79.

13. Ioannidis JPA Bernstein J, Bofetta P, et al. A network of investigator networks in human genome epidemiology. *Am J Epidemiol.* 2005;162:302–304.

14. Human Genome Epidemiology web sites. Available at: http://www.dhe.med.uoi.gr/huge_sites.php and www.dhe.med.uoi.gr/hugenet.htm (Ioannina). Accessed July 10, 2006.

15. Wacholder S, Chanock S, Garcia-Closas M, et al. Assessing the probability that a positive report is false: an approach for molecular epidemiology studies. *J Natl Cancer Inst.* 2004;96:434–442.

16. Colhoun HM, McKeigue PM, Davey Smith G. Problems of reporting genetic associations with complex outcomes. *Lancet.* 2003;361:865–872.

17. Ioannidis JPA. Why most published research findings are false. *PLoS Med.* 2005;2:e124.

18. Taioli E. International collaborative study on genetic susceptibility to environmental carcinogens. *Cancer Epidemiol Biomarkers Prev.* 1999;8:727–728.

19. Bernstein JL, Teraoka S, Haile RW, et al. WECARE Study Collaborative Group Designing and implementing quality control for multi-center screening of mutations in the ATM gene among women with breast cancer. *Hum Mutat.* 2003;21:542–550.

20. Maraganore DM, de Andrade M, Lesnick TG, et al. High-resolution whole-genome association study of Parkinson disease. *Am J Hum Genet.* 2005;77:685–693.

21. Hunter DJ, Riboli E, Haiman CA, et al. National Cancer Institute Breast and Prostate Cancer Cohort Consortium. A candidate gene approach to searching for low-penetrance breast and prostate cancer genes. *Nat Rev Cancer.* 2005;5:977–985.

22. NIH Guide for Grants and Contracts web site. Available at: http://grants.nih.gov/grants/guide/notice-files/NOT-OD-06-071.html. Accessed June 30, 2006.

23. Thomas DC. Are we ready for genome-wide association studies? *Cancer Epidemiol Biomarkers Prev.* 2006;15:595–598.

24. Raimondi S, Pedotti P, Taioli E. APIKIDS: a cohort of children born after assisted reproductive technologies. *Paediat Perinatal Epidemiol.* September 2006;20(5):411–415.

25. John EM, Hopper JL, Beck JC, et al. The Breast Cancer Family Registry: an infrastructure for cooperative multinational, interdisciplinary and translational studies of the genetic epidemiology of breast cancer. *Breast Cancer Res.* 2004;6:R375–R389.

26. NCI web site. Available at www.cancer.gov/newscenter/pressreleases/cohortconsortium. Accessed June 30, 2006.
27. Ioannidis JP, Gwinn M, Little J, et al. A road map for efficient and reliable human genome epidemiology. *Nat Genet.* 2006;38:3–5.
28. NCI web site. Available at http://epi.grants.cancer.gov/initiatives.html. Accessed June 30, 2006.
29. GENOMOS web site. Available at http://www.genomos.eu/ Accessed May 19, 2009.
30. Uitterlinden AG, Ralston SH, Brandi ML, et al. Large-scale analysis of association between common vitamin D receptor gene variations and osteoporosis: the GENOMOS Study. *Ann Intern Med.* August 15, 2006;145(4):255–264.
31. IARC web site. Available at http://inhance.iarc.fr/. Accessed June 30, 2006.
32. GenoMEL web site. Available at http://www.genomel.org/. Accessed May 19, 2009.
33. CFR web site. Available at http://epi.grants.cancer.gov/CFR/. Accessed June 30, 2006.
34. Pompanon F, Bonin A, Bellemain E, et al. Genotyping errors: causes, consequences and solutions. *Nat Rev Genet.* 2005;6:847–859.
35. Contopoulos-Ioannidis DG, Alexiou GA, Gouvias TC, et al. An empirical evaluation of multifarious outcomes in pharmacogenetics: beta2 adrenoceptor gene polymorphisms in asthma treatment. *Pharmacogenet Genomics.* October 2006;16(10):705–711.
36. Lindor NM, Rabe K, Petersen GM, et al. Lower cancer incidence in Amsterdam-I criteria families without mismatch repair deficiency: familial colorectal cancer type X. *JAMA.* 2005;293:1979–1985.
37. Ioannidis JP, Rosenberg PS, Goedert JJ, et al. International Meta-Analysis of HIV Host Genetics. Effects of CCR5-Delta32, CCR2-64I, and SDF-1 3'A alleles on HIV-1 disease progression: an international meta-analysis of individual-patient data. *Ann Intern Med.* 2001;135:782–795.
38. Rothman N, Skibola CF, Wang SS, et al. Genetic variation in TNF and IL10 and risk of non-Hodgkin lymphoma: a report from the InterLymph Consortium. *Lancet Oncol.* 2006;7:27.
39. Andrulis IL, Anton-Culver H, Beck J, et al. Cooperative Family Registry for Breast Cancer studies. Comparison of DNA- and RNA-based methods for detection of truncating BRCA1 mutations. *Hum Mutat.* 2002;20:65–73.
40. Yonan AL, Palmer AA, Gilliam TC. Hardy-Weinberg disequilibrium identified genotyping error of the serotonin transporter (SLC6A4) promoter polymorphism. *Psychiatr Genet.* 2006;16:31–34.
41. EpiSAT Project web site: DNA Repair. http://www.episat.org/episat/huge/
42. Dickersin K, Scherer R, Suci ES, et al. Problems with indexing and citation of articles with group authorship. *JAMA.* 2002;287:2772–2774.
43. NIH multi-P.I. initiative. Available at http://grants.nih.gov/grants/multi_pi/. Accessed June 27, 2006.
44. National Institutes for Health. Data Sharing Policy web site, p 17. Available at http://grants2.nih.gov/grants/policy/data_sharing/. Accessed June 10, 2006.
45. Ioannidis JP. Journals should publish all "null" results and should sparingly publish "positive" results. *Cancer Epidemiol Biomarkers Prev.* 2006;15:186.
46. GAIN initiative. Available at http://www.genome.gov/19518664. Accessed May 19, 2009.
47. NIH Roadmap interdisciplinary consortia link, p 18. Available at http://grants2.nih.gov/grants/guide/notice-files/NOT-RM-05-006.html. Accessed June 27, 2006.
48. European Community Framework. Available at http://cordis.europa.eu/fp7/. Accessed May 28, 2009.
49. Daly MB, Offit K, Li F, et al. Participation in the cooperative family registry for breast cancer studies: issues of informed consent. *J Natl Cancer Inst.* 2000;92:452–456.

50. Betancourt D, Dowling E, Seminara D, International Consortium on Prostate Cancer Genetics. Data sharing and informed consent in genetic epidemiology consortia. Poster presentation, 9th International Meeting on the Psychosocial Aspects of Genetic Testing for Hereditary Cancer, 2005:19.
51. Pan Z, Trikalinos TA, Kavvoura FK, et al. Local literature bias in genetic epidemiology: an empirical evaluation of the Chinese literature. *PLoS Med.* 2005;2:e334.
52. Ioannidis JP. Grading the credibility of molecular evidence for complex diseases. *Int J Epidemiol.* 2006;35:572–828.
53. De Angelis C, Drazen JM, Frizelle FA, et al. Clinical trial registration: a statement from the International Committee of Medical Journal Editors. *N Engl J Med.* 2004;351:1250–1251.
54. Embracing risk. *Nat Genet.* 2006;38:1.

Addendum

John P. A. Ioannidis and Daniela Seminara

In the 2 years since the Epidemiology article on "The Emergence of Networks in Human Genome Epidemiology: Challenges and Opportunities" was published, the contribution of consortia and networks to research in human genome epidemiology has become essential. In particular, the key role of consortia has become evident in the confirmation and validation of primary genome-wide association studies (GWAS) of common diseases and in the performance of the interdisciplinary research needed to begin translating GWAS results into clinical and public health applications (1). A few successful examples of this interactive approach are the Welcome Trust Case-Control Consortium, the Cancer Cohorts Consortium (CoCo), and the Genetic Association Information Network (GAIN), whose successful paradigm has been emulated in many subsequent studies (2–4). With the advent of GWAS, it has become obvious that the successful replication of emerging association signals needs very large sample sizes. Genetic effects for discovered common variants have turned up to be even smaller than previously thought and power to replicate such associations is very limited, even with very large studies (5,6). Few GWAS have hit genome-wide significance in new discovered associations immediately at the Stage 1 data (7). Consensus recommendations have pointed to the need for sizeable replication studies in similar or ethnically and geographically different populations to confirm the validity of emerging associations between SNPs and disease. Further, a number of weaker associations or associations with rarer variants may still lie below the detection threshold of initial studies due to simple power considerations (8). This has led to new, larger collaborative efforts, where data from many GWAS and/or many replication studies are merged together for extensive meta-analyses, as for example in type 2 diabetes (DIAGRAM initiative) and colon cancer (9,10). It is, therefore, fortunate that, for some common diseases, genomic data originated from more than one consortium may be available. This shows the popularity of the concept and it may stimulate healthy competition and joint scientific efforts, whenever appropriate. Given that several consortia may develop databases independently, there is a need for some synopsis of the accumulated information, as discussed in Chapter 12. Furthermore, a worldwide collaborative consortia approach will be essential in incorporating the wealth of GWAS data into gene–gene and gene–environment interaction studies.

Availability of data and biospecimens from consortia is also an issue that has shown considerable progress in the past 2 years. Several initiatives have been launched to improve on current data sharing practices (11,12). At the same time, issues of proper credit to the original investigators and protection of confidentiality need to be properly addressed (13).

Addendum References

1. Khoury MJ, Bradley L. Why should genomic medicine be more evidence-based? *Genomic Med.* 2007;1:91–93.
2. Wellcome Trust Case Control Consortium. Genome-wide association study of 14,000 cases of seven common diseases and 3,000 shared controls. *Nature.* 2007;447:661–678.
3. National Cancer Institute web site: Cohort Consortium. http://epi.grants.cancer.gov/Consortia/cohort.html. Accessed November 19, 2008.
4. Foundation for the National Institutes of Health web site. http://www.fnih.org/index.php?option=com_content&task=view&id=338&Itemid=454. Accessed November 19, 2008.
5. Moonesinghe R, Khoury MJ, Liu T, et al. Required sample size and nonreplicability thresholds for heterogeneous genetic associations. *Proc Natl Acad Sci USA.* January 15, 2008;105(2):617–622. Epub http://www.pnas.org/content/105/2/617.full. Accessed January 3, 2008.
6. Burton PR, Hansell AL, Fortier I, et al. Size matters: just how big is BIG?: quantifying realistic sample size requirements for human genome epidemiology. *Int J Epidemiol.* February 2009;38(1):263–273. Epub http://ije.oxfordjournals.org/cgi/content/full/38/1/263. Accessed August 1, 2008.
7. Manolio TA, Brooks LD, Collins FS. A HapMap harvest of insights into the genetics of common disease. J Clin Invest. 2008;118(5):1590–1605.
8. NCI-NHGRI Working Group on Replication in Association Studies, Chanock SJ, Manolio T, et al. Replicating genotype-phenotype associations. *Nature.* June 7, 2007;447(7145):655–660.
9. Zeggini E, Scott LJ, Saxena R, et al. Meta-analysis of genome-wide association data and large-scale replication identifies additional susceptibility loci for type 2 diabetes. *Nat Genet.* 2008;40(5):638–645.
10. COGENT Study, Houlston RS, Webb E, et al. The NCBI dbGaP database of genotypes and phenotypes. *Nat Genet.* 2007;39(10):1181–1186.
11. GAIN Collaborative Research Group, Manolio TA, Rodriguez LL, et al. New models of collaboration in genome-wide association studies: the Genetic Association Information Network. *Nat Genet.* 2007;39(9):1045–1051.
12. Homer N, Szelinger S, Redman M, et al. Resolving individuals contributing trace amounts of DNA to highly complex mixtures using high-density SNP genotyping microarrays. *PLoS Genet.* 2008;4(8):e1000167.
13. Zerhouni EA, Nabel EG. Protecting aggregate genomic data. *Science.* 2008;322:44.

8

Design and analysis issues in genome-wide association studies

Duncan C. Thomas

Rationale for Genome-wide Association Studies

The recent availability of commercial high-density genotyping technologies, combined with the identification of subsets of single nucleotide polymorphisms (SNPs) that are capable of "tagging" most of the common variants in the human genome from the HapMap project (1), has now made it feasible to conduct genome-wide association studies (GWAS), as first proposed about a decade ago by Risch and Merikangas (2). Many such studies are now in progress and some have already been published. Although there were a few earlier reports (3–5), it was the simultaneous publication in 2005 of the discovery of a novel association between the Complement-Factor H (*CFH*) gene and age-related macular degeneration through a GWA study using a panel of 116,204 SNPs (6), along with two independent confirmatory studies (7,8), that generated enormous enthusiasm for the potential of this approach. This finding has now been replicated over a dozen times. This enthusiasm, along with spectacular improvements in genotyping technology, has led to the availability of special funding for both methodologic research and genotyping for numerous GWAS using existing epidemiologic studies (9). Other reports are starting to appear at a rapid pace (10–14). How many of these will be replicated only time will tell, but several recent high-profile papers have included multiple replication studies (15–28). Some have not been replicated, however (29); for example, none of the 13 SNP associations identified in the Parkinson disease GWA study (10) were confirmed in a large meta-analysis (30,31).

The concept underlying the use of the GWAS approach is the so-called "common disease—common variant" (CDCV) hypothesis, which proposes that most genetic variants responsible for common diseases are relatively common, individually conferring modest relative risks (RR). Here, "common" is generally defined as having minor allele frequency (MAF) greater than 5% in the general population and "modest" RRs that are potentially detectable in epidemiologic studies of feasible size, perhaps in the range of 1.3–2.5. (With increasing sample sizes, the range of detectable RRs has been declining. For example, a recent meta-analysis (32) of three two-stage GWAS of type 2 diabetes totaling 10,000 subjects and ten replication samples totaling over 50,000 subjects identified six novel loci with RRs in the range of 1.05–1.15. Epidemiologists generally view environmental effects of such small size with great skepticism due to the potential for uncontrolled confounding, subject selection, publication, or other biases; these concerns should also be applicable to genetic associations, although perhaps in different forms such as population stratification or differential genotyping error.) It seems unlikely that there are many common variants with very large RRs that have not already been discovered. On the other hand, while there may be many rare variants with small effects, they are essentially undiscoverable by epidemiological means. Rare variants with very large RRs, like *BRCA1* for breast and ovarian cancer, are more easily detectable through family-based linkage analysis (2), since their prevalence in an unselected series of cases from the general population would still be small. Estimates of the number of common variants in the human genome are approximately 6 million (1), but an important message from HapMap is that a much smaller subset of them is sufficient because of the strong linkage disequilibrium (LD) throughout the genome. This tag SNP approach (33) is not as effective for identifying associations with rare variants, however. Although long haplotypes may effectively tag some of these, the many possible long haplotypes in a region has a detrimental effect on power. Nevertheless, it is certainly possible that a large share of common disease could be caused by multiple rare variants (34–40), a hypothesis for which there is presently no effective study design or statistical test.

It is also worth noting that a consequence of the enormous number of tests being contemplated is that there is no reason to believe that the true positive associations will be anywhere near the top of the list of the most significant ones. To illustrate this phenomenon, Zaykin and Zhivotovsky (41) pointed out that the then-replicated association of myocardial infarction with the lymphotoxin-α gene from one of the first GWAS was less significant than over 200 other associations of the 65,570 tested that were not replicated. (Ironically, subsequent meta-analysis (42) failed to confirm this association, although their methodologic point is still well taken.) They showed that in a GWA study of this size, there was only a 14% probability that a true association of this magnitude would rank in the top 200 associations and that to raise this probability to even 50% would require examining over 3,400 of the most significant associations. This happens because the probability distribution of true associations, while separated from that of null distributions by an amount that depends upon the magnitude of true associations and sample size, is essentially swamped within the tail of the null distribution. This goes to show that very large sample sizes, meticulous study design and genotyping quality control, and careful attention to the problem of multiple significance testing is essential for success.

There have now been quite a few reviews of the general principles of the design and analysis of GWAS (43–53). We focus here on some of the basic issues of multistage sampling design as they have been developed for this purpose, and some of the associated analysis issues.

Basic Principles of Design of Multistage GWAS

Most of the GWAS currently underway or already reported have used some form of multistage sampling design (54) because of the considerable savings in genotyping costs this approach offers. As the cost of commercial chips falls relative to custom genotyping, the merits of this approach will need to be reconsidered (52). The basic idea of two-stage sampling for GWAS entails genotyping part of the sample using a high-density panel (typically 300,000 to a million SNPs) and then genotyping the most promising SNPs on the remainder of the sample. A final analysis combining the information from both samples is more powerful than treating the design as a hypothesis generation followed by independent replication (55,56) because it exploits the additional information about just how significant the first stage associations were, not just the fact that they exceeded some threshold. Additional markers flanking some or all hits might also be added to better characterize the full range of genetic variation in the region (57,58). Optimization of the design entails choosing the significance levels and the allocation of samples between the two stages in such a manner as to minimize the total cost while attaining the desired genome-wide significance level and power (57–65); additional constraints on total available sample size are also possible. This optimal design is insensitive to the genetic model (mode of inheritance, relative risk, and allele frequencies) and is determined primarily by the relative cost per genotype at stages I and II, the total available sample size, and whether additional flanking markers will be tested around those selected from stage I. For example, at a cost ratio of about 17.5, with no additional SNPs being tested at stage II, the optimal design (Table 8.1) turns out to involve testing 30% of the sample in stage I at a significance level of 0.0037, and a significance level for the joint analysis of 1.6×10^{-7}; in this case, about 87% of the total cost goes to stage I genotyping, but the total cost is only 40% that of a comparably powered one-stage design. On the other hand, with five additional markers being tested for each hit, the optimal design raises the first stage sample size to 49% and reduces significance levels to 0.0005 and 0.5×10^{-7} respectively, so that 95% of the total cost goes to stage I genotyping.

Several other authors (66–68) have investigated the power of GWAS, either for a single stage or the first stage of a multistage scan, and generally concluded that sample sizes of 1,000 cases and 1,000 controls or more were sufficient to detect associations in the range of 1.7–2.0, smaller relative risks (e.g., 1.2–1.3) requiring much larger sample sizes. Table 8.2 shows such calculations (using the Quanto program (69)) for a one-stage scan; for a two-stage design with half the sample applied to stage I and half to stage II, the total sample size needed is only about 0.5% larger than shown if 1% of markers are carried forward to stage II or 2% larger if 0.2% of markers are carried forward (58).

Choice of Platform

A crucial decision to be made is the choice of genotyping platform for stage I. At the time of writing this chapter, two companies—Affymetrix and Illumina—offer

Table 8.1 Illustrative examples of optimal design parameters for two-stage GWAS, genome-wide significance level $\alpha = 0.05$ (1×10^{-7} per SNP), power $1 - \beta = 90\%$, 500,000 markers tested in stage I, minor allele frequency 20%, and genetic relative risk 1.5

	DESIGN SPECIFICATIONS				OPTIMAL DESIGN PARAMETERS		
Number of Stages	Ratio of Costs Per Genotype in Stages II/I	Number of Additional Markers Tested in Stage II	Significance Level Per Marker — Stage I	Stage II	Proportion of Total Sample Size Used in Stage I	Proportion of Total Genotyping Cost Needed for Stage I	Total Cost (Relative to One-Stage Design)
1	N.R.	N.R.	1.0×10^{-7}	N.R.	100%	100%	100%
2	5	0	0.0123	1.6×10^{-7}	26%	85%	40%
2	17.5	0	0.0037	1.6×10^{-7}	30%	87%	43%
2	17.5	5	0.0005	0.5×10^{-7}	49%	95%	87%

Table 8.2 Sample size requirements for a one-stage GWAS with 500,000 markers for different minor allele frequencies (MAF) and relative risks (RR) per allele in a multiplicative model. The corresponding population attributable risks (PAR) are given, along with the numbers (N) of cases and of controls required for genome-wide significance level $\alpha = 5\%$ and 90% power

MAF	RR	PAR	N
0.05	2.0	4.8%	1420
0.05	2.5	7.0%	483
0.05	3.0	9.1%	483
0.10	1.5	4.8%	2530
0.10	2.0	9.1%	785
0.10	2.5	13.0%	420
0.20	1.3	5.7%	3686
0.20	1.6	10.7%	1094
0.20	2.0	16.7%	482
0.40	1.2	7.4%	5397
0.40	1.4	13.8%	1576
0.40	1.6	19.4%	807

platforms ranging from 300,000 to a million SNPs. The panels differ in the way SNPs were selected and hence their coverage (r^2) of the remaining common HapMap SNPs, as well as in their laboratory performance (call rates, reproducibility, Mendelian errors, etc.). Because coverage of SNPs is highly variable across the genome and the relationship between power and r^2 is nonlinear, the average power to detect an association with a random SNP is smaller than the power based on the average r^2 (70). One cannot simply add additional sample size to cover regions with poor coverage! Thus, what is needed is to average the power for a given noncentrality parameter λ at a putative causal locus across the distribution of r^2s. Barrett and Cardon (71) have compared several panels that were available in 2006 and concluded that they generally provided similar levels of coverage (See also References 43,72–80 for further discussion of the distribution of LD across the genome and across populations and the coverage of various SNP chip sets).

Several authors have considered the trade-offs between one-stage and two-stage designs or among specific genotyping platforms (66,71,72,75). Faced with a choice between density of SNPs and sample size, it is generally agreed that it is preferable to have the largest possible sample size at the expense of less dense markers, depending upon available sample size and budget constraints. A two-stage design may, however, allow a higher density of markers to be used in stage I than would be affordable in a single-stage design, and hence improve power for regions of low LD. The ability to combine different study designs (e.g., population-based and family-based) may also favor a two-stage design. Other considerations, however, may favor a one-stage design, notably if multiple hypotheses are to be tested using these data, say multiple phenotypes in a cohort design or various subgroup analyses or interaction tests. As costs continue to drop, it is possible that two-stage designs may become obsolete. Indeed, in the NHLBI-funded STAMPEED consortium of GWAS for cardiovascular, lung, and blood disorders, none of the 13 participating centers is using a multistage design.

Prioritization of SNPs for the Next Stage
Another decision entails the selection of SNPs to be carried from stage I to stage II or to be reported as "significant" at the end of the study. Most of the literature has assumed that p-values for single SNP associations will be used for this purpose, although alternatives including using the population attributable risk (81), the False Positive Report Probability (81,82), the Bayes factors or q-values (83), empirical Bayes estimates of effect size (81), or multimarker methods like the local scan statistic (84) have been suggested. However, such approaches make no use of any external information that might suggest that some associations were more credible than others *a priori*. For example, one might wish to give greater credence to associations with SNPs located in or near genes or highly conserved regions of the genome, coding SNPs, those located under a linkage peak, or those with previously reported associations. Often such information is used informally at the conclusion of a GWAS in deciding which associations to pursue with further fine mapping or functional studies. Roeder et al. (85,86) and Whittemore (87) have proposed variants of the False Discovery Rate framework to allow a specific variable to be used to up- or down-weight the significance assigned to each association. They showed that well-chosen prior information can substantially improve the power for detecting true associations, while there was relatively little loss of power if that information proved to be uninformative. In a similar manner, Greenwood et al. (88) discussed setting different significance thresholds for SNPs on different platforms that are being used together in a single study. Each of these approaches allows only a single variable to be incorporated, with weights specified in advance. Hierarchical modeling approaches (89,90) allow multiple sources of information to be empirically weighted in models for the probability that an association is null and the expectation of the magnitude of an association given that it is not null. Simulation studies (90) showed that when there was little or no useful prior knowledge, the standard p-value ranking performed best, but when at least some of the available covariates were strongly predictive (even if one did not know which ones were truly predictive), the hierarchical Bayes ranking led to better power.

DNA pooling offers an approach that has the potential to drastically reduce the cost of genotyping for a GWA study. While the idea has been around for some time (91–94), the technical challenges in forming comparable pools and quantifying allele frequencies are formidable (95–99). It is only recently that it has proved feasible to apply this technique to high-density genotyping arrays (100–106). As currently employed, the design generally entails forming multiple small pools of cases and controls in stage I and selecting SNPs on the basis of their differences in allele frequencies. These are then retested by individual genotyping in stage II, possibly on both the original and a second sample. An obvious difficulty with DNA pooling is that it is only good for testing main effects for individual SNPs. There will be some loss of information for testing haplotype associations (107) and interactions or subgroups can be tested only if the pools have been formed based on these stratifying variables. Much remains to be done to study the best choices of design parameters (numbers of pools, sample sizes, criteria for selecting SNPs to test by individual genotyping, etc.) (108) and to estimate the statistical power and false discovery rate for this approach in practice. However, empirical applications have demonstrated that DNA pooling is capable of detecting several associations that have been discovered and established by individual genotyping in a GWA study context (109). Furthermore, several studies using this approach have reported novel associations (13,110,111), although it remains for these associations to be confirmed independently.

Gene–Environment Interactions

The NIH "Genes and Environment Initiative" has focused attention on the use of GWAS for identifying genes that modify the effects of environmental agents (112). Such studies pose additional methodologic problems, beyond the usual challenges in assessing the main effects of genes and environmental factors, such as low power (113). However, there is the opportunity to improve power by using a case-only design (114) in which G×E *interaction* is tested by testing for *association* between a gene and environmental factor among *cases*, under the assumption that this association does not exist in the general population. Such an assumption is not likely to hold for all possible SNP×E interactions in a GWA study. Testing this assumption first in controls and deciding whether to perform a case-only or conventional case-control test accordingly can lead to substantial inflation of type I error rates (115). Nevertheless, more appropriate methods for combining the inferences from case-control and case-only analyses of the same data have been described (116–120). For example, Mukherjee and Chatterjee (120) use an empirical Bayes compromise between the case-only and case-control estimators, weighted by the estimated probability of the existence of a G–E association. In the context of a GWA study, various multistage designs are possible, such as using a case-only test to screen interaction effects and then confirming that subset by a case-control test in a separate dataset. (In a single stage design, this would lead to a biased overall test unless one conditioned the case-control comparison on the case-only one being significant (121).) In practice, it is unlikely one would conduct a search for G×E interactions without also searching for main effects (thus requiring controls to be genotyped in the first stage anyway), but it would generally be more powerful to select SNPs for the second stage based on case-control comparisons of main effects and case-only comparisons of interaction effects. Use of hybrid case-only/case-control tests (121) could be even more powerful, however. More work along these lines is needed.

Other Design Issues

Family-based versus Population-based Designs
Most GWAS currently underway have adopted a traditional case-control design using unrelated individuals, in part because of its greater convenience and in part because of its greater power compared with family-based comparisons for genetic main effects (122). To further enhance power, some investigators have used cases with a positive family history to increase the expected proportion of cases carrying disease susceptibility alleles (123,124). While this device does improve power, it must be appreciated that it will lead to biased estimates of relative risk, because the frequency of the deleterious allele will be inflated in family history positive cases relative to all cases (for whom an unselected control series would have represented the appropriate source population). Likewise, it must be appreciated that any GWA study aims to be an efficient means of gene *discovery*, not *estimation* of genetic relative risks, which will tend to be exaggerated because only the largest observed effects are considered (125–127).

Another concern with case-control designs using unrelated controls is the potential for bias due to population stratification, leading to both confounding and overdispersion of test statistics due to cryptic relatedness. There are now available various statistical techniques broadly known as "genomic control" (128) (described in the analysis section below) that rely on a large number of unlinked markers to adjust for population stratification in the analysis. In a GWA study, there are more than enough markers available for use in such methods, and the chance that any truly causal association will be overadjusted by also being included in the genomic control panel (or by another SNP in that panel in strong LD with it) is miniscule.

Of course, family-based association tests (129)—case-sibling, case-parent triads, or generalized FBATs—have the attraction of being completely immune to population stratification, although they tend to be less powerful. This has led various groups to propose hybrid designs for multistage scans. For example, the NCI Cancer Family Registries' GWAS for breast and colon cancers uses cases with a positive family history and unrelated controls (unselected by family history) in the first stage for maximum power, and family-based designs in the second stage to eliminate false positives due to population stratification. The final analysis combines the information from both stages, taking account of the overlap between the case series used in each stage. Entirely family-based two-stage designs have also been proposed (130,131). A particularly clever design uses the same data in both stages, but with tests that are statistically independent (129,132,133). In its simplest form, this might involve case-parent triads, where in stage I a test based on *between-family* comparisons of parental genotypes is performed to identify loci that would have the best power for detecting association in stage II using a *within-family* test of transmission from parents to offspring. The FBAT class has recently been extended to handle multiple correlated SNPs (134,135) (as needed in a GWA study using dense markers) and copy number variants (136). Use of these methods led to the discovery of a plausible candidate gene for asthma (136). These methods are implemented in the PBAT software package (http://www.biostat.harvard.edu/~clange/default.htm). Of course, there are several disadvantages to family-based studies, including the difficulty of enrolling families, the extra cost of genotyping parents and/or additional offspring, not using between-family information efficiently, and some proportion of families being uninformative.

Populations
Another consideration is the choice of population: continental, isolated, or admixed; single or multiple. Isolated populations have the advantage of greater genetic homogeneity and, depending upon their age, could have shorter- or longer-range LD than continental populations. Recently isolated populations will tend to have broad LD, which makes them attractive for regional discovery but of limited utility for fine mapping of any disease susceptibility alleles that are segregating in that population (137,138). Old isolated populations, such as Finland, tend to have short LD and have been useful for fine mapping. Admixed populations are characterized by a lack of recombination between haplotypes coming from the source populations, and thus will have distinctive LD patterns with high correlation at long ranges between SNPs that are informative of ancestry, but lower correlation for other SNPs. Admixture studies (139–142) can be attractive for initial coarse mapping for diseases that show very different rates in their source populations, such as for hypertension or prostate cancer in African Americans or diabetes in Hispanics. On the other hand, because of their complex and generally unknown ancestries, care must be taken to allow for hidden population stratification that could generate false positives.

Some studies have exploited multiple ethnic groups, such as the Los Angeles/Hawaii Multi-Ethnic Cohort Study (143), thereby allowing tests of both an overall effect of any genetic variant (race adjusted), as well as tests of heterogeneity between ethnic groups. Using multiple ethnic groups increases the potential for fine mapping since LD structure probably differs between ethnic groups, even between those with generally high LD, that is, Europeans and Asians (as compared to Africans). Evidence for heterogeneity by racial/ethnic group may indicate the need to genotype additional markers to probe for a causal variant affecting risk in all groups, especially in regions in which some markers are related to risk in one ethnic group but other (nearby) markers are related to risk in other groups. It may even be wise to explicitly allocate some of the type I error to tests for ethnic heterogeneity in the first stage of a GWA study and to increase the marker density around such heterogeneous variants in the second stage.

Control Selection

Case-control studies can be done in the standard fashion, with controls ideally representing random samples from the source population of cases, or as nested case-control or case-cohort studies within existing cohort studies. The latter designs are likely to yield more comparable case and control groups, reduce problems with recall bias if environmental factors are to be considered, and allow simultaneous use of controls for comparison with different case groups. Nevertheless, a number of GWAS currently underway have used "convenience" control groups that may not be geographically representative of the case groups under study or could differ in other ways that could lead to spurious associations, unless appropriate measures are taken to match controls from the resource on genetic ancestry (144).

Replication and Follow-up Studies

Failure to replicate has been a recurring problem with candidate gene association studies, hence a major concern about the new generation of GWAS (29,145). True scientific replication must involve something more than a repetition of the study on a second random sampling from the same population using the same methods (145,146). Indeed, it is well known that simply splitting a sample in half and requiring significance at level α in both halves is less powerful than a single analysis of the entire sample at significance level α^2 (the two analyses having the same overall type I error rate) (55,147). Replication should thus entail some elements of different populations being studied by different investigators using different methodologies (145). Although this risks failure to replicate in the case of real heterogeneity of effects, the potential benefit in terms of insight into the generality and robustness of the association seems worth the price. In this sense, a traditional two-stage GWA study cannot be viewed as an internal replication, but simply as a more cost-efficient form of gene discovery. Many granting agencies now expect investigators to discuss plans for follow-up investigations of any associations detected and some high-profile journals are requiring replication studies as part of a single report of a genetic association (148,149). These could entail more detailed analyses of the same data, collaboration with other investigators to test the associations in different populations, bioinformatic characterization of the genomic regions identified, *in vitro* or *in vivo* functional characterization, and so on.

One question that frequently arises is whether to restrict replication claims to the same marker detected in the initial GWA scan ("exact" replication) or to test additional markers in the region and allow association with any of them (appropriately adjusted for multiple comparisons) to be treated as evidence of replication ("local" replication). While it seems intuitively appealing to use the replication step as well for the purpose of fine mapping—that is, to see whether there is another marker in the region that shows even stronger evidence for association—Clarke et al. (146) have shown theoretically and by simulation that this can be counterproductive, since the increased penalty for multiple comparisons can defeat any possible gains in power for replication. Nevertheless, the inclusion of additional markers can be advantageous in regions of relatively high LD when the original signal is weak, such as in regions where the coverage by the original panel is poor, but then any new associations discovered in the "replication" stage would require yet further confirmation. In general, they recommend deferring fine mapping to a separate sample from that used for replication in order to overcome the "winner's curse," the bias of exaggerated effect estimates in samples that have demonstrated association. In a similar vein, associations first discovered in a GWA study by imputed SNPs (as described below) should be confirmed by direct genotyping, either in the original samples, or, better yet, in independent replication samples, before a genuine association is claimed.

Analysis Issues

False Discovery Rates and Other Approaches to Multiple Comparisons
Clearly, with hundreds of thousands of tests (if not millions), the overriding statistical issue in any GWA study is the control of the false positive (type I) error rate. The traditional way of dealing with this problem is through a control of the "family-wise" error rate (FWER), the probability of making at least one false positive claim. By setting the threshold for significance extremely high, the FWER can be controlled. The simplest such approach is the Bonferroni method of dividing the genome-wide significance level α by the number of tests M to be performed to obtain the significance level for any one of them. But this is overly conservative when applied to high-density SNP chips, as there is a substantial correlation between tests due to LD, so the "effective number of tests" is substantially smaller than the number of SNPs tested. Pe'er et al. (150) have estimated the multiple testing burden from testing all HapMap SNPs (indirectly with haplotype-based tests, as described below) to be roughly equivalent to about 1 million independent tests in Caucasian populations or about 2.2 million in African populations (or for common SNPs, 500,000 in Caucasians and Asians and 1 million in Africans). Nevertheless, the concept of an "effective number of tests" has been criticized (151) as not reflecting adequately the diversity across loci in the local LD structure. While a permutation test is in principle the gold standard, it is computationally demanding on a genome-wide scale. Conneely and Boehnke (151) provide a way of estimating the multivariate normal tail probabilities that closely approximates the permutation probabilities at a fraction of the computing time. However, their method is limited to a few thousand SNPs, and hence is not applicable to a GWA study; Dudbridge and Gusnanto (152) provide an alternative approach, still relying on permutation testing, but fitting the simulated distribution of minimum p-values to a beta distribution to obtain a more accurate estimate of the "effective number of tests."

An alternative paradigm has become widely used in the gene expression field, where one expects the yield of true positive associations to be quite high; thus, one is less concerned about controlling the total number of false positives, but only as a proportion of all reported associations. This idea is captured in the False Discovery Rate (FDR) (153,154)—the expectation of the proportion of all reported associations that are truly null. Various criteria have been proposed for selecting a threshold that controls the FDR, such as a step-up algorithm that begins by selecting the most significant association at level α/M, then the next most significant at level $2\alpha/M$, and continuing in this manner until the first nonsignificant association is encountered. However, for GWAS, the expected yield of true positives is generally expected to be very low, in which case, the FDR becomes nearly identical to the FWER (155); see references 156–158 for further discussion in the context of GWAS. Using the empirical distribution of p-values to estimate the false positive rate is part of the q-value method (83,159,160). Trying to combine correction for overdispersion of p-values due to other problems such as inadequate control selection or hidden population stratification while simultaneously using the distribution of p-values to compute the FDR empirically seems challenging, however.

Efficient Methods of Significance Testing in Two-Stage Designs

Two-stage designs pose particular challenges to significance testing in the final analysis of the combined data. The basic p-value to be computed is the probability that a given SNP would have been deemed "promising" at the first stage *and* that the combined data would show significance at a genome-wide level given that it was selected for testing in the second stage, all computed under the null hypothesis that it is not in fact associated with disease. The various two-stage design papers discussed earlier have shown how to compute this probability under simplifying assumptions and thereby optimize the design, but these approximations are unreliable for analysis of real data. Among other assumptions is that of independence across SNPs, which is necessary to derive the appropriate cutoff for genome-wide significance. An obvious way to avoid having to make such assumptions is some form of a permutation test. For a single-stage design, this is straightforward: one could simply hold the genotypes fixed (thereby maintaining their LD structure) and randomly permute the phenotypes in a standard case-control design (or analogous methods for family-based studies). In a two-stage design, this is not so straightforward, however, as one must permute the entire analysis; but a random permutation of the stage I data would yield a different set of SNPs to be tested in stage II, and these genotypes are not available for permuting in stage II! Various approximations to this problem have been proposed which are computationally efficient and statistically valid (161–164). However, methods based on computing an "effective number of tests" for a given platform have typically relied on permutation tests applied to data sets (e.g., the HapMap) where very large numbers of SNPs are genotyped in relatively small numbers of subjects. There is an implicit assumption in these calculations that the null distribution of the minimum p-value for a group of tests does not depend very strongly on the number of subjects in the analysis but only on the LD pattern between the tests considered. This assumption motivates the method of Dudbridge (165), in which part of the stage

I data is reserved (when calculating the null distribution of the permutation test) for mimicking the effect of having two stages of genotyping.

Haplotype Associations and Tests for Association with Untested SNPs

Most single-SNP associations detected in a GWA study are unlikely to be causal and more likely to reflect LD with some other variant in the region (if not a false-positive). This can be tested either by adding flanking markers surrounding each hit from stage I to search for SNPs that might be more strongly associated with the trait or by conducting haplotype-based association tests (166,167). The HapMap data now makes it feasible to test the associations not just with the SNPs on the chosen platform, but with most of the roughly 6 million common SNPs in the human genome by using multimarker tags (74,168–171). (However, it remains to be seen how well such methods work in populations for which HapMap data are not available.) Several authors (172–180) have described methods for imputing HapMap SNPs based on LD patterns, in some cases augmented with haplotype inference, population genetics models, or additional resequencing data. For example, Nicolae et al. (179) use HapMap data to impute genotype probabilities for untyped SNPs based on haplotypes of flanking SNPs that have been typed; this approach is implemented in the TUNA software (180). Marchini et al. (177) use estimates of local recombination rates from HapMap and a hidden Markov model to test for association with hypothetical (unknown) variants in the region. Crucial to the validity of these approaches is to properly allow for the uncertainty in the imputed genotypes rather than simply using the most probable one; Bayesian regression approaches are sometimes used for this purpose (178), although use of the expected allele dosage yields a powerful score test with the correct type I error (181). (Nevertheless, as noted earlier, the ultimate test of an association with an imputed SNP is confirmation in an independent sample by direct genotyping.) It may also be possible to test for associations with rarer polymorphisms by using long-range haplotypes (182). As with tests of ethnic heterogeneity and GxE interactions, however, there is an obvious trade-off between the multiplicity of tests and the chances that these additional tests will yield discoveries not captured by single SNP associations. The optimal balance between the two remains a topic for further research.

Allowing for Hidden Population Structure

An early report from the Wellcome Trust Case-Control Consortium (183) highlighted the potential overdispersion that can result from population stratification, even in the relatively homogeneous population of Great Britain. The original genomic control method (128) is based on adjusting the null distribution of test statistics by an overdispersion factor that can be estimated from the distribution of a set of null markers. Structured association (184) instead uses "ancestrally informative" markers to infer the ethnic origins of each individual in the study and adjust for these estimated ancestries as confounders in the analysis of the SNPs of interest. More recently, methods based on random effects models (185), principal components (186), and Bayesian logistic regression (187) have been developed that are both computationally efficient for use on a genome-wide scale and more powerful than either traditional genomic control or structured association. At their core, the random effects and principal components methods use the genotyped SNPs to empirically estimate the relatedness between any two subjects by computing a statistic (the kinship coefficient) that summarizes how similar two subjects' SNPs are. The resulting kinship matrix is then directly used as a part of the model for the correlations between outcomes in the random effects method, or else the leading eigenvectors of the kinship matrix are extracted and used as additional fixed effects in the model for the outcomes in the principal components approach. Rakovski and Stram (personal communication) propose using the entire kinship matrix, rather than the leading principal components alone, in a modification of the Cochran-Armitage test for case-control studies; this seems to provide correction methods that encompass some of the strengths of both the original genomic control method and the principal components method.

Very large studies are capable of detecting very small RRs (recall the earlier discussion of the 1.05–1.15 RRs for diabetes (32)). However, the *magnitude* of biases due to population stratification or other sources are independent of sample size— they simply become more *significant* with larger samples. In principle, the various methods of adjustment for population stratification should perform even better in larger samples at removing bias, but only if the models are correctly specified. Very small risks are still potentially subject to residual confounding, so more and more false associations due to residual confounding will attain the significance threshold as sample sizes grow, and great caution should be exercised in interpreting very small effect sizes. Of course, the power to detect true associations will also grow with sample sizes, but not as fast as the power to detect biased associations (Table 8.3), so the false discovery rate *increases* with sample size, at a rate depending upon the prevalence and extent of uncontrolled confounding or other biases.

Gene–Gene Interactions

Analyses of GxE interactions are likely to be limited to a modest number of environmental factors already established as risk factors for the particular disease under study. This is not the case for GxG interactions, for which the purpose of the study is, after all, gene discovery. Of course, to the extent that causal genes are already known for a disease, one might wish to exclude subjects carrying mutations in these genes or to include tests of interaction of these genes with the SNPs in the scan as higher priority tests. But how should one go about prioritizing the enormous number of possible GxG interactions (125 billion pairwise interactions for a 500,000 SNP scan)? Should testing for GxG interactions be attempted at the first stage, or limited to the subset of SNPs with significant main effects in stage I? Although at first blush, it might seem both computationally and statistically efficient to limit the testing of interactions to those SNPs that showed significant main effects at some level, this strategy would fail to find interactions with little or no main effects. In a widely

Table 8.3 Variation in Type I and II error and false discovery rates with sample size for various degrees of bias in the distribution of true relative risks*

Number of Biased Associations	Mean (SD) of Biased log [log(RRs)]	Sampling SD in True log(RR)	Type I Error	Type II Error	False Discovery Rate
10,000	–3.0 (0.25)	0.4	0.0005	0.674	0.068
		0.3	0.0018	0.830	0.173
		0.2	0.0109	0.959	0.529
		0.1	0.0747	0.998	0.881
10,000	–4.0 (0.25)	0.4	0.0001	0.677	0.010
		0.3	0.0001	0.829	0.010
		0.2	0.0002	0.956	0.020
		0.1	0.0003	0.998	0.215
2,000	–3.0 (0.25)	0.4	0.0001	0.659	0.021
		0.3	0.0004	0.827	0.045
		0.2	0.0023	0.956	0.191
		0.1	0.0148	0.999	0.595
50,000	–4.0 (0.25)	0.4	0.0001	0.678	0.018
		0.3	0.0002	0.830	0.023
		0.2	0.0006	0.958	0.062
		0.1	0.0138	0.998	0.578

*Based on simulations of 100,000 markers, of which 1,000 are true with a mean log(RR) of –1.6 and SD log(RR) of 0.5, SD of biased log(RRs) 0.25, critical value $Z_{\alpha/2} = 4.055$.

quoted paper, Marchini et al. (188) demonstrated that exhaustive testing of all possible interactions was computationally feasible and more powerful than limiting the search to pairs with significant main effects across a range of interaction models. This finding was confirmed for a broader range of models by Evans et al. (189), who showed that this strategy was also more powerful than testing interactions of each significant SNP with all others. However, Kooperberg et al. (190) proposed an alternative two-stage procedure, limiting the testing of interactions to pairs of SNPs that show significant main effects and then correcting the p-value only for the number of interaction tests actually performed at the second stage; they concluded that their two-stage analyses could be considerably more powerful than single-stage scans for all possible interactions, because the search is restricted to a more parsimonious set of interactions (additive × additive) and because a less conservative adjustment for multiple comparisons is used. Newer machine learning and Bayesian search strategies also appear promising (191–193).

Exploring Multigenic Pathways

GWAS are intended primarily as a tool for gene discovery, not for testing *a priori* hypotheses. Nevertheless, given the strong prior belief that most complex diseases result from the interplay of multiple genes and multiple environmental factors acting along one or more related pathways, it is natural to ask how one should follow up on the collection of main effects and interactions that are found in a GWA study. A full treatment of this topic is beyond the scope of this chapter, but it seems obvious that biological understanding of potential mechanisms would greatly enhance the credibility of any unanticipated discoveries. While there will always be the temptation to create *post hoc* interpretations of intriguing findings, this behavior should be avoided in favor of hypothesis-driven, yet flexible, modeling strategies (194–196). For example, using the many available ontology databases that annotate genes, pathways, protein–protein interactions, and so on, one could build a hierarchical modeling strategy that incorporates such knowledge systematically as priors on the parameters of an empirical model for the epidemiologic data (105,197,198). While it might be possible to incorporate such prior knowledge in the discovery stages of a GWA study (90), the computational burden of doing so on a genome-wide scale is likely to preclude any thorough pathway-based modeling. It can, however, be done as one of the follow-up activities, once the set of plausible candidate associations and interactions has been suitably winnowed down.

In some instances, it may also be possible to gain a deeper understanding of the underlying biology by investigating multiple related phenotypes, such as asthma, lung function and related intermediate immunological phenotypes (199), colorectal polyps and cancer (200), or diabetes and related metabolic syndrome traits (28). For the latter, three reports (20,201,202) of GWAS have recently demonstrated associations of the *FTO* gene with both diabetes and obesity, suggesting a common pathway. *FTO* is expressed in the hypothalamus, a key part of the brain that influences appetite (203). Of course, there is always the risk that correlated phenotypes could generate heterogeneity in results if a gene is associated with a different trait than the one studied and the correlation between traits differs across populations (204). This appears to be the explanation for the heterogeneity of results for *FTO* and diabetes, since the effect of the gene appears to be mediated through obesity (201), and hence studies that targeted lean individuals would have little power for detecting an association with diabetes (205).

Other Issues

GWAS for High-Dimensional Phenotypes
If GWAS for a single phenotype weren't complicated enough, consider the latest generation of studies involving investigation of the genetics of gene expression on a genome-wide basis (206–211). These typically involve testing the association of tens of thousands of gene expression probes on cell lines from the HapMap subjects with hundreds of thousands of SNPs—billions (if not trillions) of significance tests in total! Clearly some more efficient methods for mining such extensive matrices of associations are needed to look for patterns that might identify *cis*- or *trans*-acting transcription factors. One such approach is based on Bayesian hierarchical modeling

of the means and covariances of expression traits in nuclear family data to test for association and linkage respectively, with the models for means and for covariances both involving mixtures of null and non-null effects in the rows (expression probes) and columns (SNPs) (212). When applied to the Morley et al. (207) data, the method identified a single SNP on chromosome 11 that appeared to control many expression traits on the same chromosome, suggesting a possible master regulatory region.

Genotyping Error

The inflated type I error rate that can result from genotyping errors in linkage and association studies has been recognized for some time and various methods of correction have been developed (see Reference 213 for a review). Clayton et al. (183) were perhaps the first to demonstrate the potential impact of genotyping error in GWAS in the context of a large study of type 1 diabetes. They showed how differences in sample handling for cases and controls could produce differential genotype misclassification, leading to seriously biased tests, and proposed an algorithm for scoring genotype calls separately in cases and controls (and stratified by center). A subsequent paper (214) showed that a refinement of their algorithm using "fuzzy" calls, rather than treating uncertain genotypes as missing data, substantially reduced the overdispersion of the test statistics.

A common practice is to test for Hardy-Weinberg equilibrium among controls and exclude from a scan any SNPs that are out of balance as an indicator of potential genotyping error. This practice has been widely recommended by various authorities and journals (e.g., References 145,148,215,216 and many others, and also see Reference 217 for a review). Nevertheless, this can be counterproductive and lead to inflated type I error rates (217). Unless genotyping error is differential, the Cochran-Armitage test for trend in proportions will retain the correct test size under misclassification, although the simple chi-square test for allelic association is to be avoided.

Software and Bioinformatics Challenges

In addition to the theoretical issues discussed above, one must consider the practical challenges in managing the enormous amount of data generated by a GWA study and the need for meticulous inspection of the raw data at every stage of the process for possible artifacts (183,214,218). Some software tailor-made for this purpose is starting to emerge (180,219–221) (http://biosun1.harvard.edu/~fbat/fbat.htm). The ENDGAME Consortium's web site (http://hgmacpro.uchicago.edu/pmwiki/pmwiki.php?n=Main.SoftwareInteroperabilityFileFormatAmpDataStandards) includes links to other relevant software and bioinformatics resources.

Data Sharing and Protection of Confidentiality

Many granting agencies—and notably in the United States, the National Institutes of Health—have adopted broad data sharing policies aimed at making the source data for publicly funded studies available to the broader research community while protecting participants' confidentiality and the original investigators' intellectual property rights (222). Needless to say, these laudable and widely accepted goals can conflict with each other, particularly for GWAS (223). For example, genotypes on a genome-wide scale are sufficient to uniquely identify any individual whose DNA may already be available in another biobank or database, such as a forensic or health insurance databank. The informed consents obtained at the time subjects originally agreed to participate in a study may not have anticipated future requirements for data sharing. In response to a recent request for public comment on the proposed data sharing policies, various organizations (224) have provided thoughtful discussions of these issues and the policies are continuing to evolve, seeking a reasonable balance.

Priorities for Allocating Limited Research Funds

By any standard, GWAS are expensive, so granting agencies obviously have an interest in funding only the most promising proposals (47,52). The NIH Center for Inherited Diseases Research, which provides genotyping services for NIH-funded studies, has enumerated a number of criteria for access (http://www.cidr.jhmi.edu/app_access_gwa.html), including

- Significance and complexity of the trait and the need for a high-throughput whole genome association study
- Quality and completeness of phenotyping and exposure measures
- Strength of the evidence for a genetic component for the trait and the anticipated size of a detectable genetic effect
- Appropriateness of the study design and population for the specific trait mapping project
- Power of the sample set to detect a genetic effect
- Plans for data management and data analysis
- Plans for follow-up studies to identify the genetic variant(s)

Clearly only time will tell whether the yield of novel and replicated findings from the public and private sectors' investment in GWAS was worth the cost, but early reports from the first generation of such studies are encouraging. As costs for this new technology continue to fall, it is reasonable to expect that the bang for the buck will continue to improve, unless, after the low-hanging fruit is harvested, a point of diminishing returns is reached. Indeed, the possibility that the two-stage design is already obsolete in light of falling chip costs is already being discussed. Newer chips are being designed to offer better coverage of copy number variants (225–229), a potentially major source of genomic variation that has only recently been investigated in terms of associations with disease (136,230–232). Even newer technologies, such as genome-wide sequencing, proteomic, metabolomic, methylomic, and other -omic technologies, are expected to soon become available at a reasonable cost and yield further insights. The "Thousand Dollar Genome" (http://grants.nih.gov/grants/guide/rfa-files/RFA-HG-04-003.html) is anticipated to be a reality before long and will doubtless make it possible to test such hypotheses as the multiple rare variants discussed earlier, which is beyond the reach of the current tag-SNP-based GWAS approach, with its focus on common variants.

Acknowledgments

Supported in part by NIH grant 5U01 ES015090. The author is grateful to James Gauderman, Juan Pablo Lewinger, Cyril Rakovski, Daniel Stram, and Heather Volk for many helpful comments on the manuscript.

References

1. Altshuler D, Brooks LD, Chakravarti A, et al. A haplotype map of the human genome. *Nature.* 2005;437:1299–1320.
2. Risch N, Merikangas K. The future of genetic studies of complex human diseases. *Science.* 1996;273:1616–1617.
3. Jonasdottir A, Thorlacius T, Fossdal R, et al. A whole genome association study in Icelandic multiple sclerosis patients with 4804 markers. *J Neuroimmunol.* 2003; 143:88–92.
4. Ophoff RA, Escamilla MA, Service SK, et al. Genomewide linkage disequilibrium mapping of severe bipolar disorder in a population isolate. *Am J Hum Genet.* 2002;71:565–574.
5. Ozaki K, Ohnishi Y, Iida A, et al. Functional SNPs in the lymphotoxin-alpha gene that are associated with susceptibility to myocardial infarction. *Nat Genet.* 2002;32:650–654.
6. Klein RJ, Zeiss C, Chew EY, et al. Complement factor H polymorphism in age-related macular degeneration. *Science.* 2005;308:385–389.
7. Haines JL, Hauser MA, Schmidt S, et al. Complement factor H variant increases the risk of age-related macular degeneration. *Science.* 2005;308:419–421.
8. Edwards AO, Ritter R, 3rd, Abel KJ, et al. Complement factor H polymorphism and age-related macular degeneration. *Science.* 2005;308:421–424.
9. Manolio TA, Rodriguez LL, Brooks L, et al. New models of collaboration in genome-wide association studies: the Genetic Association Information Network. *Nat Genet.* 2007;39:1045–1051.
10. Maraganore DM, de Andrade M, Lesnick TG, et al. High-resolution whole-genome association study of Parkinson disease. *Am J Hum Genet.* 2005;77:685–693.
11. Gudmundsson J, Sulem P, Manolescu A, et al. Genome-wide association study identifies a second prostate cancer susceptibility variant at 8q24. *Nat Genet.* 2007;39:631–637.
12. McPherson R, Pertsemlidis A, Kavaslar N, et al. A common allele on chromosome 9 associated with coronary heart disease. *Science.* 2007;316:1488–1491.
13. Spinola M, Leoni VP, Galvan A, et al. Genome-wide single nucleotide polymorphism analysis of lung cancer risk detects the KLF6 gene. *Cancer Lett.* 2007;251:311–316.
14. Duggan D, Zheng SL, Knowlton M, et al. Two genome-wide association studies of aggressive prostate cancer implicate putative prostate tumor suppressor gene DAB2IP. *J Natl Cancer Inst.* 2007;99:1836–1844.
15. Easton DF, Pooley KA, Dunning AM, et al. Genome-wide association study identifies novel breast cancer susceptibility loci. *Nature.* 2007;447:1087–1093.
16. Hunter DJ, Kraft P, Jacobs KB, et al. A genome-wide association study identifies alleles in FGFR2 associated with risk of sporadic postmenopausal breast cancer. *Nat Genet.* 2007;39:870–874.

17. Stacey SN, Manolescu A, Sulem P, et al. Common variants on chromosomes 2q35 and 16q12 confer susceptibility to estrogen receptor-positive breast cancer. *Nat Genet.* 2007;39:865–869.

18. Sladek R, Rocheleau G, Rung J, et al. A genome-wide association study identifies novel risk loci for type 2 diabetes. *Nature.* 2007;445:881–885.

19. Scott LJ, Mohlke KL, Bonnycastle LL, et al. A genome-wide association study of type 2 diabetes in Finns detects multiple susceptibility variants. *Science.* 2007;316:1341–1345.

20. Frayling TM, Timpson NJ, Weedon MN, et al. A common variant in the FTO gene is associated with body mass index and predisposes to childhood and adult obesity. *Science.* 2007;316:889–894.

21. Zeggini E, Weedon MN, Lindgren CM, et al. Replication of genome-wide association signals in U.K. samples reveals risk loci for type 2 diabetes. *Science.* 2007;316:1336–1341.

22. Duerr RH, Taylor KD, Brant SR, et al. A genome-wide association study identifies IL23R as an inflammatory bowel disease gene. *Science.* 2006;314:1461–1463.

23. Yeager M, Orr N, Hayes RB, et al. Genome-wide association study of prostate cancer identifies a second risk locus at 8q24. *Nat Genet.* 2007;39:645–649.

24. Todd JA, Walker NM, Cooper JD, et al. Robust associations of four new chromosome regions from genome-wide analyses of type 1 diabetes. *Nat Genet.* 2007;39:857–864.

25. Salonen JT, Uimari P, Aalto JM, et al. Type 2 diabetes whole-genome association study in four populations: the DiaGen consortium. *Am J Hum Genet.* 2007;81:338–345.

26. Tomlinson I, Webb E, Carvajal-Carmona L, et al. A genome-wide association scan of tag SNPs identifies a susceptibility variant for colorectal cancer at 8q24.21. *Nat Genet.* 2007;39:984–988.

27. Zanke BW, Greenwood CM, Rangrej J, et al. Genome-wide association scan identifies a colorectal cancer susceptibility locus on chromosome 8q24. *Nat Genet.* 2007;39:989–994.

28. Saxena R, Voight BF, Lyssenko V, et al. Genome-wide association analysis identifies loci for type 2 diabetes and triglyceride levels. *Science.* 2007;316:1331–1336.

29. Ioannidis JP. Non-replication and inconsistency in the genome-wide association setting. *Hum Hered.* 2007;64:203–213.

30. Elbaz A, Nelson LM, Payami H, et al. Lack of replication of thirteen single-nucleotide polymorphisms implicated in Parkinson's disease: a large-scale international study. *Lancet Neurol.* 2006;5:917–923.

31. Evangelou E, Maraganore DM, Ioannidis JP. Meta-analysis in genome-wide association datasets: strategies and application in Parkinson disease. *PLoS ONE.* 2007;2:e196.

32. Zeggini E, Scott LJ, Saxena R, et al. Meta-analysis of genome-wide association data and large-scale replication identifies additional susceptibility loci for type 2 diabetes. *Nat Genet.* 2008;40:638–645.

33. Stram DO. Tag SNP selection for association studies. *Genet Epidemiol.* 2004;27:365–374.

34. Pritchard JK. Are rare variants responsible for susceptibility to complex diseases? *Am J Hum Genet.* 2001;69:124–137.

35. Pritchard JK, Cox NJ. The allelic architecture of human disease genes: common disease-common variant...or not? *Hum Mol Genet.* 2002;11:2417–2423.

36. Kryukov GV, Pennacchio LA, Sunyaev SR. Most rare missense alleles are deleterious in humans: implications for complex disease and association studies. *Am J Hum Genet.* 2007;80:727–739.

37. Wang WY, Cordell HJ, Todd JA. Association mapping of complex diseases in linked regions: estimation of genetic effects and feasibility of testing rare variants. *Genet Epidemiol.* 2003;24:36–43.

38. Di Rienzo A. Population genetics models of common diseases. *Curr Opin Genet Dev.* 2006;16:630–636.
39. Fearnhead NS, Wilding JL, Winney B, et al. Multiple rare variants in different genes account for multifactorial inherited susceptibility to colorectal adenomas. *Proc Natl Acad Sci USA.* 2004;101:15992–15997.
40. Reich DE, Lander ES. On the allelic spectrum of human disease. *Trends Genet.* 2001;17:502–510.
41. Zaykin DV, Zhivotovsky LA. Ranks of genuine associations in whole-genome scans. *Genetics.* 2005;171:813–823.
42. Clarke R, Xu P, Bennett D, et al. Lymphotoxin-alpha gene and risk of myocardial infarction in 6,928 cases and 2,712 controls in the ISIS case-control study. *PLoS Genet.* 2006;2:e107.
43. Wang WYS, Barratt BJ, Clayton DG, et al. Genome-wide association studies: theoretical and practical concerns. *Nat Rev Genet.* 2005;6:109–118.
44. Jorgenson E, Witte JS. Genome-wide association studies of cancer. *Future Oncol.* 2007;3:419–427.
45. Amos CI. Successful design and conduct of genome-wide association studies. *Hum Mol Genet.* 2007;16 Spec No. 2:R220–R225.
46. Thomas DC, Haile RW, Duggan D. Recent developments in genomewide association scans: a workshop summary and review. *Am J Hum Genet.* 2005;77:337–345.
47. Thomas DC. Are we ready for genome-wide association studies? *Cancer Epidemiol Biomark Prev.* 2006;15:595–598.
48. Palmer LJ, Cardon LR. Shaking the tree: mapping complex disease genes with linkage disequilibrium. *Lancet.* 2005;366:1223–1234.
49. Lawrence RW, Evans DM, Cardon LR. Prospects and pitfalls in whole genome association studies. *Philos Trans R Soc Lond B Biol Sci.* 2005;360:1589–1595.
50. Hirschhorn JN, Daly MJ. Genome-wide association studies for common disease and complex traits. *Nat Rev Genet.* 2005;6:95–108.
51. Carlson CS, Eberle MA, Kruglyak L, et al. Mapping complex disease loci in whole-genome association studies. *Nature.* 2004;429:446–452.
52. Hunter DJ, Thomas G, Hoover RN, et al. Scanning the horizon: what is the future of genome-wide association studies in accelerating discoveries in cancer etiology and prevention? *Cancer Causes Control.* 2007;18:479–484.
53. Ziegler A, Konig IR, Thompson JR. Biostatistical aspects of genome-wide association studies. *Biom J.* 2008;50:8–28.
54. Satagopan JM, Verbel DA, Venkatraman ES, et al. Two-stage designs for gene-disease association studies. *Biometrics.* 2002;58:163–170.
55. Skol AD, Scott LJ, Abecasis GR, et al. Joint analysis is more efficient than replication-based analysis for two-stage genome-wide association studies. *Nat Genet.* 2006;38:209–213.
56. Yu K, Chatterjee N, Wheeler W, et al. Flexible design for following up positive findings. *Am J Hum Genet.* 2007;81:540–551.
57. Saito A, Kamatani N. Strategies for genome-wide association studies: optimization of study designs by the stepwise focusing method. *J Hum Genet.* 2002;47:360–365.
58. Wang H, Thomas DC, Pe'er I, et al. Optimal two-stage genotyping designs for genome-wide association scans. *Genet Epidemiol.* 2006;30:356–368.
59. Skol AD, Scott LJ, Abecasis GR, et al. Optimal designs for two-stage genome-wide association studies. *Genet Epidemiol.* 2007;31:776–788.
60. Muller HH, Pahl R, Schafer H. Including sampling and phenotyping costs into the optimization of two stage designs for genomewide association studies. *Genet Epidemiol.* 2007;31:844–852.

61. Kraft P, Chanock C. Study designs for genome-wide association studies. In: Rao DC, Charles Gu C, eds. *Genetic Dissection of Complex Traits*, 2nd ed. Boston: Academic Press; 2008. 465–504.
62. Service SK, Sandkuijl LA, Freimer NB. Cost-effective designs for linkage disequilibrium mapping of complex traits. *Am J Hum Genet.* 2003;72:1213–1220.
63. Kraft P. Efficient two-stage genome-wide association designs based on false positive report probabilities. *Pac Symp Biocomputing.* 2006;11:523–534.
64. Satagopan JM, Elston RC. Optimal two-stage genotyping in population-based association studies. *Genet Epidemiol.* 2003;25:149–157.
65. Satagopan JM, Venkatraman ES, Begg CB. Two-stage designs for gene-disease association studies with sample size constraints. *Biometrics.* 2004;60:589–597.
66. Nannya Y, Taura K, Kurokawa M, et al. Evaluation of genome-wide power of genetic association studies based on empirical data from the HapMap project. *Hum Mol Genet.* 2007;16:3494–3505.
67. Eberle MA, Ng PC, Kuhn K, et al. Power to detect risk alleles using genome-wide tag SNP panels. *PLoS Genet.* 2007;3:1827–1837.
68. Gail MH, Pfeiffer RM, Wheeler W, et al. Probability of detecting disease-associated single nucleotide polymorphisms in case-control genome-wide association studies. *Biostatistics.* 2008;9:201–215.
69. Gauderman WJ, Morrison JM. A computer program for power and sample size calculations for genetic-epidemiology studies, http://hydra.usc.edu/gxe. Accessed May 20, 2009.
70. Jorgenson E, Witte JS. Coverage and power in genomewide association studies. *Am J Hum Genet.* 2006;78:884–888.
71. Barrett JC, Cardon LR. Evaluating coverage of genome-wide association studies. *Nat Genet.* 2006;38:659–662.
72. de Bakker PI, Yelensky R, Pe'er I, et al. Efficiency and power in genetic association studies. *Nat Genet.* 2005;37:1217–1223.
73. Carlson CS, Eberle MA, Rieder MJ, et al. Additional SNPs and linkage-disequilibrium analyses are necessary for whole-genome association studies in humans. *Nat Genet.* 2003;33:518–521.
74. de Bakker PI, Burtt NP, Graham RR, et al. Transferability of tag SNPs in genetic association studies in multiple populations. *Nat Genet.* 2006;38:1298–1303.
75. Pe'er I, de Bakker PI, Maller J, et al. Evaluating and improving power in whole-genome association studies using fixed marker sets. *Nat Genet.* 2006;38:663–667.
76. Mueller JC, Lohmussaar E, Magi R, et al. Linkage disequilibrium patterns and tag SNP transferability among European populations. *Am J Hum Genet.* 2005;76:387–398.
77. Li M, Li C, Guan W. Evaluation of coverage variation of SNP chips for genome-wide association studies. *Eur J Hum Genet.* 2008;16:635–643.
78. Wollstein A, Herrmann A, Wittig M, et al. Efficacy assessment of SNP sets for genome-wide disease association studies. *Nucleic Acids Res.* 2007;35:e113.
79. Xu Z, Kaplan NL, Taylor JA. Tag SNP selection for candidate gene association studies using HapMap and gene resequencing data. *Eur J Hum Genet.* 2007;15:1063–1070.
80. Gu CC, Yu K, Ketkar S, et al. On transferability of genome-wide tag SNPs. *Genet Epidemiol.* 2008;32:89–97.
81. Hunter DJ, Kraft P. Drinking from the fire hose--statistical issues in genomewide association studies. *N Engl J Med.* 2007;357:436–439.
82. Samani NJ, Erdmann J, Hall AS, et al. Genomewide association analysis of coronary artery disease. *N Engl J Med.* 2007;357:443–453.
83. Wakefield J. Reporting and interpretation in genome-wide association studies. *Int J Epidemiol.* 2008;37:641–653.

84. Guedj M, Robelin D, Hoebeke M, et al. Detecting local high-scoring segments: a first-stage approach for genome-wide association studies. *Stat Appl Genet Mol Biol.* 2006;5:Article22.

85. Roeder K, Bacanu SA, Wasserman L, et al. Using linkage genome scans to improve power of association in genome scans. *Am J Hum Genet.* 2006;78:243–252.

86. Roeder K, Devlin B, Wasserman L. Improving power in genome-wide association studies: weights tip the scale. *Genet Epidemiol.* 2007;31:741–747.

87. Whittemore AS. A Bayesian false discovery rate for multiple testing. *J Appl Statist.* 2007;34:1–9.

88. Xu W, Schulze TG, DePaulo JR, et al. A tree-based model for allele-sharing-based linkage analysis in human complex diseases. *Genet Epidemiol.* 2006;30:155–169.

89. Chen GK, Witte JS. Enriching the analysis of genomewide association studies with hierarchical modeling. *Am J Hum Genet.* 2007;81:397–404.

90. Lewinger JP, Conti DV, Baurley JW, et al. Hierarchical Bayes prioritization of marker associations from a genome-wide association scan for further investigation. *Genet Epidemiol.* 2007;31:871–882.

91. Daniels J, Holmans P, Williams N, et al. A simple method for analyzing microsatellite allele image patterns generated from DNA pools and its application to allelic association studies. *Am J Hum Genet.* 1998;62:1189–1197.

92. Risch N, Teng J. The relative power of family-based and case-control designs for linkage disequilibrium studies of complex human diseases, I. DNA pooling. *Genome Res.* 1998;8:1273–1288.

93. Bansal A, van den Boom D, Kammerer S, et al. Association testing by DNA pooling: an effective initial screen. *Proc Natl Acad Sci USA.* 2002;99:16871–16874.

94. Mohlke KL, Erdos MR, Scott LJ, et al. High-throughput screening for evidence of association by using mass spectrometry genotyping on DNA pools. *Proc Natl Acad Sci USA.* 2002;99:16928–16933.

95. Barratt BJ, Payne F, Rance HE, et al. Identification of the sources of error in allele frequency estimations from pooled DNA indicates an optimal experimental design. *Ann Hum Genet.* 2002;66:393–405.

96. Pfeiffer RM, Rutter JL, Gail MH, et al. Efficiency of DNA pooling to estimate joint allele frequencies and measure linkage disequilibrium. *Genet Epidemiol.* 2002;22:94–102.

97. Sham P, Bader JS, Craig I, et al. DNA Pooling: a tool for large-scale association studies. *Nat Rev Genet.* 2002;3:862–871.

98. Feng Z, Prentice R, Srivastava S. Research issues and strategies for genomic and proteomic biomarker discovery and validation: a statistical perspective. *Pharmacogenomics.* 2004;5:709–719.

99. Zou G, Zhao H. The impacts of errors in individual genotyping and DNA pooling on association studies. *Genet Epidemiol.* 2004;26:1–10.

100. Craig DW, Huentelman MJ, Hu-Lince D, et al. Identification of disease causing loci using an array-based genotyping approach on pooled DNA. *BMC Genomics.* 2005;6:138.

101. Zuo Y, Zou G, Zhao H. Two-stage designs in case-control association analysis. *Genetics.* 2006;173:1747–1760.

102. Docherty SJ, Butcher LM, Schalkwyk LC, et al. Applicability of DNA pools on 500 K SNP microarrays for cost-effective initial screens in genomewide association studies. *BMC Genomics.* 2007;8:214.

103. Korol A, Frenkel Z, Cohen L, et al. Fractioned DNA pooling: a new cost-effective strategy for fine mapping of quantitative trait loci. *Genetics.* 2007;176:2611–2623.

104. Johnson T. Bayesian method for gene detection and mapping, using a case and control design and DNA pooling. *Biostatistics.* 2007;8:546–565.

105. Sebastiani P, Zhao Z, Abad-Grau MM, et al. A hierarchical and modular approach to the discovery of robust associations in genome-wide association studies from pooled DNA samples. *BMC Genet.* 2008;9:6.

106. Meaburn E, Butcher LM, Schalkwyk LC, et al. Genotyping pooled DNA using 100K SNP microarrays: a step towards genomewide association scans. *Nucleic Acids Res.* 2006;34:e27.

107. Wang S, Kidd KK, Zhao H. On the use of DNA pooling to estimate haplotype frequencies. *Genet Epidemiol.* 2003;24:74–82.

108. Macgregor S. Most pooling variation in array-based DNA pooling is attributable to array error rather than pool construction error. *Eur J Hum Genet.* 2007;15:501–504.

109. Pearson JV, Huentelman MJ, Halperin RF, et al. Identification of the genetic basis for complex disorders by use of pooling-based genomewide single-nucleotide-polymorphism association studies. *Am J Hum Genet.* 2007;80:126–139.

110. Kirov G, Zaharieva I, Georgieva L, et al. A genome-wide association study in 574 schizophrenia trios using DNA pooling. *Mol Psychiatry.* 2008. Available at: http://www.nature.com/mp/journal/vaop/ncurrent/abs/mp200833a.html

111. Steer S, Abkevich V, Gutin A, et al. Genomic DNA pooling for whole-genome association scans in complex disease: empirical demonstration of efficacy in rheumatoid arthritis. *Genes Immun.* 2007;8:57–68.

112. Kraft P, Yen YC, Stram DO, et al. Exploiting gene-environment interaction to detect genetic associations. *Hum Hered.* 2007;63:111–119.

113. Gauderman WJ. Sample size requirements for matched case-control studies of gene-environment interaction. *Stat Med.* 2002;21:35–50.

114. Piegorsch W, Weinberg C, Taylor J. Non-hierarchical logistic models and case-only designs for assessing susceptibility in population-based case-control studies. *Stat Med.* 1994;13:153–162.

115. Albert PS, Ratnasinghe D, Tangrea J, et al. Limitations of the case-only design for identifying gene-environment interactions. *Am J Epidemiol.* 2001;154:687–693.

116. Cheng KF. A maximum likelihood method for studying gene-environment interactions under conditional independence of genotype and exposure. *Stat Med.* 2006;25:3093–3109.

117. Chatterjee N, Carroll RJ. Semiparametric maximum likelihood estimation exploiting gene-environment independence in case-control studies. *Biometrika.* 2005;92:399–418.

118. Chatterjee N, Kalaylioglu Z, Carroll RJ. Exploiting gene-environment independence in family-based case-control studies: increased power for detecting associations, interactions and joint effects. *Genet Epidemiol.* 2005;28:138–156.

119. Mukherjee B, Zhang L, Ghosh M, et al. Semiparametric Bayesian analysis of case-control data under conditional gene-environment independence. *Biometrics.* 2007;63:834–844.

120. Mukherjee B, Chatterjee N. Exploiting gene-environment independence for analysis of case-control studies: an empirical Bayes approach to trade off between bias and efficiency. *Biometrics.* 2008;64:685–694.

121. Murcray C, Lewinger JP, Gauderman WJ. Gene-environment interaction in genome-wide association studies. *Am J Epidemiol.* 2009;169:219–226.

122. Witte JS, Gauderman WJ, Thomas DC. Asymptotic bias and efficiency in case-control studies of candidate genes and gene-environment interactions: Basic family designs. *Am J Epidemiol.* 1999;148:693–705.

123. Teng J, Risch N. The relative power of family-based and case-control designs for linkage disequilibrium studies of complex human diseases. II. Individual genotyping. *Genome Res.* 1999;9:234–241.

124. Pharoah PD, Dunning AM, Ponder BA, et al. Association studies for finding cancer-susceptibility genetic variants. *Nat Rev Cancer.* 2004;4:850–860.
125. Khoury MJ, Little J, Gwinn M, et al. On the synthesis and interpretation of consistent but weak gene-disease associations in the era of genome-wide association studies. *Int J Epidemiol.* 2007;36:439–445.
126. Garner C. Upward bias in odds ratio estimates from genome-wide association studies. *Genet Epidemiol.* 2007;31:288–295.
127. Zollner S, Pritchard JK. Overcoming the winner's curse: estimating penetrance parameters from case-control data. *Am J Hum Genet.* 2007;80:605–615.
128. Devlin B, Roeder K. Genomic control for association studies. *Biometrics.* 1999;55:997–1004.
129. Laird NM, Lange C. Family-based designs in the age of large-scale gene-association studies. *Nat Genet.* 2006;7:385–394.
130. Feng T, Zhang S, Sha Q. Two-stage association tests for genome-wide association studies based on family data with arbitrary family structure. *Eur J Hum Genet.* 2007;15:1169–1175.
131. Visscher PM, Andrew T, Nyholt DR. Genome-wide association studies of quantitative traits with related individuals: little (power) lost but much to be gained. *Eur J Hum Genet.* 2008;16:387–390.
132. Van Steen K, McQueen MB, Herbert A, et al. Genomic screening and replication using the same data set in family-based association testing. *Nat Genet.* 2005;37:683–691.
133. Ionita-Laza I, McQueen MB, Laird NM, et al. Genomewide weighted hypothesis testing in family-based association studies, with an application to a 100K scan. *Am J Hum Genet.* 2007;81:607–614.
134. Rakovski CS, Xu X, Lazarus R, et al. A new multimarker test for family-based association studies. *Genet Epidemiol.* 2007;31:9–17.
135. Xu X, Rakovski C, Laird N. An efficient family-based association test using multiple markers. *Genet Epidemiol.* 2006;30:620–626.
136. Ionita-Laza I, Perry GH, Raby BA, et al. On the analysis of copy-number variations in genome-wide association studies: a translation of the family-based association test. *Genet Epidemiol.* 2008;32:273–284.
137. Service S, DeYoung J, Karayiorgou M, et al. Magnitude and distribution of linkage disequilibrium in population isolates and implications for genome-wide association studies. *Nat Genet.* 2006;38:556–560.
138. Bonnen PE, Pe'er I, Plenge RM, et al. Evaluating potential for whole-genome studies in Kosrae, an isolated population in Micronesia. *Nat Genet.* 2006;38:214–217.
139. Patterson N, Hattangadi N, Lane B, et al. Methods for high-density admixture mapping of disease genes. *Am J Hum Genet.* 2004;74:979–1000.
140. Martinez-Marignac VL, Valladares A, Cameron E, et al. Admixture in Mexico City: implications for admixture mapping of type 2 diabetes genetic risk factors. *Hum Genet.* 2007;120:807–819.
141. Smith MW, O'Brien SJ. Mapping by admixture linkage disequilibrium: advances, limitations and guidelines. *Nat Rev Genet.* 2005;6:623–632.
142. Freedman ML, Haiman CA, Patterson N, et al. Admixture mapping identifies 8q24 as a prostate cancer risk locus in African-American men. *Proc Natl Acad Sci USA.* 2006;103:14068–14073.
143. Haiman CA, Patterson N, Freedman ML, et al. Multiple regions within 8q24 independently affect risk for prostate cancer. *Nat Genet.* 2007;39:638–644.
144. Luca D, Ringquist S, Klei L, et al. On the use of general control samples for genome-wide association studies: genetic matching highlights causal variants. *Am J Hum Genet.* 2008;82:453–463.

145. Chanock SJ, Manolio T, Boehnke M, et al. Replicating genotype-phenotype associations. *Nature.* 2007;447:655–660.

146. Clarke GM, Carter KW, Palmer LJ, et al. Fine mapping versus replication in whole-genome association studies. *Am J Hum Genet.* 2007;81:995–1005.

147. Thomas DC, Siemiatycki J, Dewar R, et al. The problem of multiple inference in studies designed to generate hypotheses. *Am J Epidemiol.* 1985;122:1080–1095.

148. Rebbeck TR, Martinez ME, Sellers TA, et al. Genetic variation and cancer: Improving the environment for publication of association studies. *Cancer Epidemiol Biomark Prev.* 2004;13:1985–1986.

149. Anonymous. Freely associating. *Nat Genet.* 1999;22:1–2.

150. Pe'er I, Yelensky R, Altshuler D, et al. Estimation of the multiple testing burden for genomewide association studies of nearly all common variants. *Genet Epidemiol.* 2008;32:381–385.

151. Conneely KN, Boehnke M. So many correlated tests, so little time! Rapid adjustment of P values for multiple correlated tests. *Am J Hum Genet.* 2007;81:1158–1168.

152. Dudbridge F, Gusnanto A. Estimation of significance thresholds for genomewide association scans. *Genet Epidemiol.* 2008;32:227–234.

153. Benjamini Y, Hochberg Y. Controlling the false discovery rate: a practical and powerful approach to multiple testing. *J Roy Statist Soc, Ser B.* 1995;57:289–300.

154. Forner K, Lamarine M, Guedj M, et al. Universal false discovery rate estimation methodology for genome-wide association studies. *Hum Hered.* 2008;65:183–194.

155. Dudoit S, Shaffer JP, Boldrick JC. Multiple hypothesis testing in microarray experiments. *Statist Sci.* 2003;18:71–103.

156. Wang H, Stram DO. Optimal two-stage genome-wide association designs based on False Discovery Rate. *Computat Statist Data Anal.* 2006;5:457–465.

157. Sun L, Crain RV, Paterson AD, et al. Stratified false discovery control for large-scale hypothesis testing with application to genome-wide association studies. *Genet Epidemiol.* 2006;30:519–530.

158. Sabatti C, Service S, Freimer N. False discovery rate in linkage and association genome screens for complex disorders. *Genetics.* 2003;164:829–833.

159. Storey JD. The positive false discovery rate: A Bayesian interpretation and the q-value. *Ann Stat.* 2003;31:2012–2035.

160. Wakefield J. A Bayesian measure of the probability of false discovery in genetic epidemiology studies. *Am J Hum Genet.* 2007;81:208–227.

161. Lin DY. Evaluating statistical significance in two-stage genomewide association studies. *Am J Hum Genet.* 2006;78:505–509.

162. Seaman SR, Muller-Myhsok B. Rapid simulation of P values for product methods and multiple-testing adjustment in association studies. *Am J Hum Genet.* 2005;76:399–408.

163. Lin DY. An efficient Monte Carlo approach to assessing statistical significance in genomic studies. *Bioinformatics.* 2005;21:781–787.

164. Dudbridge F, Koeleman BP. Efficient computation of significance levels for multiple associations in large studies of correlated data, including genomewide association studies. *Am J Hum Genet.* 2004;75:424–435.

165. Dudbridge F. A note on permutation tests in multistage association scans. *Am J Hum Genet.* 2006;78:1094–1095.

166. Huang BE, Amos CI, Lin DY. Detecting haplotype effects in genomewide association studies. *Genet Epidemiol.* 2007;31:803–812.

167. Su SY, Balding DJ, Coin LJ. Disease association tests by inferring ancestral haplotypes using a hidden markov model. *Bioinformatics.* 2008;24:972–978.

168. Stram DO, Pearce CL, Bretsky P, et al. Modeling and E-M estimation of haplotype-specific relative risks from genotype data for a case-control study of unrelated individuals. *Hum Hered.* 2003;55:179–190.

169. Evans DM, Cardon LR, Morris AP. Genotype prediction using a dense map of SNPs. *Genet Epidemiol.* 2004;27:375–384.

170. Schaid DJ. Linkage disequilibrium testing when linkage phase is unknown. *Genetics.* 2004;166:505–512.

171. Schaid DJ. Evaluating associations of haplotypes with traits. *Genet Epidemiol.* 2004;27:348–364.

172. Scheet P, Stephens M. A fast and flexible statistical model for large-scale population genotype data: applications to inferring missing genotypes and haplotypic phase. *Am J Hum Genet.* 2006;78:629–644.

173. Li N, Stephens M. Modeling linkage disequilibrium and identifying recombination hotspots using single-nucleotide polymorphism data. *Genetics.* 2003;165:2213–2233.

174. Stephens M, Scheet P. Accounting for decay of linkage disequilibrium in haplotype inference and missing-data imputation. *Am J Hum Genet.* 2005;76:449–462.

175. Browning BL, Browning SR. Efficient multilocus association testing for whole genome association studies using localized haplotype clustering. *Genet Epidemiol.* 2007;31:365–375.

176. Browning SR, Browning BL. Rapid and accurate haplotype phasing and missing-data inference for whole-genome association studies by use of localized haplotype clustering. *Am J Hum Genet.* 2007;81:1084–1097.

177. Marchini J, Howie B, Myers S, et al. A new multipoint method for genome-wide association studies by imputation of genotypes. *Nat Genet.* 2007;39:906–913.

178. Servin B, Stephens M. Imputation-based analysis of association studies: candidate regions and quantitative traits. *PLoS Genet.* 2007;3:e114.

179. Nicolae DL. Testing untyped alleles (TUNA)-applications to genome-wide association studies. *Genet Epidemiol.* 2006;30:718–727.

180. Wen X, Nicolae DL. Association studies for untyped markers with TUNA. *Bioinformatics.* 2008;24:435–437.

181. Xie R, Stram DO. Asymptotic equivalence between two score tests for haplotype-specific risk in general linear models. *Genet Epidemiol.* 2005;29:166–170.

182. Lin S, Chakravarti A, Cutler DJ. Exhaustive allelic transmission disequilibrium tests as a new approach to genome-wide association studies. *Nat Genet.* 2004;36:1181–1188.

183. Clayton DG, Walker NM, Smyth DJ, et al. Population structure, differential bias and genomic control in a large-scale, case-control association study. *Nat Genet.* 2005;37:1243–1246.

184. Pritchard JK, Stephens M, Rosenberg NA, et al. Association mapping in structured populations. *Am J Hum Genet.* 2000;67:170–181.

185. Yu J, Pressoir G, Briggs WH, et al. A unified mixed-model method for association mapping that accounts for multiple levels of relatedness. *Nat Genet.* 2005;38:203–208.

186. Price AL, Patterson NJ, Plenge RM, et al. Principal components analysis corrects for stratification in genome-wide association studies. *Nat Genet.* 2006;38:904–909.

187. Setakis E, Stimadel H, Balding D. Logistic regression protects against population structure in genetic association studies. *Gen Res.* 2006;16:290–296.

188. Marchini J, Donnelly P, Cardon LR. Genome-wide strategies for detecting multiple loci that influence complex diseases. *Nat Genet.* 2005;37:413–417.

189. Evans DM, Marchini J, Morris AP, et al. Two-stage two-locus models in genome-wide association. *PLoS Genet.* 2006;2:e157.

190. Kooperberg C, Leblanc M. Increasing the power of identifying gene x gene interactions in genome-wide association studies. *Genet Epidemiol.* 2008;32:255–263.

191. Musani SK, Shriner D, Liu N, et al. Detection of gene x gene interactions in genome-wide association studies of human population data. *Hum Hered.* 2007;63:67–84.

192. Nunkesser R, Bernholt T, Schwender H, et al. Detecting high-order interactions of single nucleotide polymorphisms using genetic programming. *Bioinformatics.* 2007;23:3280–3288.

193. Zhang Y, Liu JS. Bayesian inference of epistatic interactions in case-control studies. *Nat Genet.* 2007;39:1167–1173.

194. Thomas DC. The need for a comprehensive approach to complex pathways in molecular epidemiology. *Cancer Epidemiol Biomark Prev.* 2005;14:557–559.

195. Todd JA. Statistical false positive or true disease pathway? *Nat Genet.* 2006;38:731–733.

196. Rebbeck TR, Spitz M, Wu X. Assessing the function of genetic variants in candidate gene association studies. *Nat Rev Genet.* 2004;5:589–597.

197. Conti DV, Lewinger JP, Swan GE, Tyndale RF, Benowitz NL, Thomas PD. Using ontologies in hierarchical modeling of genes and exposures in biologic pathways. In: Swan GE, ed. *Phenotypes, Endophenotypes, and Genetic Studies of Nicotine Dependence.* Bethesda, MD: NCI Tobacco Monographs; 2009; 20:539–584.

198. Parl F, Crooke P, Conti DV, et al. Pathway-based methods in molecular cancer epidemiology. In: Rebbeck TR, Ambrosone CB, Shields PG, eds. *Fundamentals of Molecular Epidemiology.* New York: Informa Healthcare; 2008:189–204.

199. Los H, Postmus PE, Boomsma DI. Asthma genetics and intermediate phenotypes: a review from twin studies. *Twin Res.* 2001;4:81–93.

200. Croitoru ME, Cleary SP, Di Nicola N, et al. Association between biallelic and mono-allelic germline MYH gene mutations and colorectal cancer risk. *J Natl Cancer Inst.* 2004;96:1631–1634.

201. Freathy RM, Timpson NJ, Lawlor DA, et al. Common variation in the FTO gene alters diabetes-related metabolic traits to the extent expected given its effect on BMI. *Diabetes.* 2008;57:1419–1426.

202. Scuteri A, Sanna S, Chen WM, et al. Genome-wide association scan shows genetic variants in the FTO gene are associated with obesity-related traits. *PLoS Genet.* 2007;3:e115.

203. Frayling TM. Genome-wide association studies provide new insights into type 2 diabetes aetiology. *Nat Rev Genet.* 2007;8:657–662.

204. Ioannidis JP, Patsopoulos NA, Evangelou E. Heterogeneity in meta-analyses of genome-wide association investigations. *PLoS ONE.* 2007;2:e841.

205. Lindgren CM, McCarthy MI. Mechanisms of disease: genetic insights into the etiology of type 2 diabetes and obesity. *Nat Clin Pract Endocrinol Metab.* 2008;4:156–163.

206. Cheung VG, Spielman RS, Ewens KG, et al. Mapping determinants of human gene expression by regional and genome-wide association. *Nature.* 2005;437:1365–1369.

207. Morley M, Molony CM, Weber TM, et al. Genetic analysis of genome-wide variation in human gene expression. *Nature.* 2004;430:743–747.

208. Chen GK, Zheng T, Witte JS, et al. Genome-wide association analyses of expression phenotypes. *Genet Epidemiol.* 2007;31 Suppl 1:S7–S11.

209. Dixon AL, Liang L, Moffatt MF, et al. A genome-wide association study of global gene expression. *Nat Genet.* 2007;39:1202–1207.

210. Stranger BE, Forrest MS, Clark AG, et al. Genome-wide associations of gene expression variation in humans. *PLoS Genet.* 2005;1:e78.

211. Stranger BE, Nica AC, Forrest MS, et al. Population genomics of human gene expression. *Nat Genet.* 2007;39:1217–1224.

212. Pique-Regi R, Morrison J, Thomas DC. Bayesian hierchical modeling of means and covariances of gene expression data within families. *BMC Genet.* 2007;1 Suppl 1:S111.

213. Pompanon F, Bonin A, Bellemain E, et al. Genotyping errors: causes, consequences and solutions. *Nat Rev Genet.* 2005;6:847–859.
214. Plagnol V, Cooper JD, Todd JA, et al. A method to address differential bias in genotyping in large-scale association studies. *PLoS Genet.* 2007;3:e74.
215. Balding DJ. A tutorial on statistical methods for population association studies. *Nat Rev Genet.* 2006;7:781–791.
216. Weiss ST, Silverman EK, Palmer LJ. Case-control association studies in pharmacogenetics. *Pharmacogenomics J.* 2001;1:157–158.
217. Zou GY, Donner A. The merits of testing Hardy-Weinberg equilibrium in the analysis of unmatched case-control data: a cautionary note. *Ann Hum Genet.* 2006;70:923–933.
218. Moskvina V, Craddock N, Holmans P, et al. Effects of differential genotyping error rate on the type I error probability of case-control studies. *Hum Hered.* 2006;61:55–64.
219. Clayton D, Leung HT. An R package for analysis of whole-genome association studies. *Hum Hered.* 2007;64:45–51.
220. Van Steen K, Lange C. PBAT: a comprehensive software package for genome-wide association analysis of complex family-based studies. *Hum Genomics.* 2005;2:67–69.
221. Purcell S, Neale B, Todd-Brown K, et al. PLINK: a tool set for whole-genome association and population-based linkage analyses. *Am J Hum Genet.* 2007;81:559–575.
222. Foster MW, Sharp RR. Share and share alike: deciding how to distribute the scientific and social benefits of genomic data. *Nat Rev Genet.* 2007;8:633–639.
223. Boughman JA. Genomewide association studies data sharing: National Institutes of Health policy process. *Am J Hum Genet.* 2007;80:581–582.
224. International_Genetic_Epidemiology_Society. *Position Statement in response to "Request for Information (RFI): Proposed Policy for Sharing of Data obtained in NIH supported or conducted Genome-Wide Association Studies (GWAS)."* Available at http://www.genepi.org/. Accessed November 20, 2006.
225. Shen F, Huang J, Fitch KR, et al. Improved detection of global copy number variation using high density, non-polymorphic oligonucleotide probes. *BMC Genet.* 2008;9:27.
226. Lin CH, Huang MC, Li LH, et al. Genome-wide copy number analysis using copy number inferring tool (CNIT) and DNA pooling. *Hum Mutat.* 2008;29:1055–1062.
227. Kehrer-Sawatzki H. What a difference copy number variation makes. *Bioessays.* 2007;29:311–313.
228. Stranger BE, Forrest MS, Dunning M, et al. Relative impact of nucleotide and copy number variation on gene expression phenotypes. *Science.* 2007;315:848–853.
229. Skvortsov D, Abdueva D, Stitzer ME, et al. Using expression arrays for copy number detection: an example from E. coli. *BMC Bioinformatics.* 2007;8:203.
230. Estivill X, Armengol L. Copy number variants and common disorders: filling the gaps and exploring complexity in genome-wide association studies. *PLoS Genet.* 2007;3:1787–1799.
231. Sebat J, Lakshmi B, Malhotra D, et al. Strong association of de novo copy number mutations with autism. *Science.* 2007;316:445–449.
232. Franke L, de Kovel CG, Aulchenko YS, et al. Detection, imputation, and association analysis of small deletions and null alleles on oligonucleotide arrays. *Am J Hum Genet.* 2008;82:1316–1333.

9

The challenge of assessing complex gene–environment and gene–gene interactions

Peter Kraft and David J. Hunter

Introduction

Advances in the catalogs of common variation in the human genome over the past 5 years, combined with new high-throughput genotyping technologies, have dramatically improved our ability to test for associations between common genetic variation and disease risk. Genome-wide association studies (GWAS) have led to the identification of over 140 new genetic associations for over 40 diseases and phenotypes in the past 3 years alone. This burst of discovery shows no sign of abating as GWAS are conducted for additional phenotypes, and samples sizes are increased for most of the phenotypes already studied (1,2).

However, the majority of GWAS to date have tested for association between genetic markers and traits one marker at a time, averaging over variation at other loci and variation in environmental exposures. As a result, these studies may have failed to detect loci that only influence disease in the presence of a particular genetic or environmental exposure. Moreover, average measures of the effect of a functional polymorphism may obscure differences across strata defined by genetic and environmental factors that have important biologic, clinical, or public health implications.

"Gene–environment interaction" is widely accepted to be ubiquitous in the development of most complex human traits including diseases, in the broad sense that both "nature" and "nurture" contribute to the development of these traits. Similarly, the genetic influence on most common phenotypes and diseases is usually thought to result from the combined action of alleles in multiple genes ("gene–gene interaction"). In this chapter we discuss the study of gene–environment and gene–gene interactions in genetic epidemiology. We start with a review of the definition of statistical gene–environment interaction, which is what is typically measured and reported in genetic association studies, and contrast this with specific theoretical and general intuitive models for biologic interaction. We then describe how these concepts can be extended to the study of gene–gene interactions and review available study designs, with particular emphasis on estimating joint gene–environment and gene–gene effects.

Gene–Environment Interaction

Statistical Interaction

The most commonly used statistical definition of gene–environment interaction refers to departures from additivity of genetic and environmental effects on a particular outcome scale (3). For simple dichotomous genotypes (e.g., carrier $G = 1$ versus noncarrier $G = 0$) and exposures (exposed $E = 1$ versus unexposed $E = 0$), the pattern of mean trait values across the four gene–environment strata can be written as:

$$f\left(E[Y \mid G, E]\right) = \alpha + \beta_G G + \beta_E E + \beta_{GE} G \times E, \tag{9.1}$$

where $E[Y|G,E]$ denotes mean trait value conditional on G and E and $f(\cdot)$ is a link function that defines the outcome scale. For example, if Y is a binary outcome (1 if diseased, 0 if not) and $f(\cdot)$ is the identity $f(x) = x$, then Equation 9.1 models the probability of disease risk in terms of G and E on the absolute scale; if $f(\cdot)$ is the logit function $f(x) = \log(x/(1 - x))$, then Equation 9.1 models the probability of disease on the log odds scale. For a particular link $f(\cdot)$, G and E are said to interact statistically if $\beta_{GE} \neq 0$ (i.e., if $f(E[Y|G = 1,E = 1])$ is not simply the sum of the genetic effect β_G and the environmental effect β_E).

This dependence on the link function $f(\cdot)$ complicates the interpretation of formal statistical tests for "gene–environment interaction" (i.e., tests of the null hypothesis $\beta_{GE} = 0$), since different trait scales can lead to different conclusions about the presence or absence of a nonadditive interaction. For example, Figure 9.1 shows the same pattern of gene–environment effects on disease risk on two different scales: the absolute scale (left panel) and the log odds scale (right panel). In this case, there is no departure from additivity on the absolute risk scale, while there is a departure on the log odds scale. A converse example, with no departure from additivity on the log odds scale but a departure on the absolute scale, is easily constructed.

To make matters more confusing, departures from additivity on the absolute scale are often colloquially referred to as "additive interactions," and departures from additivity on the log odds or log risk scale as "multiplicative interactions." (Moreover, we note that the concept of "additive gene–environment (or gene–gene) interactions" is distinct from but related to the concept of an "additive genetic model." The latter refers to the coding of the genotype variable G in Equation 9.1: typically, when G is coded as the number of a particular allele carried (e.g., 0, 1, or 2 copies of the minor allele), the model is called additive. So as with gene–environment interactions, additivity depends on the outcome scale. In fact, different genetic models—that is, different codings for G—correspond to different *statistical* models for how alleles at the *same* locus interact. Gene–gene and gene–environment interactions refer to how alleles at *different* loci interact, or how alleles interact with exposure.)

Interaction patterns such as those presented in Figure 9.1 are sometimes called "removable" interactions, because a monotonic transformation of the outcome scale results in an additive model in G and E. There are other, "nonremovable"

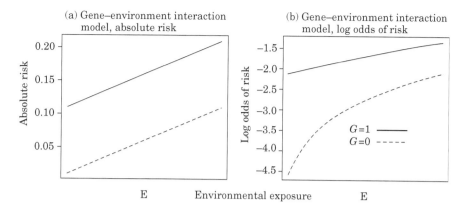

Figure 9.1   Gene–environment interaction model. The same gene–environment interaction model for a binary genotype and continuous environmental exposure on two different scales: (a) absolute risk, and (b) log odds of risk. Solid and dashed lines denote two distinct genotypes.

interactions that are not scale dependent, such as the "crossover" interaction illustrated in Figure 9.2c, or "pure interactions" where, for example, the risk genotype has no effect in unexposed individuals, but does have an effect among the exposed (Figure 9.2b). While one can test for a crossover effect explicitly (4), such interactions are quite rare in human epidemiology (5). There is no statistical test specific to pure interactions.

Biologic Interaction

On top of the confusion generated by different outcome scales potentially leading to different conclusions regarding statistical interaction, there is a disconnect between the statistical definition of interaction and notions of biologic interaction (3). Often, "biologic interaction" is not precisely defined but is based on the idea that the gene product and the exposure (or some downstream product of the exposure) physically interact. For example, carriers of the *CCR5*-delta32 mutation have lower risk of HIV infection, because the mutation changes the form of the CCR5 coreceptor, making it difficult for HIV to enter immune cells (6). It has also been hypothesized that carriers of the slow acetylator allele of the *NAT2* gene are less able to detoxify carcinogenic aromatic amines in tobacco smoke, leading to a "gene–smoking interaction" (7). However, it is very difficult to make inference about the underlying disease mechanism from the observed pattern of responses across genetic and environmental exposures, because the observed pattern will be consistent with many qualitatively different mechanisms (3,8). Strong assumptions are needed to interpret the absence or presence of statistical interaction on a particular scale as absence or presence of a biologic interaction in a specific biologic model (e.g., the "two hit" model for carcinogenesis).

Alternative definitions of "biologic interaction" are based on specific mathematical models for causality, such as the sufficient component cause or counterfactual

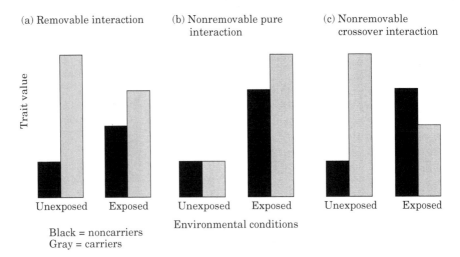

Figure 9.2   Three qualitative patterns of gene–environment interaction. The y-axis represents a trait value (e.g., mean height, disease prevalence, expected survival); the x-axis represents two environmental conditions; the black bars denote noncarriers and the gray bars represent carriers. (a) gives an example of a removable interaction. (b) and (c) are nonremovable interactions ("pure" and "crossover" interactions, respectively).

frameworks (3). Loosely, these approaches look for individuals whose response under different, counterfactual conditions (e.g., if they were born with genotype $G = 0$ instead of $G = 1$, holding all else constant) depends on both their genetic and environmental exposures. For example, the existence of individuals who would only become diseased if they were both carriers and exposed implies the presence of gene–environment interaction in this framework. For binary disease and binary genetic and environmental exposures, departures from additivity on the absolute scale imply the presence of interaction in the counterfactual sense just described (although additivity does not generally imply the absence of interactions) (3,9,10). However, the qualitative implications of detecting interactions in this sense are not clear, other than stating that for some people, both genetic and environmental risk factors play a role in disease development—something widely assumed *a priori* (in fact by definition) for complex diseases.

Allowing for Gene–Environment Interaction Without Testing for Specific Forms of Interaction

Regardless of the presence of statistical interaction or difficulties inferring biologic mechanism from epidemiologic data, it will often be useful to calculate and present stratum-specific trait summaries: for example, for continuous traits, mean values of the trait for each category of gene–environment cross-classification. For binary traits, absolute incidence rates (if available) or relative measures such as relative risks or odds ratios can be displayed. This presentation has the advantage of being "closest to the data" while allowing the reader to observe the joint action of genotype and environment (11). In the case of binary phenotypes and binary environmental and genetic exposures all the relevant data can be displayed in a 2×4 table. This presentation may be particularly helpful in evaluating the public health benefits of different screening or intervention programs (e.g., conducting genetic testing only among the exposed; only intervening to remove exposure among carriers; or a general program to remove exposure regardless of genotype) (3,12).

A similar approach that leverages potential gene–environment interaction without being tied to a particular scale (or drawing inference about gene–environment interaction *per se*) has been proposed in the context of testing large numbers of genetic variants for association with a trait (e.g., a GWAS) (13). Rather than testing each variant for association marginally (i.e., ignoring data on environmental exposures), or testing for gene–environment interaction on some scale (i.e., testing the null hypothesis that $\beta_{GE} = 0$), this approach tests the joint null of no main genetic effect or gene environment interaction ($\beta_{G} = \beta_{GE} = 0$). This test has been shown to be more powerful than either the marginal test or the standard test for "multiplicative interaction" (i.e., departure from additivity on the log odds scale) in a wide range of situations, such as when the risk variant has a modest effect among unexposed and a larger effect among exposed (13).

Analytic Issues

The scale used to define gene–environment interactions is often chosen for convenience, for example, the logistic model is typically used to analyze case-control data, making the log odds scale a natural choice. Departures from additivity on the log odds scale for two binary factors (carriers versus noncarriers, exposed versus nonexposed) are easily tested in logistic regression by including the product of the genetic and environmental exposure variables in the odds model: the statistical significance of this "interaction term" can be assessed using standard Wald, score, or likelihood ratio tests. We note that departures from additivity on the absolute scale can also be tested using case-control data using the interaction contrast ratio (3), although this approach may be particularly sensitive to the rare disease assumption (required so that odds ratios approximate relative risks) (14).

For more finely cross-classified data (multiple exposure categories, multiallelic markers such as haplotypes of linked SNPs or multiple genes), it is usually impractical to fit such saturated models, as many strata will have few observations, leading to highly variable (or inestimable) stratum-specific parameter estimates (11,15). Thus, some form of statistical modeling is necessary. For example, hierarchical modeling could be employed, treating the "first-level" stratum-specific parameters as random variables and then regressing these on "second-stage" variables (e.g., groupings of genes based on function or decompositions of environmental exposures into their biologically active components) (16,17). Additional levels of external knowledge (e.g., biochemical characteristics or predictions of the functional impact of specific types of gene variants) can be included in the "second-stage" model; these improve model fit if the details are accurate and relevant, but may harm model fit if they are not. Alternatively, a large number of potential working models based on simple "main effects plus cross-product interaction" parameterizations can be explored and summarized using Bayesian model-selection and model-averaging techniques (18).

The principal objective of both these approaches is to reduce overfitting while producing parsimonious and useful summaries of the data. Another approach ("toxicokinetic modeling") builds very detailed models for the joint action of genes and environmental exposures (e.g., by incorporating information on substrate-specific kinetics for different enzyme isoforms derived from *in vitro* experiments) (19).

Difficulties

In practice, the utility of gene–environment interaction analyses may be limited in observational studies by several factors. First, there are limits on what we can measure. Setting aside exposure measurement error and the fact that we often do not genotype the causal variant directly (20), what we observe are patterns of distribution of the gene, environmental exposure, and trait at the population level. As we discussed above, this is very different from the concept of biologic gene–environment interaction, where, for example, gene product and (some metabolite of) the exposure physically interact in some biochemical reaction.

Observational studies are also limited by our inability to assign subjects randomly to extreme exposures that rarely occur naturally (or not at all), and our inability to study subjects with genetic variants that do not occur naturally (because they have been fixed by selective pressure). In an article in the early 1970s, before the advent of dense marker maps and cheap genotyping, Richard Lewontin presented a number of plausible gene–environment interaction patterns (Figure 9.3) and discussed how they made it difficult to apportion the causes of a trait to either genes or the environment (21). His examples remain instructive now that it is possible to measure germline variants of interest directly. For example, if environmental exposure is limited to "typical" ranges as in Figure 9.3a or 9.3b, then there will either be no genetic main effect or gene–environment interaction, or these will be quite difficult to detect. If only the high extremes (>95th percentile, say) of the exposure are sampled, then for the pattern described in Figure 9.3a, there will be genetic and environmental main effects but no (or a very small) gene–environment interaction effect. On the other hand, if low and high extremes (<5th and >95th percentile) are sampled, then there will be a strong, nonremovable gene–environment interaction. The fact that we may not sample "interesting" environmental or genetic variation has implications for study design, and also for the replication of observed gene–environment interactions: if the range of exposures in the replication study does not overlap the range in the original study, it will be hard to interpret the presence or absence of a gene–environment interaction as either successful or failed replication.

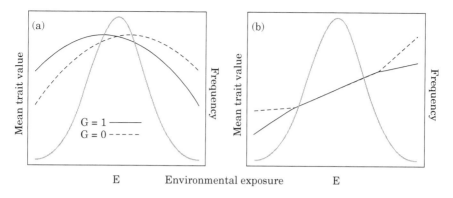

Figure 9.3 An illustration of two patterns of gene–environment interaction. The form (or presence) of gene–environment interaction depends on the range of observed environmental exposures. The y-axis represents mean trait value for subjects with two genotypes (solid and dashed lines) at different exposure levels. The gray line shows the distribution (probability density) of the environmental exposure.

When the goal of the study is to screen a number of polymorphisms for those that are associated with a trait, the relative power of the marginal genetic and gene–environment interaction analyses will depend on the true pattern of joint gene–environment effects (13). For many patterns, the marginal test will have greater power than the gene–environment interaction test, even when there is a gene–environment interaction. Finally, large sample sizes (with accurate, preferably prospectively collected environmental exposure measures) are needed to detect modest gene–environment interaction effects. This presents a serious practical challenge; gene–environment interactions are harder to demonstrate in the observational world of human epidemiology than in the experimental setting of the agricultural research station.

Despite these challenges, consideration of gene–environment interactions can be useful in the design, analysis, and interpretation of genetic association studies. In situations where a particular polymorphism with known functional effects is studied—for example, polymorphisms in drug metabolizing genes like *CYP2C9* or carcinogen metabolism genes like *NAT27*—investigators may hypothesize *a priori* that the polymorphism has a stronger effect on (or only influences) the studied trait in the presence of a certain exposure. Hence, depending on the goal of the study, investigators may wish to oversample (or even exclusively sample) subjects who have been exposed (4), or analyze genetic effects stratified by exposure. Even when there are no specific hypotheses about specific polymorphisms based on known function—as in candidate gene studies using "tagging SNPs" or genome-wide association studies—allowing for gene–environment interaction may boost power to detect polymorphisms associated with the trait (13). Often, simply describing the pattern of disease risks or trait averages across levels of genotype and environmental exposure can be very useful, regardless of testing specific hypotheses pertaining to statistical gene–environment interaction, since such information may have important clinical or public health implications.

Mendelian Randomization

If the primary scientific question is not "*how* do this gene and this environmental exposure jointly affect trait distribution?" but simply "*does* this environmental exposure affect trait distribution?" then it may occasionally suffice to test the marginal association between gene and disease—even if the principal focus is on the environmental factor. This is the concept behind "Mendelian randomization," illustrated in Figure 9.4a (22–24). If an environmental exposure influences risk of disease through an intermediate phenotype that is also influenced by variation in a known gene, then the association between the exposure and disease can be tested by examining the association between the gene variant and the disease. This approach—a form of instrumental variable analysis (25) that was first proposed to test whether the relationship between serum cholesterol and cancer is causal by studying variants in the apolipoprotein A (*APOE*) gene that alter serum cholesterol levels (26,27)—has several potential advantages. Accurate measurements of the environmental exposure may be unavailable or prohibitively expensive, and genotypes are not susceptible to recall bias and other forms of confounding that may give rise to biased exposure–disease associations, particularly in retrospective case-control studies. However, other sources of bias are possible in genetic association studies that might give rise to spurious genotype–phenotype associations (e.g., confounding by ethnicity or "population stratification") (23,28,29). Furthermore, the genetic variant may influence more than one intermediate phenotype, so the association between variation in the gene and disease may not be due to the same intermediate phenotype affected by the environmental exposure, as illustrated in Figure 9.4b; thus, an association between the genetic variant and the trait may not guarantee a causal role for the exposure. Perhaps the major limitation of the concept of Mendelian randomization is that most environmental exposures of interest do not have an intermediate phenotype that is also known to be substantially influenced by a specific genotype; thus the number of instances in which this strategy can be employed is limited.

(a) In this scenario, finding an (induced) association between the gene (G) and disease (D) supports the hypothesis for a causal relationship between environmental exposure (E) and disease.

(b) In this scenario, an association between the gene and disease gives no information about the causality of the exposure.

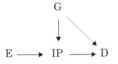
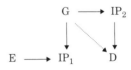

Figure 9.4   A cartoon depiction of "Mendelian randomization" after Thomas and Conti (23).

Gene–Gene Interaction

Background

Similar to the broad agreement that both "nature" and "nurture" influence most phenotypes and diseases, risk of most common diseases is thought to be influenced by variants in multiple genes, and sometimes multiple variants in each gene. Just as with gene–environment interaction, there is some confusion surrounding the term "gene–gene interaction" and the nearly synonymous term "epistasis": sometimes they are used in the sense of biologic interaction (e.g., the gene products physically interact), and sometimes they are used to refer to departures from an additive statistical model. Cordell (30) provides an excellent overview of how the term "epistasis" is used in different contexts. ("Epistasis" roughly translates as "resting upon" and refers to the dependency of one gene on the action of another "modifier" gene.)

Studies of model organisms and animal husbandry give many examples of epistatic interactions (31). For example, in 1905, Bateson et al. (32) proposed that rooster comb shape was a Mendelian trait governed by two loci, such that the effect of the first locus depended on the genotype at the second (Table 9.1). If the genotype at locus *B* is BB or Bb, then the a allele at locus *A* is recessive to the A allele and determines whether the comb shape is "walnut" or "pea." If the genotype at locus *B* is bb, however, the a allele determines whether comb shape is "rose" or "single."

We make two points here that may limit the relevance of this example (and many others from studies involving crosses of inbred strains of experimental plants or animals we could have cited) to the study of gene–gene interactions in complex human

Table 9.1 Examples of a single trait determined by the interaction of two unlinked loci: rooster comb shape and (hypothetical) risk for complex disease

Genotype	Frequency in Randomly Mating Population	Rooster Comb Shape	Disease Risk
AABB	$q_A^2 q_B^2$	Walnut	ρ
AABb	$q_A^2 2 q_B (1 - q_B)$	Walnut	ρ
AAbb	$q_A^2 (1 - q_B)^2$	Rose	$\rho\, RR_1$
AaBB	$2 q_A (1 - q_A) q_B^2$	Walnut	ρ
AaBb	$4 q_A (1 - q_A) q_B (1 - q_B)$	Walnut	ρ
Aabb	$2 q_A (1 - q_A) (1 - q_B)^2$	Rose	$\rho\, RR_1$
aaBB	$(1 - q_A)^2 q_B^2$	Pea	$\rho\, RR_2$
aaBb	$(1 - q_A)^2 2 q_B (1 - q_B)$	Pea	$\rho\, RR_2$
Aabb	$(1 - q_A)^2 (1 - q_B)^2$	Single	$\rho\, RR_3$

q_A and q_B are population allele frequencies of locus A and B respectively. ρ is baseline disease risk; the RR_i are relative risks, relative to baseline category of A-B-genotypes. Rooster comb is but one example of a two-locus interaction that interestingly has the same segregation ratios as two independently segregating recessive traits in the F_2 generation from a AABB×aabb cross (9:3:3:1). In the comb example, the a allele is recessive to A regardless of genotype at locus *B* (and similarly for the b allele). Other interaction models deviate from the classical segregation ratios (31). For example, coat color in Labrador retrievers exhibits "recessive epistasis"—the F_2 generation has on average 9/16 dogs with black coats, 4/16 with yellow, and 3/16 with brown (33).

traits. First, although more than one locus is involved, comb shape in roosters as described by Bateson et al. is a Mendelian trait with complete penetrance: genotype aabb always produces single comb shape, AABB always produces walnut, and so on. For complex human traits, the relationship between genotype and phenotype is, by definition, not so simple. If instead of comb shape, Table 9.1 described four categories of diabetes risk, we would not expect differences across strata to be strikingly large. (Based on effect sizes of replicated risk loci (34,35) the relative risk comparing the highest risk category to the lowest risk category would arguably be less than five.) This would make it difficult to identify the underlying pattern of risk in studies of modest sample size.

Second, although comb shape is determined by the interaction of loci A and B, this does not necessarily mean that locus A (or locus B) has no detectable marginal association with comb shape. For example, the probability that a rooster with aa genotype has single comb shape is q_B^2, while for Aa or AA genotypes the probability is 0. Similarly, for the hypothetical diabetes risk model, the incidence of diabetes for subjects with aa genotype is ρ $(q_B^2 RR_3 + (1 - q_B^2) RR_2)$, while for those with Aa or AA genotypes it is ρ $(q_B^2 RR_1 + (1 - q_B^2))$. Depending on the allele frequencies at locus B (and the relative risks RR_1, RR_2, and RR_3) there may be a detectable marginal association between locus A and diabetes risk. Thus, if we simply wished to know whether locus A or locus B is somehow associated with disease risk, it may suffice to test for marginal association with each locus separately. It is possible that the joint effects at the loci may "cancel out" so that there is no marginal effect at either locus—as would be the case if $q_A = q_B = 0.5$, $RR_1 = RR_2 = 0.5$, and $RR_3 = 4$. However, as with "crossover" gene–environment interactions, replicated examples of such canceling epistatic interactions are rare, and there is little evidence for such interactions from segregation studies or multilocus association studies (36–38).

Analytic Issues

Analogous to the discussion of gene–environment interactions above, the joint distribution of two dichotomized genotypes (i.e., carriers of variant A, carriers of variant B) can be displayed in a simple cross-classified table. However, once more than two or three gene variants are involved, some form of statistical modeling will almost certainly be necessary. A major difference in the study of gene–gene interactions is that the high-throughput genotyping technologies that have been such a boon to gene discovery efforts give rise to a vast number of potential two-way interactions, to say nothing of the number of three-way and higher-order interactions. At least in the two-way case for quantitative traits, however, simulation studies have shown that the problem is computationally tractable. An exhaustive search over all possible two-way interactions may have more power to detect certain types of gene–gene interaction than initially screening for marginal effects (39). The relative power of the two approaches depends on the genetic architecture of disease (allele frequencies, multilocus genotype relative risks). As sketched above, even for some joint genotype effects that we would consider "interactions" (i.e., departures from additivity on some scale) the marginal approach can be more powerful to detect one or the other locus than the joint test incorporating interaction. (A nice feature of the exhaustive two-locus scan proposed by Marchini et al. (39,40) and the analogous "joint" gene–environment test proposed by Kraft et al. (13) is that they incorporate possible gene–gene or gene–environment interactions, but are not tests of interaction *per se*. Thus they are scale-free and retain good power to detect associations between genetic loci and a trait, regardless of the form of the "interaction.")

In the context of a GWA study, an exhaustive search of higher than second-order interactions remains impractical, both due to computational limitations and the multiple testing burden. However, it may be possible to examine higher-order interactions in more focused, hypothesis-driven analyses that concentrate on a (relatively) small number of genes with a common function or on a particular metabolic pathway. Again, we caution that biologic interaction (e.g., in the sense that the product of gene *A* catalyzes the reaction transforming the products of genes *B* and *C* into metabolite D) does not imply the presence of statistical interaction on a particular scale or *vice versa* (31,41). For example, biomathematical modeling suggests that the folate metabolism pathway is quite robust to changes in the efficacy of multiple gene products along the pathway (42,43).

There are three general approaches to "pathway analysis," which we define as jointly testing whether a group of markers is associated with a trait. The first does not consider statistical interactions *per se*. Instead, it aggregates evidence for marginal association across multiple markers in the pathway, looking for an excess of modestly significant loci beyond what we would expect by chance. Examples of this approach include the Rank Truncated Product Method (44) or the Admixture Maximum Likelihood Method (45). This approach leverages the possibility that there are many genes that affect a trait, each with a subtle impact—so that although no individual marker achieves strong statistical significance, many tested loci may show suggestive evidence for association.

The second approach is similar to the first, in that it provides a test of the global null hypothesis that none of the tested markers is associated with the studied trait, but this approach allows for statistical interactions among the loci. For example, if the number of tested loci is small, this approach might entail a simple likelihood ratio test, comparing a model with additive main effects for each SNP plus all pairwise (product) interaction terms to a null model containing none of these genetic variables. (In fact, in the case of two loci, this is a variant of the approach proposed by Marchini et al.) (39) However, for more than a few loci, the large number of parameters in this model makes it impractical. More sophisticated approaches, such as U-statistics (46), Tukey's one-degree-of-freedom interaction test (47), or kernel machines (48) avoid this problem by effectively constraining the model mapping multilocus genotypes to mean trait (or risk) values, while still allowing for departures from a purely additive model across loci.

An important advantage of both these methods is that they involve only a single test for the entire pathway, eliminating the multiple-testing problem. A potential disadvantage of these techniques is that they do not identify the particular markers that are associated with the trait; they simply tell us that some (unspecified) variants in the "pathway" are associated with the disease, somehow. Alternatively, a "pathway" approach may increase power and interpretation of genetic association studies by narrowing the scope of exhaustive scans for pairwise gene–gene interaction. We note that network modeling strategies that combine information from multiple sources—for example, gene expression profiles and protein–protein interactions—may be particularly useful, as they may provide information about genetic cross talk and coregulation not contained in hand-annotated gene lists based on putative function (49). Similar techniques applied to mice resulted in the identification of gene networks that are perturbed by obesity susceptibility loci, potentially narrowing the space in which to search for gene–gene interactions (50).

Finally, data mining techniques—such as stepwise regression, Classification and Regression Trees (CART), Multivariate Adaptive Regression Splines (MARS) (51), neural networks, logic regression (52), Multifactor Dimensionality Reduction (MDR) (53), "focused interaction testing" (54), random forests (55), and so on—can be used to build explicit, typically highly nonlinear models linking genotype to phenotype. The potential advantage of these methods is that, because of their flexibility, they may be more powerful to detect nonadditive genotype–phenotype associations, and may better capture the true (statistical) relationship between genotype and phenotype. There are also important disadvantages to these methods, however:

- Many of these methods replace the strong assumption of additive effects across loci (on some scale) with other, equally strong assumptions of nonadditivity. CART, for example, can easily capture "pure" interactions but cannot easily capture additive effects. On the other hand, some of the more flexible methods (e.g., Random Forests) are "black boxes"—the final model is quite complicated and difficult to describe.
- Many of these methods are computationally intensive, so that analysis of more than a few hundred (or even a few dozen) markers becomes practically impossible.
- Evaluating statistical significance of the final model can be quite tricky, and it is easy to generate wildly exaggerated, highly statistically significant p-values if one is not careful. For example, testing the significance of the final model from a stepwise regression procedure in the same data set used to generate the model will lead to (drastic) underestimates of the corresponding p-value. Typically, some form of permutation procedure is used to ensure valid test size. (This only increases computational complexity.)
- Similarly, estimates of predictive accuracy (concordance between the predicted and actual trait values) will be overestimated if the final model is evaluated in the same data set used to construct it (the "training" data set) (56). Accuracy should ideally be estimated in an independent "test" data set, or, failing that,

using a procedure that approximates performance in a test data set, such as cross-validation (57,58).

- Although simulations have shown that these data mining tools can detect multilocus models underlying Mendelian traits (with complete penetrance and/or no phenocopies, as in the rooster comb example), it is not clear that they are as effective in detecting models that involve subtle differences in risk across genotypes.

There is a large and expanding body of literature on these methods for the analysis of genetic data. The book on statistical learning methods by Hastie, Tibshirani, and Friedman (58) provides a good introduction to general principles of data mining approaches—for example, the important distinction between training-set and test-set error—as well as particular analytic methods such as MARS and neural networks.

At the end of the day, the relative effectiveness of these different approaches to "pathway analysis" will depend on the genetic architecture of the studied trait—which we do not know *a priori*. While it may be true that the simplest answer to a problem is always wrong (59), this does not mean that simple, abstracted approaches cannot provide important, novel insights (60). It seems appropriate to "let 100 flowers bloom" and analyze multilocus genetic data using diverse approaches, each of which is sensitive to a different range of alternative hypotheses. But this ecumenical approach still requires discipline, lest too many weeds overwhelm the flowers. Initial results from multilocus analyses should be reported modestly and tentatively, both in terms of their empirical support—they will require replication in independent studies—and in terms of their qualitative, biologic interpretation (61,62).

Study Designs for Gene–Environment and Gene–Gene Interactions

Until recently, many genetic association studies have collected limited (if any) information on lifestyle and environmental exposures. Similarly, traditional epidemiologic studies have collected detailed information on exposure but have mostly not collected blood samples or other sources of DNA that would allow joint study of genes and environment. With a greater recent focus on multifactoral and common complex diseases, there is increased awareness of the need to collect high-quality information on both genes and environmental exposures in a population-based context (63).

In Table 9.2, the three main genetic association designs are summarized—family-based, retrospective case-control, and prospective cohort—in terms of characteristics relevant to the study of gene–environment interaction. These include susceptibility to population stratification bias, recall bias, survivor bias, the availability of prospectively collected plasma phenotypes (or other relevant biomarkers), and sample size. We briefly summarize these designs and their characteristics here;

Table 9.2   Select characteristics of well-established designs for gene–environment interaction

Characteristic	Study Design		
	Family-Based	Case-Control	Cohort
Potential for population stratification bias	Nil if appropriately analyzed	Varies; minimizable via good design, genomic control or principal components analysis	Varies but generally less than retrospective case-control study; minimizable via good design, genomic control or principal components analysis
Potential for recall bias	Moderate to high	Moderate to high	Nil
Potential for survivor bias	Moderate to high	Moderate to high	Nil if DNA samples obtained at baseline and disease ascertainment is complete; moderate if DNA is not obtained at baseline and participation in DNA collection low
Ability to use plasma phenotypes in cases	No	No	Yes
Required sample sizes achievable?	Common disease: yes Rare disease: yes	Common disease: yes Rare disease: yes	Common disease: yes with adequate follow-up Rare disease: no, unless multiple studies are pooled

more detailed comparisons can be found in other references (64–66). We also touch on a fourth, nontraditional design that can be used to study gene–environment or gene–gene interaction: the case-only design.

Family-Based Designs

Family-based association designs test the association between gene variants and traits by comparing cases to observed related controls or "pseudocontrols" generated from parental genotype data (67–70). By conditioning on shared genetic descent, these designs are protected against population stratification bias (if appropriately analyzed). In some situations, family-based tests of gene–environment interaction may be more powerful than tests in population-based studies (71). However, it may be more difficult to collect both genetic and environmental information on parents (especially for late-onset diseases where the parents may be deceased by the age at which their offspring develop disease) or find appropriate sibling controls (68,69). Family-based tests generally have less power for genetic main effects than an equivalent population-based case-control study with the same number of genotyped subjects.

Because information on environmental exposures (when collected at all) and genotypes is usually collected retrospectively, family-based studies share the problems of recall bias and survivor bias with retrospective case-control studies.

Case-Control Designs

In retrospective case-control studies, data on environmental exposures and DNA samples, and other biologic samples for biomarker studies, are obtained after diagnosis of disease in the cases. Selection bias may occur if the controls do not represent the source population that gave rise to the cases. Survival bias occurs if the case subjects who are interviewed and genotyped differ systematically from those who cannot be interviewed or genotyped (e.g., case subjects with a particularly lethal genetic form of the disease may die before they can be identified and enrolled in the study). Population stratification bias can arise if the allele frequencies of the variants being tested vary by ethnicity, and the ethnicity of the controls is substantially different from that of the cases. In most studies, substantial bias due to population stratification can be avoided by following basic principles of good study design and matching on self-reported ethnicity (29,72,73). This may not suffice for recently admixed populations, such as African or Hispanic Americans, however (28,74). "Genomic control" methods that test and adjust for population stratification are available, although they require subjects to be genotyped on a second panel of putatively anonymous markers (75–77)—preferably "ancestry informative markers," markers that are known to have different allele frequency in the ancestral populations, for example, Spanish, Native Americans, and Africans for Hispanic Americans (78). If large-scale genotyping data are available (as in a GWAS), then the leading principal components of genetic variation typically capture population structure and can be used as covariates in regression analyses or as stratifying variables (79,80).

The major problem in case-control studies with respect to gene–environment interactions is likely to be misclassification of information on environmental exposures. "Recall bias" arises if cases report their prediagnosis exposure histories differently after their diagnosis relative to what they would have reported prior to diagnosis. Although this differential misclassification may not actually bias the estimates of certain gene–environment interaction parameters (81), it will certainly bias the main effect estimates of environmental factors and reduce the power to detect interactions (82–84).

Finally, if biomarkers are measured in samples collected after disease diagnosis, it is difficult to assess the association of such biomarkers (which might in principle represent better measurements of long-term environmental exposure, e.g., plasma nutrient levels) with disease risk, as the biomarkers may be influenced by the disease, its treatment, or lifestyle changes made in response to diagnosis.

Cohort Designs

In prospective cohort studies, information on environmental exposures is collected at baseline (and ideally at repeated intervals during follow-up) on a large number of subjects. Preferably, DNA and biomarker information should also be collected at baseline. In prospective studies without banked samples, DNA for nested case-control studies could be obtained from cases (and matched controls) as soon as possible after diagnosis. If follow-up rates and participation rates in DNA collection are high, this minimizes the potential for selection bias, as the underlying cohort that gave rise to the cases is unambiguous, though if the interval between diagnosis and DNA collection is long, then the potential for survivor bias exists. Assuming follow-up and participation in nested case-control studies does not differ by ethnicity, the potential for population stratification bias is reduced compared with retrospective case-control studies, although it may still be a concern in some populations and require the use of appropriate statistical genomic control methods.

The principal difficulty with prospective studies is the large number of subjects who must be enrolled and followed to ensure a sufficient number of cases for an adequately powered analysis. This limits individual cohorts to the study of relatively common diseases such as myocardial infarction, diabetes, or the more common cancers such as breast, prostate, lung, and colorectal cancers. Individual prospective studies are not likely to yield sufficient power to study rare diseases, although consortia of cohorts may permit pooling of data across multiple studies in order to boost sample size. Furthermore, prospective studies may be less practical when additional subtyping of diseases is required that is not available from conventional clinical records, for example, studies of tumors with different gene expression profiles (85). These subtypes may be rare, and it may also be difficult to obtain the fresh tissue required to conduct the ancillary studies needed in order to classify cases.

Case-Only Design

The case-only design is based on the following observation: if two factors—say two genetic loci or a genetic locus and an environmental exposure—are independently distributed in the study base, and the odds ratio comparing individuals exposed to both factors with those exposed to neither is equal to the product of the odds ratios for subjects exposed to only one or the other factor, then the two factors should be independent among cases (86–88). In other words, one can test for "interaction" (specifically, departures from a log-additive odds model) simply by testing whether the two factors are associated among cases. Somewhat surprisingly, the case-only design can be more powerful than the standard case-control analysis based on logistic regression, even though the former test does not use data on controls.

In fact, it is not the case-only design *per se* that leads to the increase in efficiency, but the assumption of independence between the two factors in the study base. One can modify standard family-based and case-control analyses to incorporate this assumption (89–91). The resulting analyses achieve the same power gains as the case-only analyses, and they retain the ability to estimate main effects of either factor (which cannot be estimated in the case only analysis).

However, all of these analyses are sensitive to the assumption of independence between the two tested factors, that is, gene–gene or gene–environment independence in the study base. Even a slight association can lead to inflated type I error rates for the interaction test (87). In some situations, the assumption of gene–environment independence may be justified; in others—such as where "exposure" is a behavior or trait under genetic control, or when there is population stratification—the independence assumption may not be justified. Similarly, for many pairs of genetic markers, the assumption of independence may be justified—for example, if the markers are on different chromosomes—while for other, linked markers, it may not be. A recently proposed empirical Bayesian approach retains much of the power of the analyses based on the gene–gene or gene–environment independence assumption while retaining approximately correct type I error rates (92). It does so by weighting the results from the standard and modified analyses according to the evidence for or against the hypothesis of gene–environment independence. This approach and other analytic and design issues are reviewed in more depth in the recent article by Chatterjee and Mukherjee (4). Although the case-only design has the substantial attraction of not requiring collection of data from controls, the fact that it is only possible to test for interactions, and not main effects, is a drawback in the current era, in which we are still actively attempting to discover novel genetic and environmental main effects.

Sample Size and Power

Whether formally testing for gene–environment interaction, estimating stratum-specific parameters, or using data mining techniques to explore unsuspected gene–environment combinations, sample size is a major limiting factor in the study of gene–environment interaction. A well-known rule of thumb states that the sample size necessary to detect a departure from a multiplicative model for the joint effect of two variables (on the odds ratio or relative risk scale) is at least four times the sample size needed to evaluate the main effect of either of the variables (93). Given that environmental exposures are almost certainly measured with some error, thus attenuating estimates of both environmental main effects and gene–environment interactions, the necessary sample sizes are even larger (82–84). Small sample size is a key reason why so many genetic associations have failed to replicate and are likely to be false positives (94,95). Many recent studies have had sample sizes on the order of a few hundreds of cases, which means that only the strongest interaction effects will be replicable, and most "significant" interactions are likely to be false positives.

Because of the cost and time involved in large-scale cohort studies, case-control studies are an attractive option for the study of gene–environment interaction for rare diseases. Still, there are several long-term efforts to put together and follow new large cohorts with archived biosamples (including DNA) and information on environmental exposures (including lifestyle and anthropometric measures). The U.K. Biobank, for example, has currently enrolled over 350,000 subjects out of a target of 500,000 (96). In the short term, one way to increase the power of existing cohort studies is to pool data across multiple studies. For example, the NCI Breast and Prostate Cancer Cohort Consortium (BPC3) is currently examining gene–environment interactions in over 8,000 cases of breast cancer, and 10,000 cases of prostate cancer, pooled across ten prospective studies with over 800,000 people under follow-up and over 7 million person-years of follow-up already accrued (97).

An additional benefit of this approach is the increased coordination among participating studies, across disciplinary lines (linking genomics and epidemiology), and among the epidemiologic community in general. Combining information across multiple cohorts, provided measurements are made similarly across studies, can mitigate the main weakness of prospective studies (lack of incident cases) while capitalizing on the methodologic strengths of the prospective design.

Conclusions

Investment in studies of the joint and independent action of genes and environmental exposures may pay off in terms of increased knowledge about disease biology. Even if there are limits to inferences about biologic mechanism that can be drawn from epidemiologic studies, leveraging information about gene–environment and gene–gene interaction may lead to the discovery of loci that would not have been detected if individual genetic variants were studied in isolation. This may lead to better treatments (e.g., by suggesting drug targets) or means of chemoprevention (98). It also has been suggested that studies of gene–environment interaction may inform targeted "personalized prevention" strategies. Indeed, the assumption behind the direct-to-consumer marketing of high-dimensional genotyping from "SNP chips" is that knowledge of increased susceptibility to one or more of a range of diseases will permit personalized counseling on steps to take to reduce this risk. This scenario assumes that the relevant gene–environment interactions have been discovered and replicated, so that this advice is evidence-based (99). However, as described above, we are only at the beginning of understanding gene–environment interactions for a few diseases, and the challenges to detecting and validating hypothesized interactions are formidable (100). Affordably genotyping hundreds of thousands of SNPs or sequencing an individual's genome may be the easy part; the hard part will be making sense of it all and using this knowledge wisely.

For both gene–environment and gene–gene interactions, much larger sample sizes than are currently available are likely to be needed. For gene–environment interactions, the availability and accuracy of environmental measurements is also a major limiting factor. While statistical techniques to analyze complex pathways are likely to improve, large, well-designed studies with accurate measurements will be needed in which to employ the improved methods. Continued attention to, and funding of, appropriate epidemiologic studies will be key to unlocking the puzzle of interactions in complex diseases.

References

1. Manolio TA, Brooks LD, Collins FS. A HapMap harvest of insights into the genetics of common disease. *J Clin Invest.* 2008;118(5):1590–1605.
2. Hunter DJ, Kraft P. Drinking from the fire hose—statistical issues in genomewide association studies. *N Engl J Med.* 2007;357(5):436–439.
3. Rothman K, Greenland S. *Modern Epidemiology.* Philadelphia: Lippincott-Raven; 1998.

4. Chatterjee N, Mukherjee B. Statistical approaches to gene-gene and gene-environment interactions. In: Rebbeck TR, Ambrosone CB, Shields PG, eds. *Molecular Epidemiology: Applications in Cancer and Other Human Diseases.* New York: Informa Healthcare; 2008:145–168.

5. Weiss NS. Subgroup-specific associations in the face of overall null results: should we rush in or fear to tread? *Cancer Epidemiol Biomarkers Prev.* 2008;17(6):1297–1299.

6. de Silva E, Stumpf MP. HIV and the CCR5-Delta32 resistance allele. *FEMS Microbiol Lett.* 2004;241(1):1–12.

7. Rothman N, Wacholder S, Caporaso NE, et al. The use of common genetic polymorphisms to enhance the epidemiologic study of environmental carcinogens. *Biochim Biophys Acta.* 2001;1471(2):C1–C10.

8. Thompson W. Effect modification and the limits of biological inference from epidemiologic data. *J Clin Epidemiol.* 1991;44:221–232.

9. VanderWeele TJ, Robins JM. The identification of synergism in the sufficient-component-cause framework. *Epidemiology.*2007;18(3):329–339.

10. VanderWeele TJ, Robins JM. Four types of effect modification: a classification based on directed acyclic graphs. *Epidemiology.* 2007;18(5):561–568.

11. Botto L, Khoury M. Facing the challenge of complex genotypes and gene-environment interaction: the basic epidemiologic units in case-control and case-only designs. In: Khoury M, Little J, Burke W, eds. *Human Genome Epidemiology: A Scientific Foundation for Using Genetic Information to Improve Health and Prevent Disease.* Oxford: Oxford University Press; 2004:111–126.

12. Khoury MJ, Yang Q, Gwinn M, et al. An epidemiologic assessment of genomic profiling for measuring susceptibility to common diseases and targeting interventions. *Genet Med.* 2004;6(1):38–47.

13. Kraft P, Yen YC, Stram DO, et al. Exploiting gene-environment interaction to detect genetic associations. *Hum Hered.* 2007;63(2):111–119.

14. Kalilani L, Atashili J. Measuring additive interaction using odds ratios. *Epidemiol Perspect Innov.* 2006;3:5.

15. Robins J, Greenland S. The role of model selection in causal inference from nonexperimental data. *Am J Epidemiol.* 1986;123:392–402.

16. Hung RJ, Brennan P, Malaveille C, et al. Using hierarchical modeling in genetic association studies with multiple markers: application to a case-control study of bladder cancer. *Cancer Epidemiol Biomarkers Prev.* 2004;13(6):1013–1021.

17. Aragaki CC, Greenland S, Probst-Hensch N, et al. Hierarchical modeling of gene-environment interactions: estimating NAT2 genotype-specific dietary effects on adenomatous polyps. *Cancer Epidemiol Biomarkers Prev.* 1997;6(5):307–314.

18. Conti DV, Cortessis V, Molitor J, et al. Bayesian modeling of complex metabolic pathways. *Hum Hered.* 2003;56(1-3):83–93.

19. Cortessis V, Thomas DC. Toxicokinetic genetics: an approach to gene-environment and gene-gene interactions in complex metabolic pathways. *IARC Sci Publ.* 2004(157):127–150.

20. Hein R, Beckmann L, Chang-Claude J. Sample size requirements for indirect association studies of gene-environment interactions (G × E). *Genet Epidemiol.* 2008;32(3):235–245.

21. Lewontin RC. Annotation: the analysis of variance and the analysis of causes. *Am J Hum Genet.* 1974;26(3):400–411.

22. Clayton D, McKeigue PM. Epidemiological methods for studying genes and environmental factors in complex diseases. *Lancet.* 2001;358(9290):1356–1360.

23. Thomas DC, Conti DV. Commentary: the concept of "Mendelian Randomization." *Int J Epidemiol.* 2004;33(1):21–25.

24. Brennan P. Commentary: Mendelian randomization and gene-environment interaction. *Int J Epidemiol.* 2004;33(1):17–21.

25. Nitsch D, Molokhia M, Smeeth L, et al. Limits to causal inference based on Mendelian randomization: a comparison with randomized controlled trials. *Am J Epidemiol.* 2006;163(5):397–403.

26. Keavney B. Commentary: Katan's remarkable foresight: genes and causality 18 years on. *Int J Epidemiol.* 2004;33(1):11–14.

27. Katan MB. Commentary: Mendelian Randomization, 18 years on. *Int J Epidemiol.* 2004;33(1):10–11.

28. Thomas D, Witte J. Point: Population stratification: a problem for case-control studies of candidate gene associations? *Cancer Epidemiol Prev Biom.* 2002;11:505–512.

29. Wacholder S, Rothman N, Caporaso N. Counterpoint: bias from population stratification is not a major threat to the validity of conclusions from epidemiological studies of common polymorphisms and cancer. *Cancer Epidemiol Biomarkers Prev.* 2002;11:513–520.

30. Cordell HJ. Epistasis: what it means, what it doesn't mean, and statistical methods to detect it in humans. *Hum Mol Genet.* 2002;11(20):2463–2468.

31. Phillips PC. The language of gene interaction. *Genetics.* 1998;149(3):1167–1171.

32. Bateson W, Saunders E, Punnet R, et al. *Reports to the Evolution Committee of the Royal Society, Report II.* London: Harrison and Sons; 1905.

33. Hartwell L, Goldberg M, Reynolds A, et al. *Genetics: from Genes to Genomes.* New York: McGraw-Hill; 2006.

34. Zeggini E, Weedon MN, Lindgren CM, et al. Replication of genome-wide association signals in UK samples reveals risk loci for type 2 diabetes. *Science.* 2007;316(5829):1336–1341.

35. Frayling TM. Genome-wide association studies provide new insights into type 2 diabetes aetiology. *Nat Rev Genet.* 2007;8(9):657–662.

36. Hill WG, Goddard ME, Visscher PM. Data and theory point to mainly additive genetic variance for complex traits. *PLoS Genet.* 2008;4(2):e1000008.

37. Kathiresan S, Melander O, Anevski D, et al. Polymorphisms associated with cholesterol and risk of cardiovascular events. *N Engl J Med.* 2008;358(12):1240–1249.

38. Maller J, George S, Purcell S, et al. Common variation in three genes, including a noncoding variant in CFH, strongly influences risk of age-related macular degeneration. *Nat Genet.* 2006;38(9):1055–1059.

39. Marchini J, Donnelly P, Cardon LR. Genome-wide strategies for detecting multiple loci that influence complex diseases. *Nat Genet.* 2005;37(4):413–417.

40. Evans DM, Marchini J, Morris AP, et al. Two-stage two-locus models in genome-wide association. *PLoS Genet.* 2006;2(9):e157.

41. Hartman JLt, Garvik B, Hartwell L. Principles for the buffering of genetic variation. *Science.* 2001;291(5506):1001–1004.

42. Reed MC, Nijhout HF, Sparks R, et al. A mathematical model of the methionine cycle. *J Theor Biol.* 2004;226(1):33–43.

43. Nijhout HF, Reed MC, Budu P, et al. A mathematical model of the folate cycle: new insights into folate homeostasis. *J Biol Chem.* 2004;279(53):55008–55016.

44. Dudbridge F, Koeleman BP. Rank truncated product of *P*-values, with application to genomewide association scans. *Genet Epidemiol.* 2003;25(4):360–366.

45. Tyrer J, Pharoah PD, Easton DF. The admixture maximum likelihood test: a novel experiment-wise test of association between disease and multiple SNPs. *Genet Epidemiol.* 2006;30(7):636–643.

46. Schaid DJ, McDonnell SK, Hebbring SJ, et al. Nonparametric tests of association of multiple genes with human disease. *Am J Hum Genet.* 2005;76(5):780–793.

47. Chatterjee N, Kalaylioglu Z, Moslehi R, et al. Powerful multilocus tests of genetic association in the presence of gene-gene and gene-environment interactions. *Am J Hum Genet.* 2006;79(6):1002–1016.

48. Kwee LC, Liu D, Lin X, et al. A powerful and flexible multilocus association test for quantitative traits. *Am J Hum Genet.* 2008;82(2):386–397.

49. Tasan M, Tian W, Hill DP, et al. An en masse phenotype and function prediction system for *Mus musculus. Genome Biol.* 2008;9(Suppl 1):S8.

50. Chen Y, Zhu J, Lum PY, et al. Variations in DNA elucidate molecular networks that cause disease. *Nature.* 2008;452(7186):429–435.

51. Cook NR, Zee RY, Ridker PM. Tree and spline based association analysis of gene-gene interaction models for ischemic stroke. *Stat Med.* 2004;23(9):1439–1453.

52. Kooperberg C, Ruczinski I. Identifying interacting SNPs using Monte Carlo logic regression. *Genet Epidemiol.* 2005;28(2):157–170.

53. Ritchie MD, Hahn LW, Roodi N, et al. Multifactor-dimensionality reduction reveals high-order interactions among estrogen-metabolism genes in sporadic breast cancer. *Am J Hum Genet.* 2001;69(1):138–147.

54. Millstein J, Conti D, Gilliland F, et al. A testing framework for identifying susceptibility genes in the presence of epistasis. *Am J Hum Genet.* 2006;78:15–27.

55. Bureau A, Dupuis J, Falls K, et al. Identifying SNPs predictive of phenotype using random forests. *Genet Epidemiol.* 2005;28(2):171–182.

56. Kraft P. Curses—winner's and otherwise—in genetic epidemiology. *Epidemiology.* 2008;19(5):649–651; discussion 57–58.

57. Ioannidis JP. Microarrays and molecular research: noise discovery? *Lancet.* 2005;365(9458):454–455.

58. Hastie T, Tibshirani R, Friedman J. *The Elements of Statistical Learning.* New York: Springer; 2001.

59. Ulrich CM, Nijhout HF, Reed MC. Mathematical modeling: epidemiology meets systems biology. *Cancer Epidemiol Biomarkers Prev.* 2006;15(5):827–829.

60. Haldane JB. A defense of beanbag genetics. *Perspect Biol Med.* 1964;7:343–359.

61. Ioannidis JP. Why most published research findings are false. *PLoS Med.* 2005; 2(8):e124.

62. Ioannidis JP. Why most discovered true associations are inflated. *Epidemiology.* 2008; 19(5):640–648.

63. Thomas D. Genetic epidemiology with a capital "E." *Genet Epidemiol.* 2000; 19:289–300.

64. Garcia-Closas M, Wacholder S, Caporaso N, et al. Inference issues in cohort and case-control studies of genetic effects and gene-environment interactions. In: Khoury M, Little J, Burke W, eds. *Human Genome Epidemiology: A Scientific Foundation for Using Genetic Information to Improve Health and Prevent Disease.* Oxford: Oxford University Press; 2004:127–144.

65. Caparaso N, Rothman N, Wacholder W. Case-control studies of common alleles and environmental factors. *Monogr Natl Cancer Inst.* 1999;26:25–30.

66. Langholz B, Rothman N, Wacholder S, et als. Cohort studies for characterizing measured genes. *Monogr Natl Cancer Inst.* 1999;26:39–42.

67. Laird N, Horvath S, Xu X. Implementing a unified approach to family-based tests of association. *Genet Epidemiol.* 2000;19(Suppl1):S36–S42.

68. Weinberg C, Umbach D. Choosing a retrospective design to assess joint genetic and environmental contributions to risk. *Am J Epidemiol.* 2000;152:197–203.

69. Witte JS, Gauderman WJ, Thomas DC. Asymptotic bias and efficiency in case-control studies of candidate genes and gene-environment interactions: basic family designs. *Am J Epidemiol.* 1999;148:693–705.

70. Cordell HJ, Barratt BJ, Clayton DG. Case/pseudocontrol analysis in genetic association studies: a unified framework for detection of genotype and haplotype associations, gene-gene and gene-environment interactions, and parent-of-origin effects. *Genet Epidemiol.* 2004;26(3):167–185.
71. Gauderman W. Sample size requirements for matched case-control studies of gene-environment interaction. *Stat Med.* 2001;15:35–50.
72. Cardon LR, Palmer LJ. Population stratification and spurious allelic association. *Lancet.* 2003;361(9357):598–604.
73. Wacholder S, Rothman N, Caporaso N. Population stratification in epidemiologic studies of common genetic variants and cancer: quantification of bias. *JNCI.* 2000;92:1151–1158.
74. Kittles RA, Chen W, Panguluri RK, et al. CYP3A4-V and prostate cancer in African Americans: causal or confounding association because of population stratification? *Hum Genet.* 2002;110(6):553–560.
75. Devlin B, Roeder K. Genomic control for association studies. *Biometrics.* 1999;55:997–1004.
76. Reich D, Goldstein D. Detecting association in a case-control study while correcting for population stratification. *Genet Epidemiol.* 2001;20:4–16.
77. Pritchard J, Stephens M, Rosenberg N, et al. Association mapping in structured populations. *Am J Hum Genet.* 2000;67:170–181.
78. Bonilla C, Parra EJ, Pfaff CL, et al. Admixture in the Hispanics of the San Luis Valley, Colorado, and its implications for complex trait gene mapping. *Ann Hum Genet.* 2004;68(Pt 2):139–153.
79. Price AL, Patterson NJ, Plenge RM, et al. Principal components analysis corrects for stratification in genome-wide association studies. *Nat Genet.* 2006;38(8):904–909.
80. Luca D, Ringquist S, Klei L, et al. On the use of general control samples for genome-wide association studies: genetic matching highlights causal variants. *Am J Hum Genet.* 2008;82(2):453–463.
81. Garcia-Closas M, Thompson WD, Robins JM. Differential misclassification and the assessment of gene-environment interactions in case-control studies. *Am J Epidemiol.* 1998;147(5):426–433.
82. Garcia-Closas M, Rothman N, Lubin J. Misclassification in case-control studies of gene-environment interactions: assessment of bias and sample size. *Cancer Epidemiol Biomarkers Prev.* 1999;8(12):1043–1050.
83. Wong MY, Day NE, Luan JA, et al. The detection of gene-environment interaction for continuous traits: should we deal with measurement error by bigger studies or better measurement? *Int J Epidemiol.* 2003;32(1):51–57.
84. Wong MY, Day NE, Luan JA, et al. Estimation of magnitude in gene-environment interactions in the presence of measurement error. *Stat Med.* 2004;23(6):987–998.
85. Carr KM, Rosenblatt K, Petricoin EF, et al. Genomic and proteomic approaches for studying human cancer: prospects for true patient-tailored therapy. *Hum Genomics.* 2004;1(2):134–140.
86. Piegorsch W, Weinberg C, Taylor J. Non-hierarchical logistic models and case-only designs for assessing susceptibility in population-based case-control studies. *Stat Med.* 1994;13:153–162.
87. Liu X, Fallin MD, Kao WH. Genetic dissection methods: designs used for tests of gene-environment interaction. *Curr Opin Genet Dev.* 2004;14(3):241–245.
88. Goldstein A, Andrieu N. Detection of interaction involving identified genes: available study designs. *Monogr Natl Cancer Inst.* 1999;26:49–54.
89. Chatterjee N, Kalaylioglu Z, Carroll R. Exploiting gene-environment independence in family-based case-control studies: increased power for detecting associations, interactions and joint effects. *Genet Epidemiol.* 2005;28(2):138–156.

90. Chatterjee N, Carroll R. Semiparametric maximum likelihood estimation exploiting gene-environment independence. *Biometrika.* 2005;92:399–418.
91. Umbach D, Weinberg C. Designing and analysing case-control studies to exploit independence of genotype and exposure. *Stat Med.* 1997;16:1731–1743.
92. Mukherjee B, Ahn J, Gruber SB, et al. Tests for gene-environment interaction from case-control data: a novel study of type I error, power and designs. *Genet Epidemiol.* 2008;32(7):615–626.
93. Smith PG, Day NE. The design of case-control studies: the influence of confounding and interaction effects. *Int J Epidemiol.* 1984;13(3):356–365.
94. Wacholder S, Chanock S, Garcia-Closas M, et al. Assessing the probability that a positive report is false: an approach for molecular epidemiology studies. *J Natl Cancer Inst.* 2004;96(6):434–442.
95. Hirschhorn JN, Altshuler D. Once and again-issues surrounding replication in genetic association studies. *J Clin Endocrinol Metab.* 2002;87(10):4438–4441.
96. UK Biobank Homepage, http://www.ukbiobank.ac.uk/. Accessed August 15, 2009.
97. Hunter DJ, Riboli E, Haiman CA, et al. A candidate gene approach to searching for low-penetrance breast and prostate cancer genes. *Nat Rev Cancer.* 2005;5(12):977–985.
98. Hunter DJ, Altshuler D, Rader DJ. From Darwin's finches to canaries in the coalmine—mining the genome for new biology. *N Engl J Med.* 2008;358(26):2760–2763.
99. Haga SB, Khoury MJ, Burke W. Genomic profiling to promote a healthy lifestyle: not ready for prime time. *Nat Genet.* 2003;34(4):347–350.
100. Hunter DJ, Khoury MJ, Drazen JM. Letting the genome out of the bottle—will we get our wish? *N Engl J Med.* 2008;358(2):105–107.

10

STrengthening the REporting of Genetic
Association studies (STREGA)—an extension
of the STROBE statement

*Julian Little, Julian P. T. Higgins, John P. A. Ioannidis,
David Moher, France Gagnon, Erik von Elm, Muin J. Khoury,
Barbara Cohen, George Davey Smith, Jeremy Grimshaw,
Paul Scheet, Marta Gwinn, Robin E. Williamson,
Guang Yong Zou, Kimberley Hutchings, Candice Y. Johnson,
Valerie Tait, Miriam Wiens, Jean Golding, Cornelia
M. van Duijn, John McLaughlin, Andrew Paterson, George
Wells, Isabel Fortier, Matthew Freedman, Maja Zecevic,
Richard A. King, Claire Infante-Rivard, Alexandre Stewart,
and Nick Birkett*

Introduction

The rapidly evolving evidence on genetic associations is crucial to integrating human genomics into the practice of medicine and public health (1,2). Genetic factors are likely to affect the occurrence of numerous common diseases, and therefore identifying and characterizing the associated risk (or protection) will be important in improving the understanding of etiology and potentially for developing interventions based on genetic information. The number of publications on the associations between genes and diseases has increased tremendously; with more than 34,000 published articles, the annual number has more than doubled between 2001 and 2008 (3,4). Articles on genetic associations have been published in about 1,500 journals and in several languages.

Despite the many similarities between genetic association studies and "classical" observational epidemiologic studies (i.e., cross-sectional, case-control, and cohort) of lifestyle and environmental factors, genetic association studies present several specific challenges including an unprecedented volume of new data (5,6) and the likelihood of very small individual effects. Genes may operate in complex pathways with

Reprinted from *Annals of Internal Medicine, European Journal of Clinical Investigation, European Journal of Epidemiology, Genetic Epidemiology, Human Genetics, Journal of Clinical Epidemiology, and PLoS Medicine.*

gene–environment and gene–gene interactions (7). Moreover, the current evidence base on gene–disease associations is fraught with methodologic problems (8–10). Inadequate reporting of results, even from well-conducted studies, hampers assessment of a study's strengths and weaknesses, and hence the integration of evidence (11).

Although several commentaries on the conduct, appraisal, and/or reporting of genetic association studies have so far been published (12–39), their recommendations differ. For example, some papers suggest that replication of findings should be part of the publication (12,13,16,17,23,26,34–36) whereas others consider this suggestion unnecessary or even unreasonable (21,40–44). In many publications, the guidance has focused on genetic association studies of specific diseases (14,15,17,19,22,23,25,26,31–38) or the design and conduct of genetic association studies (13–15,17,19,20,22,23,25,30–32,35,36) rather than on the quality of the reporting.

Despite increasing recognition of these problems, the quality of reporting genetic association studies needs to be improved (45–49). For example, an assessment of a random sample of 315 genetic association studies published from 2001 to 2003 found that most studies provided some qualitative descriptions of the study participants (e.g., origin and enrolment criteria), but reporting of quantitative descriptors, such as age and sex, was variable (49). In addition, completeness of reporting of methods that allow readers to assess potential biases (e.g., number of exclusions or number of samples that could not be genotyped) varied (49). Only some studies described methods to validate genotyping or mentioned whether research staff were blinded to outcome. The same problems persisted in a smaller sample of studies published in 2006 (49). Lack of transparency and incomplete reporting have raised concerns in a range of health research fields (11,50–53) and poor reporting has been associated with biased estimates of effects in clinical intervention studies (54).

The main goal of this article is to propose and justify a set of guiding principles for reporting results of genetic association studies. The epidemiology community has recently developed the STrengthening the Reporting of OBservational studies in Epidemiology (STROBE) Statement for cross-sectional, case-control, and cohort studies (55,56). Given the relevance of general epidemiologic principles for genetic association studies, we propose recommendations in an extension of the STROBE Statement called the STrengthening the REporting of Genetic Association studies (STREGA) Statement. The recommendations of the STROBE Statement have a strong foundation because they are based on empirical evidence on the reporting of observational studies, and they involved extensive consultations in the epidemiologic research community (56). We have sought to identify gaps and areas of controversy in the evidence regarding potential biases in genetic association studies. With the recommendations, we have indicated available empirical or theoretical work that has demonstrated or suggested that a methodological feature of a study can influence the direction or magnitude of the association observed. We acknowledge that for many items, no such evidence exists. The intended audience for the reporting guideline is broad and includes epidemiologists, geneticists, statisticians, clinician scientists, and laboratory-based investigators who undertake genetic association studies. In addition, it includes "users" of such studies who wish to understand the basic premise, design, and limitations of genetic association studies in order to interpret the results. The field of genetic associations is evolving very rapidly with the advent of genome-wide association investigations, high-throughput platforms assessing genetic variability beyond common single nucleotide polymorphisms (SNPs) (e.g., copy number variants, rare variants), and eventually routine full sequencing of samples from large populations. Our recommendations are not intended to support or oppose the choice of any particular study design or method. Instead, they are intended to maximize the transparency, quality, and completeness of reporting of what was done and found in a particular study.

Methods

A multidisciplinary group developed the STREGA Statement by using literature review, workshop presentations and discussion, and iterative electronic correspondence after the workshop. Thirty-three of 74 invitees participated in the STREGA workshop in Ottawa, Ontario, Canada, in June 2006. Participants included epidemiologists, geneticists, statisticians, journal editors, and graduate students.

Before the workshop, an electronic search was performed to identify existing reporting guidance for genetic association studies. Workshop participants were also asked to identify any additional guidance. They prepared brief presentations on existing reporting guidelines, empirical evidence on reporting of genetic association studies, the development of the STROBE Statement, and several key areas for discussion that were identified on the basis of consultations before the workshop. These areas included the selection and participation of study participants, rationale for choice of genes and variants investigated, genotyping errors, methods for inferring haplotypes, population stratification, assessment of Hardy–Weinberg equilibrium (HWE), multiple testing, reporting of quantitative (continuous) outcomes, selectively reporting study results, joint effects, and inference of causation in single studies. Additional resources to inform workshop participants were the HuGENet handbook (57,58), examples of data extraction forms from systematic reviews or meta-analyses, articles on guideline development (59,60), and the checklists developed for STROBE. To harmonize our recommendations for genetic association studies with those for observational epidemiologic studies, we communicated with the STROBE group during the development process and sought their comments on the STREGA draft documents. We also provided comments on the developing STROBE Statement and its associated explanation and elaboration document (56).

Results

In Table 10.1, we present the STREGA recommendations, an extension to the STROBE checklist (55) for genetic association studies. The resulting STREGA

Table 10.1 STREGA reporting recommendations, extended from STROBE statement

Item	Item Number	STROBE Guideline	Extension for Genetic Association Studies (STREGA)
Title and Abstract	1	(a) Indicate the study's design with a commonly used term in the title or the abstract. (b) Provide in the abstract an informative and balanced summary of what was done and what was found.	
Introduction			
Background rationale	2	Explain the scientific background and rationale for the investigation being reported.	
Objectives	3	State specific objectives, including any prespecified hypotheses.	*State if the study is the first report of a genetic association, a replication effort, or both.*
Methods			
Study design	4	Present key elements of study design early in the paper.	
Setting	5	Describe the setting, locations and relevant dates, including periods of recruitment, exposure, follow-up, and data collection.	
Participants	6	(a) **Cohort study**—Give the eligibility criteria, and the sources and methods of selection of participants. Describe methods of follow-up. **Case-control study**—Give the eligibility criteria, and the sources and methods of case ascertainment and control selection. Give the rationale for the choice of cases and controls. **Cross-sectional study**—Give the eligibility criteria, and the sources and methods of selection of participants.	*Give information on the criteria and methods for selection of subsets of participants from a larger study, when relevant.*

(Continued)

Table 10.1 Continued

Item	Item Number	STROBE Guideline	Extension for Genetic Association Studies (STREGA)
		(b) **Cohort study**—For matched studies, give matching criteria and number of exposed and unexposed. **Case-control study**—For matched studies, give matching criteria and the number of controls per case.	
Variables	7	(a) Clearly define all outcomes, exposures, predictors, potential confounders, and effect modifiers. Give diagnostic criteria, if applicable.	(b) *Clearly define genetic exposures (genetic variants) using a widely used nomenclature system. Identify variables likely to be associated with population stratification (confounding by ethnic origin).*
Data sources/ measurement	8*	(a) For each variable of interest, give sources of data and details of methods of assessment (measurement). Describe comparability of assessment methods if there is more than one group.	(b) *Describe laboratory methods, including source and storage of DNA, genotyping methods and platforms (including the allele calling algorithm used, and its version), error rates and call rates. State the laboratory/center where genotyping was done. Describe comparability of laboratory methods if there is more than one group. Specify whether genotypes were assigned using all of the data from the study simultaneously or in smaller batches.*
Bias	9	(a) Describe any efforts to address potential sources of bias.	(b) *For quantitative outcome variables, specify if any investigation of potential bias resulting from pharmacotherapy was undertaken. If relevant, describe the nature and magnitude of the potential bias, and explain what approach was used to deal with this.*
Study size	10	Explain how the study size was arrived at.	
Quantitative variables	11	Explain how quantitative variables were handled in the analyses. If applicable, describe which groupings were chosen, and why.	*If applicable, describe how effects of treatment were dealt with.*

Statistical methods	12	(a) Describe all statistical methods, including those used to control for confounding.
		(b) Describe any methods used to examine subgroups and interactions.
		(c) Explain how missing data were addressed.
		(d) **Cohort study**—If applicable, explain how loss to follow-up was addressed.
		Case-control study—If applicable, explain how matching of cases and controls was addressed.
		Cross-sectional study—If applicable, describe analytical methods taking account of sampling strategy.
		(e) Describe any sensitivity analyses.
		(f) State whether Hardy–Weinberg equilibrium was considered and, if so, how.
		(g) Describe any methods used for inferring genotypes or haplotypes.
		(h) Describe any methods used to assess or address population stratification.
		(i) Describe any methods used to address multiple comparisons or to control risk of false-positive findings.
		(j) Describe any methods used to address and correct for relatedness among subjects.
Results		
Participants	13*	(a) Report the numbers of individuals at each stage of the study—e.g., numbers potentially eligible, examined for eligibility, confirmed eligible, included in the study, completing follow-up, and analyzed.
		(b) Give reasons for nonparticipation at each stage.
		(c) Consider use of a flow diagram.
		Report numbers of individuals in whom genotyping was attempted and numbers of individuals in whom genotyping was successful.

(Continued)

Table 10.1 Continued

Item	Item Number	STROBE Guideline	Extension for Genetic Association Studies (STREGA)
Descriptive data	14*	(a) Give characteristics of study participants (e.g., demographic, clinical, social) and information on exposures and potential confounders.	**Consider giving information by genotype.**
		(b) Indicate the number of participants with missing data for each variable of interest.	
		(c) **Cohort study**—Summarize follow-up time (e.g., average and total amount).	
Outcome data	15*	**Cohort study**—Report numbers of outcome events or summary measures over time.	**Report outcomes (phenotypes) for each genotype category over time.**
		Case-control study—Report numbers in each exposure category, or summary measures of exposure.	**Report numbers in each genotype category.**
		Cross-sectional study—Report numbers of outcome events or summary measures.	**Report outcomes (phenotypes) for each genotype category.**
Main results	16	(a) Give unadjusted estimates and, if applicable, confounder-adjusted estimates and their precision (e.g., 95% confidence intervals). Make clear which confounders were adjusted for and why they were included.	
		(b) Report category boundaries when continuous variables were categorized.	
		(c) If relevant, consider translating estimates of relative risk into absolute risk for a meaningful time period.	**(d) Report results of any adjustments for multiple comparisons.**

Other analyses	17	(a) Report other analyses done—e.g., analyses of subgroups and interactions, and sensitivity analyses.
		(b) If numerous genetic exposures (genetic variants) were examined, summarize results from all analyses undertaken.
		(c) If detailed results are available elsewhere, state how they can be accessed.
Discussion		
Key results	18	Summarize key results with reference to study objectives.
Limitations	19	Discuss limitations of the study, taking into account sources of potential bias or imprecision. Discuss both direction and magnitude of any potential bias.
Interpretation	20	Give a cautious overall interpretation of results considering objectives, limitations, multiplicity of analyses, results from similar studies, and other relevant evidence.
Generalizability	21	Discuss the generalizability (external validity) of the study results.
Other Information		
Funding	22	Give the source of funding and the role of the funders for the present study and, if applicable, for the original study on which the present article is based.

STREGA = STrengthening the REporting of Genetic Association studies; STROBE = STrengthening the REporting of OBservational studies in Epidemiology.

* Give information separately for cases and controls in case-control studies and, if applicable, for exposed and unexposed groups in cohort and cross-sectional studies.

checklist provides additions to 12 of the 22 items on the STROBE checklist. During the workshop and subsequent consultations, we identified five main areas of special interest that are specific to, or especially relevant in, genetic association studies: genotyping errors, population stratification, modeling haplotype variation, HWE, and replication. We elaborate on each of these areas, starting each section with the corresponding STREGA recommendation, followed by a brief outline of the issue and an explanation for the recommendations. Complementary information on these areas and the rationale for additional STREGA recommendations relating to selection of participants, choice of genes and variants selected, treatment effects in studying quantitative traits, statistical methods, relatedness, reporting of descriptive and outcome data, and issues of data volume are presented in Table 10.2.

Genotyping Errors

Recommendation for reporting of methods (Table 10.1, item 8b): Describe laboratory methods, including source and storage of DNA, genotyping methods and platforms (including the allele calling algorithm used, and its version), error rates, and call rates. State the laboratory/center where genotyping was done. Describe comparability of laboratory methods if there is more than one group. Specify whether genotypes were assigned using all of the data from the study simultaneously or in smaller batches.

Recommendation for reporting of results (Table 10.1, item 13a): Report numbers of individuals in whom genotyping was attempted and numbers of individuals in whom genotyping was successful.

Genotyping errors can occur as a result of effects of the DNA sequence flanking the marker of interest, poor quality or quantity of the DNA extracted from biological samples, biochemical artifacts, poor equipment precision or equipment failure, or human error in sample handling, conduct of the array, or handling the data obtained from the array (61). A commentary published in 2005 on the possible causes and consequences of genotyping errors observed that an increasing number of researchers were aware of the problem, but that the effects of such errors had largely been neglected (61). The magnitude of genotyping errors has been reported to vary between 0.5% and 30% (61–64). In high-throughput centers, an error rate of 0.5% per genotype has been observed for blind duplicates that were run on the same gel (64). This lower error rate reflects an explicit choice of markers for which genotyping rates have been found to be highly repeatable and whose individual polymerase chain reactions (PCR) have been optimized. Nondifferential genotyping errors, that is, those that do not differ systematically according to outcome status, will usually bias associations toward the null (65,66), just as for other nondifferential errors. The most marked bias occurs when genotyping sensitivity is poor and genotype prevalence is high (>85%) or, as the corollary, when genotyping specificity is poor and genotype prevalence is low (<15%) (65). When measurement of the environmental exposure has substantial error, genotyping errors of the order of 3% can

Table 10.2 Rationale for inclusion of topics in the STREGA recommendations

Specific Issue in Genetic Association Studies	Rationale for Inclusion in STREGA	Item(s) in STREGA	Specific Suggestions for Reporting
Main areas of special interest (see also main text).			
Genotyping errors (misclassification of exposure)	Nondifferential genotyping errors will usually bias associations toward the null (65,66). When there are systematic differences in genotyping according to outcome status (differential error), bias in any direction may occur.	8(b): Describe laboratory methods, including source and storage of DNA, genotyping methods and platforms (including the allele calling algorithm used, and its version), error rates and call rates. State the laboratory/center where genotyping was done. Describe comparability of laboratory methods if there is more than one group. Specify whether genotypes were assigned using all of the data from the study simultaneously or in smaller batches. 13(a): Report numbers of individuals in whom genotyping was attempted and numbers of individuals in whom genotyping was successful.	Factors affecting the potential extent of misclassification (information bias) of genotype include the types and quality of samples, timing of collection, and the method used for genotyping (18,61,67). When high throughput platforms are used, it is important to report not only the platform used but also the allele calling algorithm and its version. Different calling algorithms have different strengths and weaknesses ((68) and supplementary information in (69)). For example, some of the currently used algorithms are notably less accurate in assigning genotypes to single nucleotide polymorphisms with low minor allele frequencies (<0.10) than to single nucleotide polymorphisms with higher minor allele frequencies (70). Algorithms are continually being improved. Reporting the allele calling algorithm and its version will help readers to interpret reported results, and it is critical for reproducing the results of the study given the same intermediate output files summarizing intensity of hybridization. For some high-throughput platforms, the user may choose to assign genotypes using all of the data from the study simultaneously, or in smaller batches, such as by plate ((71,72) and supplementary information in (69)). This choice can affect both the overall call rate and the robustness of the calls. For case-control studies, whether genotyping was done blind to case-control status should be reported, along with the reason for this decision.

(Continued)

Table 10.2 Continued

Specific Issue in Genetic Association Studies	Rationale for Inclusion in STREGA	Item(s) in STREGA	Specific Suggestions for Reporting
Population stratification (confounding by ethnic origin)	When study subpopulations differ both in allele (or genotype) frequencies and disease risks, then confounding will occur if these subpopulations are unevenly distributed across exposure groups (or between cases and controls).	12(h): *Describe any methods used to assess or address population stratification.*	In view of the debate about the potential implications of population stratification for the validity of genetic association studies, transparent reporting of the methods used, or stating that none was used, to address this potential problem is important for allowing the empirical evidence to accrue. Ethnicity information should be presented (e.g., Winker (74)), as should genetic markers or other variables likely to be associated with population stratification. Details of case-family control designs should be provided if they are used. As several methods of adjusting for population stratification have been proposed (75), explicit documentation of the methods is needed.
Modeling haplotype variation	In designs considered in this article, haplotypes have to be inferred because of lack of available family information. There are diverse methods for inferring haplotypes.	12(g): *Describe any methods used for inferring genotypes or haplotypes.*	When discrete "windows" are used to summarize haplotypes, variation in the definition of these may complicate comparisons across studies, as results may be sensitive to choice of windows. Related "imputation" strategies are also in use (69,76,77). It is important to give details on haplotype inference and, when possible, uncertainty. Additional considerations for reporting include the strategy for dealing with rare haplotypes, window size and construction (if used), and choice of software.
Hardy–Weinberg equilibrium (HWE)	Departure from Hardy–Weinberg equilibrium may indicate errors or peculiarities in the data (73). Empirical assessments have found that 20% to 69% of genetic associations were reported with some indication about conformity with Hardy–Weinberg equilibrium, and that among some of these, there were limitations or errors in its assessment (73).	12(f): *State whether Hardy–Weinberg equilibrium was considered and, if so, how.*	Any statistical tests or measures should be described, as should any procedure to allow for deviations from Hardy–Weinberg equilibrium in evaluating genetic associations (78).

Replication	Publications that present and synthesize data from several studies in a single report are becoming more common.	3: State if the study is the first report of a genetic association, a replication effort, or both.	The selected criteria for claiming successful replication should also be explicitly documented.

Additional issues

Selection of participants	Selection bias may occur if (i) genetic associations are investigated in one or more subsets of participants (subsamples) from a particular study; or (ii) there is differential nonparticipation in groups being compared; or (iii) there are differential genotyping call rates in groups being compared.	6(a): Give information on the criteria and methods for selection of subsets of participants from a larger study, when relevant. 13(a): Report numbers of individuals in whom genotyping was attempted and numbers of individuals in whom genotyping was successful.	Inclusion and exclusion criteria, sources and methods of selection of subsamples should be specified, stating whether these were based on *a priori* or *post hoc* considerations.
Rationale for choice of genes and variants investigated	Without an explicit rationale, it is difficult to judge the potential for selective reporting of study results. There is strong empirical evidence from randomized controlled trials that reporting of trial outcomes is frequently incomplete and biased in favor of statistically significant findings (79–81). Some evidence is also available in pharmacogenetics (82).	7(b): Clearly define genetic exposures (genetic variants) using a widely used nomenclature system. Identify variables likely to be associated with population stratification (confounding by ethnic origin).	The scientific background and rationale for investigating the genes and variants should be reported. For genome-wide association studies, it is important to specify what initial testing platforms were used and how gene variants are selected for further testing in subsequent stages. This may involve statistical considerations (for example, selection of *p*-value threshold), functional or other biological considerations, fine mapping choices, or other approaches that need to be specified. Guidelines for human gene nomenclature have been published by the Human Gene Nomenclature Committee (83,84). Standard reference numbers for nucleotide sequence variations, largely but not only SNPs are provided in dbSNP, the National Center for Biotechnology Information's database of genetic variation (85). For variations not listed in dbSNP that can be described relative to a specified version, guidelines have been proposed (86,87).

(Continued)

Table 10.2 Continued

Specific Issue in Genetic Association Studies	Rationale for Inclusion in STREGA	Item(s) in STREGA	Specific Suggestions for Reporting
Treatment effects in studies of quantitative traits	A study of a quantitative variable may be compromised when the trait is subjected to the effects of a treatment (for example, the study of a lipid-related trait for which several individuals are taking lipid-lowering medication). Without appropriate correction, this can lead to bias in estimating the effect and loss of power.	9(b): *For quantitative outcome variables, specify if any investigation of potential bias resulting from pharmacotherapy was undertaken. If relevant, describe the nature and magnitude of the potential bias, and explain what approach was used to deal with this.* 11: *If applicable, describe how effects of treatment were dealt with.*	Several methods of adjusting for treatment effects have been proposed (88). As the approach to deal with treatment effects may have an important impact on both the power of the study and the interpretation of the results, explicit documentation of the selected strategy is needed.
Statistical methods	Analysis methods should be transparent and replicable, and genetic association studies are often performed using specialized software.	12(a): *State software version used and options (or settings) chosen.*	
Relatedness	The methods of analysis used in family-based studies are different from those used in studies that are based on unrelated cases and controls. Moreover, even in the studies that are based on apparently unrelated cases and controls, some individuals may have some connection and may be (distant) relatives, and this is particularly common in small, isolated populations, for example, Iceland. This may need to be probed with appropriate methods and adjusted for in the analysis of the data.	12(j): *Describe any methods used to address and correct for relatedness among subjects*	For the great majority of studies in which samples are drawn from large, nonisolated populations, relatedness is typically negligible and results would not be altered depending on whether relatedness is taken into account. This may not be the case in isolated populations or those with considerable inbreeding. If investigators have assessed for relatedness, they should state the method used (89–91) and how the results are corrected for identified relatedness.

Reporting of descriptive and outcome data	The synthesis of findings across studies depends on the availability of sufficiently detailed data.	14(a): *Consider giving information by genotype.* 15: *Cohort study—Report outcomes (phenotypes) for each genotype category over time* *Case-control study—Report numbers in each genotype category* *Cross-sectional study—Report outcomes (phenotypes) for each genotype category*	Genome-wide association studies collect information on a very large number of genetic variants concomitantly. Initiatives to make the entire database transparent and available online may supply a definitive solution to the problem of selective reporting (7). Availability of raw data may help interested investigators reproduce the published analyses and also pursue additional analyses. A potential drawback of public data availability is that investigators using the data second-hand may not be aware of limitations or other problems that were originally encountered, unless these are also transparently reported. In this regard, collaboration of the data users with the original investigators may be beneficial. Issues of consent and confidentiality (92,93) may also complicate what data can be shared, and how. It would be useful for published reports to specify not only what data can be accessed and where, but also briefly mention the procedure. For articles that have used publicly available data, it would be useful to clarify whether the original investigators were also involved and if so, how.
Volume of data	The key problem is of possible false-positive results and selective reporting of these. Type I errors are particularly relevant to the conduct of genome-wide association studies. A large search among hundreds of thousands of genetic variants can be expected by chance alone to find thousands of false-positive results (odds ratios significantly different from 1.0).	12(i): *Describe any methods used to address multiple comparisons or to control risk of false-positive findings.* 16(d): *Report results of any adjustments for multiple comparisons.* 17(b): *If numerous genetic exposures (genetic variants) were examined, summarize results from all analyses undertaken.* 17(c): *If detailed results are available elsewhere, state how they can be accessed.*	The volume of data analyzed should also be considered in the interpretation of findings. Examples of methods of summarizing results include giving distribution of p-values (frequentist statistics), distribution of effect sizes, and specifying false discovery rates.

Source: Reprinted from (94) with permission of the *Annals of Internal Medicine;* the *European Journal of Epidemiology;* the *European Journal of Clinical Investigation; Genetic Epidemiology; Human Genetics;* the *Journal of Clinical Epidemiology;* and *PLoS Medicine.*

lead to substantial underestimation of the magnitude of an interaction effect (95). When there are systematic differences in genotyping according to outcome status (differential error), bias in any direction may occur. Unblinded assessment may lead to differential misclassification. For genome-wide association studies of SNPs, differential misclassification between comparison groups (e.g., cases and controls) can occur because of differences in DNA storage, collection, or processing protocols, even when the genotyping itself meets the highest possible standards (71). In this situation, using samples blinded to comparison group to determine the parameters for allele calling could still lead to differential misclassification. To minimize such differential misclassification, it would be necessary to calibrate the software separately for each group. This is one of the reasons for our recommendation to specify whether genotypes were assigned using all of the data from the study simultaneously or in smaller batches.

Population Stratification

Recommendation for reporting of methods (Table 10.1, item 12h): Describe any methods used to assess or address population stratification.

Population stratification is the presence within a population of subgroups among which allele (or genotype, or haplotype) frequencies and disease risks differ. When the groups compared in the study differ in their proportions of the population subgroups, an association between the genotype and the disease being investigated may reflect the genotype being an indicator identifying a population subgroup rather than a causal variant. In this situation, population subgroup is a confounder because it is associated with both genotype frequency and disease risk. The potential implications of population stratification for the validity of genetic association studies have been debated (96–110). Modeling the possible effect of population stratification (when no effort has been made to address it) suggests that the effect is likely to be small in most situations (102,103,105–107). Meta-analyses of 43 gene–disease associations comprising 697 individual studies showed consistent associations across groups of different ethnic origin (107), and thus provide evidence against a large effect of population stratification, hidden or otherwise. However, as studies of association and interaction typically address moderate or small effects and hence require large sample sizes, a small bias arising from population stratification may be important (108). Study design (case-family control studies) and statistical methods (75) have been proposed to address population stratification, but so far few studies have used these suggestions (49). Most of the early genome-wide association studies used family-based designs or such methods as genomic control and principal components analysis (69,111) to control for stratification. These approaches are particularly appropriate for addressing bias when the identified genetic effects are very small (odds ratio < 1.20), as has been the situation in many recent genome-wide association studies (69,76,112–129). In view of the debate about the potential implications of population stratification for the validity of genetic association studies, we recommend transparent reporting of the methods used, or stating that none was used, to address this potential problem. This reporting will enable empirical evidence to accrue about the effects of population stratification and methods to address it.

Modeling Haplotype Variation

Recommendation for reporting of methods (Table 10.1, item 12g): Describe any methods used for inferring genotypes or haplotypes.

A haplotype is a combination of specific alleles at neighboring genes that tend to be inherited together. There has been considerable interest in modeling haplotype variation within candidate genes. Typically, the number of haplotypes observed within a gene is much smaller than the theoretical number of all possible haplotypes (130,131). Motivation for utilizing haplotypes comes, in large part, from the fact that multiple SNPs may "tag" an untyped variant more effectively than a single typed variant. The subset of SNPs used in such an approach is called "haplotype tagging" SNPs. Implicitly, an aim of haplotype tagging is to reduce the number of SNPs that have to be genotyped, while maintaining statistical power to detect an association with the phenotype. Maps of human genetic variation are becoming more complete, and large-scale genotypic analysis is becoming increasingly feasible. In consequence, it is possible that modeling haplotype variation will become more focused on rare causal variants, because these may not be included in the genotyping platforms.

In most current, large-scale genetic association studies, data are collected as unphased multilocus genotypes (i.e., which alleles are aligned together on particular segments of chromosome is unknown). It is common in such studies to use statistical methods to estimate haplotypes (132–135), and their accuracy and efficiency have been discussed (136–140). Some methods attempt to make use of a concept called haplotype "blocks" (141,142), but the results of these methods are sensitive to the specific definitions of the "blocks" (143,144). Reporting of the methods used to infer individual haplotypes and population haplotype frequencies, along with their associated uncertainties should enhance our understanding of the possible effects of different methods of modeling haplotype variation on study results as well as enabling comparison and syntheses of results from different studies.

Information on common patterns of genetic variation revealed by the International Haplotype Map (HapMap) Project (131) can be applied in the analysis of genome-wide association studies to infer genotypic variation at markers not typed directly in these studies (145,146). Essentially, these methods perform haplotype-based tests but make use of information on variation in a set of reference samples (e.g., HapMap) to guide the specific tests of association, collapsing a potentially large number of haplotypes into two classes (the allelic variation) at each marker. It is expected that these techniques will increase power in individual studies, and will aid in combining data across studies, and even across differing genotyping platforms. If imputation procedures have been used, it is useful to know the method, accuracy thresholds for acceptable imputation, how imputed genotypes were handled or weighted in the analysis, and whether any associations based on imputed genotypes were also verified on the basis of direct genotyping at a subsequent stage.

Hardy–Weinberg Equilibrium

Recommendation for reporting of methods (Table 10.1, item 12f): State whether Hardy–Weinberg equilibrium was considered and, if so, how.

Hardy–Weinberg equilibrium has become widely accepted as an underlying model in population genetics after Hardy (147) and Weinberg (148) proposed the concept that genotype frequencies at a genetic locus are stable within one generation of random mating; the assumption of HWE is equivalent to the independence of two alleles at a locus. Views differ on whether testing for departure from HWE is a useful method to detect errors or peculiarities in the data set, and also the method of testing (149). In particular, it has been suggested that deviation from HWE may be a sign of genotyping errors (73,150,151). Testing for departure from HWE has a role in detecting gross errors of genotyping in large-scale genotyping projects such as identifying SNPs for which the clustering algorithms used to call genotypes have broken down (69,70). However, the statistical power to detect less important errors of genotyping by testing for departure from HWE is low (68) and, in hypothetical data, the presence of HWE was generally not altered by the introduction of genotyping errors (78). Furthermore, the assumptions underlying HWE, including random mating, lack of selection according to genotype, and absence of mutation or gene flow, are rarely met in human populations (152,153). In 5 of 42 gene–disease associations assessed in meta-analyses of almost 600 studies, the results of studies that violated HWE significantly differed from results of studies that conformed to the model (154). Moreover, the study suggested that exclusion of HWE-violating studies may result in loss of the statistical significance of some postulated gene–disease associations and that adjustment for the magnitude of deviation from the model may also have the same consequence for some other gene–disease associations. Given the differing views about the value of testing for departure from HWE and about the test methods, transparent reporting of whether such testing was done and, if so, the method used, is important for allowing the empirical evidence to accrue.

For massive testing platforms, such as genome-wide association studies, it might be expected that many false positive violations of HWE would occur if a lenient p-value threshold were set. There is no consensus on the appropriate p-value threshold for HWE-related quality control in this setting. Hence, we recommend that investigators state which threshold they have used, if any, to exclude specific polymorphisms from further consideration. For SNPs with low minor allele frequencies, substantially more significant results than expected by chance have been observed, and the distribution of alleles at these loci has often been found to show departure from HWE.

For genome-wide association studies, another approach that has been used to detect errors or peculiarities in the data set (due to population stratification, genotyping error, HWE deviations, or other reasons) has been to construct quantile–quantile (Q/Q) plots whereby observed association statistics or calculated p-values for each SNP are ranked in order from smallest to largest and plotted against the expected null distribution (68,70). The shape of the curve can lend insight into whether or not systematic biases are present.

Replication

Recommendation: State if the study is the first report of a genetic association, a replication effort, or both (Table 10.1, item 3).

Articles that present and synthesize data from several studies in a single report are becoming more common. In particular, many genome-wide association analyses describe several different study populations, sometimes with different study designs and genotyping platforms, and in various stages of discovery and replication (68,70). When data from several studies are presented in a single original report, each of the constituent studies and the composite results should be fully described. For example, a discussion of sample size and the reason for arriving at that size would include clear differentiation between the initial group (those that were typed with the full set of SNPs) and those that were included in the replication phase only (typed with a reduced set of SNPs) (68,70). Describing the methods and results in sufficient detail would require substantial space in print, but options for publishing additional information on the study online make this possible.

Discussion

The choices made for study design, conduct, and data analysis potentially influence the magnitude and direction of results of genetic association studies. However, the empirical evidence on these effects is insufficient. Transparency of reporting is thus essential for developing a better evidence base (Table 10.2). Transparent reporting helps address gaps in empirical evidence (45), such as the effects of incomplete participation and genotyping errors. It will also help assess the impact of currently controversial issues such as population stratification, methods of inferring haplotypes, departure from HWE, and multiple testing on effect estimates under different study conditions.

The STREGA Statement proposes a minimum checklist of items for reporting genetic association studies. The statement has several strengths. First, it is based on existing guidance on reporting observational studies (STROBE). Second, it was developed from discussions of an interdisciplinary group that included epidemiologists, geneticists, statisticians, journal editors, and graduate students, thus reflecting a broad collaborative approach in terminology accessible to scientists from diverse disciplines. Finally, it explicitly describes the rationale for the decisions (Table 10.2) and has a clear plan for dissemination and evaluation.

The STREGA recommendations are available at http://www.strega-statement. org/. We welcome comments, which will be used to refine future versions of the recommendations. We note that little is known about the most effective ways to apply reporting guidelines in practice, and that therefore it has been suggested that editors and authors collect, analyze, and report their experiences in using such guidelines (155). We consider that the STREGA recommendations can be used by authors, peer reviewers, and editors to improve the reporting of genetic association studies. We invite journals to endorse STREGA, for example by including STREGA and its Web address in their Instructions for Authors and by advising authors and peer reviewers to use the checklist as a guide. It has been suggested that reporting guidelines are most helpful if authors keep the general content of the guideline items in mind as they write their initial drafts, then refer to the details of individual items as they critically appraise what they have written during the revision process (155). We emphasize that the STREGA reporting guidelines should not be used for screening submitted manuscripts to determine the quality or validity of the study being reported. Adherence to the recommendations may make some manuscripts longer, and this may be seen as a drawback in an era of limited space in a print journal. However, the ability to post information on the Web should alleviate this concern. The place in which supplementary information is presented can be decided by authors and editors of the individual journal.

We hope that the recommendations stimulate transparent and improved reporting of genetic association studies. In turn, better reporting of original studies would facilitate the synthesis of available research results and the further development of study methods in genetic epidemiology with the ultimate goal of improving the understanding of the role of genetic factors in the cause of diseases.

Summary

Making sense of rapidly evolving evidence on genetic associations is crucial to making genuine advances in human genomics and the eventual integration of this information in the practice of medicine and public health. Assessment of the strengths and weaknesses of this evidence, and hence the ability to synthesize it, has been limited by inadequate reporting of results. The STrengthening the REporting of Genetic Association (STREGA) studies initiative builds on the STrengthening the Reporting of OBservational studies in Epidemiology (STROBE) STatement and provides additions to 12 of the 22 items on the STROBE checklist. The additions concern population stratification, genotyping errors, modeling haplotype variation, Hardy–Weinberg equilibrium, replication, selection of participants, rationale for choice of genes and variants, treatment effects in studying quantitative traits, statistical methods, relatedness, reporting of descriptive and outcome data, and the volume of data issues that are important to consider in genetic association studies. The STREGA recommendations do not prescribe or dictate how a genetic association study should be designed but seek to enhance the transparency of its reporting, regardless of choices made during design, conduct, or analysis.

Acknowledgments
The authors thank Kyle Vogan and Allen Wilcox for their participation in the workshop and for their comments; Michele Cargill (Affymetrix, Inc.) and Aaron del Duca (DNA Genotek) for their participation in the workshop as observers; and the Public Population Project in Genomics (P³G), hosted by the University of Montreal and supported by Genome Canada and Genome Quebec. This article was made possible thanks to input and discussion by the P³G International Working Group on Epidemiology and Biostatistics, discussion held in Montreal, May 2007. The authors also thank the reviewers for their very thoughtful feedback, and Silvia Visentin, Rob Moriarity, Morgan Macneill, and Valery L'Heureux for administrative support. We were unable to contact Barbara Cohen to confirm her involvement in the latest version of this chapter.

References

1. Khoury MJ, Little J, Burke W. Human genome epidemiology: scope and strategies. In: Khoury MJ, Little J, Burke W, eds. *Human Genome Epidemiology: A Scientific Foundation for Using Genetic Information to Improve Health and Prevent Disease.* New York: Oxford University Press; 2004:3–16.
2. Genomics, Health and Society Working Group. *Genomics, Health and Society. Emerging Issues for Public Policy.* Ottawa: Government of Canada Policy Research Initiative; 2004.
3. Lin BK, Clyne M, Walsh M, et al. Tracking the epidemiology of human genes in the literature: the HuGE published literature database. *Am J Epidemiol.* 2006;164:1–4.
4. Yu W, Yesupriya A, Clyne M, et al. *HuGE Literature Finder.* HuGE Navigator. Available: http://www.hugenavigator.net/HuGENavigator/startPagePubLit.do/. Accessed June 19, 2009.
5. Lawrence RW, Evans DM, Cardon LR. Prospects and pitfalls in whole genome association studies. *Philos Trans R Soc Lond B Biol Sci.* 2005;360:1589–1595.
6. Thomas DC. Are we ready for genome-wide association studies? *Cancer Epidemiol Biomarkers Prev.* 2006;15:595–598.
7. Khoury MJ, Little J, Gwinn M, et al. On the synthesis and interpretation of consistent but weak gene–disease associations in the era of genome-wide association studies. *Int J Epidemiol.* 2007;36:439–445.
8. Little J, Khoury MJ, Bradley L, et al. The human genome project is complete. How do we develop a handle for the pump? *Am J Epidemiol.* 2003;157:667–673.
9. Ioannidis JP, Bernstein J, Boffetta P, et al. A network of investigator networks in human genome epidemiology. *Am J Epidemiol.* 2005;162:302–304.
10. Ioannidis JP, Gwinn M, Little J, et al. A road map for efficient and reliable human genome epidemiology. *Nat Genet.* 2006;38:3–5.
11. von Elm E, Egger M. The scandal of poor epidemiological research. *BMJ.* 2004;329:868–869.
12. Anonymous. Freely associating (editorial). *Nat Genet.* 1999;22:1–2.
13. Cardon L, Bell J. Association study designs for complex diseases. *Nat Rev Genet.* 2001;2:91–99.
14. Weiss S. Association studies in asthma genetics. *Am J Respir Crit Care Med.* 2001;164:2014–2015.

15. Weiss ST, Silverman EK, Palmer LJ. Case-control association studies in pharmacogenetics. *Pharmacogenomics*. 2001;J1:157–158.
16. Cooper DN, Nussbaum RL, Krawczak M. Proposed guidelines for papers describing DNA polymorphism-disease associations. *Hum Genet*. 2002;110:208.
17. Hegele R. SNP judgements and freedom of association. *Arterioscler Thromb Vasc Biol*. 2002;22:1058–1061.
18. Little J, Bradley L, Bray MS, et al. Reporting, appraising, and integrating data on genotype prevalence and gene–disease associations. *Am J Epidemiol*. 2002;156:300–310.
19. Romero R, Kuivaniemi H, Tromp G, et al. The design, execution, and interpretation of genetic association studies to decipher complex diseases. *Am J Obstet Gynecol*. 2002;187:1299–1312.
20. Colhoun HM, McKeigue PM, Davey Smith G. Problems of reporting genetic associations with complex outcomes. *Lancet*. 2003;361:865–872.
21. van Duijn CM, Porta M. Good prospects for genetic and molecular epidemiologic studies in the European Journal of Epidemiology. *Eur J Epidemiol* 2003;18:285–286.
22. Crossman D, Watkins H. Jesting Pilate, genetic case-control association studies, and Heart. *Heart*. 2004;90:831–832.
23. Huizinga TW, Pisetsky DS, Kimberly RP. Associations, populations, and the truth: recommendations for genetic association studies in arthritis & rheumatism. *Arthritis Rheum*. 2004;50:2066–2071.
24. Little J. Reporting and review of human genome epidemiology studies. In: Khoury MJ, Little J, Burke W, eds. *Human Genome Epidemiology: A Scientific Foundation for Using Genetic Information to Improve Health and Prevent Disease*. New York: Oxford University Press; 2004:168–192.
25. Rebbeck TR, Martinez ME, Sellers TA, et al. Genetic variation and cancer: improving the environment for publication of association studies. *Cancer Epidemiol Biomarkers Prev*. 2004;13:1985–1986.
26. Tan N, Mulley J, Berkovic S. Association studies in epilepsy: "The truth is out there." *Epilepsia*. 2004;45:1429–1442.
27. Anonymous. Framework for a fully powered risk engine. *Nat Genet*. 2005;37:1153.
28. Ehm MG, Nelson MR, Spurr NK. Guidelines for conducting and reporting whole genome/large-scale association studies. *Hum Mol Genet*. 2005;14:2485–2488.
29. Freimer NB, Sabatti C. Guidelines for association studies in human molecular genetics. *Hum Mol Genet*. 2005;14:2481–2483.
30. Hattersley AT, McCarthy MI. What makes a good genetic association study? *Lancet*. 2005;366:1315–1323.
31. Manly K. Reliability of statistical associations between genes and disease. *Immunogenetics*. 2005;57:549–558.
32. Shen H, Liu Y, Liu P, et al. Nonreplication in genetic studies of complex diseases—lessons learned from studies of osteoporosis and tentative remedies. *J Bone Miner Res*. 2005;20:365–376.
33. Vitali S, Randolph A. Assessing the quality of case-control association studies on the genetic basis of sepsis. *Pediatr Crit Care Med*. 2005;6:S74–S77.
34. Wedzicha JA, Hall IP. Publishing genetic association studies in Thorax. *Thorax*. 2005;60:357.
35. Hall IP, Blakey JD. Genetic association studies in Thorax. *Thorax*. 2005;60:357–359.
36. DeLisi LE, Faraone SV. When is a "positive" association truly a "positive" in psychiatric genetics? A commentary based on issues debated at the World Congress of Psychiatric Genetics, Boston, October 12–18, 2005. *Am J Med Genet B Neuropsychiatr Genet*. 2006;141:319–322.

37. Saito YA, Talley NJ, de Andrade M, et al. Case-control genetic association studies in gastro-intestinal disease: review and recommendations. *Am J Gastroenterol.* 2006;101:1379–1389.
38. Uhlig K, Menon V, Schmid CH. Recommendations for reporting of clinical research studies. *Am J Kidney Dis.* 2007;49:3–7.
39. NCI-NHGRI Working Group on Replication in Association Studies, Chanock SJ, Manolio T, Boehnke M, et al. Replicating genotype-phenotype associations. *Nature.* 2007;447:655–660.
40. Begg CB. Reflections on publication criteria for genetic association studies. *Cancer Epidemiol Biomarkers Prev.* 2005;14:1364–1365.
41. Byrnes G, Gurrin L, Dowty J, et al. Publication policy or publication bias? *Cancer Epidemiol Biomarkers Prev.* 2005;14:1363.
42. Pharoah PD, Dunning AM, Ponder BA, et al. The reliable identification of disease-gene associations. *Cancer Epidemiol Biomarkers Prev.* 2005;14:1362.
43. Wacholder S. Publication environment and broad investigation of the genome. *Cancer Epidemiol Biomarkers Prev.* 2005;14:1361.
44. Whittemore AS. Genetic association studies: time for a new paradigm? *Cancer Epidemiol Biomarkers Prev.* 2005;14:1359–1360.
45. Bogardus ST, Jr, Concato J, Feinstein AR. Clinical epidemiological quality in molecular genetic research. The need for methodological standards. *JAMA.* 1999;281:1919–1926.
46. Peters DL, Barber RC, Flood EM, et al. Methodologic quality and genotyping reproducibility in studies of tumor necrosis factor -308 G→A single nucleotide polymorphism and bacterial sepsis: implications for studies of complex traits. *Crit Care Med.* 2003;31:1691–1696.
47. Clark MF, Baudouin SV. A systematic review of the quality of genetic association studies in human sepsis. *Intensive Care Med.* 2006;32:1706–1712.
48. Lee W, Bindman J, Ford T, et al. Bias in psychiatric case-control studies: literature survey. *Br J Psychiatry.* 2007;190:204–209.
49. Yesupriya A, Evangelou E, Kavvoura FK, et al. Reporting of human genome epidemiology (HuGE) association studies: an empirical assessment. *BMC Med Res Methodol.* 2008;8:31.
50. Reid MC, Lachs MS, Feinstein AR. Use of methodological standards in diagnostic test research. Getting better but still not good. *JAMA.* 1995;274:645–651.
51. Brazma A, Hingamp P, Quackenbush J, et al. Minimum information about a microarray experiment (MIAME)—toward standards for microarray data. *Nat Genet.* 2001;29:356–371.
52. Pocock SJ, Collier TJ, Dandreo KJ, et al. Issues in the reporting of epidemiological studies: a survey of recent practice. *BMJ.* 2004;329:883.
53. Altman D, Moher D. Developing guidelines for reporting healthcare research: scientific rationale and procedures. *Med Clin (Barc).* 2005;125:8–13.
54. Gluud LL. Bias in clinical intervention research. *Am J Epidemiol.* 2006;163:493–501.
55. von Elm E, Altman DG, Egger M, et al. The strengthening the reporting of observational studies in epidemiology (STROBE) statement: Guidelines for reporting observational studies. *PLoS Med.* 2007;4:e296. doi:10.1371/journal.pmed.0040296.
56. Vandenbroucke JP, von Elm E, Altman DG, et al. Strengthening the reporting of observational studies in epidemiology (STROBE): explanation and elaboration. *Ann Intern Med.* 2007;147:W163–W194.
57. Little J, Higgins JPT, eds. The HuGENet™ HuGE Review Handbook, version 1.0. Available at http://www.hugenet.ca. Accessed February 28, 2006.
58. Higgins JP, Little J, Ioannidis JP, et al. Turning the pump handle: evolving methods for integrating the evidence on gene–disease association. *Am J Epidemiol.* 2007;166:863–866.

59. Altman DG, Schulz KF, Moher D, et al. The revised CONSORT statement for reporting randomized trials: explanation and elaboration. *Ann Intern Med.* 2001;134:663–694.

60. Moher D, Schultz KF, Altman D. The CONSORT statement: revised recommendations for improving the quality of reports of parallelgroup randomized trials. *JAMA.* 2001;285:1987–1991.

61. Pompanon F, Bonin A, Bellemain E, et al. Genotyping errors: causes, consequences and solutions. *Nat Rev Genet.* 2005;6:847–859.

62. Akey JM, Zhang K, Xiong M, et al. The effect that genotyping errors have on the robustness of common linkage disequilibrium measures. *Am J Hum Genet.* 2001;68:1447–1456.

63. Dequeker E, Ramsden S, Grody WW, et al. Quality control in molecular genetic testing. *Nat Rev Genet.* 2001;2:717–723.

64. Mitchell AA, Cutler DJ, Chakravarti A. Undetected genotyping errors cause apparent overtransmission of common alleles in the transmission/disequilibrium test. *Am J Hum Genet.* 2003;72:598–610.

65. Rothman N, Stewart WF, Caporaso NE, et al. Misclassification of genetic susceptibility biomarkers: implications for case-control studies and cross-population comparisons. *Cancer Epidemiol Biomarkers Prev.* 1993;2:299–303.

66. Garcia-Closas M, Wacholder S, Caporaso N, et al. Inference issues in cohort and case-control studies of genetic effects and gene environment interactions. In: Khoury MJ, Little J, Burke W, eds. *Human Genome Epidemiology: A Scientific Foundation for Using Genetic Information to Improve Health and Prevent Disease.* New York: Oxford University Press; 2004:127–144.

67. Steinberg K, Gallagher M. Assessing genotypes in human genome epidemiology studies. In: Khoury MJ, Little J, Burke W, eds. *Human Genome Epidemiology: A Scientific Foundation for Using Genetic Information to Improve Health and Prevent Disease.* New York: Oxford University Press; 2004:79–91.

68. McCarthy MI, Abecasis GR, Cardon LR, et al. Genome-wide association studies for complex traits: consensus, uncertainty and challenges. *Nat Rev Genet.* 2008;9:356–369.

69. Wellcome Trust Case Control Consortium. Genome-wide association study of 14,000 cases of seven common diseases and 3,000 shared controls. *Nature.* 2007;447:661–678.

70. Pearson TA, Manolio TA. How to interpret a genome-wide association study. *JAMA.* 2008;299:1335–1344.

71. Clayton DG, Walker NM, Smyth DJ, et al. Population structure, differential bias and genomic control in a large-scale, case-control association study. *Nat Genet.* 2005;37:1243–1246.

72. Plagnol V, Cooper JD, Todd JA, et al. A method to address differential bias in genotyping in large-scale association studies. *PLoS Genet.* 2007;3:e74. doi:10.1371/journal.pgen.0030074.

73. Salanti G, Amountza G, Ntzani EE, et al. Hardy–Weinberg equilibrium in genetic association studies: an empirical evaluation of reporting, deviations, and power. *Eur J Hum Genet.* 2005;13:840–848.

74. Winker MA. Race and ethnicity in medical research: requirements meet reality. *J Law Med Ethics.* 2006;34:520–525, 480.

75. Balding DJ. A tutorial on statistical methods for population association studies. *Nat Rev Genet.* 2006;7:781–791.

76. Scott LJ, Mohlke KL, Bonnycastle LL, et al. A genome-wide association study of type 2 diabetes in Finns detects multiple susceptibility variants. *Science.* 2007;316:1341–1345.

77. Scuteri A, Sanna S, Chen WM, et al. Genome-wide association scan shows genetic variants in the FTO gene are associated with obesity-related traits. *PLoS Genet.* 2007;3:e115. doi:10.1371/journal. pgen.0030115.

78. Zou GY, Donner A. The merits of testing Hardy–Weinberg equilibrium in the analysis of unmatched case-control data: a cautionary note. *Ann Hum Genet.* 2006;70:923–933.

79. Chan AW, Hrobjartsson A, Haahr MT, et al. Empirical evidence for selective reporting of outcomes in randomized trials: comparison of protocols to published articles. *JAMA.* 2004;291:2457–2465.

80. Chan AW, Krleza-Jeric K, Schmid I, et al. Outcome reporting bias in randomized trials funded by the Canadian Institutes of Health Research. *CMAJ.* 2004;171:735–740.

81. Chan AW, Altman DG. Identifying outcome reporting bias in randomised trials on PubMed: review of publications and survey of authors. *BMJ.* 2005;330:753.

82. Contopoulos-Ioannidis DG, Alexiou GA, Gouvias TC, et al. An empirical evaluation of multifarious outcomes in pharmacogenetics: beta-2 adrenoceptor gene polymorphisms in asthma treatment. *Pharmacogenet Genomics.* 2006;16:705–711.

83. Wain HM, Bruford EA, Lovering RC, et al. Guidelines for human gene nomenclature. *Genomics.* 2002;79:464–470.

84. Wain HM, Lush M, Ducluzeau F, et al. Genew: the human gene nomenclature database. *Nucleic Acids Res.* 2002;30:169–171.

85. Sherry ST, Ward MH, Kholodov M, et al. dbSNP: the NCBI database of genetic variation. *Nucleic Acids Res.* 2001;29:308–311.

86. Antonarakis SE. Recommendations for a nomenclature system for human gene mutations. Nomenclature working group. *Hum Mutat.* 1998;11:1–3.

87. den Dunnen JT, Antonarakis SE. Mutation nomenclature extensions and suggestions to describe complex mutations: a discussion. *Hum Mutat.* 2000;15:7–12.

88. Tobin MD, Sheehan NA, Scurrah KJ, et al. Adjusting for treatment effects in studies of quantitative traits: antihypertensive therapy and systolic blood pressure. *Stat Med.* 2005;24:2911–2935.

89. Lynch M, Ritland K. Estimation of pairwise relatedness with molecular markers. *Genetics.* 1999;152:1753–1766.

90. Slager SL, Schaid DJ. Evaluation of candidate genes in case-control studies: a statistical method to account for related subjects. *Am J Hum Genet.* 2001;68:1457–1462.

91. Voight BF, Pritchard JK. Confounding from cryptic relatedness in case-control association studies. *PLoS Genet.* 2005;1:e32. doi:10.1371/journal. pgen.0010032.

92. Homer N, Szelinger S, Redman M, et al. Resolving individuals contributing trace amounts of DNA to highly complex mixtures using high-density SNP genotyping microarrays. *PLoS Genet.* 2008;4:e1000167. doi:10.1371/journal. pgen.1000167.

93. Zerhouni EA, Nabel EG. Protecting aggregate genomic data. *Science.* 2008;322:44.

94. Little J, Higgins JPT, Ioannidis JPA, et al. STrengthening the REporting of Genetic Association Studies (STREGA)—an extension of the STROBE statement. *PLoS Med.* 2009;6(2):e1000022.

95. Wong MY, Day NE, Luan JA, et al. Estimation of magnitude in gene–environment interactions in the presence of measurement error. *Stat Med.* 2004;23:987–998.

96. Knowler WC, Williams RC, Pettitt DJ, et al. Gm3;5,13,14 and type 2 diabetes mellitus: an association in American Indians with genetic admixture. *Am J Human Genet.* 1988; 43:520–526.

97. Gelernter J, Goldman D, Risch N. The A1 allele at the D2 dopamine receptor gene and alcoholism: a reappraisal. *JAMA.* 1993;269:1673–1677.

98. Kittles RA, Chen W, Panguluri RK, et al. CYP3A4-V and prostate cancer in African Americans: causal or confounding association because of population stratification? *Hum Genet.* 2002;110:553–560.

99. Thomas DC, Witte JS. Point: population stratification: a problem for case control studies of candidate-gene associations? *Cancer Epidemiol Biomarkers Prev.* 2002;11:505–512.
100. Wacholder S, Chatterjee N, Hartge P. Joint effects of genes and environment distorted by selection biases: implications for hospital-based case-control studies. *Cancer Epidemiol Biomarkers Prev.* 2002;11:885–889.
101. Cardon LR, Palmer LJ. Population stratification and spurious allelic association. *Lancet.* 2003;361:598–604.
102. Wacholder S, Rothman N, Caporaso N. Population stratification in epidemiologic studies of common genetic variants and cancer: quantification of bias. *J Natl Cancer Inst.* 2000; 92:1151–1158.
103. Ardlie KG, Lunetta KL, Seielstad M. Testing for population subdivision and association in four case-control studies. *Am J Human Genet.* 2002;71:304–311.
104. Edland SD, Slager S, Farrer M. Genetic association studies in Alzheimer's disease research: challenges and opportunities. *Stat Med.* 2004;23:169–178.
105. Millikan RC. Re: population stratification in epidemiologic studies of common genetic variants and cancer: quantification of bias. *J Natl Cancer Inst.* 2001;93:156–157.
106. Wang Y, Localio R, Rebbeck TR. Evaluating bias due to population stratification in case-control association studies of admixed populations. *Genet Epidemiol.* 2004;27:14–20.
107. Ioannidis JP, Ntzani EE, Trikalinos TA. "Racial" differences in genetic effects for complex diseases. *Nat Genet.* 2004;36:1312–1318.
108. Marchini J, Cardon LR, Phillips MS, et al. The effects of human population structure on large genetic association studies. *Nat Genet.* 2004;36:512–517.
109. Freedman ML, Reich D, Penney KL, et al. Assessing the impact of population stratification on genetic association studies. *Nat Genet.* 2004;36:388–393.
110. Khlat M, Cazes MH, Genin E, et al. Robustness of case-control studies of genetic factors to population stratification: magnitude of bias and type I error. *Cancer Epidemiol Biomarkers Prev.* 2004;13:1660–1664.
111. Ioannidis JP. Non-replication and inconsistency in the genome-wide association setting. *Hum Hered.* 2007;64:203–213.
112. Parkes M, Barrett JC, Prescott NJ, et al. Sequence variants in the autophagy gene IRGM and multiple other replicating loci contribute to Crohn's disease susceptibility. *Nat Genet.* 2007;39:830–832.
113. Todd JA, Walker NM, Cooper JD, et al. Robust associations of four new chromosome regions from genome-wide analyses of type 1 diabetes. *Nat Genet.* 2007;39:857–864.
114. Zeggini E, Weedon MN, Lindgren CM, et al. Replication of genome-wide association signals in UK samples reveals risk loci for type 2 diabetes. *Science.* 2007;316:1336–1341.
115. Diabetes Genetics Initiative of Broad Institute of Harvard and MIT, Lund University, and Novartis Institutes of BioMedical Research, Saxena R, Voight BF, et al. Genome-wide association analysis identifies loci for type 2 diabetes and triglyceride levels. *Science.* 2007;316:1331–1336.
116. Helgadottir A, Thorleifsson G, Manolescu A, et al. A common variant on chromosome 9p21 affects the risk of myocardial infarction. *Science.* 2007;316:1491–1493.
117 McPherson R, Pertsemlidis A, Kavaslar N, et al. A common allele on chromosome 9 associated with coronary heart disease. *Science.* 2007;316:1488–1491.
118. Easton DF, Pooley KA, Dunning AM, et al. Genome-wide association study identifies novel breast cancer susceptibility loci. *Nature.* 2007;447:1087–1093.
119. Hunter DJ, Kraft P, Jacobs KB, Cox DG, et al. A genome-wide association study identifies alleles in FGFR2 associated with risk of sporadic postmenopausal breast cancer. *Nat Genet.* 2007;39:870–874.

120. Stacey SN, Manolescu A, Sulem P, et al. Common variants on chromosomes 2q35 and 16q12 confer susceptibility to estrogen receptor-positive breast cancer. *Nat Genet.* 2007;39:865–869.

121. Gudmundsson J, Sulem P, Steinthorsdottir V, et al. Two variants on chromosome 17 confer prostate cancer risk, and the one in TCF2 protects against type 2 diabetes. *Nat Genet.* 2007;39:977–983.

122. Haiman CA, Patterson N, Freedman ML, et al. Multiple regions within 8q24 independently affect risk for prostate cancer. *Nat Genet.* 2007;39:638–644.

123. Yeager M, Orr N, Hayes RB, et al. Genome-wide association study of prostate cancer identifies a second risk locus at 8q24. *Nat Genet.* 2007;39:645–649.

124. Zanke BW, Greenwood CM, Rangrej J, et al. Genome-wide association scan identifies a colorectal cancer susceptibility locus on chromosome 8q24. *Nat Genet.* 2007;39:989–994.

125. Tomlinson I, Webb E, Carvajal-Carmona L, et al. A genome-wide association scan of tag SNPs identifies a susceptibility variant for colorectal cancer at 8q24.21. *Nat Genet.* 2007;39:984–988.

126. Haiman CA, Le Marchand L, Yamamoto J, et al. A common genetic risk factor for colorectal and prostate cancer. *Nat Genet.* 2007;39:954–956.

127. Rioux JD, Xavier RJ, Taylor KD, et al. Genome-wide association study identifies new susceptibility loci for Crohn disease and implicates autophagy in disease pathogenesis. *Nat Genet.* 2007;39:596–604.

128. Libioulle C, Louis E, Hansoul S, et al. Novel Crohn disease locus identified by genome-wide association maps to a gene desert on 5p13.1 and modulates expression of PTGER4. *PLoS Genet.* 2007;3:e58. doi:10.1371/journal.pgen.0030058.

129. Duerr RH, Taylor KD, Brant SR, et al. A genome-wide association study identifies IL23R as an inflammatory bowel disease gene. *Science.* 2006;314:1461–1463.

130. Zhao LP, Li SS, Khalid N. A method for the assessment of disease associations with single-nucleotide polymorphism haplotypes and environmental variables in case-control studies. *Am J Hum Genet.* 2003;72:1231–1250.

131. International HapMap Consortium, Frazer KA, Ballinger DG, et al. A second generation human haplotype map of over 3.1 million SNPs. *Nature.* 2007;449:851–861.

132. Stephens M, Smith NJ, Donnelly P. A new statistical method for haplotype reconstruction from population data. *Am J Hum Genet.* 2001;68:978–989.

133. Qin ZS, Niu T, Liu JS. Partition-ligation-expectation-maximization algorithm for haplotype inference with single-nucleotide polymorphisms. *Am J Hum Genet.* 2002;71:1242–1247.

134. Scheet P, Stephens M. A fast and flexible statistical model for large-scale population genotype data: applications to inferring missing genotypes and haplotypic phase. *Am J Hum Genet.* 2006;78:629–644.

135. Browning SR. Missing data imputation and haplotype phase inference for genome-wide association studies. *Hum Genet.* 2008;124:439–450.

136. Huang Q, Fu YX, Boerwinkle E. Comparison of strategies for selecting single nucleotide polymorphisms for case/control association studies. *Hum Genet.* 2003;113:253–257.

137. Kamatani N, Sekine A, Kitamoto T, et al. Largescale single-nucleotide polymorphism (SNP) and haplotype analyses, using dense SNP maps, of 199 drug-related genes in 752 subjects: the analysis of the association between uncommon SNPs within haplotype blocks and the haplotypes constructed with haplotype-tagging SNPs. *Am J Hum Genet.* 2004;75:190–203.

138. Zhang W, Collins A, Morton NE. Does haplotype diversity predict power for association mapping of disease susceptibility? *Hum Genet.* 2004;115:157–164.

139. Carlson CS, Eberle MA, Rieder MJ, et al. Selecting a maximally informative set of single-nucleotide polymorphisms for association analysis using linkage disequilibrium. *Am J Hum Genet.* 2004;74:106–120.

140. van Hylckama Vlieg A, Sandkuijl LA, Rosendaal FR, et al. Candidate gene approach in association studies: Would the factor V leiden mutation have been found by this approach? *Eur J Hum Genet.* 2004;12:478–482.

141. Greenspan G, Geiger D. Model-based inference of haplotype block variation. *J Comput Biol.* 2004;11:493–504.

142. Kimmel G, Shamir R. GERBIL: Genotype resolution and block identification using likelihood. *Proc Natl Acad Sci USA.* 2005;102:158–162.

143. Cardon LR, Abecasis GR. Using haplotype blocks to map human complex trait loci. *Trends Genet.* 2003;19:135–140.

144. Ke X, Hunt S, Tapper W, et al. The impact of SNP density on fine-scale patterns of linkage disequilibrium. *Hum Mol Genet.* 2004;13:577–588.

145. Servin B, Stephens M. Imputation-based analysis of association studies: candidate regions and quantitative traits. *PLoS Genet.* 2007;3:e114. doi:10.1371/journal.pgen.0030114.

146. Marchini J, Howie B, Myers S, et al. A new multipoint method for genome-wide association studies by imputation of genotypes. *Nat Genet.* 2007;39:906–913.

147. Hardy GH. Mendelian proportions in a mixed population. *Science.* 1908;28:49–50.

148. Weinberg W. Über den nachweis der vererbung beim menschen. *Jahrhefte Des Vereines Für Vaterländische Naturkunde in Württemberg.* 1908;64:368–382.

149. Minelli C, Thompson JR, Abrams KR, et al. How should we use information about HWE in the meta-analyses of genetic association studies? *Int J Epidemiol.* 2008;37:136–146.

150. Xu J, Turner A, Little J, et al. Positive results in association studies are associated with departure from Hardy–Weinberg equilibrium: hint for genotyping error? *Hum Genet.* 2002;111:573–574.

151. Hosking L, Lumsden S, Lewis K, et al. Detection of genotyping errors by Hardy–Weinberg equilibrium testing. *Eur J Hum Genet.* 2004;12:395–399.

152. Shoemaker J, Painter I, Weir BS. A Bayesian characterization of Hardy–Weinberg disequilibrium. *Genetics.* 1998;149:2079–2088.

153. Ayres KL, Balding DJ. Measuring departures from Hardy–Weinberg: a Markov chain Monte Carlo method for estimating the inbreeding coefficient. *Heredity.* 1998;80:769–777.

154. Trikalinos TA, Salanti G, Khoury MJ, et al. Impact of violations and deviations in Hardy–Weinberg equilibrium on postulated gene–disease associations. *Am J Epidemiol.* 2006;163:300–309.

155. Davidoff F, Batalden P, Stevens D, et al. Publication guidelines for improvement studies in health care: evolution of the SQUIRE project. *Ann Intern Med.* 2008;149:670–676.

11

Integration of the evidence on gene–disease associations: methods of HuGE reviews

Julian P. T. Higgins and Julian Little

Introduction

The growing interest in genetic predisposition to common diseases, along with the rapid advances in genotyping technologies in recent years, has seen an explosion in the amount of epidemiologic evidence on gene–disease associations. Along with this growth in evidence has come an increasing need to collate and summarize the evidence in consistent, informative, and readily accessible formats. Human Genome Epidemiology (HuGE) reviews have been a cornerstone of the efforts of the Human Genome Epidemiology Network (HuGENet) to develop an online resource to house the cumulative and changing information on epidemiologic aspects of human genes (1). HuGE reviews may collate evidence on population frequencies of genetic variants, genotype–phenotype associations, interactions among genes and between genes, and environmental exposures, or a combination of these. More than 70 HuGE reviews have been completed under the auspices of HuGENet, with more than 80 in preparation at the time of writing. The majority of these reviews focus on genotype–phenotype associations, tackling evidence of association between specific genetic markers and either disease risk or quantitative traits, or both. Many similar reviews are published outside the auspices of HuGENet. In this chapter we explain what HuGE reviews aim to achieve and describe some key components of the methodology for undertaking them. The material is also directly relevant to reviews and meta-analysis of genetic association studies undertaken by groups outside of HuGENet.

What Are HuGE Association Reviews?

Genetic associations with common disease outcomes are likely to be numerous and mostly of small magnitude (2). Convincing evidence of true association therefore requires careful control over potential biases and chance effects. Control over biases is important both in study design (3) and in considering the selective availability of data on associations that have been examined (4). Large sample sizes are necessary for the detection of most associations. Furthermore, replication of findings in independent data sets is now widely regarded as a prerequisite for convincing evidence

215

Table 11.1 Characteristics of a systematic review

• Prespecification of objectives and criteria for including studies
• Comprehensive, systematic search for studies
• Reproducible methods, and duplication of tasks prone to human error
• Appraisal of included studies (including assessment of risk of bias)
• Synthesis of findings (e.g., using meta-analysis)
• Presentation of results in relation to initial objectives

of association. Thus, multiple studies are likely to exist, potentially from noncollaborating groups.

The purposes of a HuGE association review are (a) to identify all epidemiological investigations of the associations of interest; (b) to assess the reliability of the evidence; (c) to determine whether an association exists; and (d) to quantify the likely magnitude of an association if it exists. HuGE reviews are typically *systematic* reviews (see Table 11.1), aiming to identify, appraise, and synthesize evidence from all relevant existing studies on the topic in question (5). The general outline of a HuGE review is provided in Table 11.2. The strengths and limitations of systematic reviews are well established for clinical trials, largely through the efforts of The Cochrane Collaboration (6). Systematic reviews and meta-analyses are increasingly being applied to observational studies, and currently there are as many meta-analyses of observational data conducted as there are of clinical trials. The citation impact of both types of meta-analyses is equally high, the highest among all study designs in the health sciences (7). Meta-analyses of gene–disease association studies provide a key method for establishing the genetic components of complex diseases (8).

HuGE reviews cover a wide array of diseases and conditions, ranging from rare single gene disorders such as neurofibromatosis, to common conditions such as preterm birth, cancer, and heart disease (9). HuGE reviews focus on variants in a single gene, following the so-called "candidate gene" approach to identifying likely predisposing factors. Candidate genes may be chosen on the basis of either biological rationale (e.g., plausible biological pathways) or statistical evidence (e.g., findings arising from genome-wide association studies, or GWAS). However, HuGE reviews serve a different function from combined analyses (meta-analyses) of several whole genome association studies, which have a principal emphasis on detection of novel disease-associated variants. While it remains likely that a relatively limited number of variants play important roles in predisposition to common diseases (10), the collation and presentation of evidence on individual associations, and the interactions among them, through HuGE reviews, will continue to be important.

The Evolving Nature of Methodology

The rapid evolution of methodological standards for HuGE reviews is evident from the history of guidance on their conduct. They were originally proposed in 1998 by

Table 11.2 Outline of a HuGE review as recommended in the *HuGE Review Handbook*

Title
Abstract
Background
Gene(s)
Gene variants and frequency
Disease(s) or other outcomes
Objectives
Methods
Selection criteria
Identifying studies
Data collection and analysis
Results
Included studies
Quality and methodology of studies
Associations
Interactions
Discussion
Main findings
Limitations
Biology
Potential public health impact and other implications of results
(a) Potential public health impact
(b) Implications for our understanding of disease
(c) Implications for research
Potential conflicts of interest
References

Source: From Reference 11.

Khoury and Dorman (1), and more specific guidance for their content was provided in the *American Journal of Epidemiology* in 2000 (12). In January 2001 an expert panel workshop, convened by the Centers for Disease Control and Prevention (CDC) and the National Institutes of Health (NIH), led to recommendations regarding considerations that should be addressed in reporting studies of genotype prevalence in gene–disease associations, both for individual investigators and systematic reviews (3). Further experience with the HuGE review process (13) led to provision of revised guidance and formats for reviews (14). Four types of review were suggested: full reviews, association reviews, prevalence reviews, and mini-reviews. HuGE reviews continued to vary in their methodology, and particularly in the application of formal meta-analytic methods. A systematic review methodology workshop, convened by

the Cambridge Genetics Knowledge Park in November 2004, led to the more extensive guidance described in the *HuGE Review Handbook* (11,15).

We anticipate considerable further development of guidance for HuGE reviews
in the future. The field of human genome epidemiology is still relatively new and
fast-moving in terms of both technologies (the range and types of genetic variation
that can be investigated) and methodologies (study designs and statistical methods).
Evidence is accruing on the properties of these methods, particularly as a result
of improved reporting. Methods of HuGE reviews will change not only to reflect
advances in methods for review and synthesis, but particularly also as the nature
and availability of genomic data evolve over time.

Methods of HuGE Reviews

An editorial in the *American Journal of Epidemiology* offered six specific recommendations for the methodology of HuGE reviews (15). Here we elaborate on each
of these recommendations, providing an overview of some of the key considerations
in the review process. Detailed discussion of these issues, and more, is provided in
the *HuGE Review Handbook* (11). Even more detailed guidance for the conduct of
systematic reviews (particularly literature-based systematic reviews) can be found in
the *Cochrane Handbook for Systematic Reviews of Interventions* (16).

1. *Encouraging consortia of primary research investigators as the most reliable approach for performing combined analyses or meta-analyses (based
   on individual participant data)*

   HuGE reviews can be undertaken by anyone (see http://www.cdc.gov/genomics/
   hugenet/participate.htm). Literature-based systematic reviews are often prepared by researchers unconnected with the generation of the primary research
   findings. However, information in the literature may be seriously biased in favor
   of positive associations, due to selective nonpublication of uninteresting findings. Correspondence with original researchers is generally recommended in an
   attempt to tackle such problems. A substantially more reliable approach, however, is for those responsible for generating the original evidence to join forces in
   synthesizing the totality of evidence using consistent definitions of disease and
   standardized statistical methods (17); see also Chapter 7. Some possible advantages and disadvantages of different approaches to HuGE reviews are summarized in Table 11.3. In practice, HuGE reviews may compile data from a variety of
   sources, including individual participant data from some studies, aggregate data
   by correspondence from others, and summary statistics from publications for further studies. Such "conglomerate evidence" may be expected even for consortia-
   based meta-analyses (18). A trade-off may be required between focusing on the
   largest possible data set by considering all sources (thus potentially maximizing
   precision) and focusing on the "in-house" data set by using only individual participant data from the studies in the consortia (potentially minimizing bias).

Table 11.3 Data sources for meta-analysis of genetic association studies

Approach	Some Advantages and Disadvantages
Consortium-based meta-analysis with prospective genotyping	*Advantages*: complete data within the boundaries of the consortium; availability of data unrelated to findings; maximized ability to harmonize methods. *Disadvantages*: logistics of setting up a consortium; genotyping costs.
Consortium-based meta-analysis of existing data	*Advantages*: data not subject to selective availability; potential to harmonize data. *Disadvantages*: data may be incomplete; inclusion in consortium may be related to findings.
Literature-based systematic review and liaison with investigators	*Advantages*: relatively low resource requirements. *Disadvantages*: may be prone to bias due to selective availability of data.
Literature-based systematic review	*Advantages*: low resource requirements. *Disadvantages*: prone to serious bias due to selective availability of data.

2. *Adopting methods to minimize human error in the literature-based reviews, such as duplicating selection of studies and data extraction*

In literature-based reviews and meta-analyses, all reasonable attempts should be made to prevent the introduction of errors and personal biases. A key attribute of a systematic review is that criteria for including studies are clearly specified in advance. This is perhaps the most important difference between a narrative (traditional) review, in which the author is free to select data sources that fit a predetermined hypothesis, and the more objective method of systematic review. Independent duplication of steps in the review process, such as selection of studies, extraction of data, and critical assessment of methods used in the individual studies, can further reduce biases and prevent errors. Accidental omission of data, or accidental duplication of a study in a meta-analysis, may lead to spurious false-negative or false-positive findings, particularly important when effect magnitudes are likely to be small.

3. *Conducting comprehensive (yet practically realistic) searches for eligible studies, considering sources beyond MEDLINE*

The HuGE Literature Finder, within the HuGE Navigator (http://www.hugenavigator.net/), is a major source of information on gene–disease association studies, although is currently restricted to records from PubMed published after 2000 (19). A review limited to studies identified only from MEDLINE (or PubMed) may be insufficient, for two reasons. First, any review restricted to published literature is prone to publication bias, whereby only a subset comprising the most "publishable" findings is available from the totality of evidence on a particular genetic association. Second, MEDLINE is just one of several major sources of bibliographic information, and publication bias may, to some extent, be addressed by searching comprehensively for studies available through other sources. Other bibliographic databases likely to be useful in a HuGE review include EMBASE and the Science Citation Index. The overlap between these various databases is far from complete; for example, of approximately 4,800 journals indexed in EMBASE, 1,700 are not indexed in MEDLINE (20). Numerous studies in other fields have concluded that systematic reviews should search beyond MEDLINE (see Wilkins et al. (21), and other references cited in Hopewell et al. (22)) although there is a lack of evidence in the area of HuGE. Furthermore, bibliographic searches may still not retrieve all articles that are in the indexed journals (23).

The extent to which a review seeks to identify and include all evidence internationally is a further consideration. One empirical study found substantial differences between genetic associations from studies based in the People's Republic of China compared with studies done in other parts of the world (24). Limited evidence from the same study suggested that among the Chinese studies, more exciting findings tended to be reported in PubMed-indexed journals. A practical decision is often made to restrict the review to reports in English (and perhaps in other languages familiar to the review team). We suggest that a more scientifically robust strategy is to restrict the review to studies in particular geographical areas for which the literature is well covered in the databases searched (e.g., North America is well covered by PubMed and Europe is well covered by EMBASE). This would avoid the inclusion of evidence from areas in which only a minority of studies had been published in English and which, in consequence, was potentially biased.

Another potential source of information on existing studies is the increasing number of online databases, including data repositories for GWA and other association studies (25), and we anticipate that future HuGE reviews will draw extensively on such resources. For example, the database of Genotypes and Phenotypes (dbGaP; http://www.ncbi.nlm.nih.gov/gap) contains data from the Genetic Association Information Network (GAIN) among other initiatives, and the European Genotype Archive (EGA; http://www.ebi.ac.uk/ega/) contains data from the Wellcome Trust Case Control Consortium (WTCCC). In the last quarter of 2008, a paper raised concern about the possibility of identifying whether genotypic data on a specific individual was included in a publicly available database if an investigator had access to a reference database (26). This has generated a great deal of discussion and an initial response was to impose limits on the data made publicly available (27). At the time of writing, the nature and extent of such limits are still under discussion.

4. *Considering in more detail the potential for bias in individual studies and in the total body of available evidence*

The validity of a meta-analysis depends on the validity of the studies included in it, so it is important that each component study is appraised before being included in a statistical synthesis. The most important sources of bias in observational epidemiological studies are less well understood than those in some other study designs such as randomized trials. There is little empirical evidence associating study results with study characteristics for genetic association studies. Some extensive discussions of potential biases are available, however, with the principal candidates being population stratification (confounding due to subpopulations in the sample that differ both in genotype prevalence and disease risk), case definition, and methods in the collection, handling, and processing of DNA and the determination of genotypes (including blinding to case-control status) (3,28). Unfortunately, the appraisal of potential biases is difficult in practice, not only due to the uncertainty over which study characteristics are important, but also because of incomplete or variable reporting of the methods used in the studies themselves (29). Initiatives such as the STREGA statement, which offers guidelines for reporting of individual genetic association studies, may improve the situation in the future (see Chapter 10).

There is good evidence of *reporting* biases in the HuGE literature, particularly of the exaggerated effects that are often seen in the earliest reports of an association compared with subsequent attempts to replicate the finding (30). Overcoming publication bias requires the availability of all eligible data from all eligible studies (or an unbiased subset). This can only be achieved with prospective generation of the data (e.g., by a consortium), or when the reviewers are confident that all existing studies are either known or reported without bias. Unfortunately, selective reporting of only the most promising variants is a natural consequence of any attempt to summarize an association study of numerous genetic markers within the straightjacket of a traditional paper journal article. We now expect association studies to exploit the possibility of web-based publication of complete findings, but there are often obstacles to prevent this in practice.

HuGE review authors are encouraged to assess the strength of evidence that an observed association is genuine, and interim guidance for this process is available (31); see also Chapter 12. These so-called "Venice criteria," named informally after the venue of the meeting at which they were developed, assess the three domains of precision (e.g., through sample size), consistency of results across studies (e.g., through meta-analytic measures of heterogeneity), and protection from bias both within and across studies in a meta-analysis.

5. *Encouraging quantitative synthesis of results from multiple studies (meta-analysis) where appropriate*
Meta-analysis is the statistical synthesis of results from multiple studies (32). When implemented and interpreted appropriately, and applied to unbiased and correctly analyzed studies, it provides a powerful tool to understand similarities and differences between results from different studies. By exploiting the totality of evidence, meta-analyses typically offer enhanced power to detect associations, and increased precision in the estimation of their magnitude.

Meta-analyses are encouraged in HuGE reviews, and the majority of HuGE reviews in recent years have included them. Attention should always be paid to the possibility of reporting biases in reviews based on the published literature.

Most meta-analyses are undertaken simply as weighted averages of the estimates from the different studies. A metric is chosen for the analysis that ensures comparable quantities with reasonable statistical properties. For example, log odds ratios are typically combined for case-control studies, and if quantitative traits are measured using different methods across studies, they may be standardized before pooling, usually by expressing the results in terms of standard deviations. Consistency of results across studies should always be evaluated, which can be achieved using a statistical test of homogeneity or by quantifying the between-study variance (or quantities derived from these (33)). It is desirable to explore potential reasons for variation in findings across studies, although attempts at this can easily become "fishing expeditions" with unreliable consequences. Thus potential sources of variation in study results should be prespecified whenever possible, and limited in number. Methods are available to temper the statistical significance of findings based on small numbers of studies (34).

Meta-analysis methods of gene–disease association studies closely follow well-developed methodology for randomized trials (4,35,36). Due to so-called "Mendelian randomization" in the transmission of genetic material from parents to children, confounding is generally thought to be of minimal concern (although not ignorable, since it may arise through population stratification). Thus, unadjusted analyses are common in meta-analyses, even if matched studies have adjusted for matching factors such as age and sex. Special considerations in the meta-analysis of gene–disease associations include the choice of inheritance model (37,38), the treatment of Hardy-Weinberg equilibrium (39,40), and the combination of associations for markers known to be in linkage disequilibrium (41). Developments in the last area are now allowing complex syntheses of data across GWAS (42).

6. ***Encouraging incorporation of intermediate phenotypes (such as molecular markers) so that "Mendelian randomization" can be exploited to examine the causal effects of such phenotypes***
   A key development in observational epidemiology in recent years has been the recognition that nature's "randomization" of genetic material when gametes are formed can be exploited to infer causal effects of certain risk factors on disease (43); see also Chapter 21. Associations between traditional risk factors (such as lipid levels, exposures to toxins, or behaviors) are often affected by confounding (when an extraneous factor is responsible for changes in both the exposure and the outcome), or by reverse causation (when the outcome is itself responsible for modifying the exposure). However, a methodology for overcoming these problems is known as "instrumental variables" (44). An instrumental variable is one that is associated with the exposure of interest, but

not with the potential confounders. Under the assumption that the effect of the instrumental variable affects the outcome only through its effect on the exposure, the causal effect of the exposure can be deduced by examining on the one hand the association between instrumental variable and exposure, and on the other hand the association between the instrumental variable and the outcome. One example of this is the use of a polymorphism in an alcohol dehydrogenase gene (*ALDH2*) as an instrumental variable for assessing the causal effect of alcohol exposure on esophageal cancer (45). Because of their different physiological responses to drinking alcohol, individuals with different genotypes consume different amounts. However, there is little rationale (or evidence) for *ALDH2* variants to affect major confounders in the association between alcohol intake and esophageal cancer. A meta-analysis that identified an association between esophageal cancer and *ALDH2* genotype was interpreted as evidence of a causal effect of alcohol on cancer risk (45). Furthermore, a particular potential strength of the method is that by combining estimates of the gene–cancer association and gene–alcohol intake association, an indirect estimate of the causal effect of alcohol intake can be obtained.

Mendelian randomization methods will of course not solve all problems of causal inference in observational epidemiology. Strong assumptions are required for the approach to be valid. For instance, the genetic variant should not be in linkage disequilibrium with another variant involved in disease risk, and the method is problematic if there is canalization, that is, an adaptation by the body to compensate for a genuine risk conferred by the exposure. Perhaps the most important limitation, however, is the difficulty of identifying genetic variants that have real and specific effects on the exposures of interest. HuGE review authors are encouraged to consider potential intermediate phenotypes when undertaking reviews, and to collate and synthesize evidence on associations between the genotypes of interest and these intermediate phenotypes. These intermediate phenotypes may be of interest as outcomes in their own right, or may be used subsequently to explore causal relationships using Mendelian randomization methods (46). Because effects are typically small, particularly for gene–disease outcome associations, meta-analyses are likely to be necessary for many Mendelian randomization analyses.

Challenges for the Future

The transfer of systematic review methods, so well established now for synthesizing clinical trials, into the field of human genome epidemiology HuGE reviews, has met with substantial challenges. There are notable differences between genetic epidemiology evidence and clinical trial evidence. For example, precisely what constitutes an epidemiologic study can be difficult to define, and the vast numbers of variants that can now be studied mean that only a small minority of findings can be published in the traditional paper journal format. The need for large sample sizes is well recognized, and collaboration among research groups to pool the totality of relevant evidence may soon be the norm (47) while continuing to be the exception for clinical trials (48). An informatics infrastructure for the HuGE reviews has not been developed, although the reviews are well indexed and therefore easy to locate using HuGE Navigator. Major advances have been made for individual disease areas, however, particularly the comprehensive databases of studies and meta-analyses in Alzheimer disease (www.alzgene.org), Parkinson disease (www.pdgene.org), and schizophrenia (www.szgene.org) (49,50). Such databases form the basis of some of the field-wide synopses of all available evidence on genetic predisposition to major diseases described in Chapter 12 and illustrated in Part III.

The preparation of systematic (HuGE) reviews of individual associations with disease risk or quantitative traits is just one piece of a much larger jigsaw. They are key informants of field-wide synopses. On their own, however, they offer the opportunity to consider the likelihood that the totality of evidence for a particular association is available, to examine rigorously the validity of each piece of evidence, to investigate potential inconsistencies in findings across studies, and—where associations are demonstrated to be robust—to consider potential biological mechanisms and discuss implications for further research. This rigor clearly cannot be afforded to every potential association. However, while the number of associations that are established without doubt remains small, HuGE reviews have an important role to play in ensuring we are not misled unnecessarily by findings that appear to be more exciting than they are.

References

1. Khoury MJ, Dorman JS. The Human Genome Epidemiology Network. *Am J Epidemiol.* 1998;148:1–3.
2. Khoury MJ, Little J, Gwinn M, et al. On the synthesis and interpretation of consistent but weak gene-disease associations in the era of genome-wide association studies. *Int J Epidemiol.* 2007;36:439–445.
3. Little J, Bradley L, Bray MS, et al. Reporting, appraising, and integrating data on genotype prevalence and gene-disease associations. *Am J Epidemiol.* 2002;156:300–310.
4. Salanti G, Sanderson S, Higgins JPT. Obstacles and opportunities in meta-analysis of genetic association studies. *Genet Med.* 2005;7:13–20.
5. Egger M, Davey Smith G, Altman DG, eds. *Systematic Reviews in Health Care: Meta-analysis in context.* London: BMJ; 2001.
6. Chalmers I, Sandercock P, Wennberg J. The Cochrane Collaboration: Preparing, maintaining, and disseminating systematic reviews of the effects of health care. *Ann N Y Acad Sci.* 1993;703:156–165.
7. Patsopoulos NA, Analatos AA, Ioannidis JP. Relative citation impact of various study designs in the health sciences. *JAMA.* 2005;293:2362–2366.
8. Ioannidis JPA, Gwinn M, Little J, et al. A road map for efficient and reliable human genome epidemiology. *Nat Genet.* 2006;38:3–5.
9. CDC National Office of Public Health Genomics. Human Genome Epidemiology Network. Available at http://www.cdc.gov/genomics/hugenet. Accessed December 1, 2008.
10. McCarthy MI, Abecasis GR, Cardon LR, et al. Genome-wide association studies for complex traits: consensus, uncertainty and challenges. *Nat Rev Genet.* 2008;9:356–369.

11. Little J, Higgins JPT. *HuGENet HuGE Review Handbook*. Available at http://www. hugenet.ca. Accessed December 1, 2008.

12. Anonymous. Revised guidelines for submitting HuGE reviews. *Am J Epidemiol.* 2000;151:4–6.

13. Little J, Khoury MJ, Bradley L, et al. The human genome project is complete. How do we develop a handle for the pump? *Am J Epidemiol.* 2003;157:667–673.

14. Anonymous. Revised Guidelines and Format for HuGE Reviews, February 2005. Available at http://www.cdc.gov/genomics/hugenet/reviews/guidelines2.htm. Accessed December 1, 2008.

15. Higgins JPT, Little J, Ioannidis JPA, et al. Turning the pump handle: evolving methods for integrating the evidence on gene-disease association. *Am J Epidemiol.* 2007;166:863–866.

16. Higgins JPT, Green S, eds. *Cochrane Handbook for Systematic Reviews of Interventions.* Chichester: John Wiley & Sons; 2008.

17. Ioannidis JPA, Bernstein J, Boffetta P, et al. A network of investigator networks in human genome epidemiology. *Am J Epidemiol.* 2005;162:302–304.

18. Khoury MJ, Bertram L, Boffetta P, et al. Genome wide association studies, field synopses and the development of the knowledge base on genetic variation and human diseases. *Am J Epidemiol.* 2009;170:269–279.

19. Yu W, Gwinn M, Clyne M, et al. A navigator for human genome epidemiology. *Nat Genet.* 2008;40:124–125.

20. Lefebvre C, Manheimer E, Glanville J. Searching for studies. In: Higgins JPT, Green S, eds. *Cochrane Handbook for Systematic Reviews of Interventions.* Chichester: John Wiley & Sons; 2008:95–150.

21. Suarez-Almazor ME, Belseck E, Homik J, et al. Identifying clinical trials in the medical literature with electronic databases: MEDLINE alone is not enough. *Control Clin Trials.* 2000;21:476–487.

22. Wilkins T, Gillies RA, Davies K. EMBASE versus MEDLINE for family medicine searches: can MEDLINE searches find the forest or a tree? *Can Fam Physician.* 2005;51:848–849.

23. Hopewell S, Clarke M, Lefebvre C, et al. Handsearching versus electronic searching to identify reports of randomized trials. *Cochrane Database Syst Rev.* 2007;MR000001.

24. Pan Z, Trikalinos TA, Kavvoura FK, et al. Local literature bias in genetic epidemiology: an empirical evaluation of the Chinese literature. *PLoS Med.* 2005;2:e334.

25. Frodsham AJ, Higgins JPT. Online genetic databases informing human genome epidemiology: a review. *BMC Med Res Methodol.* 2007;7:31.

26. Homer N, Szelinger S, Redman M, et al. Resolving individuals contributing trace amounts of DNA to highly complex mixtures using high-density SNP genotyping microarrays. *PLoS Genet.* 2008;4:e1000167.

27. Zerhouni EA, Nabel EG. Protecting aggregate genomic data [letter]. *Science.* 2008;322:44.

28. Clayton DG, Walker NM, Smyth DJ, et al. Population structure, differential bias and genomic control in a large-scale, case-control association study. *Nat Genet.* 2005;37:1243–1246.

29. Yesupriya A, Evangelou E, Kavvoura FK, et al. Reporting of Human Genome Epidemiology (HuGE) association studies: an empirical assessment. *BMC Med Res Methodol.* 2008;8:31.

30. Ioannidis JP, Trikalinos TA. Early extreme contradictory estimates may appear in published research: the Proteus phenomenon in molecular genetics research and randomized trials. *J Clin Epidemiol.* 2005;58:543–549.

31. Ioannidis JP, Boffetta P, Little J, et al. Assessment of cumulative evidence on genetic associations: interim guidelines. *Int J Epidemiol.* 2008;37:133–135.

32. Borenstein M, Hedges LV, Higgins JPT, et al. *Introduction to Meta-analysis.* Chichester: John Wiley & Sons; 2009.

33. Higgins JPT, Thompson SG, Deeks JJ, et al. Measuring inconsistency in meta-analysis. *BMJ.* 2003;327:557–560.

34. Higgins JPT, Thompson SG. Controlling the risk of spurious findings from meta-regression. *Stat Med.* 2004;23:1663–1682.

35. Munafo MR, Flint J. Meta-analysis of genetic association studies. *Trends Genet.* 2004;20:439–444.

36. Kavvoura FK, Ioannidis JP. Methods for meta-analysis in genetic association studies: a review of their potential and pitfalls. *Hum Genet.* 2008;123:1–14.

37. Minelli C, Thompson JR, Abrams KR, et al. The choice of a genetic model in the meta-analysis of molecular association studies. *Int J Epidemiol.* 2005;34:1319–1328.

38. Salanti G, Higgins JP. Meta-analysis of genetic association studies under different inheritance models using data reported as merged genotypes. *Stat Med.* 2008;27:764–777.

39. Salanti G, Higgins JPT, Trikalinos TA, et al. Bayesian meta-analysis and meta-regression for gene-disease associations and deviations from Hardy-Weinberg equilibrium. *Stat Med.* 2007;26:553–567.

40. Minelli C, Thompson JR, Abrams KR, et al. How should we use information about HWE in the meta-analyses of genetic association studies? *Int J Epidemiol.* 2008;37:136–146.

41. Verzilli C, Shah T, Casas JP, et al. Bayesian meta-analysis of genetic association studies with different sets of markers. *Am J Hum Genet.* 2008;82:859–872.

42. Zeggini E, Scott LJ, Saxena R, et al. Meta-analysis of genome-wide association data and large-scale replication identifies additional susceptibility loci for type 2 diabetes. *Nat Genet.* 2008;40:638–645.

43. Davey Smith G, Ebrahim S. "Mendelian randomization": can genetic epidemiology contribute to understanding environmental determinants of disease? *Int J Epidemiol.* 2003;32:1–22.

44. Didelez V, Sheehan N. Mendelian randomization as an instrumental variable approach to causal inference. *Stat Methods Med Res.* 2007;16:309–330.

45. Lewis SJ, Smith GD. Alcohol, ALDH2, and esophageal cancer: a meta-analysis which illustrates the potentials and limitations of a Mendelian randomization approach. *Cancer Epidemiol Biomarkers Prev.* 2005;14:1967–1971.

46. Minelli C, Thompson JR, Tobin MD, et al. An integrated approach to the meta-analysis of genetic association studies using Mendelian randomization. *Am J Epidemiol.* 2004;160:445–452.

47. Seminara D, Khoury MJ, O'Brien TR, et al. The emergence of networks in human genome epidemiology: challenges and opportunities. *Epidemiology.* 2007;18:1–8.

48. Simmonds MC, Higgins JPT, Stewart LA, et al. Meta-analysis of individual patient data from randomized trials: a review of methods used in practice. *Clin Trials.* 2005;2:209–217.

49. Bertram L, McQueen MB, Mullin K, et al. Systematic meta-analyses of Alzheimer disease genetic association studies: the AlzGene database. *Nat Genet.* 2007;39:17–23.

50. Allen NC, Bagade S, McQueen MB, et al. Systematic meta-analyses and field synopsis of genetic association studies in schizophrenia: the SzGene database. *Nat Genet.* 2008;40:827–834.

12

Genome-wide association studies, field synopses, and the development of the knowledge base on genetic variation and human diseases

Muin J. Khoury, Lars Bertram, Paolo Boffetta,
Adam S. Butterworth, Stephen J. Chanock,
Siobhan M. Dolan, Isabel Fortier, Montserrat Garcia-Closas,
Marta Gwinn, Julian P. T. Higgins, A. Cecile J. W. Janssens,
James M. Ostell, Ryan P. Owen, Roberta A. Pagon,
Timothy R. Rebbeck, Nathaniel Rothman, Jonine L. Bernstein,
Paul R. Burton, Harry Campbell, Anand P. Chokkalingam,
Helena Furberg, Julian Little, Thomas R. O'Brien,
Daniela Seminara, Paolo Vineis, Deborah M. Winn, Wei Yu,
and John P. A. Ioannidis

The rapid growth in published genetic association studies (1) and the more recent successes of genome-wide association studies (GWAS) in finding disease susceptibility loci for several common diseases (2) present a major challenge for knowledge synthesis and dissemination. Knowledge synthesis is needed to guide further research, drug discovery efforts (3), and translational efforts for personalized risk assessment and therapy. The recent trend for direct-to-consumer advertising of whole genome analysis by several companies underscores the importance of a credible process for data synthesis and evaluation of the validity and utility of claims related to genetic prediction of disease risks (4–7).

In 2008, over 7,000 original articles were published on human genome epidemiology and the annual number has been rising rapidly (Table 12.1) (8). Furthermore, the published literature represents only a fraction of the data actually collected and analyzed. In addition, until recently, most studies have targeted one or a few gene variants (the candidate gene approach), but many new articles report the results of GWAS, and are expected to become increasingly common. More than 400 GWAS have been published total, not just since 2007,

Reprinted with modifications from the *American Journal of Epidemiology.* 2009; 170:269–279.

Table 12.1 Trends in numbers of published articles on human genome epidemiology, meta-analyses, and genome-wide association studies and numbers of genes studied, by year, 2001–2007[*]

Year	No. of Genes[†]	No. of Diseases	NO. OF ARTICLES PUBLISHED		
			Total	GWAS	Meta-Analyses[‡]
2001	633	690	2,492	0	34
2002	794	855	3,196	0	45
2003	832	880	3,476	3	65
2004	1,124	1,021	4,280	0	86
2005	1,308	1,077	5,029	5	113
2006	1,502	1,109	5,364	12	155
2007	2,142	1,292	7,222	104	208
2008	3,336	1,203	7,659	134	236

[*]HuGE Navigator query. Available at http://www.hugenavigator.net/. Accessed February 14, 2009.
[†]Genes column does not include the numbers of studied variants per gene (difficult to obtain).
[‡]Meta analyses also include HuGE reviews.
GWAS: Genome-wide association studies (individual genes not counted in genes column, unless featured in the paper).

but the pace has accelerated since 2007 (8). Only a few of these studies, however, have been deposited into accessible online databases such as the Database on Genotypes and Phenotypes (dbGAP) at the National Library of Medicine (9), the Cancer Genetic Markers of Susceptibility database (CGEMS) at the National Cancer Institute (10), and the Wellcome Trust Case Control Consortium (11). This number is expected to increase under new policies governing data sharing for GWAS (12), although type of access and confidentiality issues may continue to need careful consideration (13).

Despite a massive amount of primary data, the conclusions of genetic association studies are not always clear, requiring an evidence-based synthesis that takes into account the amount of evidence, the extent of replication, and protection from bias. Although approximately 1,000 systematic reviews and meta-analyses have been published since 2001, most have addressed only one or a few specific gene–disease associations at a time (8). Moreoever, the amount of accumulated data that needs to be integrated continues to grow rapidly, with high-throughput genotyping platforms raising the challenge exponentially.

As part of ongoing efforts in this field, we report here findings and recommendations from a multidisciplinary workshop, including geneticists, epidemiologists, journal editors, and bioinformatics experts, that was sponsored by the Human Genome Epidemiology Network (HuGENet) and held in Atlanta on January 24–25, 2008. The meeting was convened to discuss synthesis and appraisal of cumulative evidence on genetic associations and to develop a strategy for an online encyclopedia on genetic variation and common human diseases.

Progress in the HuGENet Road Map

HuGENet (14,15) is an informal global collaboration of individuals and organizations interested in accelerating the development of the knowledge base on genetic variation and human health. HuGENet has developed a "road map" (16) with several components: (i) working with genetic epidemiology study platforms (primarily consortia and networks) to improve the execution and output of these groups under the rubric of "Network of Networks" (17); (ii) promoting the publication of methodologically sound genetic association studies with transparent reporting of their methods (STrengthening the REporting of Genetic Associations or STREGA) (18) and avoidance of selective reporting; (iii) developing methods for synthesis and meta-analysis of the literature on genetic associations (the HuGE Review Handbook, version 1.0) (18); and (iv) developing "field synopses" (19) with an online encyclopedia summarizing what we know and what we do not know about genetic associations through a systematic assessment of their cumulative evidence. Such field synopses were also called for in a *Nature Genetics* 2006 editorial (20).

Field Synopses: Assessing Cumulative Evidence for Genetic Associations

An initial meeting of the Network of Networks in 2005 led to the formation of a working group on methods for assessing cumulative evidence. A workshop organized in Venice, Italy in 2006 (21) generated interim guidelines for grading the cumulative evidence in genetic associations based on three criteria: (i) the amount of evidence; (ii) the extent of replication; and (iii) protection from bias (22). The proposed scheme allows for three categories of descending credibility (A,B,C) for each of these criteria and also for a composite assessment of "strong," "moderate," or "weak" credibility (see Appendix and Reference 20 for more details). Briefly, an overall "strong" rating is reserved for a AAA rating, while an overall "weak" rating is reserved for associations with one or more C ratings. The rest are labeled as "moderate." We note that these ratings could change over time with data accruing from additional studies. The panel also discussed issues of biological and other experimental evidence and of the clinical importance of genetic associations. Pilot studies were planned in selected fields to assess cumulative evidence on gene–disease associations, calibrate the proposed guidelines, and integrate the findings into comprehensive field synopses. As of August 2009, pilot field synopses have been conducted for several diseases including Alzheimer disease, bladder cancer, schizophrenia, preterm birth, and coronary heart disease, as well as DNA repair genes and cancer phenotypes.

A field synopsis is a regularly updated snapshot of the current state of knowledge about genetic associations in a particular field of research defined by a disease (e.g., Alzheimer disease), phenotype (e.g., body mass index), or family of genes (e.g., DNA repair genes). The ideal attributes of a field synopsis are that it (a) is freely available; (b) uses online databases that are curated by researchers to develop regularly updated "online tables" on the volume of the evidence and magnitude of the associations between the disease and all genetic variants investigated; (c) uses objective and transparent criteria for grading the credibility of cumulative evidence; (d) summarizes the information in peer-reviewed articles; and (e) updates information on a regular basis. The first field synopsis—the source of AlzGene, the Alzheimer disease genetic association database (23)—was developed by Bertram, et al. and published in January 2007. This was followed by the publication of a field synopsis on schizophrenia (24) and one on DNA repair genes (25), while three other synopses are under development or peer review.

Experience with Field Synopses to Date

At the HuGENet workshop, several teams presented findings and experiences in developing field synopses, and on grading the epidemiologic evidence according to the interim Venice guidelines (22). Key features of these efforts are summarized in Table 12.2. All synopses include multiple meta-analyses involving large numbers of data sets, except for preterm birth, where evidence is sparse. Researchers performing synopses have used different thresholds or trigger points for conducting a meta-analysis. For example, in the coronary heart disease fields synopsis, investigators have considered only those associations for which at least one previous effort has been made to perform a meta-analysis. Data from GWAS have been incorporated in synopses on Alzheimer disease, schizophrenia, DNA repair genes, and bladder cancer. The preterm birth field synopsis points out the need for further research on the genetic contribution to this major public health challenge.

Many associations in the Alzheimer, schizophrenia, and two cancer-related field synopses yielded formally statistically significant results at the $p < 0.05$ level (Table 12.2). Nevertheless, only a few associations met the designation of "strong" evidence according to the Venice criteria. Similarly, in several synopses, none of the probed associations attained the status of "strong" evidence. Finally, so far, field synopses have examined only one main phenotype, except in the case of DNA repair genes. In addition to main effects, synopses have investigated genetic effects according to different genetic models, and for subgroups—for example, subgroups based on exposure, ethnic group, participant characteristics, or phenotypic subgroups. Decisions to undertake additional analyses need to be made on the basis of data availability. For example, in most field synopses, investigators were able to assess different genetic models. Often, available epidemiologic evidence may be stronger for one genetic model than for another. By contrast, there have been relatively fewer subgroup analyses based on exposures and participant characteristics, because of suboptimal reporting of these factors in genetic epidemiology studies, a deficiency that the STREGA guidance aims to address (18).

Table 12.2 Key characteristics of pilot field synopses of genetic associations

	No. of Meta-Analyses	No. of Data Sets[*](a)	Threshold[†] for Meta-Analysis	No. of Statistically Significant Associations[‡]	Strong[§] (Grade A)	World Wide Web Address
Alzheimer disease[‖]	228	1,072	4 data sets	53	NA	www.alzgene.org
Schizophrenia[#]	118	1,179	4 data sets	24	4	www.szgene.org
DNA repair genes and various cancers	241	1,087	2 independent teams	31	3	www.episat.org
Bladder cancer	36	356	3 data sets	7	1	Not yet online
Coronary heart disease	48	1,039	—	4	0	www.chdgene.com
Preterm birth	17	87	3 data sets	2	0	www.prebic.net
Major depression	22	131	3 data sets	6	2	Not yet online

[*]Total number of data sets included in the meta-analyses (not including data sets that did not undergo meta-analysis).

[†]Authors' prerequisite condition for conducting a meta-analysis.

[‡]Statistically significant ($P < 0.05$) by random-effects calculations on the default (per allele) analysis (for coronary heart disease, results are based on a meta-regression model and correspond to effects in the largest studies, while for DNA repair genes, both recessive and dominant models were investigated).

[§]Grade AAA with regard to all three Venice criteria (18).

[‖]Current on February 27, 2008.

[#]Current on April 30, 2008.

Data sets: the sum of data sets included in the meta-analyses (not including data sets that did not undergo meta-analysis); threshold: authors' prerequisite condition for conducting meta-analysis; significant: $p<0.05$ by random effects calculations on the default (per allele) analysis (for coronary heart disease, results are based on a meta-regression model and correspond to effects in the largest studies, while for DNA repair genes both recessive and dominant models were investigated); strong (grade A): grade AAA in all three Venice criteria; online address: web site for deposited data sets.

Insights from Current Field Synopses

The pilot field synopses provided detailed insight about the grading process in the three specified areas: amount of evidence, replication, and protection from bias. They identified limitations that will help refine the current approach.

Amount of Evidence

For amount of evidence, synopses have used a classification scheme based on the sample size of the minor genetic group (participants or alleles, depending on the genetic model). This is a simple measure that is readily available and has a close connection to power, Bayes factors, or false discovery rate (22). For candidate-gene variants, several postulated associations fail to reach grade A evidence (see Table 12.3). Currently, with large collaborative efforts stemming from GWAS and subsequent replication studies, this is likely to be less of a problem at least for common variants with a frequency greater than 5%–10%. For variants with lower frequency, very large sample sizes may be required. Nevertheless, some consortia have the potential of reaching even sample sizes exceeding 100,000, which means more than 1,000 for the minor allele, even for variants that occur in 0.5% of the general population. For example, the international consortium on osteoporosis (Genetic Factors for Osteoporosis, GEFOS) funded by the European Commission includes 61 studies with 133,333 participants, and for at least 14 of these studies, investigators have already conducted or plan to conduct GWAS. We may need to revisit the criteria on amount of evidence once we have a better sense of the effect sizes regularly encountered for more rare variants.

Replication

Field synopses have used I^2 to assign grades for inconsistency (amount of heterogeneity) (i.e., A for <25%, B for 25%–50%, C for >50%) across studies (23–25). One-third to one-half of the formally significant associations has moderate or large I^2 values. However, I^2 often has large uncertainty when there are only a few studies (26). Moreover, qualitative epidemiologic considerations about the presence of and potential explanation for heterogeneity would need to be taken into account in judging replication. For example, the association between *N*-acetyltransferase type 2 (*NAT2*) variants and bladder cancer risk is expected to be exposure-specific; thus, heterogeneity may readily be expected between populations with different exposures (e.g., different types of tobacco in European populations versus other populations) (27,28).

Another consideration is whether I^2 reflects heterogeneity of estimates around the null value, or heterogeneity in the magnitude of association. The former would question the presence of an association, whereas the latter would question the strength of the association. For instance, even for a consistent association such as the glutathione *S*-transferase M1 (*GSTM1*) null genotype and bladder cancer risk, there is some evidence for heterogeneity in the magnitude of the association across studies (28).

Table 12.3 Venice interim guidelines for assessing the credibility of cumulative evidence on genetic associations (Ioannidis et al., reference 22)

Criteria and Categories	Proposed Operationalization
Amount of evidence A: Large-scale evidence B: Moderate amount of evidence C: Little evidence	Thresholds may be defined on the basis of sample size, power, or false-discovery rate considerations. The frequency of the genetic variant of interest should be accounted for. As a simple rule, we suggest that category A require a sample size of more than 1,000 (total number in cases and controls, assuming a 1:1 ratio) evaluated in the least common genetic group of interest; that B correspond to a sample size of 100–1,000 evaluated in this group; and that C correspond to a sample size of less than 100 evaluated in this group (see "Discussion" section in the text and Table 12.2 for further elaboration).
Replication A: Extensive replication including at least 1 well-conducted meta-analysis with little between-study inconsistency B: Well-conducted meta-analysis with some methodological limitations or moderate between-study inconsistency C: No association; no independent replication; failed replication; scattered studies; flawed meta-analysis or large inconsistency	Between-study inconsistency entails statistical considerations (e.g., defined by metrics such as I 2, where values of 50% and above are considered large and values of 25–50% are considered moderate inconsistency) and also epidemiologic considerations for the similarity/standardization or at least harmonization of phenotyping, genotyping, and analytical models across studies. See "Discussion" section in the text for the threshold (statistical or other) required for claiming replication under different circumstances (e.g., with or without inclusion of the discovery data in situations with massive testing of polymorphisms).
Protection from bias A: Bias, if at all present, could affect the magnitude but probably not the presence of the association B: No obvious bias that may affect the presence of the association, but there is considerable missing information on the generation of evidence C: Considerable potential for or demonstrable bias that can affect even the presence or absence of the association	A prerequisite for A is that the bias due to phenotype measurement, genotype measurement, confounding (population stratification), and selective reporting (for meta-analyses) can be appraised as not being high (as shown in detail in Table 12.4)—plus, there is no other demonstrable bias in any other aspect of the design, analysis, or accumulation of the evidence that could invalidate the presence of the proposed association. In category B, although no strong biases are visible, there is no such assurance that major sources of bias have been minimized or accounted for, because information is missing on how phenotyping, genotyping, and confounding have been handled. Given that occult bias can never be ruled out completely, note that even in category A, we use the qualifier "probably."

However, such epidemiologic insight must be considered with caution, to avoid introducing subjective, speculative processes in the grading. At a minimum, considerations for upgrading or downgrading should be explicit. It may be reasonable to grade as A on this criterion associations with moderate or high heterogeneity with an extensive replication record. This replication includes a *P*-value for the summary effect (excluding the discovery data set), of $p < 10^{-7}$ even in random-effect models that account for between-study heterogeneity or have a false-positive report probability rate less than 10% or a Bayes factor less than 10^{-5}.

For example, the apparent heterogeneity in the effect of *NAT2* slow acetylation on bladder cancer risk can be explained by differences in the pattern of tobacco smoking across study populations (28). However, the presence of heterogeneity would reflect even in these cases the possibility that, bias set aside, one would need to identify the sources of heterogeneity in subsequent studies. These could include not only differential effects under different exposures, but also the possibility that the association is with a correlated phenotype and not the one tested (e.g., the fat mass and obesity-associated gene, diabetes, and obesity) (29), the impact of the different ascertainment schemes used in different studies (30), genotype misclassification (especially in isolated candidate gene studies), or a marker polymorphism that is in variable linkage disequilibrium with the causative variant across the populations (31). The latter scenario could become common in associations that emerge out of "agnostic" GWAS, where it is unlikely that the causal variant will be directly identified. In the setting of GWAS, it is easy to check whether linkage disequilibrium structures are different in different populations; in the presence of similar linkage disequilibrium structure, a cause of heterogeneity can be quickly excluded. It has been demonstrated that beyond a given threshold of inconsistency, no matter how large the studies we conduct, we may never have enough power to replicate an association (nonreplicability threshold) (32).

Another issue is the ability of the cumulative evidence to exclude an association based on lack of replication. It is notable that the Venice criteria include, under "replication C," also the possibility of "no association and failed replication," based on traditional nonsignificant results for the meta-analysis. Minute effects can never be excluded, and in fact, in GWAS, many true associations yield modest results that do not cross genome-wide association p-value thresholds or have equivalently low false report probability rates. Many true findings do not rise to the top of the single nucleotide polymorphism p-value ranks in phase 1 of a genome-wide association study (33). Despite extremely large sample sizes and cumulative meta-analyses of many GWAS, many associations may remain undiscovered and/or inconclusive. The Venice criteria should not be used to conclude that there is strong evidence for a null association.

Protection from Bias

A research finding cannot reach sufficient credibility (>50%) unless the probability of a false-positive association is less than the prestudy odds of an association's being true (34). The Venice criteria include an extensive checklist for sources of biases in different settings. The checklist has different considerations depending on whether the evidence comes from retrospective meta-analyses of published data or prospective GWAS and replication studies from collaborative consortia with harmonization of data collection and analysis.

Bias checks that have been adopted in these synopses for retrospective meta-analysis include automated checks that can be readily applied to all meta-analyses of published data. These are shown in Table 12.4, along with a list of issues that need to be considered. General checks (that can be applied automatically to all fields) have the advantage of being objective and unambiguous, but they cannot provide definitive proof for the presence or absence of bias. For instance, a small effect size (e.g., odds ratio < 1.15) could be explained by bias, but many of the confirmed associations between single nucleotide polymorphisms and chronic diseases are of this order of magnitude. Therefore, small effect sizes, if seen consistently across many studies and with no evidence for publication bias, should not be automatically penalized. For prospective evidence, such as data accumulated from one or more GWAS with prospective replication across several teams in a consortium or prospective meta-analysis of many GWAS from collaborative studies (35) the considerations are quite different. Here, the small magnitude of effect size should not be invoked as evidence of lack of protection from bias, and similarly small-study effect bias or an excess of single studies with significant findings is not an issue here, provided there is no selective reporting of results (there is no reason for such selective reporting in a consortium).

For example, in the schizophrenia synopsis (24), of the 24 associations with nominal statistical significance, 9 associations were graded as "A" and 15 as "C" for

Table 12.4 Some checks for retrospective meta-analyses in field synopses of genetic associations

General checks for the occurrence of or susceptibility to potential problems*

- Small effect size (e.g., odds ratio <1.15-fold from the null value)
- Association lost with exclusion of first study
- Association lost with exclusion of HWE-violating studies or with adjustment for HWE
- Evidence for small-study effect in an asymmetry regression test with proper type I error (*Stat Med.* 2006;25:3443–3457)
- Evidence for excess of single studies with formally statistically significant results (*Clin Trials.* 2007;4:245–253)

Topic- or subject-specific checks: Consider whether they are problems

- Unclear/misclassified phenotypes with possible differential misclassification against genotyping
- Differential misclassification of genotyping against phenotypes
- Major concerns for population stratification (need to justify for affecting odds ratio greater than 1.15-fold, not invoked to date)
- Any other reason (case-by-case basis) that would render the evidence for association highly questionable

*All general checks are likely to have only modest, imperfect sensitivity and specificity for detecting problems. In particular for effect size, a small effect size may very well reflect a true association, since many genetic associations have small effect sizes. However, if this effect has been documented in a retrospective meta-analysis that is susceptible to publication and other reporting biases, it also needs to be replicated in a prospective setting where such biases cannot operate before high credibility can be attributed to it.

"protection from bias." The main reasons for low grades were a small summary odds ratio (odds ratio < 1.15) in what are retrospective meta-analyses of published data ($n = 6$ associations), and loss of significance after excluding the initial study ($n = 6$). Less common reasons were loss of significance after excluding studies that violated Hardy-Weinberg equilibrium and significant differences in effect between small and larger studies.

Issues to Consider for Moving Forward

Defining Thresholds for Evaluating Credibility

The threshold for considering an association for further assessment must be defined in each synopsis, but it may be difficult to reach full consensus on this issue. Given that current synopses have used a large amount of evidence from candidate gene studies, most have considered for grading all probed associations that pass very lenient levels of statistical significance in meta-analysis (typically, $p < 0.05$ inferred from random-effects calculations). However, experience to date indicates that associations with grade A for the amount of evidence but p-values just below 0.05 have either very small effects (and get a C for protection from bias if a retrospective meta-analysis) or moderate/large heterogeneity (and thus get a B or C for replication consistency). Even for such associations that stem from the candidate gene era, it is uncommon to get a rating of "strong" epidemiologic evidence grading (AAA), unless the p-value for the summary effect is substantially lower. Associations that arise out of GWAS require an even more demanding threshold. Thresholds may be set based either on p-value criteria for genome-wide significance or using Bayesian approaches, of which there are several variants (36–39).

In view of the potential multiplicity of phenotypes examined and analyses performed, some authors believe that the rigorous criteria for statistical significance used in GWAS should be applied to candidate gene-derived associations. If so, p-values of 10^{-7} or lower would be required for a locus to be considered "confirmed" (40,41). Figure 12.1a shows the distribution of p-values of the loci identified by GWAS for binary outcome phenotypes and which have been included in the National Human Genome Research Institute (NHGRI) GWAS catalog as of October 14, 2008 (42,43). Of the 466 entries in the catalog, after excluding those pertaining to studies that did not reach any hits with $p < 10^{-5}$ and those that had nonbinary outcomes, 223 loci are included here. As shown, fewer than two-thirds of them (142/223) have a p-value $< 10^{-7}$ and only 39% (87/223) have a p-value $< 10^{-10}$. When several studies and data sets are combined in genome-wide investigations, typically researchers have used pooled, stratified, or simple fixed effects analyses; random effects or other approaches that also take into account the heterogeneity between data sets often would have yielded even more conservative p-values (44). This suggests that the majority of signals emerging from current GWAS and early replication efforts do not yet cross stringent levels of "genome-wide significance." This further highlights the need to include far more data from additional GWAS and replication data sets,

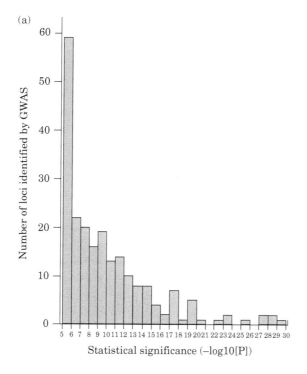

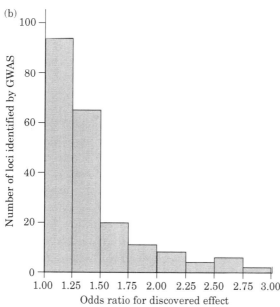

Figure 12.1 (a) Levels of statistical significance for associations of loci with p-value of 10⁻⁵ or lower identified through GWAS and entered in the catalog of GWAS as of October 14, 2008 (41,42) and limited to those that have binary phenotypes (n = 223). For details on selection of loci in the catalog see References 41 and 42. (b) Odds ratios (per allele) for the 223 associations. (c) Odds ratios for 142 of the 233 associations that have p < 10⁻⁷. Not shown are 5, 13, and 7 outliers that had values outside the depicted range in the three panels respectively.

237

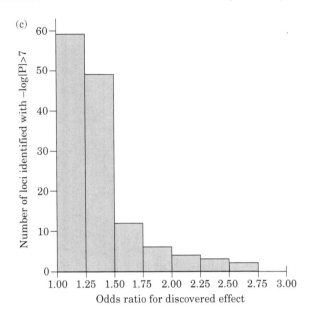

Figure 12.1 Continued.

and this can be routinely accomplished in the setting of field synopses collating all of this information.

Bayesian approaches offer the advantage of allowing different prior probabilities for an association being present based on external evidence (thus bridging agnostic and candidate approaches) (36–39). These methods also allow consideration of the impact of different assumptions about the genetic effect sizes. Empirical evidence from GWAS can offer insight about typical discovered effects. Figure 12.1b shows the distribution of the odds ratios (typically per allele, as reported in the NHGRI catalog) (42,43) in the 223 GWAS-discovered loci. As shown, the median effect corresponds to an odds ratio of 1.28, and the same median is seen for the 142 associations with $p < 10^{-7}$ (Figure 12.1c). These estimates may be inflated compared to the true effects, due to the "winner's curse" phenomenon (inflation of effects selected based on significance thresholds) (45,46). A median true odds ratio of 1.1–1.2 is therefore reasonable for these associations, and some effects many be even smaller, while exceptions of large odds ratios are probably uncommon. Nevertheless, one should acknowledge that the effect of the causal factor that is in the neighborhood of the tagging polymorphism may be larger, and we cannot yet exclude the possibility of considerably larger odds ratios for low frequency variants (47). Such variants were not assessed in the first wave of GWAS, but they are being increasingly targeted in current and future efforts (48,49).

As more synopses accrue, we can examine the stability of the Venice grading for various associations. This will help us understand whether some types of associations can change from having weak credibility to having strong credibility (and *vice versa*). As is described below, gathering empirical evidence into field synopsis databases will allow greater insight in the assessment of cumulative evidence on genetic associations.

Defining Conglomerate Evidence

It is already established practice for hypotheses about specific postulated associations to be tested using data from combinations of prospective consortia analyses stemming from GWAS and their meta-analyses and replication studies; possibly several consortia working on the same disease and phenotypes; additional scattered studies by teams that are not included in any of the consortia; and even retrospective meta-analyses encompassing some/many/all of these sources of data. Such "conglomerate evidence" from various sources of data may appear in various time sequences. The Venice criteria suggested that one should consider the highest possible level of evidence when data come from disparate sources. Perhaps the best currently available source is a well-designed prospective consortium analysis including several teams that have performed GWAS and replications. The results of such an analysis should have a much greater weight than the results of scattered smaller studies. If the consortium evidence results in "strong" evidence, it would not be reasonable to underrate this evidence because of a few small, scattered, inconclusive studies. However, the challenge will become more serious when many consortia with one or more genome-wide platforms are available, and when the scattered or retrospectively meta-analyzed data are much larger in amount than the original consortium-level data on which the reported association was based. Dealing efficiently with this situation requires transparent and comprehensive availability of the evidence from these diverse studies as discussed below.

Global Collaboration: From Data to Knowledge

After reviewing pilot field synopses, participants in the HuGENet workshop discussed how to link emerging data on genetic associations with other sources of information on the biology of genes and gene–disease relations. Clearly, the advent of GWAS in large-scale collaborative studies involving networks and consortia is a crucial first step toward the generation of large-scale data sets. Furthermore, the deposition of these data in accessible public databases can help to address the problem of publication bias commonly seen in candidate gene association studies. Nevertheless, additional efforts are needed to transform data into a knowledge base. Systematic reviews and meta-analyses represent a crucial step in building the knowledge base on genetic variation and human health. Such efforts need to be transparent and their results made available in online databases and publications. The willingness of journal editors to contribute to these efforts is critical, as investigators and systematic reviewers struggle to gain academic recognition for their work, which is often part of multinational, multiple investigator studies. Finally, the

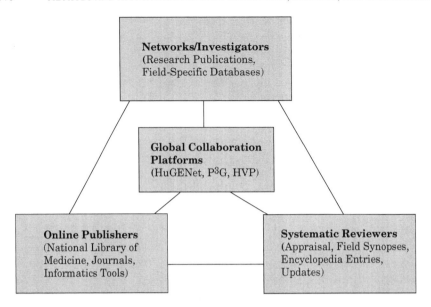

Figure 12.2 A vision for collaboration among disease- and gene-specific investigators, systematic reviewers, and online publishers. HuGENet, Human Genome Epidemiology Network; HVP, Human Variome Project; P³G, Public Population Project in Genomics

National Library of Medicine (http://www.ncbi.nlm.nih.gov/) has a leading role in linking genetic association studies with other existing databases on gene sequences, products, and linkages to disease processes (50).

At the HuGENet workshop, a vision emerged of collaboration to create a sustainable, credible knowledge base on genetic variation and human diseases. As shown in Figure 12.2, the collaboration involves research investigators, systematic reviewers, online publishers, and database developers with variable degrees of overlap among the groups. For example, investigators who are part of research consortia have their own informatics tools and databases, and they can conduct systematic reviews of their own field based on their own data or also including data from teams external to the consortium. In addition, other reviewers could contribute to these efforts, as evidenced by many previous efforts in meta-analyses and Human Genome Epidemiology (HuGE) reviews. Figure 12.2 shows the flow from generation of new data to systematic appraisal and synthesis and to online dissemination via journals and databases.

A successful example of collaboration already exists in the field of type 2 diabetes. Investigators from diverse consortia have combined efforts to conduct comprehensive meta-analyses of all GWAS and replication studies. A first meta-analysis combined three GWAS with a total of over 10,000 samples; this was followed by a second stage of replication of the most interesting signals in over 22,000 independent samples and a subsequent third stage of replication on over 57,000 samples, with data being combined by means of formal meta-analysis methods (51). Similar meta-analyses are being designed and carried out by collaborating consortia in several other fields (for example, the Psychiatric GWAS Consortium, which is conducting meta-analyses within and between five psychiatric disorders; https://pgc.unc.edu/faqs.html).

Several global collaborations focused on genotype-phenotype correlations can help support fields where large-scale studies are still in the making. For example, HuGENet sponsors the HuGE Navigator (5), a knowledge base with online tools for capturing and organizing the most up-to-date information on genetic associations and other related information. The Human Variome Project (HVP) is focused on the production and synthesis of gene- and gene-variant-centered databases with linked phenotypic outcomes (52). The Public Population Project in Genomics (P³G) (53) aims to harmonize data collected from large-scale cohort studies and biobanks around the world. Cross links among HuGENet, P³G, HVP, and other groups are crucial to convene and facilitate collective efforts in developing the knowledge base on genetic variation and human diseases. Efforts in coordinating these global collaborations are already under way through cross-linking of these enterprises. For example, P³G has an international working group in epidemiology and biostatistics that is closely related to the HuGENet movement. Another, more specialized online knowledge base development effort that can be synergistic is PharmGKB (the Pharmacogenomics Knowledge Base) (54). In addition, GeneReviews are expert-authored, peer-reviewed disease descriptions focused on the use of genetic testing in the diagnosis, management, and genetic counseling of patients and their families. GeneReviews are part of the GeneTests web site (http://www.ncbi.nlm.nih.gov/sites/GeneTests/?db=GeneTests), which also includes international directories of genetics clinics and genetics laboratories (55,56). Finally, it is important for epidemiologic efforts to be linked with biological efforts, including experimental work, assessment of endophenotypes, and functional studies in different model systems.

Schizophrenia: Field Synopsis and Example of Development of a Knowledge Base

As an example of the collaboration among primary investigators, systematic reviewers, and online publishers, Bertram et al. provide a model approach to a distributed knowledge base of genetic variants that features collaboration among the three groups outlined above. They have synthesized primary research on genetic associations in schizophrenia, and they developed a regularly updated, online SzGene database (http://www.schizophreniaforum.org/res/sczgene/default.asp), that collects and curates published results in this area. A peer-reviewed field synopsis summarizes the cumulative evidence and evaluates it according to the Venice criteria. The field synopsis is regularly updated online with updated cumulative meta-analyses. Bertram et al. have developed similar resources for Alzheimer disease (http://www.alzforum.org/res/com/gen/alzgene/default.asp).

The HuGE Navigator web site (http://www.hugenavigator.net/) serves to link field-specific efforts like SzGene with other online databases through the HuGEpedia. The HuGEpedia can be accessed by using either phenotype (Phenopedia) or a gene (Genopedia) as the starting point. For example, searching the Phenopedia for schizophrenia leads users to a page that provides an up-to-date summary of genes studied for association with schizophrenia, links to abstracts of the original publications in PubMed, meta-analyses and HuGE reviews, and abstracted meta tables. The HuGE Navigator can also be searched to locate investigators in the field and to display geographic and temporal trends in the published literature. Finally, HuGE Navigator attempts to identify and link to all published GWAS in the field, as well as to data sets deposited and available through the National Center for Biotechnology Information's (NCBI) dbGaP. Although HuGE Navigator is not a comprehensive data repository, it serves as a first stop for orientation and links to more authoritative data sources and field synopses. The highest level of data integration in this example occurs through links with NCBI databases (such as PubMed, Entrez Gene, and dbGaP). The NCBI online book, *Genes and Diseases* (57), could also expand to accommodate the most current synopses in individual fields.

Concluding Remarks

This is a crucial time in human genomics research, when advances in genome-wide analysis platforms coupled with declining costs are producing an unprecedented outpouring of replicated genetic associations with common diseases. To make the most of the research enterprise and to promote reliable and timely knowledge synthesis, the multidisciplinary working group offers the following recommendations.

First, data from GWAS should be made available for interested researchers to avoid selective positive reporting of spurious associations and to facilitate meta-analyses of particular associations. Involvement of the primary investigators of the GWAS in collaborative projects and meta-analyses should be encouraged. There is a risk of errors and misconceptions being introduced if the primary investigators who are intimately familiar with the data are not involved. Second, researchers and research networks should develop field synopses that use meta-analysis to integrate published and unpublished data and evaluate the cumulative evidence. The Venice guidelines offer interim guidance, and further empirical research is needed to assess the stability and implementation of these guidelines. Third, we encourage the development of field-specific databases, such as the SzGene database discussed above. Fourth, we encourage journal editors to publish field synopses with regular updates as called for by *Nature Genetics* in 2006 (20). Fifth, we recommend that journals and online publishers develop and make widely available databases that include standardized and systematically collected information from original research for research synthesis. The HuGE Navigator is one approach presented here, but others could emerge in the future. The rapidity of data accumulation necessitates such a systematic approach as a starting point for evaluating the gaps in our knowledge base. To succeed, these efforts depend on collaboration fueled by the availability of funding, not only for generating original research data, but also for efforts in research synthesis and dissemination. Finally, we need to ensure that epidemiologic research synthesis discussed here is accompanied by critical appraisal and synthesis of biologic research. The combination of epidemiology and biology is crucial to enhance the credibility of genetic associations and to accelerate their applications in clinical medicine and population health.

References

1. Lin B, Clyne M, Walsh M, et al. Tracking the epidemiology of human genes in the literature: the HuGE published literature database. *Am J Epidemiol.* 2006;164:1–4.
2. Topol E, Murray SS, Frazer KA. The genomics gold rush. *JAMA.* 2007;298:218–221.
3. Kingsmore SF, Lindquist IE, Mudge J, et al. Genome-wide association studies: progress and potential for drug discovery and development. *Nat Rev Drug Discov.* 2008;7:221–230.
4. Hunter DJ, Khoury MJ, Drazen JM. Letting the genome out of the bottle: will we get our wish. *N Engl J Med.* 2008;358:105–107.
5. Editorial. Risky business. *Nat Genet.* 2007;39:1415.
6. Editorial. Positively disruptive. *Nat Genet.* 2008;40:119.
7. NCI_NHGRI Working Group on Replication in Association Studies. Replicating genotype-phenotype associations. *Nature.* 2007;447:655–660.
8. Yu W, Gwinn M, Clyne M, et al. A navigator for human genome epidemiology. *Nat Genet.* 2008;40:124–125. Also available at http://www.hugenavigator.net/. Accessed February 19, 2008.
9. National Library of Medicine. Database on genotypes and phenotypes (DbGAP). Available at http://www.ncbi.nlm.nih.gov/sites/entrez?db=gap. Accessed February 19, 2008.
10. National Cancer Institute. Cancer genetic markers of susceptibility. Available at http://cgems.cancer.gov/. Accessed February 19, 2008.
11. Wellcome Trust Case-Control Consortium. Available at http://www.wtccc.org.uk/. Accessed April 19, 2008.
12. National Institutes for Health. Policy for sharing data obtained in NIH supported or conducted genome-wide association studies (GWAS). Available at http://grants.nih.gov/grants/guide/notice-files/NOT-OD-07–088.html. Accessed April 19, 2008.
13. Homer N, Szelinger S, Redman M, et al. Resolving individuals contributing trace amounts of DNA to highly complex mixtures using high-density SNP genotyping microarrays. *PLoS Genet.* 2008;4:e1000167.
14. Khoury MJ, Dorman JS. The Human Genome Epidemiology Network. *Am J Epidemiol.* 1998;148:1–3.
15. Centers for Disease Control and Prevention. The Human Genome Epidemiology Network (HuGENet). Available at http://www.cdc.gov/genomics/hugenet/default.htm. Accessed February 19, 2008.
16. Ioannidis JP, Gwinn M, Little J, et al. A road map for efficient and reliable human genome epidemiology. *Nat Genet.* 2006;38:3–5.
17. Ioannidis JP, Bernstein J, Boffetta P, et al. A network of investigator networks in human genome epidemiology. *Am J Epidemiol.* 2005;162:302–304.
18. HuGENet workshop. STrengthening the REporting of Genetic Associations (STREGA). Available at http://www.cdc.gov/genomics/hugenet/strega.htm. Accessed February 19, 2008.
19. Little J, Higgins JPT, eds. The HuGENet™ HuGE Review Handbook, version 1.0. Available at http://www.hugenet.ca. Accessed March 10, 2008.
20. Editorial. Embracing risk. *Nat Genet.* 2006;38:1.

21. HuGENet workshop on assessment of cumulative assessment of genetic associations. Available at http://www.cdc.gov/genomics/hugenet/hugewkshp_nov06.htm Accessed March 30, 2008.
22. Ioannidis JP, Boffetta P, Little J, et al. Assessment of cumulative evidence on genetic associations: interim guidelines. *Int J Epidemiol.* 2008;37:120–132.
23. Bertram L, McQueen MB, Mullin K, et al. Systematic meta-analyses of Alzheimer genetic association studies: the AlzGene database. *Nat Genet.* 2007;39:17–23.
24. Allen NC, Bagade S, McQueen MB, et al. Systematic meta-analyses and field synopsis of genetic association studies in schizophrenia: the SzGene Database. *Nat Genet.* 2008;40:827–834.
25. Vineis P, Manuguerra M, Kavvoura FK, et al. A field synopsis on low-penetrance variants in DNA repair genes and cancer susceptibility. *J Natl Cancer Inst.* 2009;101(1):24–36.
26. Ioannidis JP, Patsopoulos NA, Evangelou E. Uncertainty in heterogeneity estimates in meta-analyses. *BMJ.* 2007;335:914–916.
27. García-Closas M, Malats N, Silverman D, et al. NAT2 slow acetylation and GSTM1 null genotypes increase bladder cancer risk: results from the Spanish Bladder Cancer Study and meta-analyses. *Lancet.* 2005;366:649–659.
28. Rothman N, Garcia-Closas M, Hein DW. Commentary: reflections on G. M. Lower and colleagues' 1979 study associating slow acetylator phenotype with urinary bladder cancer: meta-analysis, historical refinements of the hypothesis, and lessons learned. *Int J Epidemiol.* 2007;36:23–28.
29. Frayling TM, Timpson NJ, Weedon MN, et al. A common variant in the FTO gene is associated with body mass index and predisposes to childhood and adult obesity. *Science.* 2007;316:889–894.
30. Burton PR, Palmer LJ, Jacobs K, et al. Ascertainment adjustment: where does it take us? *Am J Hum Genet.* 2000;67:1505–1514.
31. Ioannidis JP Non-replication and inconsistency in the genome-wide association setting. *Hum Hered.* 2007;64:203–213.
32. Moonesinghe R, Khoury MJ, Liu T, et al. Required sample size and nonreplicability thresholds for heterogeneous genetic associations. *Proc Natl Acad Sci USA.* 2008;105:617–622.
33. Thomas G, Jacobs KB, Yeager M, et al. Multiple loci identified in a genome-wide association study of prostate cancer. *Nat Genet.* 2008;40:310–315.
34. Ioannidis JP. Why most published research findings are false. *PLoS Med.* 2005;2:e124.
35. Zeggini E, Weedon MN, Lindgren CM, et al. Replication of genome-wide association signals in UK samples reveals risk loci for type 2 diabetes. *Science.* 2007;316:1336–1341.
36. Wakefield JA. Bayesian measure of the probability of false discovery in genetic epidemiology studies. *Am J Hum Genet.* 2007;81:208–227.
37. Wakefield J. Bayes factors for genome-wide association studies: comparison with P-values. *Genet Epidemiol.* July 18, 2008;33(1):79–86. [Epub ahead of print]
38. Wacholder S, Chanock S, Garcia-Closas M, et al. Assessing the probability that a positive report is false: an approach for molecular epidemiology studies. *J Natl Cancer Inst.* 2004;96:434–442.
39. Ioannidis JP. Calibration of credibility of agnostic genome-wide associations. *Am J Med Genet B Neuropsychiatr Genet.* 2008;147B:964–972.
40. Hoggart CJ, Clark TG, De Iorio M, et al. Genome-wide significance for dense SNP and resequencing data. *Genet Epidemiol.* 2008;32:179–185.
41. Pe'er I, Yelensky R, Altshuler D, Daly MJ. Estimation of the multiple testing burden for genomewide association studies of nearly all common variants. *Genet Epidemiol.* 2008;32:381–385.

42. Hindorff LA, Junkins HA, Manolio TA. A Catalog of Published Genome-Wide Association Studies. Available at www.genome.gov/26525384. Accessed October 14, 2008.

43. Manolio TA, Brooks LD, Collins FS. A HapMap harvest of insights into the genetics of common disease. *J Clin Invest.* 2008;118:1590–1605.

44. Ioannidis JP, Patsopoulos NA, Evangelou E. Heterogeneity in meta-analyses of genome-wide association investigations. *PLoS ONE.* 2007;2:e841.

45. Zollner S, Pritchard JK. Overcoming the winner's curse: estimating penetrance parameters from case-control data. *Am J Hum Genet.* 2007;80:605–615.

46. Ioannidis JP. Why most discovered true associations are inflated. *Epidemiology.* 2008;19:640–648.

47. Wright AF, Charlesworth B, Rudan I, et al. A polygenic basis for late-onset disease. *Trends Genet.* 2003;19:97–106.

48. Bodmer W, Bonilla C. Common and rare variants in multifactorial susceptibility to common diseases. *Nat Genet.* 2008;40:695–701.

49. Walsh T, McClellan JM, McCarthy SE, et al. Rare structural variants disrupt multiple genes in neurodevelopmental pathways in schizophrenia. *Science.* 2008;320:539–543.

50. National Center for Biotechnology Information Databases. Available at http://www.ncbi.nlm.nih.gov/. Accessed February 19, 2008.

51. Zeggini E, Scott LJ, Saxena R, et al. Meta-analysis of genome-wide association data and large-scale replication identifies several additional susceptibility loci for type 2 diabetes. *Nat Genet.* 2008;40:638–645.

52. Cotton RG, Appelbe W, Auerbach AD, et al. Recommendations of the 2006 Human Variome Project meeting. *Nat Genet.* 2007;39:433–436.

53. Public Population Project in Genomics (P3G). Available at http://www.p3gconsortium.org/. Accessed February 19, 2008.

54. Klein TE, Chang JT, Cho MK, et al. Integrating genotype and phenotype information: an overview of the PharmGKB project. Pharmacogenetics Research Network and Knowledge Base. *Pharmacogenomics J.* 2001;1:167–170.

55. Genereviews (genetests). Available at http://www.genetests.org/. Accessed February 19, 2008.

56. Pagon RA. GeneTests: an online genetic information resource for healthcare providers. *Med Libr Assoc.* 2006;94:343–348.

57. National Center for Biotechnology Information Genes and Diseases. Available at http://www.ncbi.nlm.nih.gov/books/bv.fcgi?call=bv.View..ShowSection&rid=gnd.preface.91. Accessed February 19, 2008.

III

CASE STUDIES: CUMULATIVE ASSESSMENT OF THE ROLE OF HUMAN GENOME VARIATION IN SPECIFIC DISEASES

13

Colorectal cancer

Harry Campbell, Steven Hawken, Evropi Theodoratou,
Alex Demarsh, Kimberley Hutchings, Candice Y. Johnson,
Lindsey Masson, Linda Sharp, Valerie Tait, and Julian Little

Introduction

Colorectal cancer is a major global public health problem, with approximately 950,000 cases newly diagnosed each year (1). Risk of developing colorectal cancer increases steeply with age and incidence is rising in many industrialized countries as life expectancy and the numbers of elderly people increase. Incidence is also rising in many developing countries, as diet and lifestyle become more similar to those in industrialized countries.

Approximately 25% of colorectal cancer cases are associated with a family history; risk is increased two to four times in first-degree relatives of a patient with colorectal cancer. A substantial proportion of the familial aggregation of colorectal cancer results from inherited susceptibility. Excess familial cancer risk can be accounted for by a combination of rare high-penetrance mutations and large numbers of common variants each conferring small genotypic risk (on the order of 1.1–2.0). These latter variants combine additively or multiplicatively to confer a range of susceptibilities in the population (2).

The relationships of genetic variants with human disease described so far largely reflect the study designs used to identify them. Linkage studies conducted among families with multiple cases of disease were successful in identifying highly penetrant variants with large effects (such as *hMLH1*, *hMSH2*, and *APC*; see below). The discovery of genes responsible for inherited colorectal cancer syndromes has been important in identifying important etiologic pathways such as the beta-catenin/APC and TGF beta/SMAD pathways. Association studies conducted in general population samples using common genetic markers typically find variants with very small effects (such as *SMAD7* and *CRAC1*; see Section "Common Low-Penetrance Variants Identified from Genome-Wide Association Studies"). Future resequencing studies are expected to identify rarer variants (e.g., prevalence 0.05–5%) with intermediate effects (3). Genome-wide studies of structural variation will likely identify deletions, amplifications, and other copy number variations influencing colorectal cancer risk.

Rare, High-Penetrance Variants

Mismatch Repair Gene Mutations (hMLH1, hMSH2, hMLH6, hPMS1, hPMS2)

The clinical syndrome due to mismatch repair gene deficiency is known as Hereditary Non-Polyposis Colorectal Cancer (HNPCC) and accounts for 2–5% of all colorectal cancer cases. Affected kindreds have an unusually high occurrence of colorectal and certain extracolonic cancers, with a relatively early age of onset.

Evidence to support a role for the mismatch repair genes *hMLH1* and *hMSH2* in the etiology of colorectal cancer has come from linkage analysis, segregation studies, and molecular–biologic analysis. The mismatch repair genes *hMLH1* and *hMSH2* are integral components of the DNA mismatch repair pathway. A HuGE review in 2002 identified 259 different pathogenic mutations (and 45 variants) in *hMLH1* and 191 different pathogenic mutations (and 55 variants) in *hMSH2* (4). In addition, deletions in mismatch repair genes appear to occur relatively commonly, particularly in *hMSH2*. HNPCC families in which mutations in *hMLH1* and *hMSH2* are not identified may harbor pathogenic mutations in other mismatch repair genes, such as *hMSH6* and *hPMS2*.

The available data do not suggest any substantial differences in the frequency of *hMLH1* or *hMSH2* mutations among populations or ethnic groups (5). The penetrance of mutations in *hMLH1/hMSH2* is incomplete and is significantly higher in men (approximately 80%) than in women (approximately 40%). A standardized incidence ratio of 68 for colorectal cancer was reported for carriers of *hMLH1* or *hMSH2* mutations compared with the general population (6). First-degree relatives of mutation carriers had a relative risk of 8.1 compared with first-degree relatives of noncarriers (7).

APC

The adenomatous polyposis coli (*APC*) gene is a tumor suppressor gene, and mutations resulting in loss of APC protein function are associated with carcinogenesis. APC protein down-regulates the Wnt signaling pathway through its binding to β-catenin and axin (8).

APC germline mutations lead to the highly penetrant, autosomal dominant neoplastic syndrome of Familial Adenomatous Polyposis Coli (FAP). This condition has an annual incidence of about 1:7,000 live births and is characterized by hundreds or thousands of colorectal adenomas, which if untreated can develop into carcinomas (9). FAP accounts for about 1% of all colorectal cancer cases.

Low-penetrance *APC* mutations have been implicated in familial colorectal cancer cases (10). The most common *APC* variants associated with inherited susceptibility are *I1307K* and *E1317Q*. At least 12 single nucleotide polymorphisms (SNPs) of *APC* have been identified, 8 of them in exon 15. The most common allele (*Asp1822Val*, frequency 10–22%) was found not to be associated with development of colorectal cancer in three studies but a positive association has been observed with two others.

MUTYH

Another familial form of colorectal cancer, *MUTYH*-associated polyposis (MAP), was first described in families with multiple colorectal adenomas or carcinomas who lacked inherited *APC* mutations (11,12). The MAP phenotype is clinically comparable to the FAP phenotype; however, it is recessively transmitted and generally results in a smaller number of adenomas and later age at onset of colorectal cancer (13).

MUTYH is a base excision repair gene. Approximately 30 mutations that alter the protein product, 52 missense variants, and 3 inframe insertions/deletions have been identified (14). The two most common *MUTYH* variants in whites account for >80% of disease-causing alleles; additional alleles have been identified in other populations.

OGG1

Base-excision repair maintains genome stability by countering oxidative DNA damage. OGG1 acts together with MYH and MTH1 to identify and remove 8-oxoguanine that has been incorporated into DNA. *OGG1* variants have been reported in association with colorectal cancer, alone or in combination with mutations in other genes (15,16).

Other Rare Variants

Several other rare, autosomal dominant disorders include increased risk of colorectal cancer. Juvenile Polyposis Syndrome, caused by mutations in *SMAD4, PTEN*, or *BMPR1A*, is associated with early onset colorectal cancer, typically before 20 years of age.

Common, Low-Penetrance Variants

Many studies have investigated associations of colorectal cancer with common variants of low-penetrance genes. Initially, most of these studies were hypothesis-driven, usually focusing on genes thought to be involved in the metabolism of particular environmental risk factors (the "candidate gene" approach). We have organized this section of the chapter around genes that operate in pathways that are thought to play a role in the causation of colorectal cancer.

We identified relevant studies by using the HuGE Navigator (available at http://www.hugenavigator.net) and extracted information using approaches we have used in HuGE reviews.

Genetic Variants Affecting Multiple Substrate Metabolism

Many studies have examined associations between colorectal cancer and variants of genes encoding enzymes involved in metabolism of carcinogens that are present in tobacco smoke or produced as a result of cooking meats. The most extensive evidence relates to the glutathione S-transferase genes *GSTM1, GSTT1*, and *GSTP1*, the cytochrome P450 1A1 gene *CYP1A1*, and the N-acteyltranferase genes *NAT1* and *NAT2*.

The glutathione S-transferases (GSTs). The glutathione S-transferases (GSTs) play a central role in the detoxification of carcinogens by catalyzing the conjugation of glutathione to potentially genotoxic compounds, including polyaromatic hydrocarbons (17). However, GSTs also conjugate isothiocyanates, which are potent inducers of enzymes that detoxify environmental mutagens, thereby diverting the isothiocyanates from the enzyme induction pathway to excretion. These two opposing potential mechanisms suggest that the role of GSTs in cancer risk is complex. GSTs also modulate the induction of the enzymes and proteins important for cellular functions such as DNA repair.

Systematic reviews and meta-analyses have been conducted examining the association between *GSTM1, GSTT1, GSTP1,* and colorectal cancer susceptibility (17–21).

GSTM1: Twenty-eight studies have investigated the association of *GSTM1* with colorectal cancer. Overall, there is evidence of a weak association of the *GSTM1* null genotype with colorectal cancer, with substantial heterogeneity.

GSTT1: Twenty-three studies have investigated the association between *GSTT1* and colorectal cancer (Table 13.1). Overall, the evidence suggests a weak association of the *GSTT1* null genotype with colorectal cancer.

GSTP1: Eleven studies have investigated the association of *GSTP1* with colorectal cancer. None of the studies supports an association.

The cytochrome P450 genes. The cytochrome P450 (CYP) family of enzymes includes over 50 characterized genes, of which the *CYP1, CYP2,* and *CYP3* families are involved in phase I metabolism of xenobiotics and drugs and also metabolism of some endogenous compounds.

CYP1A1: The *CYP1A1* gene is under the regulatory control of the aryl hydrocarbon receptor, a transcription factor that regulates gene expression. Overall, there is limited evidence for association with the *T3801C* variant, and the *Ile462Val* variant. Both studies investigating the *Thr461Asn* variant found that the *Thr/Asn* genotype was associated with significantly reduced risk of colorectal cancer compared with the *Thr/Thr* genotype.

CYP1A2: Five studies from Korea, France, Hungary, Spain, and the United Kingdom have investigated the *A164C* (rs762551) genotype in colorectal cancer, with negative or inconsistent results.

CYP1B1: Studies of European populations provide no support for association with colorectal cancer for the *C1294G* (rs1056836) or the *N453S* (rs1800440) variant.

CYP2C9: Six studies of *CYP2C9*2* genotype and colorectal cancer have had inconsistent results. None of the five studies of *CYP2C9*3* genotype found an association. Of the four studies that analyzed both *CYP2C9*2* and *CYP2C9*3* variants, three suggested an inverse association with possession of one or both variant alleles. Because these studies included only small numbers of persons with the variant

Table 13.1 Summary of studies by region and date of publication of GSTT1 null genotype and colorectal cancer

Authors	Date	Country/ Ethnicity	Gender	Description of Cases	Description of Controls	Number of Cases/ Controls	% of Controls GSTT1 null	OR (95% CI)
Abdel-Rahman et al. (22)	1999	Egypt	M/F	Newly diagnosed patients from three cancer hospitals	Healthy controls, friends of other cancer patients from the same centers, matched on age	59/51	41.2	Crude OR: 0.85 (0.37, 1.97)
Lee et al. (23)	1995	Singapore		Surgical patients	Patients with no history of neoplasms from the clinical chemistry department of a local hospital	300/183	49	Not reported
Yoshioka et al. (24)	1999	Japan		Consecutive histologically confirmed	Hospital based (routine physical exam)	106/100	41	Crude OR: 1.33 (0.77, 2.32)
Zhu et al. (25)	2002	China		Sporadic colorectal ade-nocarcinoma patients	Healthy controls	104/101	47.5	1.63 (0.94, 2.84)
Chen et al. (26)	2004	China	M/F			125/339	20.4	0.88 (0.52, 1.49)
Yeh et al. (27)	2005	China	M/F	Histologically confirmed new cases	Hospital based (presenting for routine checkup)	723/733	49.1	1.25 (1.02, 1.53)
Chenevix-Trench et al. (28)	1995	Australia		Patients with colorectal adenocarcinoma	Source not stated (n = 94) and cancer free geriatric patients (n = 54)	132/148	19 9	0.7 (0.3, 1.4) 1.5 (0.6, 4.3)
Butler et al. (29)	2001	Australia white	M/F	Queen Elizabeth Hospital, white adults	Hospital based (blood donors)	203/200	20.0	Crude OR: 2.18 (1.38, 3.43)
Zhang et al. (30)	1999	Sweden		Pathology confirmed	Population based	99/109	20%	4.49 (2.42, 8.34)

(Continued)

Table 13.1 Continued.

Authors	Date	Country/Ethnicity	Gender	Description of Cases	Description of Controls	Number of Cases/Controls	% of Controls GSTT1 null	OR (95% CI)
Laso et al. (31)	2002	Spain	M/F	Consecutive patients undergoing surgery from the University of Barcelona Hospital Clinic, Spain	Hospital based, during the same time period as case accrual	247/296	11.1	Crude OR: 1.68 (1, 2.82)
van der Hel et al. (32)	2003	Netherlands	F	Population-based screening program for early detection of breast cancer	Population based	234/765	29.3	0.91 (0.65, 1.28)
Kiss et al. (33)	2004	Hungary	M/F	Histologically confirmed	Hospital based cancer-free controls (inpatients and outpatients)	500/500	21.6	Crude OR: 1.29 (0.95, 1.74)
van der Logt et al. (34)	2004	Netherlands	M/F	Gastroenterology and general surgery patients	Recruited from local newspaper	371/415	16.6	Crude OR: 1.2 (0.84, 1.7)
Saadat and Saadat (35)	2001	Iran	M/F	Pathologically confirmed	Healthy blood donor matched to cases on age and gender	46/131	11.5	Crude OR: 1.41 (0.70, 2.88)
Ates et al. (36)	2005	Turkey	M/F	Consecutive histologically confirmed (inpatients and outpatients)	Unrelated healthy controls recruited from two hospitals in Turkey	181/204	26.0	Adjusted OR: 1.64 (1.10, 2.59)
Nascimento et al. (37)	2003	Brazil	M/F	Consecutive histologically confirmed cases	Blood donors from the same hospital	102/300	17.3	Crude OR: 0.95 (0.50, 1.80)
Seow et al. (38)	2002	Singapore	M/F	Incident cases identified through population-based Singapore Cancer Registry	Cancer-free participants of the Singapore Chinese Health Study (population based, prospective)	213/1194	40.2	Adjusted OR: 0.88 (0.64, 1.21)

Study	Year	Country	Sex	Case definition	Control definition	Cases/Controls	%	OR (95% CI)
Welfare et al. (39)	1999	U.K.	M/F	Histologically confirmed cases	Community-based controls	201/187	16.9	Adjusted OR: 1.21 (0.63, 2.0)
Loktionov et al. (40)	2001	U.K.		Histologically confirmed cases	Cancer/adenoma free participants of the ongoing UK Flexible Sigmoidoscopy Screening Trial	206/355	15.2	Crude OR: 1.43 (0.89, 2.28)
Sachse et al. (41)	2002	U.K.	M/F	Incident cases	Healthy population-based controls with no history of previous cancer	490/593	63.7	Crude OR: 0.87 (0.67, 1.13)
Rajagopal et al. (42)	2005	U.K. white	M/F	Surgical cases with operative and histological confirmation	Hospital-based cancer-free controls	361/881	17.9	Crude OR: 1.65 (1.22, 2.24)
Little et al. (43)	2006	U.K.	M/F	Histologically confirmed cases identified from the database of the pathology laboratory	Selected from the Grampian Community Health Index (list of everyone registered with a GP) matched by age and sex	264/408	17	Adjusted OR: 1.25 (0.81, 1.93) Adjusted OR: 1.23 (0.74, 2.02)
Gertig et al. (44)	1998	U.S. white	M	Cases with CRC from the prospective Physician's Health Study	White male participants not diagnosed with CRC within the prospective Physicians' Health Study	212/221	23	0.8 (0.5, 1.2)

genotypes and the associations they found were inconsistent, they provide only weak and insufficient evidence.

CYP2C19: Three studies from Spain, Turkey, and the United Kingdom investigated the association of *G681A* with colorectal cancer, with inconsistent results.

CYP2D6: Three studies from Australia, Spain, and the United Kingdom have investigated variants in this gene; however, because different gene nomenclatures were used, it is difficult to compare the results, which were inconsistent.

CYP2E1: Studies of two variants found on the c2 allele (rs3813867, rs2031920) and a variant of intron 6 (*7632T>A/Dra I*) conducted in Australia, China, France, Hungary, the Netherlands, Spain, and the United States have been negative or inconclusive.

CYP3A4: Two studies found no association of *G20230A* (rs2242480), found on the *CYP3A4*1G* or *1H* alleles, with colorectal cancer.

CYP3A5: The intronic variant *6986A>G* (rs776746), found on alleles *CYP3A5*3A* to *CYP3A5*3L*, has been investigated in two small studies of colorectal cancer. No association was found in either.

Other CYP genes: Variants of *CYP2C8*, *CYP11A1*, *CYP17A1*, *CYP19A1*, and *CYP7A1* have each been investigated in only one study, with no associations found.

The N-acetyltransferases. N-acetyltransferase 1 (NAT1) and N-acetyltransferase 2 (NAT2) function as phase II conjugating enzymes, implicated in the activation and detoxification of known carcinogens.

NAT1: The initial report of an OR of 1.9 with 95% confidence interval (95% CI 1.2–3.1) for association with possession of the *NAT1*10* allele has not been replicated in most of the subsequent studies.

NAT2: Early studies reported that the NAT2 rapid acetylation phenotype was associated with increased risk of colorectal cancer and a meta-analysis estimated the pooled OR as 1.51 (95% CI 1.07–2.12) (21). In a meta-analysis of 15 studies published before October 2001 (21), the combined risk estimate for rapid acetylators (inferred on the basis of their genotype) was 1.03 (95% CI 0.94–1.12). Most studies published since the meta-analysis have been null.

Genetic Variants Affecting Nutrient Metabolism

Virtually all epidemiologic studies of diet and colorectal cancer have been observational and subject to three potential biases: (i) diet is related to other aspects of lifestyle, which may influence risk, (ii) people eat foods rather than nutrients, and (iii) misclassification of intake, either of the food group or nutrient being investigated or of other food groups or nutrients, could dilute or bias the associations. Studying associations with genetic variants that influence nutrient metabolism might help unravel the relationship of dietary factors with colorectal cancer.

Variants of genes associated with alcohol intake and metabolism. Case-control studies have examined the associations between colorectal cancer and variants of *ALDH2*, *ADH1B* (*ADH2*), or *ADH1C* (*ADH3*). Population frequencies of the most commonly studied variants of these genes have been reviewed recently.

ALDH2: The most frequently reported associations are with a variant of *ALDH2* most prevalent in Asian populations (Table 13.2). The *ALDH2*487Lys* (rs671) variant results in reduced activity of the mitochondrial enzyme aldehyde dehydrogenase, leading to high levels of acetylaldehyde, which is thought to be carcinogenic. Because accumulation of acetaldehyde also produces unpleasant symptoms (facial flushing, increased heart rate, and nausea), persons who are homozygous or heterozygous for reduced-activity *ALDH2* variants may consume less alcohol than do those without the variant, which could lower the risk of alcohol-related diseases.

We combined the results of six case-control studies in a meta-analysis, which found the following summary ORs and 95% CIs: for heterozygotes (*ALDH2 Glu/Lys* vs. *ALDH2 Glu/Glu*), OR 0.87 (95% CI 0.73–1.04); for homozygotes (*ALDH2 Lys/Lys* vs. *ALDH2 Glu/Glu*), OR 0.73 (95% CI 0.57–0.95). Thus, the evidence suggests an inverse association of the *ALDH2*487Lys* allele with colorectal cancer in populations of north-eastern Asian ancestry.

ADH1B: Combining the results of three case-control studies, one in Europe and two in Japan, to test for heterozygous (*ADH1B Arg/His* vs. *ADH1B His/His*) or homozygous (*ADH1B Arg/Arg* vs. *ADH1B His/His*) genetic effects, we found combined ORs and 95% CIs of 1.29 (1.10, 1.52) for heterozygotes and 1.51 (1.05, 2.16) for homozygotes. It is noteworthy that this association was confined to the two Japanese studies. Although the evidence is limited, the consistency of the results across these two studies suggests that this association deserves further research attention.

ADH1C: None of the four studies of the *ADH1C Ile349Val* variant and colorectal cancer has supported an association with colorectal cancer. Combining the results of four case-control studies to test for heterozygous (*Ile/Val* vs. *ADH1C Ile/Ile*) or homozygous (*Val/Val* vs. *ADH1C Ile/Ile*) genetic effects, we found combined ORs and 95% CIs of 1.03 (0.90, 1.19) for heterozygotes and of 1.02 (0.85, 1.23) for homozygotes.

Variants related to folate and one-carbon metabolism. Folate is a B vitamin (B9) found most abundantly in vegetables and fortified grain products. Folate mediates the transfer of one-carbon units in a variety of cellular reactions, most notably in thymidine, purine, and methionine synthesis. Thymidine and purine are required for DNA synthesis and repair, whereas methionine is a precursor in reactions necessary in the maintenance of normal DNA methylation patterns (45). Hypomethylation of DNA is hypothesized to contribute to carcinogenesis through a number of mechanisms, including proto-oncogene activation, genomic instability and chromosomal structural aberrations, or uracil misincorporation during DNA synthesis.

MTHFR: MTHFR is responsible for converting 5,10-methylene-tetrahydrofolate to 5-methylenetetrahydrofolate, the principal circulating form of folate. Several studies have investigated two common variants of *MTHFR*, *C677T* and *A1298C*, in relation

Table 13.2 Summary of studies of the *ALDH2 Glu487Lys* polymorphism and cancers of the colon and/or rectum

Study/ Outcome	Year	Country/ Ethnicity	Gender	Description of Cases	Description of Controls	Number of Cases/Controls	Lys Allele Frequency	Comparison	OR (95% CI)
Yin et al. (46)	2007	Japan	M/F	Consecutive surgical admissions	Two-stage random sampling from hospital catchment areas	685/778	0.267	Lys/Lys vs Glu/Glu Lys/Glu vs Glu/Glu	0.55 (0.33–0.93) 0.89 (0.71–1.13)
Matsuo (47)	2006	Japan	M/F	Aichi Cancer Centre Hospital (ACCH)	Outpatients during same time period as case diagnoses	257/768	0.297	Lys/Lys vs Glu/Glu Lys/Glu vs Glu/Glu	0.98 (0.54–1.75) 0.99 (0.71–1.37)
Kuriki (48)	2005	Japan	M/F	Aichi Cancer Centre Hospital (ACCH)	Hospital outpatients	Men: 72/116 Women: 54/122	Men: 0.259 Women: 0.291	Lys carrier vs not	Men: 1.04 (0.53–2.06) Women: 0.87 (0.45–1.68)
Otani (49)	2005	Japan	M/F	All presenting cases identified	Hospital outpatients	107/224	0.228	Lys/Lys vs Glu/Glu Lys/Glu vs Glu/Glu	1.2 (0.49–2.9) 1.1 (0.67–1.9)

Study	Year	Country	Sex	Cases	Controls	Number	p value	Comparison	OR (95% CI)
Matsuo (50) Colon cancer	2002	Japan	M/F	Aichi Cancer Centre Hospital (ACCH)	Gastroscopy outpatients	Men: 82/118 Women: 59/123	Men: 0.263 Women: 0.293	Men: Lys/Lys vs Glu/Glu Lys/Glu vs Glu/Glu Women: Lys/Lys vs Glu/Glu Lys/Glu vs Glu/Glu	0.38 (0.10–1.51) 0.70 (0.38–1.30) 0.63 (0.16–2.48) 1.11 (0.58–2.14)
Murata (51) Colon cancer	1999	Japan	M/F	Colon cancer surgery patients	Noncancer outpatients	Men: 89/60	0.200	"Doses of mutant allele"	Men: 2.13 (0.97–4.66)
Murata (51) Rectal cancer	1999	Japan	M/F	Colon cancer surgery patients	Noncancer outpatients	Men: 74/60	0.200	"Doses of mutant allele"	Men: 1.03 (0.48–2.20)
Yokoyama (52) Colon cancer	1998	Japan	M	Consecutively admitted alcoholic males with colon cancer	Cancer-free alcoholic males consecutively admitted to same institution	46/487	0.045	Lys/Glu vs Glu/Glu	3.35 (1.51–7.45)
Jiang (53) Rectal cancer	2007	China	M/F	Incident cases	Population based	210/439	0.223	Lys/Lys vs Glu/Glu Lys/Glu vs Glu/Glu	0.72 (0.45–1.15) 0.74 (0.51–1.06)

to colorectal neoplasia; these include several meta-analyses and a HuGE review (18,19,54–57). So far, few studies have investigated the effects of combinations of variants (48).

MTHFR C677T: Twenty-nine individual studies of *MTHFR C677T* have been published, together including more than 13,000 colorectal cancer cases. In general, the risk of colorectal cancer appears to be lower in persons with the *TT* genotype, compared with the *CC* genotype (Table 13.3). We performed an updated meta-analysis for this chapter and found the summary OR 0.83 (95% CI 0.76–0.91) for persons with the *TT* versus the *CC* genotype. Some evidence suggests that the apparently protective effect of the *TT* genotype may be negated in persons with low folate or methionine intake and in persons who consume large quantities of alcohol.

MTHFR A1298C: Seventeen studies of *MTHFR A1298C* have been published, together including more than 7,000 colorectal cancer cases. Most studies found that *CC* homozygotes were at moderately reduced risk of colorectal cancer compared with *AA* homozygotes. Our updated, random-effects meta-analysis of these 17 studies found a summary OR 0.80 (95% CI 0.7–0.93) for persons with the *CC* versus the *AA* genotype. The *C677T* and *A1298C* variants appear to be in strong linkage disequilibrium, suggesting that studies of the *A1298C* and *C677T* variants are measuring the same association with colorectal cancer.

Methionine synthase (MTR): Ten studies of *MTR A2756G* have been published, together including more than 9,000 colorectal cancer cases. Our meta-analysis of all the available studies found a null summary effect, as well as evidence of statistical heterogeneity. Further investigation is required to determine whether population differences in environmental exposures (e.g., alcohol, diet) could help explain this heterogeneity.

Methionine synthase reductase (MTRR): The *GG* genotype of the *A66G* variant has been inconsistently associated with moderately reduced risk of colorectal cancer.

Cystathionine-β-synthase (CBS): Three studies have examined a 68 base-pair insertion in exon 8 of the *CBS* gene in relation to colorectal cancer. An Australian study found that the 68bp insertion was less frequent in subjects with proximal tumors, suggesting a possible protective effect. Two additional studies in the United States and United Kingdom found no evidence of an association.

Thymidylate synthase (TS): The *TS* enhancer region contains a series of 28 base-pair tandem repeats, most commonly 2 repeats (2rpt) or 3 repeats (3rpt); the 3rpt variant produces a nearly threefold increase in *TS* expression. The five studies comparing 2rpt genotypes with non-2rpt genotypes in relation to colorectal cancer suggest a protective effect for 2rpt variants, although not all reached statistical significance.

Variants of iron metabolism genes. Iron is a key element in cellular processes (58) and may have a role in the etiology of cancer (59), including colorectal cancer (60).

Table 13.3 Summary of features of studies of *MTHFR C677T* polymorphism and colorectal cancer

Study	Year	Country/Ethnicity	Gender	Description of Cases	Description of Controls	% TT in Controls	Number of Cases/Controls
Chen et al. (61)	1996	U.S. white	M	Health Professionals Followup Study (HPFS)	HPFS	13.4	144/627
Ma et al. (62)*	1997	U.S. white	M	Physicians' Health Study (PHS)	PHS	15.0	202/326
Slattery et al. (63)†	1999	U.S. >90% white	M/F	Kaiser Permanente Medical Care Program (KPMCP)	Population	11.4	1,467/1,821
Park et al. (64)	1999	Korea	M/F	Hospital series	Hospital	16.1	200/460
Ryan et al. (65)	2001	Ireland	M/F	Hospital series	Hospital	9.8	136/848
Chen et al. (66)*‡	2002	U.S. white	M	PHS	PHS	15.0	202/326
Shannon et al. (67)	2002	Australia	M/F	Hospital series	Population	9.4	501/1,207
Keku et al. (68)‡	2002	U.S. white	M/F	North Carolina Colon Cancer Study (NCCCS)	Population	9.5	308/539
		U.S. black				1.8	244/329
Le Marchand et al. (69)‡	2002	U.S. Japanese	M/F	Hawaii Tumor Registry (HTR)	Population	19.4	322/397
		U.S. white				14.0	149/171
		U.S. Hawaiian				3.4	77/88
Matsuo et al. (70)‡	2002	Japan	M/F	Hospital series	Hospital	14.9	142/241
Sachse et al. (41)	2002	U.K. white	M/F	Hospital series	Hospital	8.3	490/592
Toffoli et al. (71)‡	2003	Italy	M/F	Hospital series	Population	20.1	276/279
Heijmans et al. (72)	2003	Netherlands	M	Zutphen Elderly Study (ZES) cohort	ZES cohort	7.9	18/7,933§
Plaschke et al. (73)‡	2003	Germany	M/F	Hospital series	Hospital	11.0	287/346
Pufulete et al. (74)‡	2003	U.K.	M/F	Hospital series	Hospital	7.9	28/76
Kim et al. (75)	2004	Korea	M/F	Hospital series	Hospital	14.7	243/225

(Continued)

Table 13.3 Continued

Study	Year	Country/Ethnicity	Gender	Description of Cases	Description of Controls	% TT in Controls	Number of Cases/Controls
Curtin et al. (76)[†][‡]	2004	U.S. >90% white	M/F	KPMCP	Population	11.5	1,608/1,972
Yin et al. (77)[‡]	2004	Japan	M/F	Hospital series	Population	17.1	685/778
Ulvik et al. (78)	2004	Norway	M/F	JANUS cohort	JANUS cohort	9.7	2,159/2,190
Le Marchand et al. (79)	2005	U.S. mixed	M/F	Multiethnic cohort	Population	12.6	822/2,021
Otani et al. (49)[‡]	2005	Japan	M/F	Hospital series	Hospital	25.7	106/222
Matsuo et al. (80)[‡]	2005	Japan	M/F	Hospital series	Hospital	17.4	256/771
Jiang et al. (81)[‡]	2005	China	M/F	Screening cohort	Screening cohort	18.3	196/980
Wang et al. (82)[‡]	2006	India	M/F	Hospital series	Population	0	302/291
Webb et al. (83)	2006	U.K. white	M/F	Hospital series	Population	12.1	2,556/2,692
Koushik et al. (84)[‡]	2006	U.S. 97% white	M/F	Nurses Health Study(NHS)/HPFS	NHS/HPFS	14.1	349/794
Murtaugh et al. (85)[‡]	2007	U.S. 84% white	M/F	KPMCP	Population	11.5	742/970
Sharp et al. (86)[‡]	2007	U.K. 98% white	M/F	Grampian Health Board Registry	Population	11.9	264/408
Theodoratou (87)[‡]	2008	U.K. >99% white	M/F	Hospital series	Population	11.5	999/1,010

[*]Data for same subjects, used later publication in meta-analysis (66).
[†]Data for same subjects, used later publication in meta-analysis (76).
[‡]Also looked at A1298C.
[§]Prospective cohort study.

HFE: HFE is an MHC-Class I molecule involved in the uptake of iron in the small intestine. Two *HFE* mutations, *C282Y* and *H63D*, are associated with hereditary hemochromatosis in populations of European origin. Both mutations are associated with elevated transferrin saturation and serum ferritin levels, with variable biochemical penetrance that may be modified by several factors (see Section "Gene–Environment Interaction in the Etiology of Colorectal Cancer").

We identified seven case-control studies that investigated associations of the *C282Y* and *H63D* variants with colorectal cancer. The frequency of the *Y282* allele rarely exceeds 0.10 and these studies were underpowered to assess its effect. Two studies also investigated the *S142G* variant (rs3817672) in the transferrin receptor gene (*TFRC*) as a potential modifier of association with the *C282Y* and *H63D* variants of *HFE*. These seven studies offer little evidence to support an association of the *C282Y* variant with colorectal cancer; the four studies that examined association with the *H63D* variant gave inconsistent results.

Variants influencing vitamin D and calcium metabolism. ***VDR:*** 1α, 25-dihydroxy vitamin D_3 [$1\alpha,25(OH)_2D_3$], the active form of vitamin D, is synthesized from both dietary vitamin D and skin-derived precursors through the action of ultraviolet sunlight. In addition to its role in regulating calcium absorption and blood calcium concentration, vitamin D may have anticarcinogenic activity via its binding to the vitamin D receptor (VDR) (88). Vitamin D could affect colorectal cancer risk by influencing cell proliferation and differentiation, apoptosis, and angiogenesis (89,90) or by affecting insulin resistance (91).

Several variants of the *VDR* gene have been identified. A poly-A repeat at the $3'$ untranslated region of the gene has been found to be associated with increased mRNA expression; it is in linkage disequilibrium with four restriction fragment length variants (RFLPs) known as *Bsm*I (rs1544410), *Apa*I (rs7975232), *Taq*I (rs731236), and *Tru9*I. An RFLP (*Fok*I, rs10735810) at the first potential start site of the gene (ATG to ACG) results in a long version of the VDR protein (T-allele or the "f" allele) or a protein shortened by three amino acids (C-allele or the "F" allele).

Several case-control studies have investigated the associations of *VDR* variants with colorectal cancer (91); some have reported a positive association with the "f" allele (rs10735810). Our meta-analysis of four studies of *Fok*I found OR 0.94 (95% CI 0.58–1.53); our meta-analysis of three studies of *Bsm*I found OR 1.18 (95% CI 1.04–1.33).

Lipid metabolism. ***APOE:*** The apolipoprotein E *(APOE)* gene has three alleles: *APOE ε2*, *APOE ε3*, and *APOE ε4*. These alleles arise due to two missense SNPs, rs429358 and rs7412, which result in T/C base substitution, and corresponding *Cys/Arg* amino acid changes at residues 112 and 158, respectively. *APOE* may influence colorectal cancer development through three possible pathways: cholesterol and bile metabolism, triglyceride and insulin regulation, and inflammation (92).

Five studies have examined *APOE* variants in relation to colorectal cancer. One study found that *APOE* ε4 was associated with significantly reduced risk of proximal colon cancer (OR 0.35, 95% CI 0.14–0.86). A study conducted in the United Kingdom found that persons with the ε2/ε3 genotype had a 90% increased risk of colorectal cancer compared with the ε3/ε3 genotype; no association was found with the ε4 genotype. A U.S. study found that the absence of an *APOE* ε3 allele significantly increased the risk of colon cancer (OR 1.37 95% CI 1.00–1.87), especially among those diagnosed at greater than 64 years of age; in this study, *APOE* genotype was not associated with rectal cancer.

Physical activity, obesity, and insulin-related variants. More than 40 case-control or cohort studies have examined physical activity and the risk of colorectal cancer (93). These studies provide consistent evidence that physical activity is associated with a reduced risk of colon cancer, with relative risks for the highest category of activity compared with the lowest in the range 0.4–0.9 (94). The risk decreases in a dose–response fashion with increasing levels of activity (93). Excess weight raises risk of developing colon cancer (but not rectal cancer), with an increase of 15% in risk for an overweight person and 33% for an obese person (95,96). The similarity of risk factors for colon cancer and diabetes, and the observation that insulin promotes the growth of colon cells *in vitro* and colon tumors *in vivo,* suggested that hyperinsulinaemia and insulin resistance could lead to colorectal cancer through the growth-promoting effects of elevated levels of insulin, glucose, or triglycerides.

IGF: One mechanism by which raised insulin levels could affect cancer risk is by increasing the bioactivity of insulin-like growth factor-1 (IGF-1) and inhibiting production of two main binding proteins, IGFBP-1 and IGFBP-2 (97). IGF-1 has mitogenic effects on normal and neoplastic cells, inhibiting apoptosis and stimulating cell proliferation (97). The machinery of the IGF complex is comprised of peptide ligands (IGF-I and IGF-II), as well as their respective receptors, binding proteins (IGFBP-1–6), and IGFBP proteases. The combination of a Western-style diet, sedentary lifestyle, and obesity might lead to an increase in circulating insulin levels, which could trigger elevation of IGF-I bioavailability through insulin-mediated changes in IGFBP concentrations (98).

Four prospective studies of colorectal cancer have observed a greater than two-fold increased risk amongst those in the highest quintile of circulating *IGF-1* levels, compared with those in the lowest quintile. However, one of the four studies looked separately at rectal cancer and found a statistically nonsignificant ($p = 0.09$) inverse trend, which provides some weak evidence that this relationship may not hold for rectal cancer. One prospective study observed an inverse relationship between IGFBP-1 and IGFBP-2 levels and colorectal cancer, but two others were null.

One study reported that a genetic variant at position 1663 in the human growth hormone-1 (*GH1*) gene reduced colorectal cancer risk. Another study reported that variants in genes encoding the insulin receptor substrates (*IRS-1, IRS-2*) increased colon cancer risk; this study also reported that variants in the *IGF-1* and *IGFBP-3* genes were not independently related to cancer but appeared to act together with *IRS-1* to influence risk. *IRS-1* and *IGF-1* variants have been reported to be associated with an increased risk of colon cancers with specific *KRAS2* and *TP53* mutations. All of these findings require replication.

Genetic Variants Affecting Inflammation and Immune Response

Prostaglandin-endoperoxide synthase (PTGS), also known as cyclo-oxygenase (COX), is involved in the biosynthesis of the prostanoids. It has two isozymes, a constitutive PTGS1, and an inducible PTGS2. PTGS2 is involved in inflammation and mitogenesis.

PTGS1/COX1. No associations with colorectal cancer were found in three studies of variants in the *PTGS1/COX1* gene; however, the rarity of the minor variants necessitates larger, population-based studies.

PTGS2/COX2. A large study in Beijing found positive associations with variants at *-1195* and *-765*; however, two other studies found no association with the *-765* variant. Two studies of the *Val511Ala* variant (rs5273) found no association with colorectal cancer.

PPARD and PPARG. Peroxisome proliferator-activated receptors (*PPARs*) are a group of nuclear receptor proteins that function as transcription factors regulating gene expression. *PPARG* is expressed in high levels in normal colonic mucosa, colorectal adenoma, and colon cancer cell lines; it has been implicated as a potential mediator of colorectal cancer risk in animal studies. An association study of *PPARG Pro12Ala* (rs1801282) reported the following OR (95% CI): 0.83 (0.69–1.01) for proximal tumors, 1.00 (0.83–1.21) for distal tumors, and 1.04 (0.86–1.25) for rectal tumors. No association with this variant was observed in two other studies. Single studies found no association of *PPARG C1431* or an unspecified rare variant of *PPARD* with colorectal cancer. A single study of the *PPARG C478T* variant suggested that the TT genotype might be associated with reduced risk.

Cytokine genes. Cytokines include the interleukins, lymphokines, and cell signal molecules, such as tumor necrosis factor and the interferons. IL-1, IL-6, and IL-8 proteins are generally considered proinflammatory and IL-4, IL-4R, and IL-10 antiinflammatory in effect.

Interleukin-1β: The three most commonly studied SNPs in *IL-1β* are *T-31C* (rs1143627), *C-511T* (rs16944), and *+3954C/T* (rs1143634); the first two are in close linkage disequilibrium and may influence gene expression. Three studies of *T-31C* found no significant association with colorectal cancer. Two studies that examined the *C-511T* variant in *H. pylori* positive persons found that risk of colorectal cancer was reduced in those carrying the T-allele.

Interleukin-6: Studies of the *IL-6 -174G/C* variant (rs1800795) have produced conflicting results.

Interleukin-8: No clear association has been found for the *IL-8 T-251A* variant (rs4073) with colorectal cancer.

Interleukin-4: In a study reporting a significant inverse association of the *IL-4 -584T* allele (rs2243250) with colorectal cancer, Hardy-Weinberg equilibrium was violated in the control samples and this association was not replicated in a subsequent study.

Interleukin-10: Two studies found no association with colorectal cancer for any of three variants in the promoter region of the *IL-10* gene: *-1082G/A* (rs1800871), *-592C/A* (rs1800872), and *-819C/T* (rs1800871).

Interleukin-1RN: Two small studies investigating the association of an 86 base-pair VNTR variant in intron 2 of the *IL-1RN* gene (interleukin-1 receptor antagonist) with colorectal cancer reported conflicting results. A population-based study in Germany found no association of the *IL-1RN A9589T* variant (rs454078) with colorectal cancer.

Interleukins-12A and 18: In a single study of colorectal cancer and variants of *IL12A*, no association was observed. In a small single study of *IL18*, a positive association was found with the *607A* variant.

Tumor necrosis factor-α (TNFα): None of five studies investigating the association of the *-308G/A* variant (rs1800629) with colorectal cancer found significant associations. Investigations of a *TNFα* microsatellite dinucleotide repeat polymorphism have had conflicting results.

Toll-like receptors (TLRs). Toll-like receptors are a key component of the innate immune system and inflammatory response to pathogens through activation of the NF-κB and mitogen-associated protein (MAP) kinase signaling pathways (99). Toll-like receptor 4 (TLR4) is of particular interest with respect to gastrointestinal malignancies (99,100).

Three studies have examined the association of colorectal cancer with variants in the *TLR4* gene. Positive results from a small study in Croatia were not replicated in two larger studies. The Croatian study also reported an association of a *GT* dinucleotide repeat microsatellite variant (intron 2) in the *TLR2* gene but no association with the *Arg753Gln* variant (rs5743708).

Other inflammation-related or immunoregulatory genes. *HRAS (Harvey Rat Sarcoma Virus Proto-oncogene): H-ras1*, a proto-oncogene that encodes a protein involved in mitogenic signal transduction and differentiation, is highly polymorphic in humans (19). Several studies have evaluated the association between *HRAS1-VNTR* rare alleles and colorectal cancer. Two systematic reviews that included pooled analyses of *HRAS1-VNTR* rare alleles (frequencies in controls ranging from 1% to 6%) reported the following OR (95% CI): 2.5 (1.54–4.05) and 2.67 (1.47–4.85).

NF-kappaB (*NFKB1*): Nuclear factor-kappaB (NF-kappaB) is an inducible transcription factor that plays a major role in the regulation of genes involved in immune and inflammatory response. Studies of an insertion/deletion variant (*-94ins/delATTG*) in the promoter region of the *NFKB1* gene have had variable results. The insertion/deletion variant was not associated with colorectal cancer survival. Another study reported a significant association with sporadic colorectal cancer in a Swedish study population with ORs and 95% CIs of 7.73 (3.06–19.57) for heterozygote deletion and 6.58 (2.35–18.43) for homozygote deletion; no association was found among Swedish patients with a family history of colorectal cancer or in a Chinese population.

LTA/TNFβ: Lymphotoxin alpha (*LTA*), a member of the *TNF* superfamily, is also known as *TNFβ*. A single study has reported association with colorectal cancer for a haplotype in the major histocompatibility locus region containing SNPs of *TNFα*, *RAGE*, *HSP70-2*, and *LTA*. Another study suggested an association with the *NcoI* RFLP of *TNFβ*.

NOS2: A single study found no association of *NOS2* tetra-repeat and penta-repeat polymorphisms with colorectal cancer. Another study found no association with the *NOS2A +524T>C* variant.

Genetic Variation and Exogenous Hormones

Exogenous estrogens such as hormone replacement therapy (HRT) might be associated with colorectal tumors. In two large randomized controlled trials of the possible health benefits of HRT in postmenopausal women (101), the incidence of colorectal cancer was reduced by about a third (pooled RR = 0.64, 95% CI 0.45–0.92) (102). Information is limited on the potential genetic modifiers of this apparent protective effect (see Section "Gene–Environment Interaction in the Etiology of Colorectal Cancer").

Estrogen-metabolizing genes: Seven variants in ten estrogen-metabolizing genes were studied for association with colorectal cancer risk: *COMT (Val158Met, rs4680), HSD17 (vIV), CYP17 (rs743572), CYP19 (Arg264Cys, rs70051; C1558T), CYP1A1 (Ile462Val, rs1048943; MspI RFLP), CYP1B1 (Leu432Val, rs1056836)*, and estrogen receptor (*ER*) α *IVSI (C401T, rs2234693)*. No associations were found.

Estrogen and androgen receptors: A single study investigated the role of variants in the *ERα (A351G, rs9340799), ERβ (G1082A, rs1256049*, and a *CA* repeat variant in intron 5), and androgen receptor (*AR, CAG* repeat variant) genes. The risk of colorectal cancer was increased in women with at least 25 *CA* repeats on both alleles in *ER* β (OR 2.13, 95% CI 1.24–3.64) and in men with increasing numbers of AR *CAG* repeats (OR 1.28, 95% CI 1.06–1.54). These studies have not been replicated.

Genetic Variants Associated with Adhesion Molecules and Extracellular Matrix Remodeling

Tumor cell–stromal cell interactions and remodeling of the extracellular matrix (ECM) have implications for the progression and spread of cancer (103,104).

CDH1: Of the many cell–cell adhesion molecules, E-cadherin (encoded by *CDH1*l) has so far received the greatest attention in relation to colorectal cancer. A systematic review of colorectal cancer in association with *CDH1*160A* reported a pooled OR 1.15 (95% CI 0.89–1.5). Two subsequent studies reported that the A-allele was not associated with colorectal cancer. A systematic review of association with the *870A* variant reported OR 1.19 (95% CI 1.06–1.34).

ICAM1: A single study reported no associations with colorectal cancer for variants in the *ICAM1* gene (*G241R*, rs1799969; *K469E*, rs5498).

MMP variants: Matrix metalloproteinases, a family of 23 enzymes in humans, are important for proteolysis of the extracellular matrix but also for cell growth, regulation of apoptosis, and cell motility (105,106). Nine studies have investigated associations between variants in this family of genes and colorectal cancer. Several small studies suggested that the homozygous *MMP-1 1607G* genotype is associated with colorectal cancer, but this was not replicated in larger studies. In one of these studies, a *MMP-3* variant causing lower enzyme activity was associated with colorectal cancer (OR = 2.1; 95% CI = 1.2–3.8). No consistent pattern of association between *MMP-2, -3,* or *-9* promoter variants and colorectal cancer has been found.

Genetic Variants Affecting Angiogenesis

Angiogenesis is a key process in the development and progression of cancer (107). Signaling by vascular endothelial growth factor (VEGF) is an important rate-limiting step in angiogenesis (107). Four members of the *VEGF* family have been identified—VEGF-A, VEGF-B, VEGF-C, and VEGF-D (now designated FIGF, c-fos induced growth factor). VEGF-A is the most abundant in colorectal tissues, where increased *VEGF-A* expression has been observed (108,109). Increased expression of *VEGF-A* and *VEGF-C* has also been reported in colorectal cancer (108).

No associations with colorectal cancer have been found for any of three *VEGF-A* variants: *-2578C/A, -634G/C,* and *+936C/T*).

Very limited evidence is available to assess the importance of other genes thought to be implicated in angiogenesis and related inflammatory pathways in the development of colorectal cancer. Two studies reported no association with colorectal cancer of the *G801A* variant (rs1801157) of *CXCL12*.

Associations of colorectal cancer with variation in two other angiogenesis-related genes (*PTGS2/COX2, IL-8*) are reviewed in Sections "*PTGS2/COX2*" and "*Cytokine genes.*"

Genetic Variants Affecting Inhibition of Cell Growth

TGF-beta signaling pathway. TGF-β is a cell growth inhibitor that acts by binding to type I (TGFBR1) and type II (TGFBR2) transmembrane receptors to form a heteromeric complex, TGFBR1/TGFBR2. TGFBR2 phosphorylates TGFBR1, which in turn activates TGFBR1 kinase. Defects in this mechanism can lead to unrestricted cell growth due to the loss of growth inhibitory activity.

TGFB1: Two studies reported no association of variants in the *TGFB1* gene (transforming growth factor-β1) with colorectal cancer.

TGF-beta receptors (TGFBR1, TGFBR2): A meta-analysis comprising 12 case-control studies of colorectal cancer, with a combined 1,585 cases and 4,399 controls, reported an association of *TGFBR1*6A* with colorectal cancer (OR 1.20, 95% CI 1.01–1.43). Germline mutations of *TGFBR2* may predispose to the development of HNPCC.

Cell cycle regulatory genes (*CCND1*). Cyclin D1, encoded by the *CCND1* gene, has a key role in the cell cycle. A recent meta-analysis comprising 12 case-control studies and a total of 8,260 cases reported a small but significant positive association of the *G870A* variant (rs603965) with colorectal cancer (OR = 1.19, 95% CI 1.06–1.34) (110). In a subsequent study, risk of familial (but not sporadic) colorectal cancer was increased in persons with homozygous *AA* genotypes, compared with *GG* homozygotes.

Common Low-Penetrance Variants Identified from Genome-Wide Association Studies

Recently, the increasing availability of multigene chips and microarrays has prompted a move toward "scanning" large numbers of SNPs for possible associations with disease. In this section, we briefly summarize genome-wide association studies (GWAS) of colorectal cancer that had been reported at the time of writing.

Known rare, high-penetrance germline mutations account for less than 5% of cases of colorectal cancer. Recent findings from GWAS have identified common genetic variants at six loci, increasing the proportion of colorectal cancer that can be associated with specific genetic risk factors. ORs are typically in the range of 1.1–1.4 for heterozygous carriers of the risk allele and 1.6–1.7 for homozygotes. The associations of these six loci with colorectal cancer tend to be consistent among studied populations in different parts of the world.

The first of these six loci, on chromosome 8q24, is close to *POU5F1P1*, a known transcription factor, and 340,873 bp telomeric to the oncogene *MYC* (111–113). Variants from several regions at this locus, separated by sites of recombination, confer independent risk and have also been shown to be associated with prostate and breast cancer risk.

The second locus, on chromosome 15q13.3, is known as *CRAC1* or *HMPS* (hereditary mixed polyposis syndrome) (114). One SNP is located in the 3′ UTR of *GREM1*, which codes a bone morphogenetic protein (BMP) involved in the TGF-beta/BMP pathway that is causally involved in juvenile polyposis.

The third locus, *SMAD7*, on chromosome 18q21, is involved in TGF-beta and Wnt signaling (115). *SMAD7* acts as an intracellular antagonist of TGF-beta signaling and changes in its expression have been shown to influence progression of colorectal cancer.

A fourth locus, at 8q23, contains the gene *EIF3H*, for which amplification and overexpression have been described in breast, prostate, and hepatocellular cancers (116). No causal gene has been identified at the fifth locus at 10p14 (116). The sixth locus, at 11q23, contains four open reading frames and a polymorphic binding site for micro-RNAs (117).

The six loci identified so far by GWAS account for <5% of excess familial colorectal cancer risk. Given the limited power of these studies to detect the least common variants, it seems likely that many (perhaps 50–100) additional common variants remain to be discovered. Although their individual effects on risk are small, the combined effects of several variants could produce much larger risks and so could be clinically useful in directing prevention strategies. Further development of risk profiling using common variants will require the identification of additional variants in larger GWAS and through meta-analysis of GWAS. Large, multinational cohort studies will be needed to validate such genetic risk predictive models.

Gene–Environment Interaction in the Etiology of Colorectal Cancer

Investigation of potential gene–environment interactions has focused on candidate genes with a role in metabolism of dietary, drug, and environmental constituents associated with risk of colorectal cancer. Studies have investigated interactions of variants of *GSTM1*, *GSTT1*, and *CYP1A1* with tobacco smoking; *APC* variants with diet (intake of total fat and specific fat types) and lifestyle factors (taking hormone replacement therapy [HRT]); *HFE C282Y* and *H63D* with age, gender, ethnic group, other genes, smoking, alcohol intake and dietary intake of iron; *CYP1A1*, *NAT1*, and *NAT2* with meat intake; variants of *GSTM1*, *GSTT1*, and *CYP1A1* with vegetable intake; variants of *MTHFR, MTR, MTRR,* and *CBS* with intake of folate and related nutrients; variants of *COX2 (PTGS2), PPARD, UGT1A6, CYP2C8, CYP2C9,* and genes encoding the interleukins with NSAID use; and genes thought to influence hormone metabolism with HRT use.

Overall, consistent evidence of gene–environment interaction has not been observed. Although investigating the complex interplay of genes and environment is widely considered to offer much promise for improving our understanding of the etiology of complex diseases, including colorectal cancer, research in this area is challenging (118). Many studies of gene–environment interaction and colorectal cancer have lacked statistical power to detect interaction. For example, of four studies that assessed interactions of *CYP1A1* variants with different levels of smoking and consumption of meat, vegetables, and fruit, two studies included only about 200 cases. The methods used to test for interaction have varied among studies, making it difficult to integrate and summarize the evidence. For example, some studies have classified persons as "smokers" or "nonsmokers" (or "smokers," "former smokers," or "nonsmokers"); however, others have collected detailed information concerning the number of cigarettes smoked per day, age when individuals started smoking, and number of years smoked. Furthermore, although the metabolism of any exposure is likely to depend on the balance among the relative activities of all enzymes active within the metabolic pathway, few studies have investigated interactions of exposures with combinations of genes (or SNPs) operating in such pathways. New analytical approaches for exploring gene pathways in disease etiology are under development but their performance characteristics and properties are not yet well understood.

Conclusions

Inherited genetic factors play an important role in the etiology of colorectal cancer. Rare high-penetrance mutations account for a small proportion of disease but their identification plays an important role in the clinical management of the high-risk families in which these mutations segregate. The results of most candidate gene association studies of colorectal cancer have not been replicated consistently. Many results can be considered false positives; others may represent very small effects, which will require replication in larger studies before firm conclusions can be reached.

More recently, genome-wide association studies have discovered many common, low-penetrance genetic variants associated with risk of colorectal cancer. These studies have been conducted by large-scale, international collaborations (see Chapter 6). Further research is required to identify causal variants and to investigate pathophysiological pathways. Before tests for multiple common variants are used for risk profiling (e.g., to guide prevention and treatment strategies), prospective studies in several populations will be needed to validate risk estimates and to demonstrate improved health outcomes.

References

1. IARC. Globocan. cancer incidence, mortality and prevalence worldwide. *IARC database 2000*. Available at www.who.int. Accessed January 2009.
2. Houlston RS, Peto J. The search for low-penetrance cancer susceptibility alleles. *Oncogene*. 2004;23:6471–6476.
3. Campbell H, Manolio T. Commentary: rare alleles, modest genetic effects and the need for collaboration. *Int J Epidemiol*. 2007;36:445–448.
4. Mitchell RJ, Farrington SM, Dunlop MG, et al. Mismatch repair genes hMLH1 and hMSH2 and colorectal cancer: a HuGE review. *Am J Epidemiol*. 2002;156:885–902.
5. Dunlop MG, Farrington SM, Nicholl I, et al. Population carrier frequency of hMSH2 and hMLH1 mutations. *Br J Cancer*. 2000;83:1643–1645.

6. Aarnio M, Sankila R, Pukkala E, et al. Cancer risk in mutation carriers of DNA-mismatch-repair genes. *Int J Cancer*. 1999;81:214–218.

7. Millar AL, Pal T, Madlensky L, et al. Mismatch repair gene defects contribute to the genetic basis of double primary cancers of the colorectum and endometrium. *Hum Mol Genet*. 1999;8:823–829.

8. Senda T, Iizuka-Kogo A, Onouchi T, et al. Adenomatous polyposis coli (APC) plays multiple roles in the intestinal and colorectal epithelia. *Med Mol Morphol*. 2007;40:68–81.

9. Segditsas S, Tomlinson I. Colorectal cancer and genetic alterations in the wnt pathway. *Oncogene*. 2006;25:7531–7537.

10. Xu Y, Pasche B. TGF-beta signaling alterations and susceptibility to colorectal cancer. *Hum Mol Genet*. 2007;16 Spec No 1:R14–R20.

11. Al-Tassan N, Chmiel NH, Maynard J, et al. Inherited variants of MYH associated with somatic G:C-->T:A mutations in colorectal tumors. *Nat Genet*. 2002;30:227–232.

12. Sieber OM, Lipton L, Crabtree M, et al. Multiple colorectal adenomas, classic adenomatous polyposis, and germ-line mutations in MYH. *N Engl J Med*. 2003;348:791–799.

13. Kury S, Buecher B, Robiou-du-Pont S, et al. The thorough screening of the MUTYH gene in a large French cohort of sporadic colorectal cancers. *Genet Test*. 2007;11(4):373–9.

14. Cheadle JP, Sampson JR. MUTYH-associated polyposis—from defect in base excision repair to clinical genetic testing. *DNA Repair (Amst)*. 2007;6:274–279.

15. Kim IJ, Ku JL, Kang HC, et al. Mutational analysis of OGG1, MYH, MTH1 in FAP, HNPCC and sporadic colorectal cancer patients: R154H OGG1 polymorphism is associated with sporadic colorectal cancer patients. *Hum Genet*. 2004;115:498–503.

16. Moreno V, Gemignani F, Landi S, et al. Polymorphisms in genes of nucleotide and base excision repair: risk and prognosis of colorectal cancer. *Clin Cancer Res*. 2006;12:2101–2108.

17. Cotton SC, Sharp L, Little J, et al. Glutathione S-transferase polymorphisms and colorectal cancer. *Am J Epidemiol*. 2000;151:7–32.

18. Houlston RS, Tomlinson IPM. Polymorphisms and colorectal tumor risk. *Gastroenterology*. 2001;121:282–301.

19. de Jong MM, Nolte IM, te Meerman GJ, et al. Low-penetrance genes and their involvement in colorectal cancer susceptibility. *Cancer Epidemiol Biomarkers Prev*. 2002;11:1332–1352.

20. Smits KM, Gaspari L, Weijenberg MP, et al. Interaction between smoking, GSTM1 deletion and colorectal cancer: results from the GSEC study. *Biomarkers*. 2003;8:299–310.

21. Ye Z, Parry JM. Meta-analysis of 20 case-control studies on the N-acetyltransferase 2 acetylation status and colorectal cancer risk. *Med Sci Monit*. 2002;8:CR558–CR565.

22. Abdel-Rahman SZ, Soliman AS, Bondy ML, et al. Polymorphism of glutathione S-transferase loci GSTM1 and GSTT1 and susceptibility to colorectal cancer in Egypt. *Cancer Lett*. 1999;142:97–104.

23. Lee EJ, Wong JY, Yeoh PN, et al. Glutathione S-transferase-theta (GSTT1) genetic polymorphism among Chinese, Malays and Indians in Singapore. *Pharmacogenetics*. 1995;5:332–334.

24. Yoshioka M, Katoh T, Nakano M, et al. Glutathione S-transferase (GST) M1, T1, P1, N-acetyltransferase (NAT) 1 and 2 genetic polymorphisms and susceptibility to colorectal cancer. *J UOEH*. 1999;21:133–147.

25. Zhu Y, Deng C, Zhang Y, et al. The relationship between GSTM1, GSTT1 gene polymorphisms and susceptibility to sporadic colorectal adenocarcinoma. *Zhonghua Nei Ke Za Zhi*. 2002;41:538–540.

26. Chen K, Jiang QT, Ma XY, et al. Associations between genetic polymorphisms of glutathione S-transferase M1 and T1, smoking and susceptibility to colorectal cancer: A case-control study. *Zhonghua Zhong Liu Za Zhi*. 2004;26:645–648.

27. Yeh CC, Hsieh LL, Tang R, et al. Vegetable/fruit, smoking, glutathione S-transferase polymorphisms and risk for colorectal cancer in Taiwan. *World J Gastroenterol.* 2005;11:1473–1480.

28. Chenevix-Trench G, Young J, Coggan M, et al. Glutathione S-transferase M1 and T1 polymorphisms: susceptibility to colon cancer and age of onset. *Carcinogenesis.* 1995;16:1655–1657.

29. Metabolic genotypes and risk for colorectal cancer. *J Gastroenterol Hepatol.* 2001;16:631–635.

30. Zhang H, Ahmadi A, Arbman G, et al. Glutathione S-transferase T1 and M1 genotypes in normal mucosa, transitional mucosa and colorectal adenocarcinoma. *Int J Cancer.* 1999;84:135–138.

31. Laso N, Lafuente MJ, Mas S, et al. Glutathione S-transferase (GSTM1 and GSTT1)-dependent risk for colorectal cancer. *Anticancer Res.* 2002;22:3399–3403.

32. van der Hel OL, Bueno-de-Mesquita HB, Roest M, et al. No modifying effect of NAT1, GSTM1, and GSTT1 on the relation between smoking and colorectal cancer risk. *Cancer Epidemiol Biomarkers Prev.* 2003;12:681–682.

33. Kiss I, Nemeth A, Bogner B, et al. Polymorphisms of glutathione-S-transferase and arylamine N-acetyltransferase enzymes and susceptibility to colorectal cancer. *Anticancer Res.* 2004;24:3965–3970.

34. van der Logt EM, Bergevoet SM, Roelofs HM, et al. Genetic polymorphisms in UDP-glucuronosyltransferases and glutathione S-transferases and colorectal cancer risk. *Carcinogenesis.* 2004;25:2407–2415.

35. Saadat I, Saadat M. Glutathione S-transferase M1 and T1 null genotypes and the risk of gastric and colorectal cancers. *Cancer Lett.* 2001;169:21–26.

36. Ates NA, Tamer L, Ates C, et al. Glutathione S-transferase M1, T1, P1 genotypes and risk for development of colorectal cancer. *Biochem Genet.* 2005;43:149–163.

37. Nascimento H, Costa FF, Coy CSR, et al. Possible influence of glutathione S-transferase GSTT1 null genotype on age of onset of sporadic colorectal adenocarcinoma. *Dis Colon Rectum.* 2003;46:510–515.

38. Seow A, Yuan JM, Sun CL, et al. Dietary isothiocyanates, glutathione S-transferase polymorphisms and colorectal cancer risk in the Singapore Chinese Health Study. *Carcinogenesis.* 2002;23:2055–2061.

39. Welfare M, Adeokun AM, Bassendine MF, et al. Polymorphisms in GSTP1, GSTM1, and GSTT1 and susceptibility to colorectal cancer. *Cancer Epidemiol Biomarkers Prev.* 1999;8:289–292.

40. Loktionov A, Watson MA, Gunter M, et al. Glutathione-S-transferase gene polymorphisms in colorectal cancer patients: interaction between GSTM1 and GSTM3 allele variants as a risk-modulating factor. *Carcinogenesis.* 2001;22:1053–1060.

41. Sachse C, Smith G, Wilkie MJV, et al. A pharmacogenetic study to investigate the role of dietary carcinogens in the etiology of colorectal cancer. *Carcinogenesis.* 2002;23:1839–1849.

42. Rajagopal R, Deakin M, Fawole AS, et al. Glutathione S-transferase T1 polymorphisms are associated with outcome in colorectal cancer. *Carcinogenesis.* 2005;26:2157–2163.

43. Little J, Sharp L, Masson LF, et al. Colorectal cancer and genetic polymorphisms of CYP1A1, GSTM1 and GSTT1: a case-control study in the Grampian region of Scotland. *Int J Cancer.* 2006;119:2155–2164.

44. Gertig DM, Stampfer M, Haiman CH, et al. Glutathione S-transferase GSTM1 and GSTT1 polymorphisms and colorectal cancer risk: a prospective study. *Cancer Epidemiol Biomarkers Prev.* 1998;7:1001–1005.

45. Choi SW, Mason JB. Folate status: effects on pathways of colorectal carcinogenesis. *J Nutr.* 2002;132:2413S–2418S.

46. Yin G, Kono S, Toyomura K, et al. Alcohol dehydrogenase and aldehyde dehydrogenase polymorphisms and colorectal cancer: the Fukuoka colorectal cancer study. *Cancer Sci.* 2007;98:1248–1253.
47. Matsuo K, Wakai K, Hirose K, et al. A gene-gene interaction between ALDH2 Glu487Lys and ADH2 His47Arg polymorphisms regarding the risk of colorectal cancer in Japan. *Carcinogenesis.* 2006;27:1018–1023.
48. Kuriki K, Hamajima N, Chiba H, et al. Relation of the CD36 gene A52C polymorphism to the risk of colorectal cancer among Japanese, with reference to the aldehyde dehydrogenase 2 gene Glu487Lys polymorphism and drinking habit. *Asian Pac J Cancer Prev.* 2005;6:62–68.
49. Otani T, Iwasaki M, Hanaoka T, et al. Folate, vitamin B6, vitamin B12, and vitamin B2 intake, genetic polymorphisms of related enzymes, and risk of colorectal cancer in a hospital-based case-control study in Japan. *Nutr Cancer.* 2005;53:42–50.
50. Matsuo K, Hamajima N, Hirai T, et al. Aldehyde dehydrogenase 2 (ALDH2) genotype affects rectal cancer susceptibility due to alcohol consumption. *J Epidemiol.* 2002;12:70–76.
51. Murata M, Tagawa M, Watanabe S, et al. Genotype difference of aldehyde dehydrogenase 2 gene in alcohol drinkers influences the incidence of Japanese colorectal cancer patients. *Jap J Cancer Res.* 1999;90:711–719.
52. Yokoyama A, Muramatsu T, Ohmori T, et al. Alcohol-related cancers and aldehyde dehydrogenase-2 in Japanese alcoholics. *Carcinogenesis.* 1998;19:1383–1387.
53. Jiang A, Gao CM, Wu JZ, et al. Association between ADH2/ALDH2 genetic polymorphism and habit of alcohol drinking and the susceptibility of rectal cancer. *Chinese Journal of Cancer Prevention and Treatment.* 2007;14:1445–1449.
54. Kono S, Chen K. Genetic polymorphisms of methylenetetrahydrofolate reductase and colorectal cancer and adenoma. *Cancer Sci.* 2005;96:535–542.
55. Huang Y, Han S, Li Y, et al. Different roles of MTHFR C677T and A1298C polymorphisms in colorectal adenoma and colorectal cancer: a meta-analysis. *J Hum Genet.* 2007;52:73–85.
56. Sharp L, Little J. Polymorphisms in genes involved in folate metabolism and colorectal neoplasia: a HuGE review. *Am J Epidemiol.* 2004;159:423–443.
57. Hubner RA, Houlston RS. MTHFR C677T and colorectal cancer risk: a meta-analysis of 25 populations. *Int J Cancer.* 2007;120:1027–1035.
58. Wintergerst ES, Maggini S, Hornig DH. Contribution of selected vitamins and trace elements to immune function. *Ann Nutr Metab.* 2007;51:301–323.
59. Huang X. Iron overload and its association with cancer risk in humans: evidence for iron as a carcinogenic metal. *Mutat Res.* 2003;533:153–171.
60. Nelson RL. Iron and colorectal cancer risk: human studies. *Nutr Rev.* 2001;59:140–148.
61. Chen J, Giovannucci E, Kelsey K, et al. A methylenetetrahydrofolate reductase polymorphism and the risk of colorectal cancer. *Cancer Res.* 1996;56:4862–4864.
62. Ma J, Stampfer MJ, Giovannucci E, et al. Methylenetetrahydrofolate reductase polymorphism, dietary interactions, and risk of colorectal cancer. *Cancer Res.* 1997;57:1098–1102.
63. Slattery ML, Potter JD, Samowitz W, et al. Methylenetetrahydrofolate reductase, diet, and risk of colon cancer. *Cancer Epidemiol Biomarkers Prev.* 1999;8:513–518.
64. Park KS, Mok JW, Kim JC. The 677>T mutation in 5,10-methylenetetrahydrofolate reductase and colorectal cancer risk. *Genet Test.* 1999;3:233–236.
65. Ryan BM, Molloy AM, McManus R, et al. The methylenetetrahydrofolate reductase (MTHFR) gene in colorectal cancer: role in tumor development and significance of allelic loss in tumor progression. *Int J Gastrointest Cancer.* 2001;30:105–111.

66. Chen J, Ma J, Stampfer MJ, et al. Linkage disequilibrium between the 677C>T and 1298A>C polymorphisms in human methylenetetrahydrofolate reductase gene and their contributions to risk of colorectal cancer. *Pharmacogenetics.* 2002;12: 339–342.

67. Shannon B, Gnanasampanthan S, Beilby J, et al. A polymorphism in the methylenetetra-hydrofolate reductase gene predisposes to colorectal cancers with microsatellite instability. *Gut.* 2002;50:520–524.

68. Keku T, Millikan R, Worley K, et al. 5,10-methylenetetrahydrofolate reductase codon 677 and 1298 polymorphisms and colon cancer in African Americans and whites. *Cancer Epidemiol Biomarkers Prev.* 2002;11:1611–1621.

69. Le Marchand L, Donlon T, Hankin JH, et al. B-vitamin intake, metabolic genes, and colorectal cancer risk (United States). *Cancer Causes Control.* 2002;13:239–248.

70. Matsuo K, Hamajima N, Hirai T, et al. Methionine synthase reductase gene A66G polymorphism is associated with risk of colorectal cancer. *Asian Pac J Cancer Prev.* 2002;3:353–359.

71. Toffoli G, Gafa R, Russo A, et al. Methylenetetrahydrofolate reductase 677 C-->T polymorphism and risk of proximal colon cancer in north Italy. *Clin Cancer Res.* 2003;9:743–748.

72. Heijmans BT, Boer JMA, Suchiman HED, et al. A common variant of the methyle-netetrahydrofolate reductase gene (1p36) is associated with an increased risk of cancer. *Cancer Res.* 2003;63:1249–1253.

73. Plaschke J, Schwanebeck U, Pistorius S, et al. Methylenetetrahydrofolate reductase poly-morphisms and risk of sporadic and hereditary colorectal cancer with or without micro-satellite instability. *Cancer Lett.* 2003;191:179–185.

74. Pufulete M, Al-Ghnaniem R, Leather AJ, et al. Folate status, genomic DNA hypomethy-lation, and risk of colorectal adenoma and cancer: a case control study. *Gastroenterology.* 2003;124:1240–1248.

75. Kim D, Ahn Y, Lee B, et al. Methylenetetrahydrofolate reductase polymorphism, alcohol intake, and risks of colon and rectal cancers in Korea. *Cancer Lett.* 2004;216:199–205.

76. Curtin K, Bigler J, Slattery ML, et al. MTHFR C677T and A1298C polymor-phisms: diet, estrogen and risk of colon cancer. *Cancer Epidemiol Biomarkers Prev.* 2004;13:285–292.

77. Yin G, Kono S, Toyomura K, et al. Methylenetetrahydrofolate reductase C677T and A1298C polymorphisms and colorectal cancer: the Fukuoka colorectal cancer study. *Cancer Sci.* 2004;95:908–913.

78. Ulvik A, Vollset SE, Hansen S, et al. Colorectal cancer and the methylenetetrahydrofo-late reductase 677C -> T and methionine synthase 2756A -> G polymorphisms: a study of 2,168 case-control pairs from the JANUS cohort. *Cancer Epidemiol Biomarkers Prev.* 2004;13:2,175–2180.

79. Le Marchand L, Wilkens LR, Kolonel LN, et al. The MTHFR C677T polymorphism and colorectal cancer: the multiethnic cohort study. *Cancer Epidemiol Biomarkers Prev.* 2005;14:1198–1203.

80. Matsuo K, Ito H, Wakai K, et al. One-carbon metabolism related gene polymorphisms interact with alcohol drinking to influence the risk of colorectal cancer in Japan. *Carcinogenesis.* 2005;26:2164–2171.

81. Jiang Q, Chen K, Ma X, et al. Diets, polymorphisms of methylenetetrahydrofolate reductase, and the susceptibility of colon cancer and rectal cancer. *Cancer Detect Prev.* 2005;29:146–154.

82. Wang J, Gajalakshmi V, Jiang J, et al. Associations between 5,10-methylenetetrahydro-folate reductase codon 677 and 1298 genetic polymorphisms and environmental factors

with reference to susceptibility to colorectal cancer: a case-control study in an Indian population. *Int J Cancer.* 2006;118:991–997.

83. Webb EL, Rudd MF, Sellick GS, et al. Search for low penetrance alleles for colorectal cancer through a scan of 1467 non-synonymous SNPs in 2575 cases and 2707 controls with validation by kin-cohort analysis of 14 704 first-degree relatives. *Hum Mol Genet.* 2006;15:3263–3271.

84. Koushik A, Kraft P, Fuchs CS, et al. Nonsynonymous polymorphisms in genes in the one-carbon metabolism pathway and associations with colorectal cancer. *Cancer Epidemiol Biomarkers Prev.* 2006;15:2408–2417.

85. Murtaugh MA, Curtin K, Sweeney C, et al. Dietary intake of folate and co-factors in folate metabolism, MTHFR polymorphisms, and reduced rectal cancer. *Cancer Causes Control.* 2007;18:153–163.

86. Sharp L, Little J, Brockton NT, et al. Polymorphisms in the methylenetetrahydrofolate reductase (MTHFR) gene, intakes of folate and related B vitamins and colorectal cancer: a case-control study in a population with relatively low folate intake. *Br J Nutr.* February 2008;99(2):379–389.

87. Theodoratou E, Farrington SM, Tenesa A, et al. Dietary vitamin B6 intake and the risk of colorectal cancer. *Cancer Epidemiol Biomarkers Prev.* 2008;17:171–182.

88. Jimenez-Lara AM. Colorectal cancer: potential therapeutic benefits of vitamin D. *Int J Biochem Cell Biol.* 2007;39:672–677.

89. Park SY, Murphy SP, Wilkens LR, et al. Calcium and vitamin D intake and risk of colorectal cancer: the multiethnic cohort study. *Am J Epidemiol.* 2007;165:784–793.

90. Gross MD. Vitamin D and calcium in the prevention of prostate and colon cancer: new approaches for the identification of needs. *J Nutr.* 2005;135:326–331.

91. Slattery ML, Neuhausen SL, Hoffman M, et al. Dietary calcium, vitamin D, VDR genotypes and colorectal cancer. *Int J Cancer.* 2004;111:750–756.

92. Slattery ML, Sweeney C, Murtaugh M, et al. Associations between apoE genotype and colon and rectal cancer. *Carcinogenesis.* 2005;26:1422–1429.

93. Friedenreich CM. Physical activity and cancer prevention: from observational to intervention research. *Cancer Epidemiol Biomarkers Prev.* 2001;10:287–301.

94. McTiernan A, Ulrich C, Slate S, et al. Physical activity and cancer etiology: associations and mechanisms. *Cancer Causes Control.* 1998;9:487–509.

95. Bergstrom A, Pisani P, Tenet V, et al. Overweight as an avoidable cause of cancer in Europe. *Int J Cancer.* 2001;91:421–430.

96. IARC Working Group. *IARC Handbooks of Cancer Prevention Vol 6: The Role of Weight Control and Physical Activity in Cancer Prevention.* Vol 6. Lyon: IARC; 2002.

97. Kaaks R. Nutrition, insulin, IGF-1 metabolism and cancer risk: a summary of epidemiological evidence. *Novartis Found Symp.* 2004;262:247–260.

98. Heavey PM, McKenna D, Rowland IR. Colorectal cancer and the relationship between genes and the environment. *Nutr Cancer.* 2004;48:124–141.

99. Fukata M, Abreu MT. Role of toll-like receptors in gastrointestinal malignancies. *Oncogene.* 2008;27:234–243.

100. El-Omar EM, Ng MT, Hold GL. Polymorphisms in toll-like receptor genes and risk of cancer. *Oncogene.* 2008;27:244–252.

101. Rossouw JE, Anderson GL, Prentice RL, et al. Risks and benefits of estrogen plus progestin in healthy postmenopausal women: principal results from the Women's Health Initiative randomized controlled trial. *JAMA.* 2002;288:321–333.

102. Beral V, Banks E, Reeves G. Evidence from randomised trials on the long-term effects of hormone replacement therapy. *Lancet.* 2002;360:942–944.

103. Duffy MJ, McGowan PM, Gallagher WM. Cancer invasion and metastasis: changing views. *J Pathol.* 2008;214:283–293.

104. Clark JC, Thomas DM, Choong PF, et al. RECK—a newly discovered inhibitor of metastasis with prognostic significance in multiple forms of cancer. *Cancer Metastasis Rev.* 2007;26:675–683.

105. Clark IM, Swingler TE, Sampieri CL, et al. The regulation of matrix metalloproteinases and their inhibitors. *Int J Biochem Cell Biol.* 2007;40(6–7):1362–1378.

106. Decock J, Paridaens R, Ye S. Genetic polymorphisms of matrix metalloproteinases in lung, breast and colorectal cancer. *Clin Genet.* 2008;73:197–211.

107. Costa C, Incio J, Soares R. Angiogenesis and chronic inflammation: cause or consequence? *Angiogenesis.* 2007;10:149–166.

108. Hanrahan V, Currie MJ, Gunningham SP, et al. The angiogenic switch for vascular endothelial growth factor (VEGF)-A, VEGF-B, VEGF-C, and VEGF-D in the adenoma-carcinoma sequence during colorectal cancer progression. *J Pathol.* 2003;200:183–194.

109. Yamamori M, Sakaeda T, Nakamura T, et al. Association of VEGF genotype with mRNA level in colorectal adenocarcinomas. *Biochem Biophys Res Commun.* 2004. 2004;325:144–150.

110. Tan XL, Nieters A, Kropp S, et al. The association of cyclin D1 G870A and E-cadherin C-160A polymorphisms with the risk of colorectal cancer in a case control study and meta-analysis. *Int J Cancer.* 2008;122:2573–2580.

111. Haiman CA, Le ML, Yamamato J, et al. A common genetic risk factor for colorectal and prostate cancer. *Nat Genet.* 2007;39:954–956.

112. Tomlinson I, Webb E, Carvajal-Carmona L, et al. A genome-wide association scan of tag SNPs identifies a susceptibility variant for colorectal cancer at 8q24.21. *Nat Genet.* 2007;39:984–988.

113. Zanke BW, Greenwood CM, Rangrej J, et al. Genome-wide association scan identifies a colorectal cancer susceptibility locus on chromosome 8q24. *Nat Genet.* 2007;39:989–994.

114. Jaeger E, Webb E, Howarth K, et al. Common genetic variants at the CRAC1 (HMPS) locus on chromosome 15q13.3 influence colorectal cancer risk. *Nat Genet.* 2008;40:26–28.

115. Broderick P, Carvajal-Carmona L, Pittman AM, et al. A genome-wide association study shows that common alleles of SMAD7 influence colorectal cancer risk. *Nat Genet.* 2007;39:1315–1317.

116. Tomlinson IP, Webb E, Carvajal-Carmona L, et al. A genome-wide association study identifies colorectal cancer susceptibility loci on chromosomes 10p14 and 8q23.3. *Nat Genet.* 2008;40(5):623–630.

117. Tenesa A, Farrington SM, Prendergast JG, et al. Genome-wide association scan identifies a colorectal cancer susceptibility locus on 11q23 and replicates risk loci at 8q24 and 18q21. *Nat Genet.* 2008;40(5):631–637.

118. Hunter DJ. Gene-environment interactions in human diseases. *Nat Rev Genet.* 2005;6:287–298.

14

Childhood leukemias

Anand P. Chokkalingam and Patricia A. Buffler

Introduction

The term "leukemia" refers broadly to cancer of the white blood cells, or leuko-cytes. As a group, leukemias are the most common cancer among people under 15 years of age, accounting for 32% of all childhood malignancies. Age-standardized annual incidence rates worldwide range from 1.2 to 7.6 per 100,000 (1). In the United States, rates are 4.5 per 100,000, with an estimated 2,500 new childhood leukemia (CL) cases diagnosed annually (2). The highest incidence rates are in the 1–4-year-old age subgroup (2).

The etiology of childhood leukemias is believed to be distinct from that of adults, due largely to the clearer role for early life exposures, including those *in utero*. However, few risk factors have been established. Those that have been established include ionizing radiation, chemotherapeutic agents, and specific genetic abnormal-ities; these explain less than 10% of incidence, leaving at least 90% of cases with an unresolved etiologic mechanism (3,4). A number of exogenous risk factors have been suggested, including immunological factors, environmental factors, and maternal and child dietary factors. In addition, a heritable component has been suggested (5).

It is becoming increasingly clear that "childhood leukemia" actually refers to a group of diseases, composed immunophenotypically of ~80% childhood acute lymphoblastic leukemia (ALL) and ~17% childhood acute myeloblastic leukemia (AML), with the remainder including chronic myeloblastic and chronic lymphoblas-tic leukemias. Furthermore, even finer subgroupings can be made on the basis of affected precursor cell type (e.g., B-cell ALL), cytogenetic factors (e.g., TEL-AML1, hyperdiploidy), age of onset (e.g., infant leukemia, 0–12 months), and combinations thereof (common B-cell ALL [c-ALL], diagnosed between ages 2 and 5 years and expressing surface antigens CD10 and CD19). It is likely that the etiology of each of these immunophenotypic subtypes is distinct.

The early age of onset of childhood leukemias strongly suggests the role of genetic factors. However, much of the dramatic excess risk observed among mono-zygotic versus dizygotic twins of ALL patients has been attributed in good part to intraplacental metastasis, rather than a highly penetrant inherited risk allele (5), sug-gesting that for ALL, as with other multifactorial diseases (6), inherited risk alleles are likely to be low-penetrance susceptibility alleles that may interact with environmental factors to modulate disease risk. Indeed, common ALL chromosomal rearrangements are found in ~1% of healthy children (7), and *in vitro* and animal studies have shown that while expression of the TEL-AML1 fusion protein is sufficient to establish a covert preleukemic clone, it is not sufficient to transform hematopoietic cell lines into leukemic cells (8). Rearrangements alone are insufficient for disease onset, and there may be a strong role for genetic susceptibility, via main effects of genes or interaction with other factors, in at least one of the two or more "hits" (from Greaves' "two-hit hypothesis") (9) required for onset of ALL.

Genetically influenced mechanisms including immunity and response to infection, as well as one-carbon metabolism, are designed to protect against various external threats. Other mechanisms are involved as well, such as membrane transport; detoxification and biotransformation of reactive intermediates derived from environmental carcinogens; trapping or decomposition of reactive oxygen species (ROS); and DNA repair enzymes. Functionally significant inherited polymorphisms in genes involved at critical junctions along these pathways may alter the way in which a child responds to environmental threats and may lead to an increased risk of developing childhood leukemias. A growing number of primary studies and meta-analyses (10,11) have been published linking variants in these genes with risk of childhood ALL or AML.

The purpose of this review is to summarize the total body of literature on the genetic epidemiology of childhood leukemias, focusing specifically on main effects of gene variants, highlighting conclusions that can be drawn based on the work to date, and emphasizing challenges and future directions.

Methods

Study Identification and Eligibility

We searched PubMed (National Library of Medicine, Bethesda, MD) using the following search strategy: (childhood OR childre* OR pediatri* OR paediatri*) AND (leukemia [ti] OR leukemias [ti] OR leukaemia [ti] OR leukaemias [ti]) AND (polymorphi* OR (genetic AND varian*)). The last search was run on October 17, 2007. We included studies that reported on ALL and/or AML, provided the results for each type were reported separately. We excluded news reports, studies of treatment response (i.e., not of disease risk), studies of gene–environment interactions in which the gene main effects could not be discerned separately, studies which did not report results separately for children, case-only gene–environment interaction studies, and studies not reported in English.

Data Extraction

We reviewed each paper, noting year of publication, country of origin, study design (single study, meta-analysis), numbers of cases and controls, ages, use of child controls, genetic contrast(s), and effect size(s). Among overlapping studies, only the largest was retained. When a well-conducted meta-analysis of variant/disease associations was available, that study served as a summary of all included single studies, and we extracted summary data from the meta-analysis as well as any subsequent single studies. We considered a meta-analysis to be well-conducted if it performed a comprehensive literature search, clearly explained its inclusion and exclusion criteria, and performed appropriate statistical analyses, including fixed- and random-effects models, assessment of heterogeneity, and publication bias. Meta-analyses that did not meet these criteria were excluded from this synopsis.

Assessment of Evidence

We followed the Venice criteria (12) in assessing the quality of the evidence for genetic associations with childhood ALL and AML. Briefly, we assigned letter scores (A, B, or C) for each variant-disease association for each of the following areas: amount of evidence, replication, and protection from bias. For example, an association that shows consistent results in a well-conducted meta-analysis with over 1,000 cases (with low heterogeneity), and with a few other individual studies generally reporting the same effect, would garner a "B" in the area of amount, and "B" in the area of replication. (If null effects, that is, odds ratios close to 1, were reported in most studies, these too were considered replicated.) In contrast, a meta-analysis of over 10,000 cases with low heterogeneity followed by multiple individual studies across numerous populations reporting the same effect would warrant an "A" in the area of amount and an "A" in the area of replication. If there was no reason to suspect a strong effect of population stratification or notable genotyping error, the association would garner a "B" in the area of protection from bias; strong evidence of design-based and/or analytical methods to address these concerns would warrant an "A." Finally, the lowest individual area score was assigned as the overall summary score (12). We strove to report variants by RefSeq numbers, and where possible, their allele frequencies in the various HapMap populations (http://www.hapmap. org) and the SNP500 control group (http://snp500cancer.nci.nih.gov/).

Results

Using the search strategy and exclusion criteria noted above, we identified 57 studies for inclusion (10,13–69). Of these, 22 primary papers (13–22,29–34,41,46–49,69) were included in three well-conducted meta-analyses (10,11,68), and thus were not extracted separately. The literature to date reflects an examination of 67 variants in 36 genes in childhood leukemia etiology (Figure 14.1). These genes can generally be divided into the following pathways: folate metabolism, xenobiotic metabolism, immune function, DNA repair, and other. The evidence for each variant-disease association was assessed as described above, and the results are summarized in Table 14.1, organized by disease entity (i.e., ALL or AML) and by gene pathway. Below, we describe each of the pathways and results and the status of evidence in each.

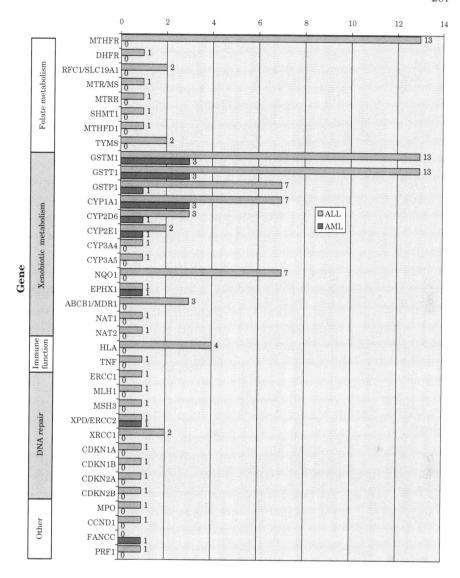

*Figure 14.1 Count of primary childhood leukemia genetic epidemiology reports, by ALL/
AML and Gene as of October 17, 2007.*

Folate Metabolism

Folate, an essential micronutrient, plays a central role in preserving the balance
between fidelity of DNA synthesis and availability of methyl groups for DNA
methylation (14). Deficiency in folate induces chromosomal damage and formation of fragile chromosomal sites, which are often associated with carcinogenesis
(70), and there is suggestive evidence that maternal folate supplementation during pregnancy reduces risk of ALL in children (71). Furthermore, hyperdiploid

Table 14.1 Summary of evidence for genetic associations with childhood acute lymphoblastic leukemia (ALL) and acute myeloblastic leukemia (AML)

			POLYMORPHISM					ALL			
			Variant AF					Evidence assessment[†]			
Pathway/ Gene	Name(s)[*]	RefSeq number (if avail)	CEU	HCB	JPT	YRI	SNP500 Controls	Amt	Replic'n	Protected from bias	OVERALL
Folate metabolism											
MTHFR	677C>T, A222V	rs1801133	0.242	0.511	0.364	0.108	0.284	B	B	A	B
	1298A>C, E429A	rs1801131	0.358	0.2	0.178	0.102	0.265	B	C	A	C
DHFR	3' UTR 829C>T	not found	—	—	—	—	—	C	C	B	C
RFC1/ SLC19A1	80G>A (R27H)	not found	—	—	—	—	—	C	C	B	C
MTR/MS	D919G, 2756A>G, Ex26-20A>G	rs1805087	0.167	0.067	0.233	0.3	0.206	C	C	B	C
MTRR	66A>G, I49M, Ex2-64A>G	rs1801394	0.448	0.25	0.302	0.233	0.426	C	C	B	C
	524C>T, S202L, Ex5+123C>T	rs1532268	0.733	0.878	0.967	0.792	0.309	C	C	B	C
	1049A>G, K377R, Ex7-9A>G	rs162036	0.233	0.233	0.102	0.449	N/A	C	C	B	C
	1783C>T, H622Y, Ex14+14C>T	rs10380	0.2	0.2	0.111	0.375	0.191	C	C	B	C
SHMT1	L474F, 1420C>T	rs1979277	0.342	0.078	0.044	0.4	0.25	C	C	B	C
MTHFD1	401G>A, R134K, Ex6+24A>G	rs1950902	0.792	0.778	0.773	0.892	0.837	C	C	B	C
	1958G>A, R653Q, Ex20-39G>A	rs2236225	0.458	0.222	0.261	0.2	N/A	C	C	B	C
TYMS	2R>3R 5'UTR 28bp repeat	None	—	—	—	—	—	C	C	B	C
	1494del6 3' UTR 6bp deletion	rs16430	N/A	N/A	N/A	N/A	0.53	C	C	B	C
Xenobiotic metabolism											
GSTM1	Deletion in Ex4	None	—	—	—	—	—	B	B	B	B
GSTT1	Deletion in Ex5	None	—	—	—	—	—	B	B	B	B
GSTP1	I105V, GSTP1*B, BsmaI	rs1695	0.625	0.822	0.889	0.642	0.672	B	B	B	B

Association, Comments	Evidence assessment[†]				Association, Comments
	Amt	Replic'n	Protected from bias	OVERALL	
Meta-analysis (10 studies, through 4/06) shows no significant decrease in risk in 1,914 cases. Of three subsequent studies, two are null and one showed significantly decreased risk.	—	—	—	—	—
Meta-analysis (10 studies, through 4/06) shows no association with risk in 1,710 cases. Of two subsequent studies, one shows significant risk increase, while other shows significant risk reduction.	—	—	—	—	—
No association, one study	—	—	—	—	—
No association, two studies	—	—	—	—	—
No association, one study	—	—	—	—	—
Significant association, one study	—	—	—	—	—
No association, one study	—	—	—	—	—
No association, one study	—	—	—	—	—
No association, one study	—	—	—	—	—
No association, one study	—	—	—	—	—
No association, one study	—	—	—	—	—
No association, one study	—	—	—	—	—
No association, two studies	—	—	—	—	—
No association, one study	—	—	—	—	—
Meta analysis (seven studies, through 7/04) shows no association. Of six subsequent studies, three showed significant risk increase, one showed borderline increase, and two were null.	C	C	B	C	Mixed results: of three studies, two were null and one showed significant risk increase.
Meta-analysis (seven studies, through 7/04) shows no association. Of six subsequent studies, three showed non-significant increases, and three were null.	C	C	B	C	No association, three studies.
Meta-analysis (four studies, through 7/04) shows no association. Of three subsequent studies, one showed a significant increase and two were null.	C	C	C	C	No association, one study.

(Continued)

283

Table 14.1 Continued

Pathway/ Gene	Name(s)[a]	RefSeq number (if avail)	POLYMORPHISM — Variant AF CEU	HCB	JPT	YRI	SNP500 Controls	ALL — Evidence assessment[b] Amt	Replic'n	Protected from bias	OVERALL
CYP1A1	6235T>C, MspI, CYP1A1*2A, m1	rs4646903	N/A	N/A	N/A	N/A	0.316	C	C	C	C
	CYP1A1*2C, CYP1A1*2B, m2, 1462V, 4889A>G	rs1048943	0.067	0.256	0.2	0	0.118	C	C	C	C
	CYP1A1*4, m4, T461N, 4887C>A	rs1799814	0.025	0	0	0	0.029	C	C	C	C
CYP2D6	CYP2D6*3, 1bp del at 2637, BstNI	rs45593132	N/A	N/A	N/A	N/A	N/A	C	C	C	C
	CYP2D6*4, HpaII, 1934G>A	rs3892097	N/A	N/A	N/A	N/A	0.108	C	C	C	C
CYP2E1	CYP2E1*5, -1259G>C	rs3813867	0.067	0.289	0.205	0.067	0.049	C	C	C	C
	CYP2E1*3, -1019C>T, PstI	rs2031920	0.059	0.289	0.205	0	0.049	C	C	C	C
CYP3A4	CYP3A4*1B, -391A>G	rs2740574	0.025	0	0	0.746	0.157	C	C	C	C
CYP3A5	CYP3A5*3	None	—	—	—	—	—	C	C	C	C
NQO1	P187S, Ex6+40C>T, 609 ex6	rs1800566	0.217	0.522	0.389	0.192	0.265	B	B	A	B
	R139W, Ex4-3C>T, 465C>T	rs4986998	0.008	0.022	0.034	0	0.02	C	C	B	C
EPHX1	Ex3-28T>C, Y113H	rs1051740	0.325	0.467	0.444	0.1	0.358	C	C	B	C
	Ex4+52A>G, H139R	rs2234922	0.175	0.056	0.111	0.383	0.203	C	C	B	C
ABCB1/ MDR1	3435C>T	rs1045642	0.542	0.4	0.478	0.117	0.417	C	C	B	C
	2352G>A	not found	—	—	—	—	—	C	C	B	C
	934A>G	not found	—	—	—	—	—	C	C	B	C
	692T>C	not found	—	—	—	—	—	C	C	B	C
	-129T>C	None	—	—	—	—	—	C	C	B	C
	1236C>T	rs1128503	0.392	0.689	0.578	0.123	N/A	C	C	B	C
	2677G>T,A	rs2032582	0.398	N/A	N/A	0	A = 0.039 T = 0.353	C	C	B	C
NAT1	≥ 1 copy of *10	N/A	—	—	—	—	—	C	C	B	C
NAT2	slow/slow phenotype	N/A	—	—	—	—	—	C	C	B	C

Association, Comments	Evidence assessment*				Association, Comments
	Amt	Replic'n	Protected from bias	OVERALL	
Mixed results—four of seven show some effect (consistent allele) while rest are null. There is inconsistency in reporting of CYP1A1 alleles.	C	C	C	C	No association, three studies.
Mixed results—one of three shows association, other two are null. There is inconsistency in reporting of CYP1A1 alleles.	—	—	—	—	—
No association in two studies.	—	—	—	—	—
No association in two studies, *3 allele is rare. There is inconsistency in reporting of CYP2D6 alleles.	C	C	C	C	No association in one study, *3 allele is rare. There is inconsistency in reporting of CYP2D6 alleles.
No association in three studies, *4 allele is not common. There is inconsistency in reporting of CYP2D6 alleles.	C	C	C	C	No association in one study, *4 allele is not common. There is inconsistency in reporting of CYP2D6 alleles.
Significant association, two studies.	C	C	C	C	Significant association, one study.
No association, one study.	—	—	—	—	—
No association, one study. Rare variant.	—	—	—	—	—
No association, one study.	—	—	—	—	—
Meta-analysis (seven studies, through 10/07) shows no association. Reporting of *2 allele inconsistent among primary studies.	—	—	—	—	—
No association, two studies.	—	—	—	—	—
No association, one study.	C	C	C	C	No association, one study.
No association, one study.	C	C	C	C	No association, one study.
Mixed results: of three studies, two support elevated risk with T allele, while one shows null results.	—	—	—	—	—
No association, one study.	—	—	—	—	—
No association, one study.	—	—	—	—	—
No association, one study.	—	—	—	—	—
No association, one study.	—	—	—	—	—
No association, one study.	—	—	—	—	—
No association, one study.	—	—	—	—	—
No association, one study.	—	—	—	—	—
Significant association, one study.	—	—	—	—	—

(Continued)

285

Table 14.1 Continued

Pathway/ Gene	Name(s)*	RefSeq number (if avail)	Variant AF					Evidence assessment†			
			CEU	HCB	JPT	YRI	SNP500 Controls	Amt	Replic'n	Protected from bias	OVERALL
Immune function											
HLA	DR53/DRB4	N/A	—	—	—	—	—	C	C	B	C
	DQB1*05	N/A	—	—	—	—	—	C	C	C	C
	DPB1*0201	N/A	—	—	—	—	—	C	C	B	C
TNF	-850C>T	rs4248158	—	—	—	—	—	C	C	C	C
DNA repair											
ERCC1	8092C>A	not found	—	—	—	—	—	C	C	B	C
	19007G>A	not found	—	—	—	—	—	C	C	B	C
MLH1	1219V, Ex8-23A>G	rs1799977	0.333	0.044	0.078	0.042	0.147	C	C	B	C
MSH3	R-940E	not found	—	—	—	—	—	C	C	B	C
	T-1036A	not found	—	—	—	—	—	C	C	B	C
XPD/ ERCC2	D312N	rs1799793	0.314	0.067	0.102	0.068	0.176	C	C	B	C
	K751Q, Ex23+61A>C	rs13181	0.625 (t)	0.678	0.633	0.658	0.211	C	C	B	C
XRCC1	R194W	rs1799782	0.092	0.244	0.278	0.083	0.129	C	C	B	C
	R280H	rs25489	0.033	N/A	N/A	0.025	N/A	C	C	B	C
	R399Q	rs25487	N/A	0.274	0.279	0.1	0.353	C	B	B	C
CDKN1A	-1284T>C	rs733590	0.392	N/A	N/A	N/A	N/A	C	C	B	C
	-899T>G	rs762624	N/A	N/A	N/A	N/A	N/A	C	C	B	C
	-791T>C	rs2395655	0.608	0.533	0.378	0.225	N/A	C	C	B	C
CDKN1B	-1857C>T	rs3759217	0.058	0.056	0.07	0.05	N/A	C	C	B	C
	-1608G>A	None	—	—	—	—	—	C	C	B	C
	-373G>T	None	—	—	—	—	—	C	C	B	C
CDKN2A	-222T>A	None	—	—	—	—	—	C	C	B	C
CDKN2B	-1270C>T	None	—	—	—	—	—	C	C	B	C
	-593A>T,C	None	—	—	—	—	—	C	C	B	C
	-287G>C	None	—	—	—	—	—	C	C	B	C
Other											
MPO	-642G>A, (463 promoter variant)	rs2333227	N/A	N/A	N/A	N/A	0.245	C	C	B	C
CCND1	Ex4-1G>A, P241P	rs603965	0.517	0.544	0.389	0.158	0.431	C	C	C	C
FANCC	S26F	rs1800361	N/A	N/A	N/A	N/A	N/A	—	—	—	—
PRF1	A91V, 272C>A	rs35947132	N/A	N/A	N/A	N/A	N/A	B	C	C	C

*Marker naming conventions: [amino acid][position][amino acid], e.g., R139W; or [position][base]>[base], e.g., 465C>T.
†Venice criteria (Ioannidis et al., 2007).

Association, Comments	Evidence assessment[†]				Association, Comments
	Amt	Replic'n	Protected from bias	OVERALL	
Significant association, one study.	—	—	—	—	—
Significant association, one study.	—	—	—	—	—
Significant association, two studies.	—	—	—	—	—
Significant association, one study.	—	—	—	—	—
Signficant association, one study.	—	—	—	—	—
No association, one study.	—	—	—	—	—
No association, one study.	—	—	—	—	—
No association, one study.	—	—	—	—	—
No association, one study.	—	—	—	—	—
No association, one study.	—	—	—	—	—
No association, one study.	C	C	C	C	No association, one study.
Mixed results: of two studies, one showed null effect, one showed reduced risk with variant.	—	—	—	—	—
No association, two studies.	—	—	—	—	—
Significant association, two studies in varied populations (elevated risk).	—	—	—	—	—
No association, one study.	—	—	—	—	—
No association, one study.	—	—	—	—	—
No association, one study.	—	—	—	—	—
No association, one study.	—	—	—	—	—
No association, one study.	—	—	—	—	—
No association, one study.	—	—	—	—	—
Significant association, one study.	—	—	—	—	—
No association, one study.	—	—	—	—	—
No association, one study.	—	—	—	—	—
No association, one study.	—	—	—	—	—
No association, one study.	—	—	—	—	—
Significant association, one study.	—	—	—	—	—
—	C	C	C	C	Significant association, one study.
No association, one large study (>2000 cases)	—	—	—	—	—

287

cases, whose lymphocytes often have multiple copies of chromosome 21, are particularly responsive to methotrexate, the folate pathway inhibitor whose receptor is encoded on chromosome 21 (72). Variants in the more than a dozen genes, including those encoding the methylene tetrahydrofolate reductase (*MTHFR*), dihydrofolate reductase (*DHFR*), reduced folate carrier (*SLC19A1*), methionine synthase (*MTR*), 5-methyltetrahydrofolate-homocysteine methyltransferase reductase (*MTRR*), serine hydroxymethyltransferase 1 (*SHMT1*), methylenetetrahydrofolate dehydrogenase 1 (*MTHFD1*), and thymidylate synthetase (*TYMS*), may alter folate metabolism and therefore risk of childhood leukemia.

The most studied gene in the folate pathway is *MTHFR*, which has two low-function polymorphisms: *677C>T* (rs1801133) and *1298A>C* (rs1801131). A recent meta-analysis (10) of ten studies (13–22) concluded that there was no significant association of *677C>T* with ALL risk, and three subsequent studies indicate either no association or a reduced risk associated with the variant (23–25); on balance, results indicate a modestly decreased risk or no effect of this marker, an effect that was consistent across most studies. The evidence was given an overall rating of "B." In contrast, the *1298A>C* marker of *MTHFR* was found in the same meta-analysis to be unassociated with childhood ALL risk (10): individual studies were heterogeneous in their findings, an effect mirrored by two subsequent studies (24,25), one of which reported a significant risk increase while the other reported a significant risk decrease. Overall evidence for this marker was rated at "C," given the absence of consistent replication.

With the exception of *MTHFR*, all the other genes in the folate pathway have shown null results for ALL, were studied in a single study, or both (23,26–28). Overall evidence for each of these was ranked as "C." No results have been published for childhood AML risk and folate genes.

Xenobiotic Metabolism

In order to exert their effects, potentially harmful chemicals must first gain entry into target cells, and then undergo cellular metabolic processes that might alter activity. Membrane transporters such as those encoded by the multiple drug resistance (*ABCB1/MDR1*) gene act as efflux pumps to expel compounds from the cell and are strategically expressed in regions of the body that act as epithelial barriers or perform excretory functions (73). In addition, enzymes involved in phase I (bioactivation) and phase II (detoxification) metabolism maintain a critical balance of activation and inactivation of a wide range of chemical exposures of relevance to CL, including drugs, chemical carcinogens, insecticides, petroleum products, nitrosamines, PAHs, and other environmental pollutants (74). Major metabolic enzyme families include the phase I cytochrome P450 (CYP) and the phase II glutathione-S-transferase (GST) and N-acetyl transferase (NAT) enzymes.

In childhood leukemia, the most commonly studied xenobiotic metabolism genes are those in the *GST* family, specifically, *GST-mu-1* (*GSTM1*), *GST-theta-1* (*GSTT1*), and *GST-pi-1* (*GSTP1*). *GSTM1* detoxifies polycyclic aromatic hydrocarbons, and *GSTT1* metabolizes epoxides and halomethanes; common deletions in both of these genes result in the loss of enzyme function (75). In contrast, the most commonly studied variant in *GSTP1* is a single nucleotide polymorphism: I105V. A meta-analysis (11) of seven studies published through July 2004 (15,29–34) revealed no overall association of the *GSTM1* and *GSTT1* deletions with risk of childhood ALL, and six subsequent studies (35–40) showed null results to modestly increased risks for the *GSTM1* marker and null results for the *GSTT1* marker, suggesting no association overall. For *GSTP1* and ALL, a meta-analysis (11) including four studies published through July 2004 (15,33,34,43) showed no overall association, a finding supported by three subsequent studies (35,40,42). Overall evidence for each of these *GSTs* in childhood ALL risk was assessed at "B."

Variants in the *GSTs* have also been examined in risk of childhood AML; however, far fewer studies have been conducted than for childhood ALL, and sometimes just one study has been conducted (15,38,40,44). Evidence for *GSTs* in childhood AML was assessed at an overall ranking of "C."

There are a large number of enzymes in the CYP superfamily of hemoproteins, which are primarily membrane-bound enzymes involved in phase I xenobiotic metabolism. CYP enzymes can metabolize multiple substrates, playing an important role in hepatic metabolism of drugs and toxic compounds, as well as extrahepatic synthesis and metabolism of cholesterol and hormones. Epidemiologic studies have examined genes encoding five of these enzymes in association with childhood leukemias (*CYP1A1, CYP2D6, CYP2E1, CYP3A4,* and *CYP3A5*). However, there is some inconsistency with regard to reporting of variant alleles of several *CYP* genes, notably *CYP1A1* and *CYP2D6*. This inconsistency stems from the occasional grouping of multiple SNPs into multi-SNP alleles that are akin to haplotypes; however, not all studies regularly genotype all of the variants needed to adequately classify these multi-SNP alleles, and the description of the genotyping and allele classification methods is often inadequate to allow verification that the alleles were classified correctly. As a result, in this synopsis, we focus on the effects of each individual SNP, rather than the multi-SNP alleles.

Results from the seven individual studies that have examined the *6235T>C* variant in *CYP1A1* with regard to childhood ALL risk are inconsistent, with four showing some evidence of association with the same allele (29,34,36,38), while the other three showed no effect (15,39,40). Fewer childhood ALL studies reported on the other two *CYP1A1* variants: just three reported on the *4889A>G* (29,36,39), and two reported on the *4887T>A* variant (29,39). Overall, evidence for *CYP1A1* markers in ALL risk was rated at "C," with no consistent effect. A meta-analysis for *CYP1A1* is warranted; however, it would have to address the potential inconsistencies in allele reporting, as noted above. For remaining *CYP* genes, including *CYP2D6, CYP2E1, CYP3A4,* and *CYP3A5*, there were only one or two reports for each variant (29,34,36,38,39,43). Overall evidence for these remaining *CYP* genes in childhood ALL risk was rated at "C."

There are limited reports of *CYP* genes in childhood AML risk; the most often reported is the *6235T>C* variant of *CYP1A1*, and three individual studies found no association (15,38,40). However, the amount of evidence here is small, and overall evidence thus garnered a "C." Few reports have been published for other *CYP* gene variants in childhood AML (38).

Several reports of the NAD(P)H dehydrogenase, quinone 1 (*NQO1*) in childhood ALL risk have been published to date. This phase II enzyme detoxifies quinones and acts as an antioxidant, reducing the exposure of DNA to reactive oxygen species. Seven reports published through October 2007 (40,41,46–49,69) were summarized in a recent meta-analysis (68), which found no childhood ALL association of rs1800566, a loss-of-function variant. Results across these individual studies were moderately consistent, and thus the evidence for this *NQO1* variant in childhood ALL risk is rated as "B" overall. However, it should be noted that, as with the *CYP* alleles, there is some inconsistency in the reporting of these alleles. Another variant in the *NQO1* gene, rs4986998, has been reported in only two studies (48,69), both reporting no association. Evidence for this *NQO1* marker in childhood ALL etiology is rated "C" overall. No studies of *NQO1* variants and childhood AML have been reported.

With the exception of *ABCB1/MDR1*, for which there are three inconsistent reports on the *3435C>T* variant in childhood ALL risk (51–53), there are scattered single reports for the remaining genes in the xenobiotic metabolism pathway and risk of either childhood ALL (40,50) or childhood AML (40). Where evidence is available for any of these genes it is rated "C" overall.

Immune Function

As a malignancy of lymphocytes, ALL is likely to be influenced by elements of the immune system's normal function, which is to protect against infectious agents and tumor growth. However, despite biological plausibility for a role of immune function genes in the genetic epidemiology of childhood leukemias, few reports have been published to date. The human leukocyte antigen (HLA) is an obvious target, due to its critical role in presentation of specific antigenic peptides derived from infectious agents. However, the major histocompatibility complex (MHC) is complicated, and traditional methods of assessing HLA types are time-consuming and costly, and therefore prohibitive for large epidemiologic studies. Nevertheless, three *HLA* loci have been examined. *HLA-DRB4* and *HLA-DQB1* were found to be significantly-associated with risk in individual studies (54,55). Another locus, the *HLA-DPB1* locus, was found to be associated with childhood ALL in two UK studies (56,57). Finally, a single study of tumor necrosis factor (*TNF*) with risk of childhood ALL found no association (58). Owing to the small number of studies published to date, the evidence for all genes involved in immune function in childhood ALL is rated "C" overall. No studies have examined these genes in childhood AML.

DNA Repair

DNA is regularly assaulted by a variety of endogenous processes and exogenous factors, including cigarette smoke, dietary factors, ROSs, and chemicals, all of which can cause varying degrees of DNA damage and lead to DNA mutation, which can in turn contribute to cancer development (76). DNA repair mechanisms defend against these exogenous insults, correcting DNA damage as well as normal replication errors. Base excision repair removes simple base modifications, including single-strand breaks, oxidative DNA damage, and alkylation and nonbulky adducts (77). Nucleotide excision repair removes larger lesions, which often result from environmental damage, including UV radiation and external carcinogens (78). Alkyltransferases directly reverse DNA damage by transferring alkyl groups from damaged DNA onto a transferase enzyme (79). Double-stranded DNA breaks are repaired through several mechanisms including the homologous recombination repair pathway (80). In addition to involvement in susceptibility, functional changes in DNA repair may play a specific role in facilitating some of the chromosomal rearrangements that are the hallmark of ALL and are often considered the first of a two (or more) hit etiological hypothesis (81).

Three different variants in the X-ray cross-complementary group 1 (*XRCC1*) gene have been studied with regard to childhood ALL. Results from just two studies were consistent for rs25489 (no association) and rs25487 (increased risk associated with variant allele), and mixed for rs1799782 (59,60). The evidence is rated as "C" given the small number of studies. Eight other genes in the DNA repair pathway have also been examined; however, just a single study has been published for variants in each (59,61–63,65). Overall evidence for involvement of DNA repair genes in childhood ALL is rated as "C." No studies of these genes have been published for childhood AML.

Other Genes

A handful of other genes that do not fit into one of the pathways above have also been examined with respect to childhood ALL or AML, including myeloperoxidase (*MPO*), cyclin D1 (*CCND1*), Fanconi's anemia group C (*FANCC*), and perforin (*PRF1*). These genes have all been examined in single reports, and with the exception of *PRF1*, which included >2,500 cases (64), all studies were of moderate size (<200 cases) (41,66,67). Thus, evidence for all these genes is rated overall as "C"; little can be said regarding their involvement in risk of childhood leukemia.

Summary and Future Directions

There is a growing amount of evidence for associations of gene variants in childhood leukemia etiology, particularly for ALL. However, when assessed by the Venice criteria (12), this evidence is insufficient for most genes. No genes had evidence rated "A." Of the five genes where evidence for one or more variants ranked "B" (*MTHFR, GSTM1, GSTT1, GSTP1*, and *NQO1*), none was found to show a significant association, and most were indicative of a null effect. However, overall, few genes have been studied to date for ALL, and many high-probability candidates remain unexamined or unreplicated. Even fewer genes have been studied for AML.

In addition, entire pathways with strong biological plausibility, such as the immune function and DNA repair pathways, remain poorly studied.

For gene variants where there are six or more individual studies, all but one were included in a well-conducted meta-analysis. There are currently eight individual studies of the *CYP1A1 6235T>C* variant (rs4646903). A meta-analysis will soon be warranted for this marker and others in the *CYP1A1* gene, and will require careful scrutiny of the individual studies to ensure that the variant alleles are reported consistently.

It is important to note that the effects of genes occur within the context of exposure to other risk factors, including both environmental and genetic factors. While gene–gene and gene–environment interactions are beyond the scope of the current synopsis, the gene main effects observed in the included studies of childhood leukemia are likely to be masked or otherwise influenced by such interactions.

As a summary of genetic variants associated with "childhood" disease, this synopsis posed some unique challenges. For one, because childhood leukemia is a somewhat rare and therefore difficult-to-study disease, the sample size in most individual reports is modest, usually 100 to 200 cases. Such a sample size is insufficient to properly examine risk associated with variants that are present at 5–10% frequency. Thus, analyses combining data across multiple studies are perhaps more relevant for childhood leukemia than for other, more common diseases. In addition, the age-based definition of childhood varies across many studies. In some, it is <15 years, while in others it is <21 years. For a summary such as this chapter, it is not feasible to drill down further within each individual study to focus on certain age groups—such an effort would, however, be appropriate for a pooled analysis or meta-analysis of a single association. Another consideration is that many studies utilize adult controls compared to child cases. This may lead to potential bias, in that observed associations may in fact be related to longevity rather than childhood leukemia. Provided these associations hold up in other studies that use child controls, such longevity concerns can be allayed; however, it is important that this issue be considered in pooled and meta-analyses.

There were a number of general challenges as well. One was that we restricted inclusion to English-language articles. Five articles were thus excluded; all were in Chinese. However, a review of their English abstracts indicated that these articles often merged childhood and adult leukemias, or failed to report AML and ALL separately; thus, it is likely that these papers would have been excluded from this synopsis on other grounds. In addition, it is unknown how many reports we may have missed by restricting our literature search to PubMed. However, this number of reports is unlikely to be large, and given the nature of this synopsis, the overall conclusions would unlikely be impacted. The naming of variants, too, was not always straightforward. Naming conventions have been standardized only recently. As a result, for some studies, particularly older ones that often refer to polymorphisms by a restriction enzyme, it is not always clear whether the reported polymorphism is the same as in more recent reports. Furthermore, as noted earlier in this synopsis, the naming of multi-SNP variant alleles poses a challenge for reporting and pooling, as investigators have not been consistent in their naming conventions for such alleles. For example, while two unique variants are required in order to possess the *2 allele in one study, another study may require just one of those variants to characterize the *2 allele. However, such challenges are to be expected in a rapidly evolving field such as genetic epidemiology, and with many naming conventions now widely accepted it will be easier to merge results going forward.

One new initiative in the area of childhood leukemia research is evolution of the Childhood Leukemia International Consortium (CLIC, http://clic.berkeley.edu). Started in 2006, this international consortium is open to all investigators who have or are developing an epidemiologic study of childhood leukemias. Participation in this consortium will enable individual investigators to conduct coordinated analysis and/or publish results for individual markers and/or genes, permitting rapid replication of both positive and null results with sufficient sample sizes. Indeed, as noted above, for childhood leukemias, the acquisition of sufficient sample sizes will require collaboration between study groups, particularly for AML, and even finer subgroups defined by cytogenetic and epigenetic factors.

Another exciting development is the advent of large-scale genotyping and whole genome scans. Such approaches involve interesting new analytical and statistical challenges, including power, multiple comparisons, and false-positives. However, the availability of large, standardized panels from such companies as Illumina (San Diego, CA) and Affymetrix (Santa Clara, CA) will also permit uniformity of genotyping across studies, allowing ready pooling of data and replication of findings. Per-sample costs for these panels continue to decrease, and it is thus becoming increasingly feasible to implement these in childhood leukemia epidemiology studies. In the future, synopses such as this will take advantage of applications of these large-scale genotyping panels across successive groups of cases and controls, so that novel genes will be revealed from the data. This is in contrast to the current candidate gene approach, which has been useful so far, but suffers from a slow pace of results and replication, as well as the already-noted inconsistencies in genotyping approaches and naming conventions.

In summary, the literature for genetic associations with childhood leukemia is small but growing, and much remains to be done. While the best-studied genes to date show no overall association, there are a number of highly likely candidate genes and entire pathways that remain under-studied. Evolving efforts, including the development of the Childhood Leukemia International Consortium and the application of large-scale genotyping technologies to epidemiology studies, hold much promise for this field. The next five years will see enormous growth in our knowledge of the genetic epidemiology of childhood leukemias.

Acknowledgments
We wish to thank Simon Chu for assistance with assembling papers and tables, and Neela Guha and Jeffrey Chang for assistance with extracting data from papers.

References

1. Parkin DM, Whelan SL, Ferlay J, et al. *Cancer Incidence in Five Continents, Vol. I–VIII.* IARC CancerBase No. 7, Lyon: International Agency for Research on Cancer; 2005.
2. U.S. Cancer Statistics Working Group. United States Cancer Statistics 2002 Incidence and Mortality. U.S. Department of Health and Human Services, Centers for Disease Controls and Prevention and National Cancer Institute, Atlanta, 2005.
3. Greaves MF and Alexander F. An infectious etiology for common acute lymphoblastic leukemia in childhood? *Leukemia.* 1993;7:349–360.
4. Buffler PA, Kwan M, Reynolds P, et al. Environmental and genetic risk factors for childhood leukemia: appraising the evidence. *Cancer Invest.* 2005;23:60–75.
5. Greaves MF, Maia AT, Wiemels JL, et al. Leukemia in twins: lessons in natural history. *Blood.* 2003;102:2321–2333.
6. Hunter DJ. Gene-environment interactions in human diseases. *Nat Rev Genet.* 2005;6:287–298.
7. Mori H, Colman SM, Xiao Z, et al. Chromosome translocations and covert leukemic clones are generated during normal fetal development. *Proc Natl Acad Sci USA.* 2002;99:8242–8247.
8. Andreasson P, Schwaller J, Anastasiadou E, et al. The expression of ETV6/CBFA2 (TEL/AML1) is not sufficient for the transformation of hematopoietic cell lines in vitro or the induction of hematologic disease in vivo. *Cancer Genet Cytogenet.* 2001;130:93–104.
9. Greaves M. Aetiology of acute leukaemia. *Lancet.* 1997;349:344–349.
10. Pereira TV, Rudnicki M, Pereira AC, et al. 5,10-Methylenetetrahydrofolate reductase polymorphisms and acute lymphoblastic leukemia risk: a meta-analysis. *Cancer Epidemiol Biomarkers Prev.* 2006;15:1956–1963.
11. Ye Z and Song H. Glutathione s-transferase polymorphisms (GSTM1, GSTP1 and GSTT1) and the risk of acute leukaemia: a systematic review and meta-analysis. *Eur J Cancer.* 2005;41:980–989.
12. Ioannidis JP, Boffetta P, Little J, et al. Assessment of cumulative evidence on genetic associations: interim guidelines. *Int J Epidemiol.* February 2008;37(1):120–132.
13. Franco RF, Simoes BP, Tone LG, et al. The methylenetetrahydrofolate reductase C677T gene polymorphism decreases the risk of childhood acute lymphocytic leukaemia. *Br J Haematol.* 2001;115:616–618.
14. Wiemels JL, Smith RN, Taylor GM, et al. Methylenetetrahydrofolate reductase (MTHFR) polymorphisms and risk of molecularly defined subtypes of childhood acute leukemia. *Proc Natl Acad Sci USA.* 2001;98:4004–4009.
15. Balta G, Yuksek N, Ozyurek E, et al. Characterization of MTHFR, GSTM1, GSTT1, GSTP1, and CYP1A1 genotypes in childhood acute leukemia. *Am J Hematol.* 2003;73:154–160.
16. Chiusolo P, Reddiconto G, Cimino G, et al. Methylenetetrahydrofolate reductase genotypes do not play a role in acute lymphoblastic leukemia pathogenesis in the Italian population. *Haematologica.* 2004;89:139–144.
17. Krajinovic M, Lamothe S, Labuda D, et al. Role of MTHFR genetic polymorphisms in the susceptibility to childhood acute lymphoblastic leukemia. *Blood.* 2004;103:252–257.
18. Chatzidakis K, Goulas A, Athanassiadou-Piperopoulou F, et al. Methylenetetrahydrofolate reductase C677T polymorphism: association with risk for childhood acute lymphoblastic leukemia and response during the initial phase of chemotherapy in Greek patients. *Pediatr Blood Cancer.* 2006;47:147–151.

19. Oliveira E, Alves S, Quental S, et al. The MTHFR C677T and A1298C polymorphisms and susceptibility to childhood acute lymphoblastic leukemia in Portugal. *J Pediatr Hematol Oncol.* 2005;27:425–429.

20. Schnakenberg E, Mehles A, Cario G, et al. Polymorphisms of methylenetetrahydrofolate reductase (MTHFR) and susceptibility to pediatric acute lymphoblastic leukemia in a German study population. *BMC Med Genet.* 2005;6:23.

21. Thirumaran RK, Gast A, Flohr T, et al. MTHFR genetic polymorphisms and susceptibility to childhood acute lymphoblastic leukemia. *Blood.* 2005;106:2591–2592.

22. Zanrosso CW, Hatagima A, Emerenciano M, et al. The role of methylenetetrahydrofolate reductase in acute lymphoblastic leukemia in a Brazilian mixed population. *Leuk Res.* 2006;30:477–481.

23. Giovannetti E, Ugrasena DG, Supriyadi E, et al. Methylenetetrahydrofolate reductase (MTHFR) C677T and thymidylate synthase promoter (TSER) polymorphisms in Indonesian children with and without leukemia. *Leuk Res.* January 2008;32(1):19–24.

24. Reddy H, Jamil K. Polymorphisms in the MTHFR gene and their possible association with susceptibility to childhood acute lymphocytic leukemia in an Indian population. *Leuk Lymphoma.* 2006;47:1333–1339.

25. Kim NK, Chong SY, Jang MJ, et al. Association of the methylenetetrahydrofolate reductase polymorphism in Korean patients with childhood acute lymphoblastic leukemia. *Anticancer Res.* 2006;26:2879–2881.

26. Gast A, Bermejo JL, Flohr T, et al. Folate metabolic gene polymorphisms and childhood acute lymphoblastic leukemia: a case-control study. *Leukemia.* 2007;21:320–325.

27. Whetstine JR, Gifford AJ, Witt T, et al. Single nucleotide polymorphisms in the human reduced folate carrier: characterization of a high-frequency G/A variant at position 80 and transport properties of the His(27) and Arg(27) carriers. *Clin Cancer Res.* 2001;7:3416–3422.

28. Goto Y, Yue L, Yokoi A, et al. A novel single-nucleotide polymorphism in the 3'-untranslated region of the human dihydrofolate reductase gene with enhanced expression. *Clin Cancer Res.* 2001;7:1952–1956.

29. Krajinovic M, Labuda D, Richer C, et al. Susceptibility to childhood acute lymphoblastic leukemia: influence of CYP1A1, CYP2D6, GSTM1, and GSTT1 genetic polymorphisms. *Blood.* 1999;93:1496–1501.

30. Saadat I and Saadat M. The glutathione S-transferase mu polymorphism and susceptibility to acute lymphocytic leukemia. *Cancer Lett.* 2000;158:43–45.

31. Alves S, Amorim A, Ferreira F, et al. The GSTM1 and GSTT1 genetic polymorphisms and susceptibility to acute lymphoblastic leukemia in children from north Portugal. *Leukemia.* 2002;16:1565–1567.

32. Davies SM, Bhatia S, Ross JA, et al. Glutathione S-transferase genotypes, genetic susceptibility, and outcome of therapy in childhood acute lymphoblastic leukemia. *Blood.* 2002;100:67–71.

33. Barnette P, Scholl R, Blandford M, et al. High-throughput detection of glutathione s-transferase polymorphic alleles in a pediatric cancer population. *Cancer Epidemiol Biomarkers Prev.* 2004;13:304–313.

34. Canalle R, Burim RV, Tone LG, et al. Genetic polymorphisms and susceptibility to childhood acute lymphoblastic leukemia. *Environ Mol Mutagen.* 2004;43:100–109.

35. Zielinska E, Zubowska M, Bodalski J. Polymorphism within the glutathione S-transferase P1 gene is associated with increased susceptibility to childhood malignant diseases. *Pediatr Blood Cancer.* 2004;43:552–559.

36. Joseph T, Kusumakumary P, Chacko P, et al. Genetic polymorphism of CYP1A1, CYP2D6, GSTM1 and GSTT1 and susceptibility to acute lymphoblastic leukaemia in Indian children. *Pediatr Blood Cancer.* 2004;43:560–567.
37. Wang J, Zhang L, Feng J, et al. Genetic polymorphisms analysis of glutathione S-transferase M1 and T1 in children with acute lymphoblastic leukemia. *J Huazhong Univ Sci Technolog Med Sci.* 2004;24:243–244.
38. Aydin-Sayitoglu M, Hatirnaz O, Erensoy N, et al. Role of CYP2D6, CYP1A1, CYP2E1, GSTT1, and GSTM1 genes in the susceptibility to acute leukemias. *Am J Hematol.* 2006;81:162–170.
39. Pakakasama S, Mukda E, Sasanakul W, et al. Polymorphisms of drug-metabolizing enzymes and risk of childhood acute lymphoblastic leukemia. *Am J Hematol.* 2005;79:202–205.
40. Clavel J, Bellec S, Rebouissou S, et al. Childhood leukaemia, polymorphisms of metabolism enzyme genes, and interactions with maternal tobacco, coffee and alcohol consumption during pregnancy. *Eur J Cancer Prev.* 2005;14:531–540.
41. Krajinovic M, Sinnett H, Richer C, et al. Role of NQO1, MPO and CYP2E1 genetic polymorphisms in the susceptibility to childhood acute lymphoblastic leukemia. *Int J Cancer.* 2002;97:230–236.
42. Gatedee J, Pakakassama S, Muangman S, et al. Glutathione s-transferase p1 genotypes, genetic susceptibility and outcome of therapy in Thai childhood acute lymphoblastic leukemia. *Asian Pac J Cancer Prev.* 2007;8:294–296.
43. Krajinovic M, Labuda D, Sinnett D. Glutathione S-transferase P1 genetic polymorphisms and susceptibility to childhood acute lymphoblastic leukaemia. *Pharmacogenetics.* 2002;12:655–658.
44. Liu QX, Chen HC, Liu XF, et al. Study on the relationship between polymorphisms of Cyp1A1, GSTM1, GSTT1 genes and the susceptibility to acute leukemia in the general population of Hunan province. *Zhonghua Liu Xing Bing Xue Za Zhi.* 2005;26:975–979.
45. Krajinovic M, Labuda D, Mathonnet G, et al. Polymorphisms in genes encoding drugs and xenobiotic metabolizing enzymes, DNA repair enzymes, and response to treatment of childhood acute lymphoblastic leukemia. *Clin Cancer Res.* 2002;8:802–810.
46. Kracht T, Schrappe M, Strehl S, et al. NQO1 C609T polymorphism in distinct entities of pediatric hematologic neoplasms. *Haematologica.* 2004;89:1492–1497.
47. Sirma S, Agaoglu L, Yildiz I, et al. NAD(P)H: quinone oxidoreductase 1 null genotype is not associated with pediatric de novo acute leukemia. *Pediatr Blood Cancer.* 2004;43:568–570.
48. Eguchi-Ishimae M, Eguchi M, Ishii E, et al. The association of a distinctive allele of NAD(P)H:quinone oxidoreductase with pediatric acute lymphoblastic leukemias with MLL fusion genes in Japan. *Haematologica.* 2005;90:1511–1515.
49. Lanciotti M, Dufour C, Corral L, et al. Genetic polymorphism of NAD(P)H:quinone oxidoreductase is associated with an increased risk of infant acute lymphoblastic leukemia without MLL gene rearrangements. *Leukemia.* 2005;19:214–216.
50. Sinnett D, Krajinovic M, Labuda D. Genetic susceptibility to childhood acute lymphoblastic leukemia. *Leuk Lymphoma.* 2000;38:447–462.
51. Hattori H, Suminoe A, Wada M, et al. Regulatory polymorphisms of multidrug resistance 1 (MDR1) gene are associated with the development of childhood acute lymphoblastic leukemia. *Leuk Res.* December 2007;31(12):1633–1640.
52. Jamroziak K, Mlynarski W, Balcerczak E, et al. Functional C3435T polymorphism of MDR1 gene: an impact on genetic susceptibility and clinical outcome of childhood acute lymphoblastic leukemia. *Eur J Haematol.* 2004;72:314–321.
53. Urayama KY, Wiencke JK, Buffler PA, et al. MDR1 gene variants, indoor insecticide exposure, and the risk of childhood acute lymphoblastic leukemia. *Cancer Epidemiol Biomarkers Prev.* 2007;16:1172–1177.

54. Dorak MT, Owen G, Galbraith I, et al. Nature of HLA-associated predisposition to childhood acute lymphoblastic leukemia. *Leukemia.* 1995;9:875–878.

55. Dearden SP, Taylor GM, Gokhale DA, et al. Molecular analysis of HLA-DQB1 alleles in childhood common acute lymphoblastic leukaemia. *Br J Cancer.* 1996;73:603–609.

56. Taylor GM, Dearden S, Payne N, et al. Evidence that an HLA-DQA1-DQB1 haplotype influences susceptibility to childhood common acute lymphoblastic leukaemia in boys provides further support for an infection-related aetiology. *Br J Cancer.* 1998;78:561–565.

57. Taylor GM, Dearden S, Ravetto P, et al. Genetic susceptibility to childhood common acute lymphoblastic leukaemia is associated with polymorphic peptide-binding pocket profiles in HLA-DPB1*0201. *Hum Mol Genet.* 2002;11:1585–1597.

58. Fidani L, Athanassiadou-Piperopoulou F, Goulas A, et al. An association study of the tumor necrosis factor alpha C-850T polymorphism and childhood acute lymphoblastic leukemia in a population from northern Greece. *Leuk Res.* 2004;28:1053–1055.

59. Pakakasama S, Sirirat T, Kanchanachumpol S, et al. Genetic polymorphisms and haplotypes of DNA repair genes in childhood acute lymphoblastic leukemia. *Pediatr Blood Cancer.* January 2007;48(1):16–20.

60. Joseph T, Kusumakumary P, Chacko P, et al. DNA repair gene XRCC1 polymorphisms in childhood acute lymphoblastic leukemia. *Cancer Lett.* 2005;217:17–24.

61. Wang SL, Zhao H, Zhou B, et al. Polymorphisms in ERCC1 and susceptibility to childhood acute lymphoblastic leukemia in a Chinese population. *Leuk Res.* November 2006;30(11):1341–1345.

62. Mathonnet G, Krajinovic M, Labuda D, et al. Role of DNA mismatch repair genetic polymorphisms in the risk of childhood acute lymphoblastic leukaemia. *Br J Haematol.* 2003;123:45–48.

63. Healy J, Belanger H, Beaulieu P, et al. Promoter SNPs in G1/S checkpoint regulators and their impact on the susceptibility to childhood leukemia. *Blood.* January 15, 2007;109(2):683–692.

64. Mehta PA, Davies SM, Kumar A, et al. Perforin polymorphism A91V and susceptibility to B-precursor childhood acute lymphoblastic leukemia: a report from the Children's Oncology Group. *Leukemia.* 2006;20:1539–1541.

65. Mehta PA, Alonzo TA, Gerbing RB, et al. XPD Lys751Gln polymorphism in the etiology and outcome of childhood acute myeloid leukemia: a Children's Oncology Group report. *Blood.* 2006;107:39–45.

66. Barber LM, McGrath HE, Meyer S, et al. Constitutional sequence variation in the Fanconi anaemia group C (FANCC) gene in childhood acute myeloid leukaemia. *Br J Haematol.* 2003;121:57–62.

67. Hou X, Wang S, Zhou Y, et al. Cyclin D1 gene polymorphism and susceptibility to childhood acute lymphoblastic leukemia in a Chinese population. *Int J Hematol.* 2005;82:206–209.

68. Guha N, Chang JS, Chokkalingam AP, et al. NQO1 polymorphisms and de novo childhood leukemia: a HuGE review and meta-analysis. *Am J Epidemiol.* December 1, 2008;168(11):1221–1232.

69. Wiemels JL, Pagnamenta A, Taylor GM, et al. A lack of a functional NAD(P)H:quinone oxidoreductase allele is selectively associated with pediatric leukemias that have MLL fusions. United Kingdom Childhood Cancer Study Investigators. *Cancer Res.* 1999;59:4095–4099.

70. Blount BC, Mack MM, Wehr CM, et al. Folate deficiency causes uracil misincorporation into human DNA and chromosome breakage: implications for cancer and neuronal damage. *Proc Natl Acad Sci USA.* 1997;94:3290–3295.

71. Thompson JR, Gerald PF, Willoughby ML, et al. Maternal folate supplementation in pregnancy and protection against acute lymphoblastic leukaemia in childhood: a case-control study. *Lancet.* 2001;358:1935–1940.

72. Pui CH, Relling MV, Downing JR. Acute lymphoblastic leukemia. *N Engl J Med.* 2004; 350:1535–1548.

73. Brockmoller J, Cascorbi I, Henning S, et al. Molecular genetics of cancer susceptibility. *Pharmacology.* 2000;61:212–227.

74. Strange RC, Fryer AA. The glutathione S-transferases: influence of polymorphism on cancer susceptibility. *IARC Sci Publ.* 1999;148:231–249.

75. Coles BF, Kadlubar FF. Detoxification of electrophilic compounds by glutathione S-transferase catalysis: determinants of individual response to chemical carcinogens and chemotherapeutic drugs? *Biofactors.* 2003;17:115–130.

76. Berwick M, Vineis P. Markers of DNA repair and susceptibility to cancer in humans: an epidemiologic review. *J Natl Cancer Inst.* 2000;92:874–897.

77. Thompson LH, West MG. XRCC1 keeps DNA from getting stranded. *Mutat Res.* 2000;459:1–18.

78. Sancar A, Tang MS. Nucleotide excision repair. *Photochem Photobiol.* 1993;57:905–921.

79. Inoue R, Abe M, Nakabeppu Y, et al. Characterization of human polymorphic DNA repair methyltransferase. *Pharmacogenetics.* 2000;10:59–66.

80. Kanaar R, Hoeijmakers JH, van Gent DC. Molecular mechanisms of DNA double strand break repair. *Trends Cell Biol.* 1998;8:483–489.

81. Greaves M. Childhood leukaemia. *Br Med J.* 2002;324:283–287.

15

Bladder cancer

*Jonine D. Figueroa, Montserrat Garcia-Closas,
and Nathaniel Rothman*

Background

Bladder carcinogenesis is an excellent model for the evaluation of genetic susceptibility and gene–environment interactions because of the relatively homogeneous
histology, the well-established causes of bladder cancer, including tobacco and
occupational aromatic amine (AA) exposure, and the considerable interindividual
variation in carcinogen metabolizing and DNA repair genes relevant for aromatic
amine-induced cancer. There have been numerous studies investigating the association of genetic polymorphisms and bladder cancer risk. Initial reports carried
out in the 1980s were often small, with limited power to detect associations with
risk. More recently, larger studies have become prominent and meta-analyses and
pooled analyses summarizing the literature have provided strong evidence for associations between common genetic variants and bladder cancer risk. The majority
of these reports have been on polymorphisms in candidate genes that are involved
in processes thought to mediate bladder carcinogenesis such as carcinogen metabolism, DNA repair, inflammation, cell cycle control, apoptosis, oxidative stress,
and methylation. In addition to the study of candidate genes and pathways, several genome-wide association studies (GWAS) are in progress, using an agnostic
approach to identify novel common susceptibility loci with dense genetic markers
that capture the majority of common variation across the genome. For this chapter,
we performed a literature search using the HuGE Navigator with the term "bladder cancer" and PubMed searches with the terms "bladder cancer polymorphisms"
and "bladder cancer risk variants" through September, 2008 for the purpose of performing systematic meta-analysis (Figueroa, et al., in progress). Publications that
did not have controls that were related to outcomes other than bladder cancer risk
(e.g., survival), or were performed in special populations (e.g., nonsmokers), were
excluded. From this search we identified 32 SNPs reported on in three or more studies (Table 15.1) and we summarize here the current evidence for the role of common
genetic variation in the etiology of bladder cancer.

Table 15.1 Summary table of SNPs reported on in three or more studies with frequency data and total number of cases and controls available for meta-analysis

Pathway	Gene	Chromosomal Location	Polymorphism (dbSNP rs number)	Position	Additional Information	Minor Allele or the Nonrisk Allele	MAF	Studies (N)	Cases (N)	Controls (N)	References
CMET	GSTM1	1p13.3	null/present	Ex4+10+>−	Gene deletion	Present	NA	36	6,913	9,586	(1–9)[*]
CMET	GSTP1	11q13	rs1695	Ex5-24A>G	I105V	G (Val)	0.29	8	1,912	2,358	(10)[*]
CMET	GSTT1	22q11.23	null/present	Ex5-49+>−	Gene deletion	Present	NA	26	5,861	7,478	(1–7,9,11–27)[*]
CMET	NAT1	8p23.1-p21.3	rs1057126	Ex3-177A>T	3'UTR	Fast acetylation[†]	NA	10	2,759	3,108	(3,5,28–35)[*,†]
CMET	NAT1	8p23.1-p21.3	rs15561	Ex3-170A>C	3'UTR	Fast acetylation[†]	NA	10	2,759	3,108	(3,5,28–35)[*,†]
CMET	NAT2	8p22	rs1208	Ex2-367G>A	R268K	Fast acetylation[†]	NA	41	6,363	11,805	(1–5,36–39)[*]
CMET	NAT2	8p22	rs1799930	Ex2-580G>A	R197Q	Fast acetylation[†]	NA	41	6,363	11,805	(1–5,36–39)[*]
CMET	NAT2	8p22	rs1799931	Ex2-313G>A	G286E	Fast acetylation[†]	NA	41	6,363	11,805	(1–5,36–39)[*]
CMET	NAT2	8p22	rs1801279	Ex2+197G>A	R64Q	Fast acetylation[†]	NA	41	6,363	11,805	(1–5,36–39)[*]
CMET	NAT2	8p22	rs1801280	Ex2+347T>C	I114T	Fast acetylation[†]	NA	41	6,363	11,805	(1–5,36–39)[*]
CMET	NQO1	16q22.1	rs1800566	Ex6+40C>T	P187S	T (Ser)	0.25	8	2,603	2,694	(2,12,13,22,40–44)
CMET	SULT1A1	16p12.1	rs9282861	Ex9+44G>A	R213H	A (His)	0.49	3	1,083	1,189	(12,45,46)
DNA repair	APEX1	14q11.2-q12	rs1130409	Ex5+5T>G	D148E	C (Glu)	0.47	5	2,334	2,522	(47–51)
DNA repair	ERCC2	19q13.3	rs1799793	Ex10-16G>A	D312N	A (Asn)	0.34	5	2,399	2,668	(2,47,52–54)
DNA repair	ERCC2	19q13.3	rs13181	Ex23+61A>C	K751Q	C (Gln)	0.34	9	3,377	3,638	(2,8,13,29,47,52–55)
DNA repair	ERCC5	13q33	rs17655	Ex15-344G>C	D1104H	C (His)	0.25	3	2,055	2,020	(13,47,52)
DNA repair	NBN	8q21	rs1805794	Ex6-32G>C	E185Q	C (Gln)	0.31	5	2,798	2,835	(2,13,47,56,57)
DNA repair	OGG1	3p26.2	rs1052133	Ex6-315C>G	S326C	G (Cys)	0.26	4	1,953	1,871	(47,48,58,59)
DNA repair	XPC	3p25	rs2228000	Ex9-377C>T	A499V	T (Val)	0.25	4	2,310	2,419	(2,47,52,60)

DNA repair	XPC	3p25	rs2279017	IVS12-6A>C		+	0.37	3	1,222	1,336	(2,47,60)
DNA repair	XPC	3p25	rs2228001	Ex16+211C>A	K939Q	C (Gln)	0.40	4	2,592	2,557	(13,47,52,60)
DNA repair	XRCC1	19q13.2	rs1799782	Ex6-22C>T	R194W	T (Trp)	0.07	6	3,072	3,206	(47,48,53,54,61,62)
DNA repair	XRCC1	19q13.2	rs25489	Ex9+16G>A	R280H	A (His)	0.05	3	1,808	1,771	(48,61,62)
DNA repair	XRCC1	19q13.2	rs25487	Ex10-4A>G	Q399R	A (Gln)	0.35	10	3,693	3,931	(2,13,47,48,53–55, 58,61,62)*
DNA repair	XRCC2	7q36.1	rs3218536	Ex3+442G>A	R188H	A (His)	0.10	3	1,899	1,833	(47,54,56)
DNA repair	XRCC3	14q32.3	rs1799796	IVS7-14A>G		G	0.33	3	967	1,055	(2,47,54)
DNA repair	XRCC3	14q32.3	rs861539	Ex8-53C>T	T241M	T (Met)	0.37	8	3,173	3,302	(2,13,47,53–56,63)*
DNA repair	XRCC4	5q13-q14	rs1805377	IVS7-1G>A	Splice site	A	0.10	3	1,742	1,756	(2,47,56)
Methylation	MTHFR	1p36.3	rs1801133	Ex5+79C>T	A222V	T (Val)	0.36	7	2,492	2,638	(13,22,64–68)
Methylation	MTHFR	1p36.3	rs1801131	Ex8-62A>C	E429A	C (Ala)	0.29	6	2,356	2,513	(13,22,64–67)
Methylation	MTR	1q43	rs1805087	Ex26-20A>G	D919G	G (Gly)	0.19	3	685	689	(65,66,68)
Cell Cycle	CCND1	11q13	rs9344	Ex4-1G>A	Splice site at codon 241	A	0.46	4	1,656	1,774	(13,69–71)
Cell Cycle	TP53	17p13.1	rs1042522	Ex4+119C>G	R72P	C (Pro)	0.25	3	712	731	(71–73)
Inflammation	IL1B	2q14	rs1143634	Ex5+14C>T	F105F	T	0.20	3	876	887	(74–76)
Inflammation	IL1B	2q14	rs16944	-1060T>C		T	0.35	3	866	882	(74–76)
Apoptosis	TNF	6p21.3	rs1800629	-487A>G		A	0.14	3	916	984	(59,76,77)
Oxidative stress	SOD2	6q25.3	rs4880	Ex2+24T>C	V16A	T (Val)	0.62	3	649	637	(78–80)

*Denotes that a meta-analysis has been performed for this SNP and is listed in the references.

†SNPs listed for NAT1 and NAT2 are all needed in order to determine the haplotypes and fast or slow acetylation activity as reviewed in references (81,82).

CMET = Carcinogen metabolism pathway; MAF = Average minor allele frequency among the available studies; NA = Not applicable since the composite haplotype is what is reported on for NAT1 and NAT2 acetylator genotypes.

Epidemiology of Bladder Cancer

It is estimated that in the United States about 57,000 cases of cancer of the urinary bladder are diagnosed and 12,500 deaths from the disease occur each year (83). Bladder cancer in the United States accounts for 6% of all new cancer cases among men and 2% of new cancer cases among women. Bladder cancer is a relatively homogeneous disease within industrialized countries and transitional cell carcinomas constitute 93–95% of malignant tumors of the urinary bladder (84). The other 5–7% of nontransitional cell carcinomas includes squamous cell carcinomas, adenocarcinomas, undifferentiated carcinomas, and other rare histological types (85). Heterogeneity of disease often requires the subclassification of tumors resulting in reduced power to detect associations within distinct subtypes. Thus, the relative homogeneity of bladder tumors facilitates investigations of genetic susceptibility compared to other more heterogeneous diseases.

Tobacco smoking and occupational exposure to AA are known bladder cancer risk factors that explain a large proportion of the disease (86). Because of the critical role of AA and perhaps other chemical carcinogens in tobacco smoke in the etiology of bladder cancer, common variation in carcinogen metabolizing genes and DNA repair mechanisms have been the most prominent genetic candidates studied to date.

Inherited Susceptibility to Bladder Cancer

Family History of Cancer and Bladder Cancer Risk

Reports of familial clustering of early onset bladder cancer provide evidence for a genetic component in bladder cancer (87–92). Studies examining familial risk have found relative risks ranging from 1.2 to 4.0 for subjects with at least one first-degree relative diagnosed with bladder cancer (93). Bladder cancer may also occur more frequently in certain familial syndromes. For instance, hereditary nonpolyposis colon cancer has been reported to increase the risk of bladder cancer (94), although the finding is not fully consistent (95). In addition, a recent study found increased bladder cancer risk among hereditary retinoblastoma cases (96). However, to date, there are no established high-penetrance mutations in genes associated with bladder cancer. Overall, there is little evidence to suggest the existence of a major hereditary form of bladder cancer.

Common Genetic Polymorphisms and Bladder Cancer Risk

Many studies have evaluated genetic polymorphisms and bladder cancer risk, but most early studies had limited statistical power to detect moderate to weak associations, particularly when the prior probability of association is low, or for the evaluation of gene–environment interactions (97). Systematic meta-analyses and pooled analyses of data from individual studies are important means to identify associations unlikely to be false-positives. Here, we review the rationale and findings from association studies of bladder cancer by biologic pathways, and present updated meta-analyses for the four most commonly studied polymorphisms in bladder cancer: N-acetyl transferase2 *(NAT2)*, N-acetyl transferase1 *(NAT1)*, glutathione S-transferase M1 *(GSTM1)*, and glutathione S-transferase T1 *(GSTT1)*.

Carcinogen Metabolism

N-acetyl transferases (NAT1 and NAT2). The *NAT1* and *NAT2* genes are both located on chromosome 8, *NAT1* on 8p21.3–23.1 and *NAT2* on 8p21.3–23.1 and 8p22 (81,98). NATs can metabolize aromatic and heterocyclic amines, which are known carcinogens that can produce tumors in animal models (99). Activation and detoxification pathways for bladder carcinogens such as AA have been implicated in bladder cancer etiology (100–102). The capability to detoxify aromatic mono-amines by N-acetylation, including 4-aminobiphenyl, which has been implicated in tobacco-related bladder carcinogenesis, is polymorphic in human populations. A number of *NAT2* alleles have been identified (http://louisville.edu/medschool/pharmacology/NAT2.html). The effects of *NAT2* polymorphisms and the combina-torial haplotypes or allelic types and their molecular genetics have been reviewed extensively (82). Recombinant expression systems have been the primary means of data to show that *NAT2* allelic variants have reduced substrate affinity, catalytic activities, or altered protein stability, which result in slow or fast/intermediate acety-lator phenotypes (81,98). The alleles for *NAT2* rapid-acetylator alleles are *NAT2*4, NAT2*11A, NAT2*12A, NAT2*12B, NAT2*12C, NAT2*13*; about 50% of Caucasian, and a lower percentage of African (30%) and Asian (15%) populations, are homozy-gous for a mutated *NAT2* responsible for decreased enzyme activity (slow acetyla-tors) (98,103,104).

Lower et al. first hypothesized in 1979 that individuals with the NAT2 slow acety-lation phenotype would be at higher risk of bladder cancer if they were exposed to AA (105). A relatively large number of studies were carried out subsequently to evaluate this hypothesis. The majority of studies have been in Caucasian populations where the frequency of the slow acetylator phenotype is so prevalent that the genetic models have most commonly evaluated the risk associated with the slow acetyla-tor phenotype compared to fast/intermediate acetylators and bladder cancer risk. Pooling and meta-analyses have shown compelling evidence for an increased risk of bladder cancer among *NAT2* slow acetylators (1,36,37). We have updated previous meta-analyses to include five additional studies (2–5,38), shown in Figure 15.1. This meta-analysis included 41 studies with a total of 6,363 cases and 11,805 controls, and provides further evidence for an increased risk of bladder cancer for *NAT2* slow acetylators compared with fast/intermediate acetylators (overall *p*-value = 3×10^{-8}). The association is strongest among European Caucasians in whom a majority of the studies have been carried out (20 total [OR and 95% CI for European Caucasians 1.42 (1.29–1.56)]; Figure 15.1). The meta-analyses showed evidence of significant heterogeneity of relative risk estimates across studies, as determined by the I^2 sta-tistic. The heterogeneity was reduced when analyses were restricted to Caucasians

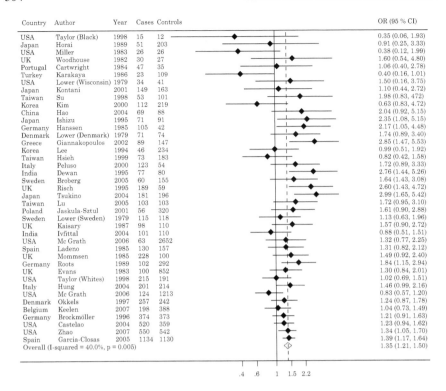

Country	Author	Year	Cases	Controls	OR (95 % CI)
USA	Taylor (Black)	1998	15	12	0.35 (0.06, 1.93)
Japan	Horai	1989	51	203	0.91 (0.25, 3.33)
USA	Miller	1983	26	26	0.38 (0.12, 1.99)
UK	Woodhouse	1982	30	27	1.60 (0.54, 4.80)
Portugal	Cartwright	1984	47	35	1.06 (0.40, 2.78)
Turkey	Karakaya	1986	23	109	0.40 (0.16, 1.01)
USA	Lower (Wisconsin)	1979	34	41	1.50 (0.16, 3.75)
Japan	Kontani	2001	149	163	1.10 (0.44, 2.72)
Taiwan	Su	1998	53	101	1.98 (0.83, 472)
Korea	Kim	2000	112	219	0.63 (0.83, 4.72)
China	Hao	2004	69	88	2.04 (0.92, 5.15)
Japan	Ishizu	1995	71	91	2.35 (1.08, 5.15)
Germany	Hanssen	1985	105	42	2.17 (1.05, 4.48)
Denmark	Lower (Denmark)	1979	71	74	1.74 (0.89, 3.40)
Greece	Giannakopoulos	2002	89	147	2.85 (1.47, 5.53)
Korea	Lee	1994	46	234	0.99 (0.51, 1.92)
Taiwan	Hsieh	1999	73	183	0.82 (0.42, 1.58)
Italy	Peluso	2000	123	54	1.72 (0.89, 3.33)
India	Dewan	1995	77	80	2.76 (1.44, 5.26)
Sweden	Broberg	2005	60	155	1.64 (1.43, 3.08)
UK	Risch	1995	189	59	2.60 (1.43, 4.72)
Japan	Tsukino	2004	181	196	2.99 (1.65, 5.42)
Taiwan	Lu	2005	103	103	1.72 (0.95, 3.10)
Poland	Jaskula-Sztul	2001	56	320	1.61 (0.90, 2.88)
Sweden	Lower (Sweden)	1979	115	118	1.13 (0.63, 1.96)
UK	Kaisary	1987	98	110	1.57 (0.90, 2.72)
India	Ivfittal	2004	101	110	0.88 (0.51, 1.51)
USA	Mc Grath	2006	63	2652	1.32 (0.77, 2.25)
Spain	Ladeno	1985	130	157	1.31 (0.82, 2.12)
UK	Mommsen	1985	228	100	1.49 (0.92, 2.40)
Germany	Roots	1989	102	292	1.84 (1.15, 2.94)
UK	Evans	1983	100	852	1.30 (0.84, 2.01)
USA	Taylor (Whites)	1998	215	191	1.02 (0.69, 1.51)
Italy	Hung	2004	201	214	1.46 (0.99, 2.16)
USA	Mc Grath	2006	124	1213	0.83 (0.57, 1.20)
Denmark	Okkels	1997	257	242	1.24 (0.87, 1.78)
Belgium	Keelen	2007	198	388	1.04 (0.73, 1.49)
Germany	Brockmöller	1996	374	373	1.21 (0.91, 1.63)
USA	Castelao	2004	520	359	1.23 (0.94, 1.62)
USA	Zhao	2007	550	542	1.34 (1.05, 1.70)
Spain	Garcia-Closas	2005	1134	1130	1.39 (1.17, 1.64)
Overall (I-squared = 40.0%, p = 0.005)					1.35 (1.21, 1.50)

.4   .6   1   1.5 2.2

	Cases (N)	Controls (N)	Studies (N)	OR	95% CI		pval	I pval	I²
All ethnicities	6,363	11,805	41	1.35	1.21	1.50	3×10^{-8}	0.005	40.0
Caucasians only	5,262	10,022	28	1.33	1.20	1.47	9×10^{-8}	0.064	30.6
European Caucasians	3,707	4,889	20	1.42	1.29	1.56	4×10^{-13}	0.540	0.0
USA Caucasians	1,532	5,024	7	1.12	0.92	1.36	0.25	0.157	35.5
Asians	908	1,581	10	1.43	1.02	2.00	0.04	0.041	48.7

Figure 15.1   NAT2 slow acetylation and bladder cancer risk. Association between NAT2 and bladder cancer risk. Odds ratios (OR) and 95% confidence intervals (CI) are for NAT2 slow versus intermediate/fast acetylators. Studies are weighted and presented by rank according to the inverse of the variance of the log OR estimate. I² statistic and corresponding p-values are used to assess heterogeneity of ORs across studies. There was also no evidence for an excess of statistically significant findings (p = 0.85).

from Europe and the United States, and increased among the ten Asian studies (Figure 15.1). There was no evidence of potential bias from the Harbord's test ($p = 0.95$; see Appendix A for more details).

Previous analyses have also shown evidence of an interaction between smoking status and *NAT2* genotype (1,37). We have updated our previous case-only meta-analysis and show evidence for interaction using data from 4,503 cases in 23 studies (Figure 15.2). This association was present only among European Caucasians, and was not observed in Asian studies or in studies carried out among Caucasians in

Author	Year	Country	Cases		OR (95% CI)
Horai	1989	Japan	50		0.74 (0.06, 8.71)
Lower	1979	Sweden	67		0.95 (0.08, 11.12)
Karakaya	1986	Turkey	23		0.13 (0.02, 0.98)
Miller	1983	USA	26		0.82 (0.13, 5.08)
Romkes	2000	UK	91		2.80 (0.62, 12.52)
Jaskula-Sztul	2001	Poland	59		0.97 (0.24, 3.87)
Dewan	1995	India	77		2.52 (0.65, 9.80)
Kontani	2001	Japan	149		0.35 (0.10, 1.28)
Ishizu	1995	Japan	47		0.71 (0.21, 2.42)
Roots	1989	Germany	101		0.83 (0.26, 2.62)
Hung	2004	Italy	201		0.63 (0.21, 1.87)
Ladero	1985	Spain	130		1.10 (0.42, 2.90)
Hanssen	1985	Germany	105		1.06 (0.41, 2.73)
Kaisary	1987	UK	98		1.11 (0.49, 2.48)
Mittal	2004	India	101		1.12 (0.51, 2.47)
Okkels	1997	Denmark	253		1.93 (0.90, 4.15)
Risch	1995	UK	178		1.72 (0.81, 3.65)
Taylor (Whites)	1998	USA	215		0.74 (0.35, 1.53)
Mommsen	1985	UK	149		1.84 (0.89, 3.80)
Tsukino	2004	Japan	325		1.02 (0.51, 2.06)
Brockmöller	1996	Germany	374		1.51 (0.96, 2.37)
Zhao H	2007	USA	550		1.15 (0.78, 1.71)
Garcia-Closas	2004	Spain	1134		1.36 (0.96, 1.92)
Overall (I-squared = 0.0%, p = 0.540)					1.21 (1.04, 1.42)

0.4 0.6 1 1.5 2.2

	Cases (N)	Studies (N)	Interaction OR	95% CI		*p*val	*I* pval	I^2
All ethnicities	4,503	23	1.21	1.04	1.42	0.02	0.540	0.0
Caucasians only	3,731	16	1.28	1.08	1.52	0.005	0.834	0.0
European Caucasians	2,940	13	1.38	1.13	1.68	0.002	0.886	0.0
USA Caucasians	791	3	1.03	0.73	1.45	0.86	0.555	0.0
Asians	571	4	0.78	0.46	1.34	0.37	0.556	0.0

Figure 15.2 Case-only meta-analysis of the interaction between NAT2 and smoking on bladder cancer risk. Interaction between NAT2, smoking, and bladder cancer risk. Odds ratios (OR) and 95% confidence intervals (CI) for multiplicative interaction using a case-only design. Studies are weighted and presented by rank according to the inverse of the variance of the log OR estimate. I² statistic and corresponding p-values are used to assess heterogeneity of interaction ORs across studies.

the United States. This may suggest differences in the interaction by geographic region, which could be correlated with other factors such as tobacco type (blond vs. black tobacco); however, there are notably fewer studies on Asians and United States Caucasians, and further data are needed to determine if an interaction exists (Figure 15.2). In addition, a recent Bayesian meta-analysis of *NAT2* genotype/phenotype also supports a stronger risk of bladder cancer associated with the *NAT2* slow acetylation among smokers, using methods that accommodate evidence from studies where some exposure variables have been reported differently or omitted (106). Since tobacco smoking is a primary source of exposure to AA in the general population and *NAT2* slow acetylators have a decreased capacity to detoxify aromatic monoamines, this gene–environment interaction has strong biological plausibility (98). Further evidence supporting the interaction includes a report where smokers with the *NAT2* slow polymorphism had higher levels of 4-aminobiphenyl hemoglobin adducts in peripheral red blood cells than smokers with the *NAT2* rapid polymorphism (107). However, additional studies in diverse geographic regions are still required to confirm this interaction.

Most studies discussed above were conducted in the general population, without specific occupational or environmental exposures to bladder carcinogens. Studies among subjects occupationally exposed to AA also tend to show associations between *NAT2* slow acetylation and increased bladder cancer risk (108,109). For example, in a groundbreaking paper, Cartwright et al. reported that individuals in the United Kingdom with occupational exposure to aromatic amines were at very high risk of bladder cancer. Furthermore, Cartwright et al. observed that slow acetylator status could be used to identify susceptible individuals in potentially hazardous occupations (OR = 16.7, 95% CI = 2.2–129.1) (110). In contrast, a study of *NAT2* genotype and phenotype and bladder cancer in participants from a cohort of workers with well-documented occupational exposure to benzidine, a potent bladder carcinogen, found that *NAT2* slow acetylation was protective, with a pooled estimate from two studies carried out in the same population of OR = 0.3 (95% CI = 0.1–1.0) (111,112). Further, experimental studies have shown that the N-acetylation of benzidine, an aryldiamine, produces a far better substrate for subsequent oxidation to its hydroxylamine (113). In addition, a study of workers exposed to benzidine or benzidine-based dyes supported the experimental observation that N-acetylation is an activation step for benzidine by demonstrating that the predominant DNA adduct in exfoliated urothelial cells was N-acetylated (114). This body of work suggests that in contrast to arylmonoamines, such as 4-aminobiphenyl and 2-naphthylamine from tobacco smoke, N-acetylation of aryldiamines such as benzidine is an activation rather than a detoxification step. Further complicating the situation is that benzidine is a better substrate for *NAT1* than *NAT2* (113). Taken together, it would seem that the *NAT2* slow acetylation does not increase risk for bladder cancer among workers exposed to benzidine and may indeed be protective.

The *NAT1* gene codes for an enzyme involved in the activation of aromatic amines by O-acetylation (98). NAT1 shows selectivity for p-amino-benzoic acid and p-phenylene-diamine and there are 26 alleles for *NAT1* identified in humans (see http://louisville.edu/medschool/pharmacology/Human.NAT1.pdf). The *NAT1*10* genotype, has been associated with higher levels of NAT1 activity and DNA adducts in human bladder tissue (115). There is, however, inconsistent evidence for an association between bladder cancer risk and *NAT1*10* allele alone or in combination with *NAT2* slow acetylation (1,28,39). We conducted a meta-analysis of ten published studies including a total of 2,759 cases and 3,108 controls, and estimated a summary relative risk for *NAT1*10* "at risk" allele compared with *NAT1*4* of OR = 1.02 (95% CI = 0.85–1.23), *p*-value = 0.82 (Table 15.2). There was evidence of significant heterogeneity across studies from the I^2 statistic (see Appendix A for more details). There was also some evidence for an excess of statistically significant findings. Therefore, current evidence does not support an overall association

Table 15.2 Meta-analysis of *GSTT1* and *NAT1* polymorphisms and bladder cancer risk

Gene	Polymorphism		Cases (N)	Controls (N)	Studies (N)	OR	95% CI		pval	I^2 pval	I^2
NAT1	Slow vs Fast	All ethnicities	2,759	3,108	10	1.02	0.85	1.23	0.82	0.012	57.4
		Caucasians Only	2,578	2,815	8	1.06	0.87	1.28	0.57	0.017	59.0
		European Caucasians	1,874	2,133	6	1.13	0.89	1.43	0.32	0.029	59.9
		European Caucasians (with atleast 100 cases)	1,761	1,668	4	1.26	0.98	1.62	0.07	0.048	62.1
GSTT1	null vs present	All ethnicities	5,861	7,478	26	1.07	0.94	1.22	0.27	0.009	44.0
		Caucasians Only	4,694	5,808	19	1.10	0.95	1.28	0.21	0.048	38.0
		European Caucasians	2,651	2,940	10	1.12	0.86	1.46	0.40	0.010	58.5
		European Caucasians (with atleast 100 cases)	2,425	2,391	7	1.13	0.85	1.51	0.40	0.017	61.2
		USA Caucasians	1,703	2,506	5	1.03	0.87	1.22	0.75	0.462	0.0
		Asians	961	1,224	5	0.89	0.71	1.12	0.32	0.158	39.4

Notes: Association between *GSTT1*, *NAT1*, and bladder cancer risk. Odds ratios (OR) and 95% confidence intervals (CI) are for *GSTT1* null versus present genotypes; and *NAT1*10* at risk allele compared with the *NAT1*4* allele. I^2 statistic and corresponding *p*-values are used to assess heterogeneity of ORs across studies.

between *NAT1* polymorphisms and bladder cancer risk. It has been recently suggested by Sanderson et al. that there may be an interaction between *NAT1*, *NAT2*, and smoking; however, this needs to be further corroborated in additional epidemiology studies (39).

Glutathione S-transferases (GSTM1, GSTT1, and GSTP1). The cytosolic glutathione transferases (GST) are a superfamily of phase II enzymes that conjugate electrophilic substrates with the nucleophilic tripeptide glutathione (116). The *GSTM1* gene codes for the cytosolic mu class of glutathione S-transferases, an enzyme involved in detoxification of a range of carcinogens, including aflatoxin B, aryl halides, polycyclic aromatic hydrocarbons (PAHs), and reactive oxygen species (117,118). A common homozygous deletion (null genotype) polymorphism of *GSTM1* is associated with lack of enzyme activity (119), which is present in about 50% of Caucasians. Meta-analyses have consistently reported that the *GSTM1* null genotype increases risk of bladder cancer (1,120). We present an updated meta-analysis in Figure 15.3 that includes eight additional studies (2–9) and one updated report (11) in addition to the studies included in our previous publication (1). The meta-analysis of 36 studies shows a consistent association with bladder cancer risk for the *GSTM1* null compared with present genotype across all ethnicities (OR ranging from 1.26 to 1.47, depending on geographic region) (Figure 15.3). There is evidence from I^2 of significant heterogeneity of relative risk estimates across studies; however, as the plot shows, this heterogeneity is not around the null value of 1.0, but rather around the point estimate of 1.43. There was no evidence of potential bias from the Harbord's test ($p = 0.27$, see Appendix A for more details). It has been previously shown by Garcia-Closas et al., 2005 (1) that the relative risk for *GSTM1* null genotype and bladder cancer is similar for smokers and never smokers, suggesting that the *GSTM1* activity protects equally against tobacco-related and non-tobacco-related bladder cancers, and may reduce the risk of bladder cancer through mechanisms that are not specific to the detoxification of PAHs in tobacco smoke. We present an updated case-only analysis of *GSTM1* (Figure 15.4) that is consistent with what has been previously reported (1), with an interaction OR of 1.01 (0.87–1.16) and a p-value for interaction = 0.94. The biologic basis for this consistent association, which is present in studies carried out in Europe, the United States, and Asia, has not yet been clarified. Other hypothesized mechanisms of action for *GSTM1* are protection from oxidative damage through metabolism of reactive oxygen species (118).

The *GSTT1* gene has been identified as encoding a specific glutathione transferase activity that can catalyze the glutathione conjugation of dichloromethane and epoxides and can be carcinogenic (121,122). This enzyme also displays a gene deletion in about 10–20% of Caucasian individuals. The *GSTT1* deletion has been investigated in 26 studies of bladder cancer; however there is no evidence for an association in our meta-analysis of 5,861 cases and 7,478 controls (Table 15.2). Meta-analysis of *GSTT1* suggests significant heterogeneity around the null, unlike *GSTM1*, where meta-analyses show consistent associations with increased risk.

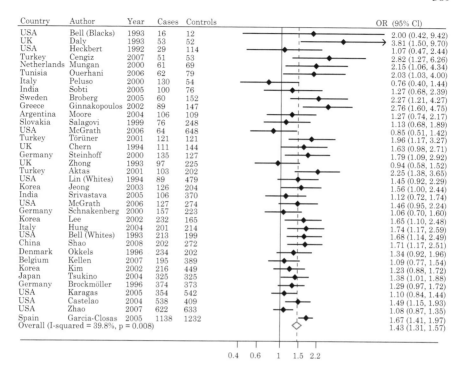

Country	Author	Year	Cases	Controls	OR (95% CI)
USA	Bell (Blacks)	1993	16	12	2.00 (0.42, 9.42)
UK	Daly	1993	53	52	3.81 (1.50, 9.70)
USA	Heckbert	1992	29	114	1.07 (0.47, 2.44)
Turkey	Cengiz	2007	51	53	2.82 (1.27, 6.26)
Netherlands	Mungan	2000	61	69	2.15 (1.06, 4.34)
Tunisia	Ouerhani	2006	62	79	2.03 (1.03, 4.00)
Italy	Peluso	2000	130	54	0.76 (0.40, 1.44)
India	Sobti	2005	100	76	1.27 (0.68, 2.39)
Sweden	Broberg	2005	60	152	2.27 (1.21, 4.27)
Greece	Ginnakopoulos	2002	89	147	2.76 (1.60, 4.75)
Argentina	Moore	2004	106	109	1.27 (0.74, 2.17)
Slovakia	Salagovi	1999	76	248	1.13 (0.68, 1.89)
USA	McGrath	2006	64	648	0.85 (0.51, 1.42)
Turkey	Törüner	2001	121	121	1.96 (1.17, 3.27)
UK	Chern	1994	111	144	1.63 (0.98, 2.71)
Germany	Steinhoff	2000	135	127	1.79 (1.09, 2.92)
UK	Zhong	1993	97	225	0.94 (0.58, 1.52)
Turkey	Aktas	2001	103	202	2.25 (1.38, 3.65)
USA	Lin (Whites)	1994	89	479	1.45 (0.92, 2.29)
Korea	Jeong	2003	126	204	1.56 (1.00, 2.44)
India	Srivastava	2005	106	370	1.12 (0.72, 1.74)
USA	McGrath	2006	127	274	1.46 (0.95, 2.24)
Germany	Schnakenberg	2000	157	223	1.06 (0.70, 1.60)
Korea	Lee	2002	232	165	1.65 (1.10, 2.48)
Italy	Hung	2004	201	214	1.74 (1.17, 2.59)
USA	Bell (Whites)	1993	213	199	1.68 (1.14, 2.49)
China	Shao	2008	202	272	1.71 (1.17, 2.51)
Denmark	Okkels	1996	234	202	1.34 (0.92, 1.96)
Belgium	Kellen	2007	195	389	1.09 (0.77, 1.54)
Korea	Kim	2002	216	449	1.23 (0.88, 1.72)
Japan	Tsukino	2004	325	325	1.38 (1.01, 1.88)
Germany	Brockmöller	1996	374	373	1.29 (0.97, 1.72)
USA	Karagas	2005	354	542	1.10 (0.84, 1.44)
USA	Castelao	2004	538	409	1.49 (1.15, 1.93)
USA	Zhao	2007	622	633	1.08 (0.87, 1.35)
Spain	Garcia-Closas	2005	1138	1232	1.67 (1.41, 1.97)
Overall (I-squared = 39.8%, p = 0.008)					1.43 (1.31, 1.57)

0.4   0.6   1   1.5 2.2

	Cases (N)	Controls (N)	Studies (N)	OR	95% CI		*p*val	*I* pval	I^2
All ethnicities	6,913	9,586	36	1.45	1.31	1.60	3×10^{-13}	0.001	49.3
Caucasians only	5,590	7,713	28	1.47	1.29	1.66	2×10^{-9}	0.0001	58.5
European Caucasians	3,111	3,851	15	1.50	1.25	1.80	2×10^{-5}	0.0004	63.6
USA Caucasians	2,036	3,298	8	1.26	1.08	1.46	2×10^{-3}	0.215	26.7
Asians	1,101	1,415	5	1.46	1.24	1.72	6×10^{-6}	0.689	0.0

Figure 15.3   GSTM1 null genotype and bladder cancer risk. Association between GSTM1 and bladder cancer risk. Odds ratios (OR) and 95% confidence intervals (CI) are for GSTM1 null versus present genotypes. Studies are weighted and presented by rank according to the inverse of the variance of the log OR estimate. I^2 statistic and corresponding p-values are used to assess heterogeneity of ORs across studies. There was also no evidence for an excess of statistically significant findings (p = 0.99).

These results do not support *GSTT1* null deletion as an important susceptibility factor for bladder cancer.

GSTP1b allele is a nonsynonymous polymorphism (rs1695) that converts the 105 amino acid to valine; it has been shown to possess an elevated enzymatic activity toward certain substrates like chrysene-1,2-diol-3,4-epoxide, ethacrynic acid, and bromosulfophthalein, whereas *GSTP1a* allele has an isoleucine at position 105 and has been shown to possess an elevated enzymatic activity for substances like 3,4-dichloro-1-nitrobenzene and 1-chloro-2, 4-dinitrobenzene. The *GSTP1 Ile105Val* (rs1695) valine form has been thought to be the at risk allele (118,123,124). A recent

Author	Year	Country	Cases		OR (95% CI)
Heckbert	1992	USA	29		3.20 (0.26, 40.06)
Daly	1993	UK	53		2.00 (0.46, 8.75)
Ouerhani	2006	Tunisia	62		1.89 (0.48, 7.40)
Chern	1994	UK	95		0.85 (0.24, 3.01)
Cengiz	2007	Turkey	51		0.68 (0.21, 2.28)
Hung	2004	Italy	201		1.05 (0.37, 2.96)
Peluso	2000	Italy	130		3.23 (1.19, 8.79)
Moore	2004	Argentina	114		1.42 (0.59, 3.42)
Sobti	2005	India	100		0.44 (0.18, 1.03)
Törüner	2001	Turkey	121		1.24 (0.53, 2.93)
Srivastava	2004	India	106		1.34 (0.60, 2.96)
Lee	2002	Korea	232		0.85 (0.39, 1.89)
Aktas	2001	Turkey	103		0.72 (0.33, 1.58)
Kang	1999	Korea	174		0.85 (0.39, 1.86)
Okkels	1996	Denmark	234		0.96 (0.44, 2.07)
Bell (Whites)	1993	USA	213		1.32 (0.65, 2.67)
Shao	2008	China	202		1.07 (0.61, 1.88)
Karagas	2005	USA	354		1.04 (0.61, 1.77)
Tsukino	2004	Japan	325		1.11 (0.69, 1.78)
Brockmöller	1996	Germany	374		1.06 (0.68, 1.66)
Garcìa-Closas	2004	Spain	1226		0.77 (0.54, 1.11)
Zhao	2007	USA	622		1.00 (0.70, 1.43)
Overall (I-squared = 0.0%, p = 0.708)					1.01 (0.87, 1.16)

.4 .6   1 1.5 2.2

	Cases (N)	Studies (N)	Interaction OR	95% CI		pval	I pval	I²
All ethnicities	5,121	22	1.01	0.87	1.16	0.94	0.708	0.0
Caucasians only	3,644	13	1.02	0.85	1.21	0.84	0.542	0.0
European Caucasians	2,426	9	1.03	0.78	1.37	0.82	0.305	15.4
USA Caucasians	1,218	4	1.06	0.81	1.40	0.65	0.750	0.0
Asians	933	4	1.01	0.75	1.37	0.93	0.908	0.0

Figure 15.4   Case-only meta-analysis of the interaction between GSTM1, smoking, and bladder cancer risk. Interaction between GSTM1, smoking, and bladder cancer risk. Odds ratios (OR) and 95% confidence intervals (CI) are for multiplicative interaction using a case-only design. Studies are weighted and presented by rank according to the inverse of the variance of the log OR estimate. I² statistic and corresponding p-values are used to assess heterogeneity of interaction ORs across studies.

pooled analysis of the *GSTP1 Ile105Val* and bladder cancer risk suggested the *Ile/ Val Val/Val* genotypes were significantly associated with bladder cancer risk, compared with the *GSTP1 Ile/Ile* genotype OR = 1.54 (95% CI = 1.21, 1.99; $p < 0.001$) for *Ile/Val*, OR = 2.17 (95% CI = 1.27, 3.71; $p = 0.005$), respectively. The association appeared to be the strongest in Asian countries. When the analysis was limited to European Caucasians (nine studies), the summary OR decreased (OR = 1.24, 95% CI = 1.00–1.52) (10). There was evidence of unexplained heterogeneity of these associations and the cause of this is unclear. Therefore additional studies are needed to clarify the relationship between genetic variants in *GSTP1* and bladder cancer risk.

Cytochrome P450s, sulfotransferases, NAD(P)H dehydrogenase quinone. Other enzymes that could affect the risk of bladder cancer include cytochrome P450

enzymes such as CYP1A1, CYP1B1, CYP2C19, CYP2D6, CYP2E1, sulfotransferases (SULT) involved in the activation of aromatic amines, and NAD(P)H
dehydrogenase quinone 1 (*NQO1*). Cytochrome P450 *CYP1A2* is involved in the
activation of aromatic amines by N-hydroxylation, and is polymorphic in human
populations; however, the functional relevance of the genetic variants is not well
characterized (125), and to date it is unclear whether they play a role in bladder
cancer. In a recent report by Figueroa et al. (40) two nonredundant SNPs in the
CYP1A1 gene in the promoter and 3′ of the STP codon were associated with bladder cancer risk: *CYP1A1* rs2472299 and *CYP1A1* rs2198843. In addition, one SNP
in the promoter of the *CYP1B1* gene (rs162555) and a rare SNP *Y62F* (rs4987024) in
SULT1A2, a gene involved in the activation of aromatic amines (126), were associated with bladder cancer risk (40). Furthermore, a nonsynonymous SNP in *SULT1A1*
rs9282861(*R213H*) has been consistently observed to be inversely associated with
bladder cancer risk in three studies (4,12,45). All of these findings require replication in additional studies. The nonsynonymous SNPs in *CYP1A1* rs1048943 (*I462V*)
and *CYP1B1* rs1056836 (*V432L*) have been shown to be associated with altered
enzymatic activity; however, there is little evidence to suggest their association with
bladder cancer risk (40,127).

NQO1's activity has been found to have detoxifying properties by reducing the
presence of hydroquinones that can be excreted, but activates nitroaromatic amines
present in tobacco smoke (41,128–130). The variant allele of *NQO1* rs1800566
(*P187S*) has been shown to have reduced quinone reductase activity from *in vitro*
studies (131–133). A recent meta-analysis of six bladder cancer studies of 1,410
cases and 1,485 controls in Caucasian populations suggest an increased risk for the
rs1800566 (*P187S*) CT/TT genotype of 1.20 (1.00–1.43) (41). However, this association was not confirmed in a large case-control study in Spain (40) and relative risk
estimates suggested an inverse relationship with risk.

DNA repair. A complex network of complementary DNA repair mechanisms exists
to prevent the detrimental consequences of DNA damage caused by endogenous and
exogenous exposures, and genetic variation in DNA repair genes may alter repair
function and contribute to cancer risk (134). There are four main types of DNA
repair pathways: nucleotide-excision repair (NER), base-excision repair (BER),
double-strand break repair (DSBR), and mismatch repair (MMR). Of the different
DNA repair pathways, genetic polymorphisms in NER, BER, and DSBR have been
investigated in multiple studies of bladder cancer.

Nucelotide-excision repair genes. The main pathway involved in the repair of bulky
chemical adducts produced by aromatic amines and other carcinogens in tobacco
smoke is the nucleotide-excision repair (NER) pathway (135). Epidemiologic studies suggest that genetic variation in NER genes could affect bladder cancer risk
(29,52,60,136,137). There is evidence from five studies that two correlated polymorphisms, in *ERCC2*, (*D312N*) rs1799793 and *ERCC2* (*K751Q*) rs13181, exhibit a
modest association with bladder cancer risk. However, additional evidence is needed
to establish these associations. The *XPC* gene is involved in damage recognition in

NER, and two SNPs have been evaluated in multiple studies rs2228000 (*A499V*) and rs2228001 (*K939Q*). The *XPC* rs2228000 (*A499V*) SNP was evaluated in four studies, which suggest a recessive association with risk with the TT (*Val/Val*) genotype (13,52,60,136). In contrast, there is little evidence to suggest an association with risk in these four studies for the *XPC* rs2228001 (*K939Q*) SNP. Lastly, there was little evidence from three studies that a SNP in the endonuclease *ERCC5* gene, rs17655 (*D1104H*), was associated with bladder cancer (13,47,52).

In summary, the NER is a promising candidate pathway for bladder cancer and current studies suggest the presence of weak associations between common genetic variation in this pathway and risk. Ongoing collaborative studies will be critical in providing the additional evidence required to confirm or rule out these associations.

Base-excision repair genes. BER plays a key role in DNA repair by removing DNA damaged by oxidation, deamination, and ring fragmentation (138). Exposure to tobacco smoking can increase production of reactive oxygen species (ROS), which have the potential to induce oxidative damage (139), so BER ability might be associated with bladder cancer risk. BER is primarily responsible for repairing single nucleotides and consists of four steps: (i) excising the damaged base by glycosylases (*OGG1* and *MUTYH*); (ii) incising the DNA backbone by an endonuclease (*APEX1*, also known as *APE*); (iii) filling the nucleotide gap by polymerases (*POLB* and *POLD*) coordinated by the *XRCC1* scaffold protein, the protein-modifying poly ADP ribose proteins (e.g., *PARP1*), and the replication component *PCNA* for long base repair patches; and (iv) ligating the remaining nick by ligases (*LIG1* and *LIG3*) (139,140). A SNP in *OGG1* *S326C* (rs1052133) has been evaluated in four studies, three of which found inverse associations with risk among the homozygote variant carriers (47–49,58,141), compared with the CC genotype; however, more data from other studies are needed to confirm or deny the potential recessive effects of this polymorphism.

Bladder cancer risk and *XRCC1* genetic variation have been the focus of a number of studies (2,13,48–50,53–55,58,61–63,141–148). The *XRCC1* gene encodes the major coordinating protein of BER and interacts with PARP1, LIG3, and POLB. The *XRCC1* rs25487 (*Q399R*) variant results in an amino acid substitution in the region of *XRCC1* responsible for interacting with PARP1 (147). However, meta-analyses including a total of 2,900 cases and 2,893 controls from our study population and six previously published studies (13,47,55,62,141,143) showed no significant overall association with bladder cancer risk , with ORs of 1.08 (0.94–1.23) and 0.99 (0.83–1.19) for heterozygote and homozygote variants, respectively (48). Associations with bladder cancer risk for CT/TT genotypes for a relatively rare nonsynonymous polymorphism in *XRCC1* rs1799782 (*R194W*) have been inconsistent compared with the CC genotype in four studies (47,48,62,148). Lastly, variants for the *APEX1* rs3136820 (*D148E*) SNP (47–49,58,141,148) have been suggested to potentially have a moderate decrease in bladder cancer risk among homozygous variant carriers and evidence for an interaction with smoking was suggested (51) but was not confirmed (48), and requires additional studies. In summary, the current literature provides weak evidence for associations between common variation in BER and bladder cancer risk, and suggested associations require confirmation in future studies.

Double-strand break repair genes. DSBR is important in maintaining genomic stability and deficiency can result in susceptibility to cancer. DNA double-strand breaks (DSBs) can promote genomic instability resulting in chromosomal abnormalities (149–152), which can arise from a variety of exogenous and endogenous exposures including ionizing radiation and tobacco smoke (151,153–155). Given the importance of DSBR in cellular genomic maintenance, interindividual variation in DSBR pathway genes that sense and repair this damage could contribute to bladder cancer risk. Recent evidence suggests that DSBs could be relevant for bladder cancer, and include reports of somatic mutations and altered expression of DNA damage response pathway genes *ATM* and *CHK2* (156), and DSBR nonhomologous end joining (NHEJ) mechanisms that have been reported to be more error prone in bladder tumors (157). The *XRCC3* nonsynonymous SNP *T241M* (rs861539) has been related to bladder cancer risk in previous studies and a recent meta-analysis of seven studies including 2,003 cases and 2,140 controls suggests a weak increase in risk (OR 1.17, 95% CI = 1.00–1.36) (48). Additional DSBR SNPs evaluated in relation to bladder cancer risk include the *NBN* rs1805794 (*E185Q*) and a rare SNP in *XRCC2* rs3218536 (*R188H*) and will require additional evidence to determine if they are associated with risk (47,54,56). The DSBR genes have some promising findings that could be susceptibility factors, and more evidence is needed to confirm these leads.

Other pathways and genes. Genetic polymorphisms in cell cycle control genes, inflammation, methylation, and apoptosis have also been evaluated in relation to bladder cancer risk with promising but unconfirmed findings (47,64,158). The *CDH1* Cadherin gene, which is commonly methylated in bladder cancers, is one of the most promising, as there is evidence that polymorphisms in this gene may be associated with risk (14,159), but these have been evaluated in very few studies, and further evidence is needed. In the future, these pathways, which are hypothesized to be important for many cancers, may represent novel risk factors.

Summary. In summary, the current literature provides consistent evidence for an association with bladder cancer risk and common variants in two key carcinogen metabolizing genes, *NAT2* and *GSTM1*; however, the current evidence for other putative functional variants in candidate genes is weak. Although weak to modest associations, associations with variants in these genes, or gene–gene or gene–environment interactions are possible, they will require very large collaborative studies to be established. The International Consortium of Bladder Cancer (http://dceg. cancer.gov/icbc/) has been established to facilitate these large-scale analyses with adequate power to detect weak associations and interactions, using both candidate gene and genome-wide approaches. Although most studies to date have evaluated only a few variants in each candidate gene, advances in genotyping technology and SNP databases are allowing more comprehensive evaluation of common variants in pathways of interest, as well as exploratory analyses using genome-wide scans, and it is expected that in the coming years new regions associated with bladder cancer risk will be identified.

Functional Susceptibility Assays

Integrative assays that reflect multiple biologic influences in carcinogenic pathways such as germline variation, epigenetic changes, and regulation of gene expression and protein activity are promising biomarkers of susceptibility. For instance, assays that measure the capacity to repair DNA after exposure to carcinogens in cultured peripheral lymphocytes have been used as an integrative measure of susceptibility to carcinogenic exposures. Mutagen sensitivity assays are an indirect measure of DNA repair capacity, and it is known that different mutagens elicit different DNA repair pathways. Evidence to support this hypothesis comes from two reports where bladder cancer cases had a greater tendency to have DNA damage caused by benzo(a)pyrene diol epoxide (160), and to have decreased capacity to repair DNA damage induced by 4-aminobiphenyl in lymphocyte cultures (161). Future studies are needed to support these findings in other populations, particularly in prospective studies with collection of blood samples prior to the diagnosis of bladder cancer. Although these are markers of susceptibility, these are complex and expensive assays and thus difficult to use in large epidemiology studies.

Telomeres, the termini of linear chromosomes, consist of large but variable numbers of DNA oligomer repeats embedded in a nucleoprotein complex (162) and have also been reported to be associated with aging diseases such as cancer (163). Telomere shortening has been inversely associated with age, and telomere length can vary in human peripheral blood lymphocytes and buffy coats from individuals with the same age (162,163). It is hypothesized that individuals with telomere dysfunction may be at a higher risk for bladder cancer because of elevated likelihood for genetic instability. Data to support this hypothesis come from studies showing evidence for an association between shorter telomeres and an increase in bladder cancer risk (2,164,165). Changes in patterns of DNA methylation at promoter CpG-islands in tumor tissue frequently occur, and global hypomethylation of DNA is thought to contribute to carcinogenesis by the induction of genome instability and gene-specific hypomethylation (166). Recently, a report by Moore (167) showed that leukocyte DNA hypomethylation is associated with increased risk of developing bladder cancer, and this association was independent of smoking and other risk factors. This suggests that the amount of global methylation in genomic DNA could provide a useful biomarker of susceptibility to certain cancer types. Telomere length assays and methylation assays are attractive because they are thought to reflect both genetic and environmental influences. Future work needs to be done to follow up on these findings, which have been mostly performed in case-control studies, using prospective cohorts with samples taken at multiple time points in order to rule out reverse causality.

Future Directions

Genome-wide association studies are currently underway and it is expected that these studies will identify new loci associated with bladder cancer risk, and yield new insights into gene–gene and gene–environmental interactions. Using the current platforms, dense genotyping for both SNPs and copy number variants are expected to provide important information on risk of bladder cancer by stage, grade, and molecular subtypes, and response to treatment (particularly treatment with Bacillus Calmette-Guerin [BCG], which stimulates an immune response within the bladder to help destroy any remaining cancer cells), recurrence, and ultimately survival.

Appendix A

Meta-analysis methods

We updated previously published meta-analysis of *NAT2* and *NAT1* slow acetylators compared with fast acetylators, and *GSTM1* and *GSTT1* null carriers compared with present carriers (1,37). We conducted a HuGE Navigator literature finder database search and a PubMed literature search of peer reviewed studies published on or before September 2008 in English. A random-effect model was used to estimate summary ORs and 95% CIs by weighing each study result by a within- and between-study variance (168). Homogeneity of study results was assessed by the I-squared statistic (169). For *GSTM1* and *NAT2* polymorphisms that showed significant associations, the Harbord's test (170), which tests the relationship between the magnitude of the association and the precision of the estimate, was used as a possible indication of publication or related biases. Lastly, for these two SNPs, we performed an additional diagnostic test that can detect whether there is an excess of statistically significant single studies (171). Statistical analyses were performed with STATA Version 9.1, Special Edition (STATA Corporation, College Station, TX).

References

1. Garcia-Closas M, Malats N, Silverman D, et al. NAT2 slow acetylation, GSTM1 null genotype, and risk of bladder cancer: results from the Spanish Bladder Cancer Study and meta-analyses. *Lancet*. 2005;366(9486):649–659.
2. Broberg K, Bjork J, Paulsson K, et al. Constitutional short telomeres are strong genetic susceptibility markers for bladder cancer. *Carcinogenesis*. 2005;26(7):1263–1271.
3. Castelao JE, Yuan JM, Gago-Dominguez M, et al. Carotenoids/vitamin C and smoking-related bladder cancer. *Int J Cancer*. 2004;110(3):417–423.
4. Kellen E, Zeegers M, Paulussen A, et al. Does occupational exposure to PAHs, diesel and aromatic amines interact with smoking and metabolic genetic polymorphisms to

increase the risk on bladder cancer? The Belgian case control study on bladder cancer risk. *Cancer Lett.* 2007;245(1–2):51–60.

5. McGrath M, Michaud D, De Vivo I. Polymorphisms in GSTT1, GSTM1, NAT1 and NAT2 genes and bladder cancer risk in men and women. *BMC Cancer.* 2006;6:239.

6. Cengiz M, Ozaydin A, Ozkilic AC, et al. The investigation of GSTT1, GSTM1 and SOD polymorphism in bladder cancer patients. *Int Urol Nephrol.* 2007;39(4):1043–1048.

7. Ouerhani S, Tebourski F, Slama MR, et al. The role of glutathione transferases M1 and T1 in individual susceptibility to bladder cancer in a Tunisian population. *Ann Hum Biol.* 2006;33(5–6):529–535.

8. Shao J, Gu M, Xu Z, et al. Polymorphisms of the DNA gene XPD and risk of bladder cancer in a Southeastern Chinese population. *Cancer Genet Cytogenet.* 2007;177(1):30–36.

9. Sobti RC, Al-Badran AI, Sharma S, et al. Genetic polymorphisms of CYP2D6, GSTM1, and GSTT1 genes and bladder cancer risk in North India. *Cancer Genet Cytogenet.* 2005;156(1):68–73.

10. Kellen E, Hemelt M, Broberg K, et al. Pooled analysis and meta-analysis of the gluta-thione S-transferase P1 Ile 105Val polymorphism and bladder cancer: a HuGE-GSEC review. *Am J Epidemiol.* 2007;165(11):1221–1230.

11. Zhao H, Lin J, Grossman HB, et al. Dietary isothiocyanates, GSTM1, GSTT1, NAT2 polymorphisms and bladder cancer risk. *Int J Cancer.* 2007;120(10):2208–2213.

12. Hung RJ, Boffetta P, Brennan P, et al. GST, NAT, SULT1A1, CYP1B1 genetic polymor-phisms, interactions with environmental exposures and bladder cancer risk in a high-risk population. *Int J Cancer.* 2004;110(4):598–604.

13. Sanyal S, Festa F, Sakano S, et al. Polymorphisms in DNA repair and metabolic genes in bladder cancer. *Carcinogenesis.* 2004;25(5):729–734.

14. Tsukino H, Kuroda Y, Nakao H, et al. E-cadherin gene polymorphism and risk of urothe-lial cancer. *Cancer Lett.* 2003;195(1):53–58.

15. Brockmoller J, Cascorbi I, Kerb R, et al. Combined analysis of inherited polymorphisms in arylamine N-acetyltransferase 2, glutathione S-transferases M1 and T1, microsomal epoxide hydrolase, and cytochrome P450 enzymes as modulators of bladder cancer risk. *Cancer Res.* 1996;56(17):3915–3925.

16. Chen YC, Xu L, Guo YL, et al. Polymorphisms in GSTT1 and p53 and urinary tran-sitional cell carcinoma in south-western Taiwan: a preliminary study. *Biomarkers.* 2004;9(4–5):386–394.

17. Giannakopoulos X, Charalabopoulos K, Baltogiannis D, et al. The role of N-acetyltransferase-2 and glutathione S-transferase on the risk and aggressiveness of bladder cancer. *Anticancer Res.* 2002;22(6B):3801–3804.

18. Jong Jeong H, Jin Kim H, Young Seo I, et al. Association between glutathione S-transferase M1 and T1 polymorphisms and increased risk for bladder cancer in Korean smokers. *Cancer Lett.* 2003;202(2):193–199.

19. Karagas MR, Park S, Warren A, et al. Gender, smoking, glutathione-S-transferase variants and bladder cancer incidence: a population-based study. *Cancer Lett.* 2005;219(1):63–69.

20. Kim WJ, Kim H, Kim CH, et al. GSTT1-null genotype is a protective factor against bladder cancer. *Urology.* 2002;60(5):913–918.

21. Lee SJ, Cho SH, Park SK, et al. Combined effect of glutathione S-transferase M1 and T1 genotypes on bladder cancer risk. *Cancer Lett.* 2002;177(2):173–179.

22. Moore LE, Wiencke JK, Bates MN, et al. Investigation of genetic polymorphisms and smok-ing in a bladder cancer case-control study in Argentina. *Cancer Lett.* 2004;211(2):199–207.

23. Peluso M, Airoldi L, Magagnotti C, et al. White blood cell DNA adducts and fruit and vegetable consumption in bladder cancer. *Carcinogenesis.* 2000;21(2):183–187.

24. Salagovic J, Kalina I, Habalova V, et al. The role of human glutathione S-transferases M1 and T1 in individual susceptibility to bladder cancer. *Physiol Res.* 1999;48(6):465–471.

25. Srivastava DS, Mishra DK, Mandhani A, et al. Association of genetic polymorphism of glutathione S-transferase M1, T1, P1 and susceptibility to bladder cancer. *Eur Urol.* 2005;48(2):339–344.

26. Steinhoff C, Franke KH, Golka K, et al. Glutathione transferase isozyme genotypes in patients with prostate and bladder carcinoma. *Arch Toxicol.* 2000;74(9):521–526.

27. Toruner GA, Akyerli C, Ucar A, et al. Polymorphisms of glutathione S-transferase genes (GSTM1, GSTP1 and GSTT1) and bladder cancer susceptibility in the Turkish population. *Arch Toxicol.* 2001;75(8):459–464.

28. Gu J, Liang D, Wang Y, et al. Effects of N-acetyl transferase 1 and 2 polymorphisms on bladder cancer risk in Caucasians. *Mutat Res.* 2005;581(1–2):97–104.

29. Stern MC, Johnson LR, Bell DA, et al. XPD codon 751 polymorphism, metabolism genes, smoking, and bladder cancer risk. *Cancer Epidemiol Biomarkers Prev.* 2002;11(10 Pt 1):1004–1011.

30. Taylor JA, Umbach DM, Stephens E, et al. The role of N-acetylation polymorphisms in smoking-associated bladder cancer: evidence of a gene-gene-exposure three-way interaction. *Cancer Res.* 1998;58(16):3603–3610.

31. Cascorbi I, Roots I, Brockmoller J. Association of NAT1 and NAT2 polymorphisms to urinary bladder cancer: significantly reduced risk in subjects with NAT1*10. *Cancer Res.* 2001;61(13):5051–5056.

32. Okkels H, Sigsgaard T, Wolf H, et al. Arylamine N-acetyltransferase 1 (NAT1) and 2 (NAT2) polymorphisms in susceptibility to bladder cancer: the influence of smoking. *Cancer Epidemiol Biomarkers Prev.* 1997;6(4):225–231.

33. Hsieh FI, Pu YS, Chern HD, et al. Genetic polymorphisms of N-acetyltransferase 1 and 2 and risk of cigarette smoking-related bladder cancer. *Br J Cancer.* 1999;81(3):537–541.

34. Jaskula-Sztul R, Sokolowski W, Gajecka M, et al. Association of arylamine N-acetyltransferase (NAT1 and NAT2) genotypes with urinary bladder cancer risk. *J Appl Genet.* 2001;42(2):223–231.

35. Brockmoller J, Cascorbi I, Kerb R, et al. Polymorphisms in xenobiotic conjugation and disease predisposition. *Toxicol Lett.* 1998;102–103:173–183.

36. Marcus PM, Vineis P, Rothman N. NAT2 slow acetylation and bladder cancer risk: a meta-analysis of 22 case-control studies conducted in the general population. *Pharmacogenetics.* 2000;10(2):115–122.

37. Rothman N, Garcia-Closas M, Hein DW. Commentary: Reflections on G. M. Lower and colleagues' 1979 study associating slow acetylator phenotype with urinary bladder cancer: meta-analysis, historical refinements of the hypothesis, and lessons learned. *Int J Epidemiol.* 2007;36(1):23–28.

38. Hao GY, Zhang WD, Chen YH, et al. Relationship between genetic polymorphism of NAT2 and susceptibility to urinary bladder cancer. *Zhonghua Zhong Liu Za Zhi.* 2004;26(5):283–286.

39. Sanderson S, Salanti G, Higgins J. Joint effects of the N-acetyltransferase 1 and 2 (NAT1 and NAT2) genes and smoking on bladder carcinogenesis: a literature-based systematic HuGE review and evidence synthesis. *Am J Epidemiol.* 2007;166(7):741–751.

40. Figueroa JD, Malats N, Garcia-Closas M, et al. Bladder cancer risk and genetic variation in AKR1C3 and other metabolizing genes. *Carcinogenesis.* October 2008;29(10):1955–1962.

41. Chao C, Zhang ZF, Berthiller J, et al. NAD(P)H:quinone oxidoreductase 1 (NQO1) Pro187Ser polymorphism and the risk of lung, bladder, and colorectal cancers: a meta-analysis. *Cancer Epidemiol Biomarkers Prev.* 2006;15(5):979–987.

42. Choi JY, Lee KM, Cho SH, et al. CYP2E1 and NQO1 genotypes, smoking and bladder cancer. *Pharmacogenetics.* 2003;13(6):349–355.

43. Park SJ, Zhao H, Spitz MR, et al. An association between NQO1 genetic polymorphism and risk of bladder cancer. *Mutat Res.* 2003;536(1–2):131–137.

44. Schulz WA, Krummeck A, Rosinger I, et al. Increased frequency of a null-allele for NAD(P)H: quinone oxidoreductase in patients with urological malignancies. *Pharmacogenetics.* 1997;7(3):235–239.

45. Zheng L, Wang Y, Schabath MB, et al. Sulfotransferase 1A1 (SULT1A1) polymorphism and bladder cancer risk: a case-control study. *Cancer Lett.* 2003;202(1):61–69.

46. Kellen E, Zeegers M, Paulussen A, et al. Fruit consumption reduces the effect of smoking on bladder cancer risk. The Belgian case control study on bladder cancer. *Int J Cancer.* 2006;118(10):2572–2578.

47. Wu X, Gu J, Grossman HB, et al. Bladder cancer predisposition: a multigenic approach to DNA-repair and cell-cycle-control genes. *Am J Hum Genet.* 2006;78(3):464–479.

48. Figueroa JD, Malats N, Real FX, et al. Genetic variation in the base excision repair pathway and bladder cancer risk. *Hum Genet.* 2007;121(2):233–242.

49. Huang M, Dinney CP, Lin X, et al. High-order interactions among genetic variants in DNA base excision repair pathway genes and smoking in bladder cancer susceptibility. *Cancer Epidemiol Biomarkers Prev.* 2007;16(1):84–91.

50. Andrew AS, Karagas MR, Nelson HH, et al. DNA repair polymorphisms modify bladder cancer risk: a multi-factor analytic strategy. *Hum Hered.* 2008;65(2):105–118.

51. Terry PD, Umbach DM, Taylor JA. APE1 genotype and risk of bladder cancer: evidence for effect modification by smoking. *Int J Cancer.* 2006;118(12):3170–3173.

52. Garcia-Closas M, Malats N, Real FX, et al. Genetic variation in the nucleotide excision repair pathway and bladder cancer risk. *Cancer Epidemiol Biomarkers Prev.* 2006;15(3):536–542.

53. Andrew AS, Nelson HH, Kelsey KT, et al. Concordance of multiple analytical approaches demonstrates a complex relationship between DNA repair gene SNPs, smoking and bladder cancer susceptibility. *Carcinogenesis.* 2006;27(5):1030–1037.

54. Matullo G, Guarrera S, Sacerdote C, et al. Polymorphisms/haplotypes in DNA repair genes and smoking: a bladder cancer case-control study. *Cancer Epidemiol Biomarkers Prev.* 2005;14(11 Pt 1):2569–2578.

55. Shen M, Hung RJ, Brennan P, et al. Polymorphisms of the DNA repair genes XRCC1, XRCC3, XPD, interaction with environmental exposures, and bladder cancer risk in a case-control study in northern Italy. *Cancer Epidemiol Biomarkers Prev.* 2003;12(11 Pt 1):1234–1240.

56. Figueroa JD, Malats N, Rothman N, et al. Evaluation of genetic variation in the double-strand break repair pathway and bladder cancer risk. *Carcinogenesis.* 2007;28(8):1788–1793.

57. Choudhury A, Elliott F, Iles MM, et al. Analysis of variants in DNA damage signalling genes in bladder cancer. *BMC Med Genet.* 2008;9:69.

58. Karahalil B, Kocabas NA, Ozcelik T. DNA repair gene polymorphisms and bladder cancer susceptibility in a Turkish population. *Anticancer Res.* 2006;26(6C):4955–4958.

59. Kim EJ, Jeong P, Quan C, et al. Genotypes of TNF-alpha, VEGF, hOGG1, GSTM1, and GSTT1: useful determinants for clinical outcome of bladder cancer. *Urology.* 2005;65(1):70–75.

60. Sak SC, Barrett JH, Paul AB, et al. Comprehensive analysis of 22 XPC polymorphisms and bladder cancer risk. *Cancer Epidemiol Biomarkers Prev.* 2006;15(12):2537–2541.

61. Sak SC, Barrett JH, Paul AB, et al. DNA repair gene XRCC1 polymorphisms and bladder cancer risk. *BMC Genet.* 2007;8:13.

62. Stern MC, Umbach DM, van Gils CH, et al. DNA repair gene XRCC1 polymorphisms, smoking, and bladder cancer risk. *Cancer Epidemiol Biomarkers Prev* 2001;10(2):125–131.

63. Stern MC, Umbach DM, Lunn RM, et al. DNA repair gene XRCC3 codon 241 polymorphism, its interaction with smoking and XRCC1 polymorphisms, and bladder cancer risk. *Cancer Epidemiol Biomarkers Prev.* 2002;11(9):939–943.

64. Moore LE, Malats N, Rothman N, et al. Polymorphisms in one-carbon metabolism and trans-sulfuration pathway genes and susceptibility to bladder cancer. *Int J Cancer.* 2007;120(11):2452–2458.

65. Lin J, Spitz MR, Wang Y, et al. Polymorphisms of folate metabolic genes and susceptibility to bladder cancer: a case-control study. *Carcinogenesis.* 2004;25(9):1639–1647.

66. Ouerhani S, Oliveira E, Marrakchi R, et al. Methylenetetrahydrofolate reductase and methionine synthase polymorphisms and risk of bladder cancer in a Tunisian population. *Cancer Genet Cytogenet.* 2007;176(1):48–53.

67. Karagas MR, Park S, Nelson HH, et al. Methylenetetrahydrofolate reductase (MTHFR) variants and bladder cancer: a population-based case-control study. *Int J Hyg Environ Health.* 2005;208(5):321–327.

68. Kimura F, Florl AR, Steinhoff C, et al. Polymorphic methyl group metabolism genes in patients with transitional cell carcinoma of the urinary bladder. *Mutat Res.* 2001;458(1–2):49–54.

69. Cortessis VK, Siegmund K, Xue S, et al. A case-control study of cyclin D1 CCND1 870A→G polymorphism and bladder cancer. *Carcinogenesis.* 2003;24(10):1645–1650.

70. Wang L, Habuchi T, Takahashi T, et al. Cyclin D1 gene polymorphism is associated with an increased risk of urinary bladder cancer. *Carcinogenesis.* 2002;23(2):257–264.

71. Ye Y, Yang H, Grossman HB, et al. Genetic variants in cell cycle control pathway confer susceptibility to bladder cancer. *Cancer.* 2008;112(11):2467–2474.

72. Mabrouk I, Baccouche S, El-Abed R, et al. No evidence of correlation between p53 codon 72 polymorphism and risk of bladder or breast carcinoma in Tunisian patients. *Ann N Y Acad Sci.* 2003;1010:764–770.

73. Soulitzis N, Sourvinos G, Dokianakis DN, et al. p53 codon 72 polymorphism and its association with bladder cancer. *Cancer Lett.* 2002;179(2):175–183.

74. Bid HK, Manchanda PK, Mittal RD. Association of interleukin-1Ra gene polymorphism in patients with bladder cancer: case control study from North India. *Urology.* 2006;67(5):1099–1104.

75. Tsai FJ, Chang CH, Chen CC, et al. Interleukin-4 gene intron-3 polymorphism is associated with transitional cell carcinoma of the urinary bladder. *BJU Int.* 2005;95(3):432–435.

76. Yang H, Gu J, Lin X, et al. Profiling of genetic variations in inflammation pathway genes in relation to bladder cancer predisposition. *Clin Cancer Res.* 2008;14(7):2236–2244.

77. Ahirwar D, Kesarwani P, Manchanda PK, et al. Anti- and proinflammatory cytokine gene polymorphism and genetic predisposition: association with smoking, tumor stage and grade, and bacillus Calmette-Guerin immunotherapy in bladder cancer. *Cancer Genet Cytogenet.* 2008;184(1):1–8.

78. Hung RJ, Boffetta P, Brennan P, et al. Genetic polymorphisms of MPO, COMT, MnSOD, NQO1, interactions with environmental exposures and bladder cancer risk. *Carcinogenesis.* 2004;25(6):973–978.

79. Ichimura Y, Habuchi T, Tsuchiya N, et al. Increased risk of bladder cancer associated with a glutathione peroxidase 1 codon 198 variant. *J Urol.* 2004;172(2):728–732.

80. Terry PD, Umbach DM, Taylor JA. No association between SOD2 or NQO1 genotypes and risk of bladder cancer. *Cancer Epidemiol Biomarkers Prev.* 2005;14(3):753–754.

81. Hein DW, Doll MA, Fretland AJ, et al. Molecular genetics and epidemiology of the NAT1 and NAT2 acetylation polymorphisms. *Cancer Epidemiol Biomarkers Prev.* 2000;9(1):29–42.

82. Hein DW. N-acetyltransferase 2 genetic polymorphism: effects of carcinogen and haplotype on urinary bladder cancer risk. *Oncogene.* 2006;25(11):1649–1658.

83. Jemal A, Murray T, Samuels A, et al. Cancer statistics, 2003. *CA Cancer J Clin.* 2003;53(1):5–26.

84. Surveillance Research Program. In: National Cancer Institute. SEER*Stat software version 5.0.19.2003.

85. Hans-Olov Adami DH, Dimitrios Trichopoulos, eds. *Textbook of Cancer Epidemiology,* 2nd ed. Oxford: Oxford University Press; 2008.

86. Schottenfeld D. and Fraumeni J.F. Jr., *Cancer Epidemiology and Prevention,* 3rd edition, Oxford University Press; 2006.

87. Aben KK, Witjes JA, Schoenberg MP, et al. Familial aggregation of urothelial cell carcinoma. *Int J Cancer.* 2002;98(2):274–278.

88. Cartwright RA. Genetic association with bladder cancer. *Br Med J.* 1979;2(6193):798.

89. Kantor AF, Hartge P, Hoover RN, et al. Familial and environmental interactions in bladder cancer risk. *Int J Cancer.* 1985;35(6):703–706.

90. Kunze E, Chang-Claude J, Frentzel-Beyme R. Life style and occupational risk factors for bladder cancer in Germany. A case-control study. *Cancer.* 1992;69(7):1776–1790.

91. Piper JM, Matanoski GM, Tonascia J. Bladder cancer in young women. *Am J Epidemiol.* 1986;123(6):1033–1042.

92. Kiemeney LA, Schoenberg M. Familial transitional cell carcinoma. *J Urol.* 1996; 156(3):867–872.

93. Plna K, Hemminki K. Familial bladder cancer in the National Swedish Family Cancer Database. *J Urol.* 2001;166(6):2129–2133.

94. Lindor NM, Greene MH. The concise handbook of family cancer syndromes. Mayo Familial Cancer Program. *J Natl Cancer Inst.* 1998;90(14):1039–1071.

95. Watson P, Lynch HT. Extracolonic cancer in hereditary nonpolyposis colorectal cancer. *Cancer.* 1993;71(3):677–685.

96. Fletcher O, Easton D, Anderson K, et al. Lifetime risks of common cancers among retinoblastoma survivors. *J Natl Cancer Inst.* 2004;96(5):357–363.

97. Deitz AC, Rothman N, Rebbeck TR, et al. Impact of misclassification in genotype-exposure interaction studies: example of N-acetyltransferase 2 (NAT2), smoking, and bladder cancer. *Cancer Epidemiol Biomarkers Prev.* 2004;13(9):1543–1546.

98. Hein DW. Molecular genetics and function of NAT1 and NAT2: role in aromatic amine metabolism and carcinogenesis. *Mutat Res.* 2002;506–507:65–77.

99. Layton DW, Bogen KT, Knize MG, et al. Cancer risk of heterocyclic amines in cooked foods: an analysis and implications for research. *Carcinogenesis.* 1995;16(1):39–52.

100. Pelucchi C, Bosetti C, Negri E, et al. Mechanisms of disease: the epidemiology of bladder cancer. *Nat Clin Pract Urol.* 2006;3(6):327–340.

101. Silverman DT, Hartge P, Morrison AS, et al. Epidemiology of bladder cancer. *Hematol Oncol Clin North Am.* 1992;6(1):1–30.

102. Vineis P, Pirastu R. Aromatic amines and cancer. *Cancer Causes Control.* 1997;8(3):346–355.

103. Vatsis KP, Martell KJ, Weber WW. Diverse point mutations in the human gene for polymorphic N-acetyltransferase. *Proc Natl Acad Sci USA.* 1991;88(14):6333–6337.

104. Weber WW. Populations and genetic polymorphisms. *Mol Diagn.* 1999;4(4):299–307.

105. Lower GM, Jr., Nilsson T, Nelson CE, et al. N-acetyltransferase phenotype and risk in urinary bladder cancer: approaches in molecular epidemiology. Preliminary results in Sweden and Denmark. *Environ Health Perspect.* 1979;29:71–79.

106. Salanti G, Higgins JP, White IR. Bayesian synthesis of epidemiological evidence with different combinations of exposure groups: application to a gene-gene-environment interaction. *Stat Med.* 2006;25(24):4147–4163.
107. Yu MC, Skipper PL, Taghizadeh K, et al. Acetylator phenotype, aminobiphenyl-hemoglobin adduct levels, and bladder cancer risk in white, black, and Asian men in Los Angeles, California. *J Natl Cancer Inst.* 1994;86(9):712–716.
108. Hein DW. Acetylator genotype and arylamine-induced carcinogenesis. *Biochim Biophys Acta.* 1988;948(1):37–66.
109. Vineis P, Marinelli D, Autrup H, et al. Current smoking, occupation, N-acetyltransferase-2 and bladder cancer: a pooled analysis of genotype-based studies. *Cancer Epidemiol Biomarkers Prev.* 2001;10(12):1249–1252.
110. Cartwright RA, Glashan RW, Rogers HJ, et al. Role of N-acetyltransferase phenotypes in bladder carcinogenesis: a pharmacogenetic epidemiological approach to bladder cancer. *Lancet.* 1982;2(8303):842–845.
111. Carreon T, Ruder AM, Schulte PA, et al. NAT2 slow acetylation and bladder cancer in workers exposed to benzidine. *Int J Cancer.* 2006;118(1):161–168.
112. Hayes RB, Bi W, Rothman N, et al. N-acetylation phenotype and genotype and risk of bladder cancer in benzidine-exposed workers. *Carcinogenesis.* 1993;14(4):675–678.
113. Zenser TV, Lakshmi VM, Hsu FF, et al. Metabolism of N-acetylbenzidine and initiation of bladder cancer. *Mutat Res.* 2002;506–507:29–40.
114. Rothman N, Bhatnagar VK, Hayes RB, et al. The impact of interindividual variation in NAT2 activity on benzidine urinary metabolites and urothelial DNA adducts in exposed workers. *Proc Natl Acad Sci USA.* 1996;93(10):5084–5089.
115. Badawi AF, Hirvonen A, Bell DA, et al. Role of aromatic amine acetyltransferases, NAT1 and NAT2, in carcinogen-DNA adduct formation in the human urinary bladder. *Cancer Res.* 1995;55(22):5230–5237.
116. Thier R, Bruning T, Roos PH, et al. Markers of genetic susceptibility in human environmental hygiene and toxicology: the role of selected CYP, NAT and GST genes. *Int J Hyg Environ Health.* 2003;206(3):149–171.
117. Hayes JD, Flanagan JU, Jowsey IR. Glutathione transferases. *Annu Rev Pharmacol Toxicol.* 2005;45:51–88.
118. Hayes JD, Strange RC. Glutathione S-transferase polymorphisms and their biological consequences. *Pharmacology.* 2000;61(3):154–166.
119. Seidegard J, Pero RW. The genetic variation and the expression of human glutathione transferase mu. *Klin Wochenschr.* 1988;66(Suppl 11):125–126.
120. Engel LS, Taioli E, Pfeiffer R, et al. Pooled analysis and meta-analysis of glutathione S-transferase M1 and bladder cancer: a HuGE review. *Am J Epidemiol.* 2002;156(2):95–109.
121. Pemble S, Schroeder KR, Spencer SR, et al. Human glutathione S-transferase theta (GSTT1): cDNA cloning and the characterization of a genetic polymorphism. *Biochem J.* 1994;300(Pt 1):271–276.
122. Schroder KR, Wiebel FA, Reich S, et al. Glutathione-S-transferase (GST) theta polymorphism influences background SCE rate. *Arch Toxicol.* 1995;69(7):505–507.
123. Hu X, O'Donnell R, Srivastava SK, et al. Active site architecture of polymorphic forms of human glutathione S-transferase P1–1 accounts for their enantioselectivity and disparate activity in the glutathione conjugation of 7beta,8alpha-dihydroxy-9-alpha,10alpha-ox y-7,8,9,10-tetrahydrobenzo(a)pyrene. *Biochem Biophys Res Commun.* 1997;235(2):424–428.

124. Hu X, Ji X, Srivastava SK, et al. Mechanism of differential catalytic efficiency of two polymorphic forms of human glutathione S-transferase P1–1 in the glutathione conjugation of carcinogenic diol epoxide of chrysene. *Arch Biochem Biophys*. 1997;345(1):32–38.

125. Landi MT, Sinha R, Lang NP, et al. Human cytochrome P4501A2. *IARC Sci Publ*. 1999;148:173–195.

126. Meinl W, Meerman JH, Glatt H. Differential activation of promutagens by alloenzymes of human sulfotransferase 1A2 expressed in *Salmonella typhimurium*. *Pharmacogenetics*. 2002;12(9):677–689.

127. Vineis P, Veglia F, Garte S, et al. Genetic susceptibility according to three metabolic pathways in cancers of the lung and bladder and in myeloid leukemias in nonsmokers. *Ann Oncol*. 2007;18(7):1230–1242.

128. Joseph P, Jaiswal AK. NAD(P)H:quinone oxidoreductase1 (DT diaphorase) specifically prevents the formation of benzo[a]pyrene quinone-DNA adducts generated by cytochrome P4501A1 and P450 reductase. *Proc Natl Acad Sci USA*. 1994;91(18):8413–8417.

129. Joseph P, Xie T, Xu Y, et al. NAD(P)H:quinone oxidoreductase1 (DT-diaphorase): expression, regulation, and role in cancer. *Oncol Res*. 1994;6(10–11):525–532.

130. Sachse C, Smith G, Wilkie MJ, et al. A pharmacogenetic study to investigate the role of dietary carcinogens in the etiology of colorectal cancer. *Carcinogenesis*. 2002;23(11):1839–1849.

131. Kuehl BL, Paterson JW, Peacock JW, et al. Presence of a heterozygous substitution and its relationship to DT-diaphorase activity. *Br J Cancer*. 1995;72(3):555–561.

132. Misra V, Grondin A, Klamut HJ, et al. Assessment of the relationship between genotypic status of a DT-diaphorase point mutation and enzymatic activity. *Br J Cancer*. 2000;83(8):998–1002.

133. Siegel D, McGuinness SM, Winski SL, et al. Genotype-phenotype relationships in studies of a polymorphism in NAD(P)H: quinone oxidoreductase 1. *Pharmacogenetics*. 1999;9(1):113–121.

134. Goode EL, Ulrich CM, Potter JD. Polymorphisms in DNA repair genes and associations with cancer risk. *Cancer Epidemiol Biomarkers Prev*. 2002;11(12):1513–1530.

135. Friedberg EC. How nucleotide excision repair protects against cancer. *Nat Rev Cancer*. 2001;1(1):22–33.

136. Zhu Y, Lai M, Yang II, et al. Genotypes, haplotypes and diplotypes of XPC and risk of bladder cancer. *Carcinogenesis*. 2007;28(3):698–703.

137. Schabath MB, Delclos GL, Grossman HB, et al. Polymorphisms in XPD exons 10 and 23 and bladder cancer risk. *Cancer Epidemiol Biomarkers Prev*. 2005;14(4):878–884.

138. Frosina G. Commentary: DNA base excision repair defects in human pathologies. *Free Radic Res*. 2004;38(10):1037–1054.

139. Wilson DM, 3rd, Sofinowski TM, McNeill DR. Repair mechanisms for oxidative DNA damage. *Front Biosci*. 2003;8:d963–d981.

140. Fan J, Wilson DM, 3rd. Protein-protein interactions and posttranslational modifications in mammalian base excision repair. *Free Radic Biol Med*. 2005;38(9):1121–1138.

141. Matullo G, Guarrera S, Carturan S, et al. DNA repair gene polymorphisms, bulky DNA adducts in white blood cells and bladder cancer in a case-control study. *Int J Cancer*. 2001;92(4):562–567.

142. Matullo G, Dunning AM, Guarrera S, et al. DNA repair polymorphisms and cancer risk in non-smokers in a cohort study. *Carcinogenesis*. 2006;27(5):997–1007.

143. Kelsey KT, Park S, Nelson HH, et al. A population-based case-control study of the XRCC1 Arg399Gln polymorphism and susceptibility to bladder cancer. *Cancer Epidemiol Biomarkers Prev*. 2004;13(8):1337–1341.

144. Damaraju S, Murray D, Dufour J, et al. Association of DNA repair and steroid metabolism gene polymorphisms with clinical late toxicity in patients treated with conformal radiotherapy for prostate cancer. *Clin Cancer Res.* 2006;12(8):2545–2554.

145. Matullo G, Palli D, Peluso M, et al. XRCC1, XRCC3, XPD gene polymorphisms, smoking and (32)P-DNA adducts in a sample of healthy subjects. *Carcinogenesis.* 2001;22(9):1437–1445.

146. Stern MC, Conway K, Li Y, et al. DNA repair gene polymorphisms and probability of p53 mutation in bladder cancer. *Mol Carcinog.* September 2006;45(9):715–719.

147. Wang Y, Spitz MR, Zhu Y, et al. From genotype to phenotype: correlating XRCC1 polymorphisms with mutagen sensitivity. *DNA Repair (Amst).* 2003;2(8):901–908.

148. Andrew AS, Nelson HH, Kelsey KT, et al. Concordance of multiple analytical approaches demonstrates a complex relationship between DNA repair gene SNPs, smoking, and bladder cancer susceptibility. *Carcinogenesis.* May 2005 ;27(5):1030–1037.

149. Catto JW, Meuth M, Hamdy FC. Genetic instability and transitional cell carcinoma of the bladder. *BJU Int.* 2004;93(1):19–24.

150. Ferguson DO, Alt FW. DNA double strand break repair and chromosomal translocation: lessons from animal models. *Oncogene.* 2001;20(40):5572–5579.

151. Jeggo PA, Lobrich M. Contribution of DNA repair and cell cycle checkpoint arrest to the maintenance of genomic stability. *DNA Repair (Amst).* 2006;5(9–10):1192–1198.

152. Yamamoto Y, Matsuyama H, Kawauchi S, et al. Biological characteristics in bladder cancer depend on the type of genetic instability. *Clin Cancer Res.* 2006;12(9):2752–2758.

153. Khanna KK, Jackson SP. DNA double-strand breaks: signaling, repair and the cancer connection. *Nat Genet.* 2001;27(3):247–254.

154. Nakayama T, Kaneko M, Kodama M, et al. Cigarette smoke induces DNA single-strand breaks in human cells. *Nature.* 1985;314(6010):462–464.

155. Pryor WA, Hales BJ, Premovic PI, et al. The radicals in cigarette tar: their nature and suggested physiological implications. *Science.* 1983;220(4595):425–427.

156. Bartkova J, Horejsi Z, Koed K, et al. DNA damage response as a candidate anti-cancer barrier in early human tumorigenesis. *Nature.* 2005;434(7035):864–870.

157. Bentley J, Diggle CP, Harnden P, et al. DNA double strand break repair in human bladder cancer is error prone and involves microhomology-associated end-joining. *Nucleic Acids Res.* 2004;32(17):5249–5259.

158. Leibovici D, Grossman HB, Dinney CP, et al. Polymorphisms in inflammation genes and bladder cancer: from initiation to recurrence, progression, and survival. *J Clin Oncol.* 2005;23(24):5746–5756.

159. Kiemeney LA, van Houwelingen KP, Bogaerts M, et al. Polymorphisms in the E-cadherin (CDH1) gene promoter and the risk of bladder cancer. *Eur J Cancer.* 2006;42(18):3219–3227.

160. Schabath MB, Spitz MR, Grossman HB, et al. Genetic instability in bladder cancer assessed by the comet assay. *J Natl Cancer Inst.* 2003;95(7):540–547.

161. Lin J, Kadlubar FF, Spitz MR, et al. A modified host cell reactivation assay to measure DNA repair capacity for removing 4-aminobiphenyl adducts: a pilot study of bladder cancer. *Cancer Epidemiol Biomarkers Prev.* 2005;14(7):1832–1836.

162. De Meyer T, Rietzschel ER, De Buyzere ML, et al. Studying telomeres in a longitudinal population based study. *Front Biosci.* 2008;13:2960–2970.

163. Aubert G, Lansdorp PM. Telomeres and aging. *Physiol Rev.* 2008;88(2):557–579.

164. Wu X, Amos CI, Zhu Y, et al. Telomere dysfunction: a potential cancer predisposition factor. *J Natl Cancer Inst.* 2003;95(16):1211–1218.

165. McGrath M, Wong JY, Michaud D, et al. Telomere length, cigarette smoking, and bladder cancer risk in men and women. *Cancer Epidemiol Biomarkers Prev.* 2007;16(4):815–819.

166. Esteller M, Herman JG. Cancer as an epigenetic disease: DNA methylation and chromatin alterations in human tumours. *J Pathol.* 2002;196(1):1–7.

167. Moore LE, Pfeiffer RM, Poscablo C, et al. Genomic DNA hypomethylation as a biomarker for bladder cancer susceptibility in the Spanish Bladder Cancer Study: a case-control study. *Lancet Oncol.* 2008;9(4):359–366.

168. Laird NM, Mosteller F. Some statistical methods for combining experimental results. *Int J Technol Assess Health Care.* 1990;6(1):5–30.

169. Higgins JP, Thompson SG. Quantifying heterogeneity in a meta-analysis. *Stat Med.* 2002;21(11):1539–1558.

170. Harbord RM, Egger M, Sterne JA. A modified test for small-study effects in meta-analyses of controlled trials with binary endpoints. *Stat Med.* 2006;25(20):3443–3457.

171. Ioannidis JP, Trikalinos TA. An exploratory test for an excess of significant findings. *Clin Trials.* 2007;4(3):245–253.

16

Type 2 diabetes

Eleftheria Zeggini and Mark I. McCarthy

Introduction

Type 2 diabetes (T2D) represents one of the most important causes of global morbidity and mortality. On current projections, the prevalence of this condition will double within a generation, with most of this increase occurring in the countries least well equipped to deal with the social and economic consequences (1). These rapid changes in prevalence clearly reflect global shifts in lifestyle (greater caloric intake and reduced energy expenditure) that are closely linked to rising rates of obesity. Nevertheless, twin and family studies have repeatedly demonstrated that individual predisposition to T2D has a substantial genetic component (2). Identification of the genes and variants responsible for these predisposition effects provides valuable insights into pathogenesis; these should, in turn, spur translational advances in clinical care, including development of novel therapeutic and diagnostic approaches. In addition, it may well become increasingly possible to use personal genetic profile information as a means toward more targeted, individualized clinical management.

Genetics of Type 2 Diabetes: The Past

Until the current phase of rapid advances in the identification of variants influencing individual risk of multifactorial type 2 diabetes (see Section Genetics of Type 2 Diabetes: The Present), progress in this field had been tentative. Putting aside type 1 diabetes (which we do not consider in this chapter—for an up-to-date review see Reference 3), success in diabetes genetics was mostly restricted to studies of highly penetrant monogenic and syndromic forms of nonautoimmune diabetes such as maturity onset diabetes of the young (MODY) and neonatal diabetes (NDM).

Monogenic and Syndromic Forms of Diabetes

The cardinal features of MODY (autosomal dominant family history, early-onset nonautoimmune diabetes) meant this condition was readily amenable to linkage-based positional-cloning approaches applied to segregating pedigrees (4). Clinical suspicions about phenotypic heterogeneity (5) were substantiated by gene-mapping efforts that revealed a number of distinct genetic causes for MODY. On most counts, seven genes have been implicated (4,6), with the principal phenotypic differences noted between those instances of MODY attributable to defects in glucose-sensing due to mutations in the glucokinase gene (7,8), and those resulting from mutations in islet-transcription factors (9,10). While the former have a modest increase in fasting glucose levels detectable at birth and stable thereafter, the latter result in a progressive form of diabetes in which serious diabetes-related complications are much more likely. Because there are important prognostic and therapeutic differences between these different molecular etiologies of diabetes—patients with transcription factor mutations are notably sensitive to sulfonylureas (11), while those with glucose-sensing defects usually respond well to diet—this is an area where molecular diagnostics and individual genetic profiling are already a feature of standard clinical care (12).

There is a similar story with neonatal diabetes mellitus, which, as the name suggests, is characterized by diabetes onset in the first few months of life. Historically, this condition was categorized on clinical grounds into transient and permanent forms, the former characterized by remission during childhood but with a recurrence of T2D later in life. Identification of genes harboring mutations responsible for this largely sporadic condition has demonstrated that these subtypes lie on a continuum. Although imprinting defects on chr6 are a common cause of transient NDM (13), and *INS* mutations of permanent NDM (6), mutations in the genes encoding the two components of the beta-cell K_{ATP} channel (*KCNJ11* and *ABCC8*) can cause either, with clinical severity largely mirroring the extent to which the mutation concerned abrogates channel function (14). Indeed, when the mutations are particularly severe, the phenotypic consequences can extend to involvement of other tissues (e.g., brain) in which these genes are expressed (15). Crucially, evidence that the adverse effect of many *KCNJ11* mutations on channel closure is restricted to physiological, and not pharmacological, stimuli has allowed many individuals diagnosed with NDM (who conventionally had been treated with insulin) to achieve much improved metabolic control on oral medication (11).

As well as these examples, gene discovery efforts conducted in the many rare Mendelian syndromes which include diabetes among their clinical features, have identified many other genes harboring causal mutations with the capacity to disturb glucose homeostasis (16,17). These genetic abnormalities extend to the mitochondrial genome, where heteroplasmic mutations at position 3243 (in a gene encoding a transfer RNA) have been shown to result in a syndrome of maternally inherited diabetes and deafness (18).

Although all of these conditions are relatively rare (in combination, they account for only a few percent of all nonautoimmune diabetes), they provide several lessons relevant to the subsequent discussion of multifactorial diabetes. First, these studies demonstrate that diabetes can result from defects in many different processes, though most affect in various ways the capacity of the pancreatic beta cell to maintain adequate glucose-stimulated insulin secretion in the face of advancing age or insulin resistance. Second, precisely because the prognostic implications of each specific diagnosis for the subject and the subject's relatives are so diverse, and because the benefits of optimizing therapy to the specific molecular diagnosis are so clear, there has been a steady increase in the use of clinical genetic approaches to ensure that, wherever possible, each subject obtains an accurate molecular diagnosis (4).

Multifactorial diabetes.   In comparison, progress in finding the genes involved in individual predisposition to more common, late-onset, multifactorial forms of nonautoimmune diabetes has, until recently, been slow. This difference in pace reflects the obvious fact that much of the success in identifying genes causal for monogenic or syndromic diabetes was predicated on exploiting the strong genotype–phenotype correlations that define such conditions. In multifactorial diabetes, predisposition is the consequence of multiple contributory factors (both genetic and environmental) and the effect of any single variant accordingly modest. This has serious repercussions in terms of power and interpretation (19) that are only now being overcome (see following text).

Through the late 1990s and the early part of this decade, two predominant approaches to gene discovery for T2D were in play. The linkage approach sought to locate chromosomal regions that, within families, displayed unusual patterns of cosegregation with diabetes. These studies exploited a variety of experimental designs: sometimes the focus was on large multiplex pedigrees, at other times on collections of nuclear families or affected sib pairs. The linkage approach is powerful when, as with MODY, the causal variants are penetrant, but it becomes much less attractive when penetrances are low and there is substantial locus heterogeneity, both of which are likely to prevail in T2D. Although more than 40 linkage scans for T2D have been performed, the overall picture has been one of multiple modest signals, few of which show much evidence of replication (20,21). These studies have made it clear that, as far as T2D is concerned, there are no common variants of large effect (equivalent, for example, to HLA in type 1 diabetes). Efforts to fine-map the causal variants within replicated linkage signals continue, but have in most cases been superseded, for reasons of cost and efficiency, by genome-wide association (GWA) approaches. However, a desire to identify associated variants within the replicating linkage signal on chromosome 10 contributed to the discovery of *TCF7L2* as a T2D susceptibility locus in 2006 (22) (Figure 16.1). Although this signal has been widely replicated (23), and these variants have the largest effect size of any common T2D-susceptibility variant identified, those effect sizes are far too small to account for the observed linkage signal. It seems therefore that the discovery of *TCF7L2* by fine-mapping was serendipitous.

The complementary approach to multifactorial T2D gene discovery has focused on association mapping in sets of unrelated individuals (typically, cases and controls). Although this approach is paying dividends now that it is being applied genome wide (see following text), previously the cost and throughput of genotyping technologies restricted such analyses to consideration of only modest numbers of variants. Not surprisingly, therefore, these efforts focused on subsets of variants selected because they were considered particularly likely to influence individual risk

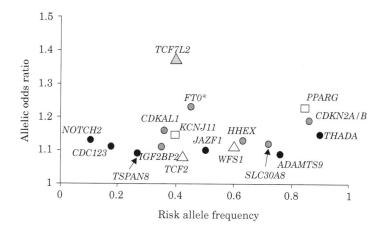

*Figure 16.1   Atlas of established type 2 diabetes susceptibility variants showing 17 loci with an established role in T2D susceptibility. Rectangles denote susceptibility variants identified through candidate gene approaches. Triangles denote susceptibility variants identified through large-scale pathway-based or fine-mapping approaches. Circles denote susceptibility variants identified through genome-wide association scans (green for individual scans, red for GWA meta-analysis). *FTO increases risk of type 2 diabetes through its effect on obesity.*

of T2D (16). Usually, such selection focused on "candidate" genes, plucked from the genome on the basis of some perceived fit between their known or presumed function and the mechanisms thought to be involved in diabetes pathogenesis. This approach, although it did generate two notable successes (*PPARG* and *KCNJII*), was blighted by three main factors. First, poor understanding of T2D pathogenesis (the very reason why genetic studies were being done in the first place), meant that candidate gene selection was an imprecise art: even the most promising candidates still had low prior odds of harboring variants affecting disease predisposition, especially because most studies provided only patchy coverage of the variants contained within such a gene (16,24). Second, the prevalent use of small sample sizes meant that, for realistic models of locus effect size, the power of any given study to detect an association, even if it existed, was typically poor. And third, an understandable desire to declare "positive" associations on the basis of nominally significant findings (without due allowance for all the statistical tests performed), resulted in the promulgation of a large number of completely spurious claims of causal association. Because the chances of detecting real signals were low and the opportunities for declaring false-positive associations legion, the inevitable consequence was that although many associations were claimed, very few of these were genuine and, naturally, failures of replication were the order of the day (24,25).

There were two notable exceptions to this pattern. Common variants in two candidates (*PPARG* and *KCNJII*) were, in a series of studies of ever-increasing size, shown to be robustly associated with T2D risk (26–28) (Figure 16.1). In each case, the genes involved represented particularly compelling candidates (each encodes a protein, which in turn forms the target for one of the established classes of diabetes therapeutic agents, thiazolidinediones and sulphonylureas, respectively). The variants studied were—as nonsynonymous coding substitutions for which there was empirical evidence of a functional effect—a cut above the average in terms of their biological credentials. Both variants had only modest effect sizes (per-allele odds ratios of ~1.2), and it was only through aggregation of data from multiple data sets that the association signals became entirely convincing. Both variants have been independently detected in the GWA studies which have appeared more recently (29–35). There have also been two recent additions to the list of T2D susceptibility genes (*WFS1* and *TCF2*), identified through large-scale pathway-based approaches (36–38) (Figure 16.1).

Genetics of Type 2 Diabetes: The Present

Advances in high-throughput genotyping technologies, a better understanding of human sequence variation, and the availability of large-scale sample sets have culminated in the feasibility of GWA scans. Over the past 18 months, the field of T2D genetics has seen tremendous progress with six large-scale GWA scans published (29–35). This gene-agnostic approach to disease gene hunting has overcome the problem of selecting a target on the basis of assigned biological candidacy. Furthermore, by probing several hundreds of thousands of single nucleotide polymorphisms (SNPs) genome wide (defined by commercial genotyping platform content), these studies capture a large proportion of common variation, thereby addressing the issue of restricted marker selection. In addition, the field is now much wiser in terms of declaring association, with stringent statistical thresholds observed, and with adherence to the gold standard of replication a strict prerequisite for proclaiming that an associated locus plays a role in disease susceptibility. Advances in statistical methods for handling, analyzing, and interpreting large-scale data have furthermore enabled researchers to tackle pragmatic problems such as those of population stratification, the delineation of intervals most likely to harbor associated disease variants, and the accurate inference of association signals at variants that have not been directly assayed.

The era of GWA scans has already been extremely successful in identifying additional T2D susceptibility loci. In addition to confirming the five loci identified through more targeted approaches (*TCF7L2, PPARG, KCNJ11, TCF2,* and *WFS1*), the T2D GWA scans published during 2007 detected another set of six independent, robustly replicating signals, bringing the total to eleven (including one locus that was subsequently shown to mediate its effect on T2D through obesity) (Figure 16.1). These studies were all carried out in individuals of European descent. The study designs, however, varied across scans, mainly in terms of genotyping platform, case and control ascertainment, sample size, and the approaches taken in the follow-up of novel signals.

The first scan to be published (33) made use of two commercially available platforms, genotyping a moderately sized sample on the Illumina HumanHap300 and Infinium Human1 arrays. T2D cases, from France, were preferentially selected to have a positive family history of T2D, early age at onset, and to be lean. By following up interesting signals in a larger independent sample, also from France, this scan confirmed *TCF7L2* and identified four putative T2D susceptibility loci, of which two (*SLC30A8*, and *HHEX/IDE*) have since been widely replicated. Three further groups undertaking GWA scans for T2D recognized the power gains to be afforded by collaboration and combined efforts to detect additional disease variants (29–32). Together, these studies (comprising the three GWA scans and large-scale follow-up sample sets) confirmed known associations at *TCF7L2*, *PPARG*, *KCNJ11*, *SLC30A8*, and *HHEX/IDE* and identified four novel loci (in and around the *CDKAL1*, *CDKN2A/2B*, *FTO,* and *IGF2BP2* genes). The Diabetes Genetics Initiative (DGI) scan used the Affymetrix 500k chip to genotype T2D cases (partially enriched for family history) and controls from Finland and Sweden, and reviewed interesting findings in large-scale samples of European descent (29). The Wellcome Trust Case Control Consortium scan is the largest scan to be carried out to date, genotyping 2,000 T2D cases (enriched for family history and early onset), and 3,000 controls, all from the United Kingdom, on the 500k Affymetrix platform (31). The large-scale replication set samples for this study also came from the United Kingdom (32). The Finland-United States Investigation of NIDDM genetics (FUSION) scan employed the Illumina HumanHap300 to genotype T2D cases (partially enriched for family history) and controls, and followed up interesting signals in an independent set of individuals, all from Finland (30). A further T2D GWA scan focused on T2D cases and controls from Iceland, genotyped on the Illumina HumanHap300 platform, with signals of interest pursued in independent samples from Europe, Hong Kong, and West Africa (35). This study provided independent identification of the *CDKAL1* signal and confirmed several of the previously identified T2D loci. Finally, a smaller-scale scan carried out in individuals of European descent used the HumanHap300 platform, a replication set from France to follow up promising signals, and confirmed *TCF7L2* as a T2D risk locus, but lacked the power to detect further novel signals (32).

These discoveries have generated new insights into established and putative new etiological pathways in T2D. Examination of variants in the *HHEX/IDE*, *SLC30A8*, and *CDKAL1* susceptibility regions demonstrated associations with reduced pancreatic beta-cell function (35,39). *IGF2BP2* codes for insulin-like growth factor 2 binding protein 2, and, among other things, regulates translation of IGF2 (which has known effects on both insulin secretion and action). The *FTO* locus is now well established as the first robustly replicating obesity risk variant (40). Finally, the *CDKAL1* and *CDKN2A* and *CDKN2B* genes are involved in cell-cycle regulation: finding that these variants influence T2D risk through an effect on beta-cell proliferation and regeneration, if confirmed, will help to address longstanding controversies regarding the contribution of reduced beta-cell mass to the pathogenesis of T2D.

Importantly, these newly identified signals are most likely to represent proxies of the truly causal variants. Extensive fine-mapping and resequencing experiments will be necessary to pinpoint the most probable locations of the variants that are directly causal for disease; extensive functional and physiological studies will be required to elucidate the exact role of these risk loci in T2D etiopathogenesis. The success of GWA scans has provided us with additional insights into the genetic architecture of common disease in general. Although rarer variants are also likely to contribute to disease risk (see Section Genetics of Type 2 Diabetes: The Future?), the variants identified so far are common (mainly owing to the SNP content of available arrays) and have modest effect sizes. In fact, the allelic odds ratios of previously established T2D susceptibility genes (such as *PPARG*) are so modest that single GWA scans failed to detect them on the basis of statistical genome-wide significance. Clearly, further increases in statistical power are necessary if we are to achieve more comprehensive detection of T2D-susceptibility loci. The combination of genome-wide scans in a meta-analysis framework is one way of achieving this.

Taking this natural next step, the DGI, FUSION, and WTCCC groups undertook a meta-analysis of the three respective scans, under the auspices of the Diabetes Genetics Replication and Meta-Analysis (DIAGRAM) Consortium (41). The chances of identifying additional T2D risk loci were further enhanced by following imputation approaches (42) to infer genotypes at untyped variants across the HapMap. A total of ~2.2 million SNPs passing stringent genotype quality control were combined across 10,128 samples, and promising novel signals were followed up in large-scale replication samples, all of European descent. Six novel T2D risk loci were confirmed (in and around the *JAZF1*, *CDC123/CAMK1D*, *TSPAN8/LGR5*, *THADA*, *ADAMTS9*, and *NOTCH2* genes) (Figure 16.1). These findings highlight the value of increased GWA sample size, imputation approaches, and replication typing in several tens of thousands of samples. They also define novel pathways involved in glucose homeostasis and diabetes pathogenesis. The effect sizes at all six new T2D loci were modest or small (with allelic odds ratio estimates as low as 1.09), indicating that efforts on an even larger scale will be required to identify additional common risk variants, which are likely to be of smaller or equal effect size. As with the previously established T2D susceptibility loci, these discoveries represent only a first, but crucial, step in gaining a better understanding of T2D etiology.

Genetics of Type 2 Diabetes: The Future?

Despite these successes in identifying variants influencing diabetes susceptibility and improving our understanding of the pathogenesis of T2D, it is evident that these loci explain only a small proportion of the variance in individual predisposition.

There are several ways of arriving at such measures, but here we consider just two. In terms of familial aggregation, the combined sibling relative risk attributable to all the known common susceptibility variants for diabetes is ~1.07. This compares unfavorably with epidemiologic estimates of the total extent of familial aggregation (~3 in Europeans) (43). If we look instead at measures of discriminative accuracy (such as those derived from receiver operating characteristic curves (44)), the picture is similar. Although it is possible to define small numbers of individuals who, by dint of inheriting very few or very many of the known susceptibility variants, have widely divergent risks of diabetes, most individuals will fall in the middle of the distribution of risk-allele counts, and depart only modestly from "average" risk (44). As a result, the discriminative accuracy (the area under the receiver operating characteristic curve) achievable with the known variants comes to only ~60%, a value that suffers in comparison with that achievable (~80%) using a group of "traditional" risk factors (e.g., age, BMI, ethnicity). The extent to which genetic and traditional risk factors provide independent, orthogonal information on individual predisposition is, as yet, unclear; it seems likely, however, that there will be considerable overlap.

Although these findings certainly suggest that the opportunities for individual risk-prediction are, at present, rather limited, they raise a very interesting question. If the known common variants are NOT responsible for the familial aggregation and heritability of T2D observed in epidemiologic studies, what is?

Inevitably, other common SNP variants will be found and will boost the overall variance explained; however, they are likely to have only modest effects if they have not been found by now. Similarly, efforts to fine-map the association signals (which will in some cases reveal untyped variants with substantially larger effects) and to understand nonadditive interactions may help to bridge this "hcritability" gap, as will efforts to examine other types of variants (notably structural variants such as CNVs) that are poorly tagged on existing GWA platforms, and to understand the role of epigenetic modifications.

It now seems likely that the best boost to predictive power may well come from efforts to determine the extent to which T2D predisposition is influenced by intermediate penetrance variants (45,46). It is clear from T2D linkage studies that such variants cannot be common as well as penetrant (as otherwise we would have detected them), but low-frequency, intermediate-penetrance variants will typically have escaped attention by the approaches that have dominated gene discovery so far, neither penetrant enough to be detected using classical monogenic linkage approaches, nor common enough to be captured by GWA studies. Higher penetrance means tighter genotype–phenotype correlations and much greater predictive power. For example, a variant with a minor allele frequency of 1% and genotype relative risk of 3 has a greater locus-specific sibling relative risk than the known variants in *TCF7L2*. Only ~30 such loci distributed across the genome would suffice to explain the observed sibling relative risk for diabetes, and to match traditional risk factors on tests of discriminative accuracy. The advent of new high-throughput resequencing techniques provides the first opportunity for researchers to seek out such variants in a systematic way. The degree to which these efforts succeed will have an important bearing on the potential for individual prediction as a tool for improved management of multifactorial T2D.

Of course, prediction of disease at the level of the individual is not the only way in which present and future genetic discoveries can contribute to improved clinical management and prevention of diabetes. The biology revealed by these discoveries offers new opportunities for development of novel therapeutic and even preventative approaches. Perhaps the best prospects for the latter to date follow from the illustration, through genetics, that variants in the *SLC30A8* gene influence diabetes susceptibility (33). *SLC30A8* encodes a zinc transporter central to the normal function of insulin-containing secretory granules in the pancreatic beta cell. This observation has rekindled interest in possible relationships between dietary zinc exposure and diabetes risk. If future studies were to prove that zinc exposure represents a modifiable risk factor for T2D, appropriate public health measures could be contemplated.

In addition, although the specificity and sensitivity of the predisposing genetic variants may be insufficient to merit their use for individual prediction, this does not preclude their potential to identify (perhaps in combination with classical, nongenetic risk factors) *groups* of individuals at particularly high risk of developing T2D. Such "high-risk" groups are particularly attractive recruits to intervention trials, because the high baseline rate of disease progression should enhance power, reduce costs, and provide more efficient resolution of important public health questions. In all of these ways, genetic discoveries can provide the keys to unlock future public health advances in the management of diabetes.

References

1. Zimmet P, Alberti KGMM, Shaw J. Global and societal implications of the diabetes epidemic. *Nature*. 2001;414:782–787.
2. Stumvoll M, Goldstein BJ, van Haeften TW. Type 2 diabetes: principles of pathogenesis and therapy. *Lancet*. 2005;365:1333–1346.
3. Todd JA, Walker NM, Cooper JD, et al. Robust associations of four new chromosome regions from genome-wide analyses of type 1 diabetes. *Nat Genet*. 2007;39:857–864.
4. Stride A, Hattersley AT. Different genes, different diabetes: lessons from maturity-onset diabetes of the young. *Ann Med*. 2002;34:207–216.
5. Tattersall RB, Mansell PI. Maturity onset-type diabetes of the young (MODY): one condition or many? *Diabet Med*.1991;8:402–410.
6. Stoy J, Edghill EL, Flanagan SE, et al. Insulin gene mutations as a cause of permanent neonatal diabetes. *Proc Natl Acad Sci USA*. 2007;104:15040–15044.
7. Froguel P, Vaxillaire M, Sun F, et al. Close linkage of glucokinase locus on chromosome 7p to early-onset non-insulin-dependent diabetes mellitus. *Nature*. 1992;356:162–165.
8. Hattersley AT, Turner RC, Permutt MA, et al. Linkage of type 2 diabetes to the glucokinase gene. *Lancet*. 1992;339:1307–1310.
9. Yamagata K, Furuto H, Oda N, et al. Mutations in the hepatocyte nuclear factor-4α gene in maturity-onset diabetes of the young (MODY1). *Nature*. 1996;384:458–460.
10. Yamagata K, Oda N, Kaisaki PJ, et al. Mutations in the hepatocyte nuclear factor-1α gene in maturity-onset diabetes of the young (MODY3). *Nature*. 1996;384:455–458.
11. Pearson ER, Starkey BJ, Powell RJ, et al. Genetic cause of hyperglycaemia and response to treatment in diabetes. *Lancet*. 2003;362:1275–1281.

12. McCarthy MI, Hattersley AT. Molecular diagnostics in monogenic and multifactorial forms of type 2 diabetes. *Expert Rev Mol Diagn.* 2001;1:403–412.

13. Gardner RJ, Mackay DJG, Mungall AJ, et al. An imprinted locus associated with transient neonatal diabetes mellitus. *Hum Mol Genet.* 2000;9:589–596.

14. Gloyn AL, Pearson ER, Artcliff AL, et al. Activating mutations in the gene encoding the ATP-sensitive potassium-channel subunit Kir6.2 and permanent neonatal diabetes. *N Engl J Med.* 2004;350:1838–1849.

15. Gloyn AL, Diatloff ZC, Edghill EL, et al. KCNJ11 activating mutations are associated with developmental delay, epilepsy and neonatal diabetes syndrome and other neurological features. *Eur J Hum Genet.* 2006;14:824–830.

16. McCarthy MI. Progress in defining the molecular basis of type 2 diabetes mellitus through susceptibility-gene identification. *Hum Mol Genet.* 2004;13:R33–R41.

17. Owen K, Hattersley AT. Maturity-onset diabetes of the young: from clinical description to molecular genetic characterization. *Best Pract Res Clin Endocrinol Metab.* 2001;15:309–323.

18. Kadowaki T, Kadowaki H, Mori Y, et al. A subtype of diabetes mellitus associated with a mutation of mitochondrial DNA. *N Engl J Med.* 1994;330:962–968.

19. Hattersley AT, McCarthy MI. A question of standards: what makes a good genetic association study? *Lancet.* 2005;366:1315–1323.

20. McCarthy MI. Growing evidence for diabetes susceptibility genes from genome scan data. *Curr Diab Rep.* 2003;3:159–167.

21. Guan W, Pluzhnikov A, Cox NJ, Boehnke M for the International Type 2 Diabetes Linkage Analysis Consortium. Meta-analysis of 23 Type 2 diabetes linkage studies from the International Type 2 Diabetes Linkage Analysis Consortium. *Hum Hered.* 2008;66:35–49.

22. Grant SFA, Thorleifson G, Reynisdottir I, et al. Variant of transcription factor 7-like 2 (TFC7L2) gene confers risk of type 2 diabetes. *Nat Genet.* 2006;38:320–323.

23. Groves CJ, Zeggini E, Minton J, et al. Association analysis of 6,736 U.K. subjects provides replication and confirms TCF7L2 as a type 2 diabetes susceptibility gene with a substantial effect on individual risk. *Diabetes.* 2006;55:2640–2644.

24. Wacholder S, Chanock S, Garcia-Closas M, et al. Assessing the probability that a positive report is false: an approach for molecular epidemiology studies. *J Natl Cancer Inst.* 2004;96:434–442.

25. Lohmueller KE, Pearce CL, Pike M, et al. Meta-analysis of genetic association studies supports a contribution of common variants to susceptibility to common disease. *Nat Genet.* 2003;33:177–182.

26. Altshuler D, Hirschhorn JN, Klarmemark M, et al. The common PPARgamma Pro12Ala polymorphism is associated with decreased risk of type 2 diabetes. *Nat Genet.* 2000;26:76–80.

27. Gloyn AL, Weedon MN, Owen KR, et al. Large-scale association studies of variants in genes encoding the pancreatic beta-cell KATP channel subunits Kir6.2 (KCNJ11) and SUR1 (ABCC8) confirm that the KCNJ11 E23K variant is associated with type 2 diabetes. *Diabetes.* 2003;52:568–572.

28. Nielsen ED, Hansen L, Carstensen K, et al. The E23K variant of Kir6.2 associates with impaired post-OGTT serum insulin response and increased risk of type 2 diabetes. *Diabetes.* 2003;52:573–577.

29. Saxena R, Voight BV, Lyssenko V, et al. Genome-wide association analysis identifies loci for type 2 diabetes and triglyceride levels. *Science.* 2007;316:1331–1335.

30. Scott LJ, Mohlke KL, Bonnycastle LL, et al. A genome-wide association study of type 2 diabetes in Finns detects multiple susceptibility variants. *Science.* 2007;316:1341–1345.

31. Wellcome Trust Case Control Consortium. Genome-wide association study of 14,000 cases of seven common diseases and 3,000 shared controls. *Nature.* 2007;447:661–678.

32. Zeggini E, Weedon MN, Lindgren C, et al. Replication of genome-wide association signals in UK samples reveals risk loci for type 2 diabetes. *Science.* 2007;316:1336–1341.

33. Sladek R, Rocheleau G, Rung J, et al. A genome-wide association study identifies novel risk loci for type 2 diabetes. *Nature.* 2007;445:881–885.

34. Salonen JT, Uimari P, Aalto JM, et al. Type 2 diabetes whole-genome association study in four populations: the DiaGen consortium. *Am J Hum Genet.* 2007;81:338–345.

35. Steinsthorsdottir V, Thorleifsson G, Reynisdottir I, et al. A variant in CDKAL1 influences insulin response and risk of type 2 diabetes. *Nat Genet.* 2007;39:770–775.

36. Sandhu MS, Weedon MN, Fawcett MA, et al. WFS1 is a type 2 diabetes susceptibility gene. *Nat Genet.* 2007;39:951–953.

37. Winckler W, Weedon MN, Graham RR, et al. Evaluation of common variants in the six known MODY genes for association with Type 2 Diabetes. *Diabetes.* 2007;56:685–693.

38. Gudmundsson J, Sulem P, Steinthorsdottir V, et al. Two variants on chromosome 17 confer prostate cancer risk, and the one in TCF2 protects against type 2 diabetes. *Nat Genet.* 2007;39:977–983.

39. Pascoe L, Tura A, Patel SK, et al. Common variants of the novel type 2 diabetes genes, CDKAL1 and HHEX/IDE, are associated with decreased pancreatic beta-cell function. *Diabetes.* 2007;56:3101–3104.

40. Frayling TM, Timpson NJ, Weedon MN, et al. A common variant in the FTO gene is associated with body mass index and predisposes to childhood and adult obesity. *Science.* 2007;316:889–894.

41. Zeggini E, Scott LJ, Saxena R, et al. Meta-analysis of genome-wide association data and large-scale replication identifies additional susceptibility loci for type 2 diabetes. *Nat Genet.* 2008;40:638–645.

42. Marchini J, Howie B, Myers S, et al. A new multipoint method for genome-wide association studies by imputation of genotypes. *Nat Genet.* 2007;39:906–913.

43. Köbberling J, Tillil H. Empirical risk figures for first degree relatives of non-insulin-dependent diabetics. In Köbberling J, Tattersall R, eds. *The Genetics of Diabetes Mellitus.* London: Academic Press; 1982:201–209.

44. Janssens ACJW, Pardo MC, Steyerberg EW, van Duijn CM. Revisiting the clinical validity of multiplex genetic testing in complex diseases. *Am J Hum Genet.* 2004;74:585–588.

45. Stratton MR, Rahman N. The emerging landscape of breast cancer susceptibility. *Nat Genet.* 2008;40:17–22.

46. Romeo S, Pennacchio LA, Fu Y, et al. Population-based resequencing of ANGPTL4 uncovers variations that reduce triglycerides and increase HDL. *Nat Genet.* 2007;39:513–516.

17

Osteoporosis

*André G. Uitterlinden, Joyce B. J. van Meurs,
and Fernando Rivadeneira*

Abstract

Osteoporosis is—together with osteoarthritis—the most common locomotor disease, and its clinical sequela, including fractures, cause substantial disease burden and costs. It has strong genetic influences, and identification of the underlying DNA variants can help in understanding the disease process and might benefit development of interventions and diagnostics. Yet, its complex genetic architecture, that is, with larger effects for rare risk alleles and small effects of more common risk alleles, has just begun to be revealed but leave the majority of risk alleles still unidentified. Of the different approaches used, genetic association analysis followed by replication and prospective, multicentred meta-analysis has proven successful to identify genetic markers for osteoporosis. To accomplish this, the GENOMOS and GEFOS consortia have been established, using large collections of DNA samples from subjects with osteoporosis phenotypes that use standardized methodology and definitions. These collaborative consortia have identified—and refuted—associations of well-known candidate genes, and also play an important role in validation of risk alleles from genome-wide association studies (GWAS) for osteoporosis. Together with studies on rare variants, the GWA approach, in combination with the GENOMOS/GEFOS consortia, will help in clarifying the genetic architecture of complex bone traits such as bone mineral density (BMD), and—eventually—in understanding the genetics of fracture risk, the clinically more relevant but biologically more challenging endpoint in osteoporosis. Such genetic insights will be useful in understanding biology and are likely to also find applications in clinical practice.

Osteoporosis Has Genetic Influences

Osteoporosis is defined by decreased BMD and degenerative microarchitectural changes of bone tissue, and consequently an increased fracture risk. In the absence of molecular insights into the cause of the disease, definitions remain vague and descriptive. The main emphasis in this definition is on aspects of bone while the clinically relevant endpoint in osteoporosis, that is, fracture risk, is only in part

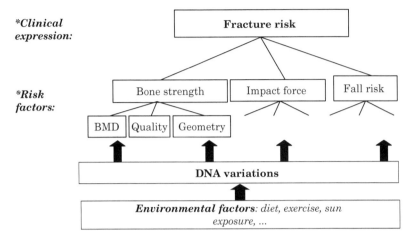

Figure 17.1 Schematic depiction of the genetic architecture of osteoporosis as a complex trait.

determined by bone characteristics. Also, other anthropometric and physiological parameters contribute to the risk of suffering fractures, such as falling risk (determining trauma, which involves cognitive function and muscle control) and obesity (that can dampen the impact of a fall) (see Figure 17.1). Thus, the genetic analysis of osteoporosis will include the genetics of bone characteristics, such as BMD, but also needs to address the genetics of cognition, muscle strength, and so on and other factors related to risk of falling.

Many aspects of osteoporosis have been found to have strong genetic influences (Table 17.1). This can be derived, for example, from genetic epidemiologic analyses, which showed that, in women, a maternal family history of fracture is positively related to fracture risk (1). Most evidence, however, has come from twin studies on BMD (2–6). For BMD the heritability has been estimated to be high: 50–80% (2–5). Thus, although twin studies can overestimate the heritability, a considerable part of the variance in BMD values might be explained by genetic factors, while the remaining part could be due to environmental factors and/or to gene–environment interactions. This also implicates that there are "bone density" genes, variants of which will result in BMD levels that are different between individuals. These differences can become apparent in different ways, for example, as peak BMD or as differences in the rates of bone loss at advanced age. While this notion has resulted in much attention being paid to the genetics of BMD in the field of osteoporosis, it is likely that this attention is also due simply to the widespread availability of devices to measure BMD. This does not necessarily imply that BMD is the most important biological parameter of bone strength to consider or the most important genetic factor in osteoporosis. At the same time, it is important to realize that (low) BMD is but one of many risk factors for osteoporotic fracture, the clinically most relevant endpoint of the disease.

Table 17.1 Heritability estimates of osteoporosis-related phenotypes

Phenotype	Heritability (h^2)
Bone mineral density	50–80%
Bone turnover/biochemical markers	40–70%
Bone geometry	70–85%
Quantitative ultrasound parameters	80%
Height	80–90%
Age-at-menopause	60%
Body mass index	60–70%
Hip fracture risk	3–68%
Wrist fracture risk	54%

Heritability estimates of fracture risk have been—understandably—much more limited due to the scarcity of good studies allowing precise estimates. Andrew et al. (5) studied 6,570 white healthy UK female volunteer twins between 18 and 80 years of age, and identified and validated 220 nontraumatic wrist fracture cases. They estimated a heritability of 54% for the genetic contribution to liability of wrist fracture in these women. Interestingly, while BMD was also highly heritable, the statistical models showed very little overlap of shared genes between the two traits in this study. Michaelsson et al. (6) studied 33,432 Swedish twins (including 6,021 twins with any fracture, 3,599 with an osteoporotic fracture, and 1,055 with a hip fracture after the age of 50 years) and concluded that heritability of hip fracture overall was 48% but was 68% in twins younger than 69 years, and decreased to 3% in elderly twins 79 years and older. Indeed, another Finnish study of elderly twins showed very little heritability for risk of fracture (7).

Altogether, this suggests that fracture risk is genetically determined, but that at older age other, perhaps environmental, factors become more important in explaining variance in fracture risk, and may be in modifying the effect of genetic predisposition. Gene–environment interactions one can think of, in this respect, include diet, exercise, and exposure to sunlight (for vitamin D metabolism). While genetic predisposition will be constant during life, environmental factors tend to change during the different periods of life resulting in different "expression levels" of the genetic susceptibility. The complex aggregate phenotype of aging is associated with a general functional decline resulting in, for example, less exercise, less time spent outdoors, changes in diet, and so on. This gene–environment interaction can result in diminished expression of these genotype factors in the final phenotype ("the penetrance") for particular genetic susceptibilities or, alternatively, their being revealed only later on in life after a period during which they go unnoticed due to sufficient exposure to one or more environmental factors. Given the Human Genome Project and its sequela, most attention in the analysis of gene–environment interactions has gone to the genes (also referred to as the "genocentric" approach). The idea behind this is that once we know which gene variants are involved, it will be more straightforward to analyze the contribution of environmental factors and their interplay with genetic factors.

Risk Gene Identification in Complex Genetic Diseases

Most common diseases such as diabetes, osteoporosis, and cardiovascular diseases, as well as many disease-related so-called intermediate traits or endophenotypes such as cholesterol levels, glucose levels, and bone mineral density, have strong genetic influences, meaning that genetic variants that contribute to this heritability will exist. Yet, the identification of genetic factors underlying these disorders and traits and clarifying their genetic architecture has been very problematic, given the complex nature of the phenotypes and the limited molecular tools available at the time to identify the underlying genetic factors. Complex diseases are typically influenced by many genetic variants, of which common ones have modest effect sizes and the rare ones more substantial, while the variability in expression of the disease phenotype is also influenced by environmental factors in interaction with the genetic factors. Figure 17.2 shows the molecular genetic approaches most commonly used in the past two decades to identify genetic susceptibility factors for such complex diseases: the top-down genome-wide approaches and the bottom-up candidate gene approaches. It is safe to say now that linkage approaches in related subjects have

Type of approach	Resolution	Effectiveness	
		Common risk alleles	Rare risk alleles
"Top-down"/hypothesis free			
* **Genome wide <u>linkage</u> analysis**	5–20 million bp	–	+/–
- Pedigrees			
- Sib-pairs			
- Human, mouse			
* **Genome wide <u>association</u> (GWA) analysis**	5–50 thousand bp	+	–
- 100K–2000K SNP analysis in cases/controls			
* **Genome wide sequencing**	1 bp	(+)	(+)
- full genome not yet feasible on large scale			
"Bottom-up"/up-front hypothesis			
* **<u>Association</u> analyses of candidate gene polymorphisms** (based on biology)	1 bp	+/–	+/–
* **Candidate sequencing**	1 bp	+	+
- Selected regions (e.g., exons, gene regions)			

Figure 17.2 Some characteristics of the most commonly used molecular approaches to identify susceptibility alleles for complex disorders. "Resolution" indicates the size of the chromosomal area, which is identified as being linked/associated to the phenotype of interest, and which can vary from one base pair to many millions of base pairs. "Effectiveness" indicates the success rate of the method to identify risk alleles for complex genetic diseases and phenotypes, either common or rare, as derived from publications.

been unsuccessful in identifying common genetic factors in complex disease. This is most likely due to the low power of this approach to detect the subtle effects and to the low "genetic resolution," meaning that very large chromosomal areas were potentially identified but with many possible candidate genes in each. On the other hand, the candidate gene approach in association studies has frequently suffered from irreproducible results, mostly due to limited samples size and lack of standardization in phenotyping and genotyping. In the field of osteoporosis genetics, the GENOMOS consortium and, more recently, the GEFOS consortium, were started to address the problems in the candidate gene association analysis in particular, and in the genome-wide association studies (GWAS).

Novel approaches based on large-scale and high-throughput sequencing are now emerging, which will generate a complete catalog of all variants present in a given sequence, rare and common, rather than having to rely on markers and patterns of linkage disequilibrium. These sequencing techniques are now being used for deep sequence analysis of selected areas (e.g., hits from GWAS), but are not yet able to provide the complete human genome sequences in large collections of samples. Yet hopes are high, and the expectation is that within a few years this will be possible at acceptable costs and on a large scale. This will result in a second surge of genetic association studies generating comprehensive collections of sequence variations, common and (very) rare, including *de novo* events in individuals. Nevertheless, also for these studies, the large consortia such as GENOMOS/GEFOS will play a crucial role, given the requirements for large samples sizes to detect the effects and the infrastructure for proper association studies with standardization and replication.

We will first briefly discuss the classical association study design, followed by a description of the GENOMOS consortium, the recent GWAS on osteoporosis, and the GEFOS project.

Association Analysis of Candidate Gene Polymorphisms

The *bottom-up* approach to identify genetic risk factors for osteoporosis builds upon biology, that is, the known involvement of a particular gene in aspects of osteoporosis, for example, bone metabolism. This gene is then referred to as a "candidate gene." The candidacy of such a gene can be established by several lines of evidence:

1. Cell biological and molecular biological experiments, indicating, for example, bone cell-specific expression of the gene.
2. Animal models in which a gene has been mutated (e.g., natural mouse mutants), over-expressed (transgenic mice), or deleted (knock-out mice), and which result in a bone-phenotype.
3. Naturally occurring mutations of the human gene, resulting in monogenic Mendelian diseases with a bone phenotype.
4. More recently, any "hit" from a GWA study.

Subsequently, such genes are scrutinized for sequence variants, which lead to (subtle) differences in level and/or function of the encoded protein. We distinguish mutations, rare variants, and polymorphisms purely on the basis of frequency: polymorphisms occur in at least 1% of the population, rare variants in less than 1% of the general population, while mutations occur in particular pedigrees and are usually linked to a monogenetic disease. The DNA sequence variant that is currently mostly being studied is the Single Nucleotide Polymorphism or SNP, which is the most common type of variation in the human genome. Of course, several other types of sequence variation need consideration, such as variable number of tandem repeats (VNTR) and copy number variations (CNV). Yet, especially the CNVs require specialized analytical tools and reference data to study in large populations, which are now being generated. Therefore, assessing their role in complex disease in a comprehensive way will have to wait for further studies, whereas for SNPs, most technology is now in place, resulting in many studies on SNPs in relation to complex diseases.

Several databases are now available, which contain information on DNA sequence variation, especially on the common variants in any gene of the Human Genome (e.g., dbSNP from, NCBI, Celera, HapMap, and several more specialized databases such as from the program for genomic analysis (PGA)). Common DNA sequence variations were usually regarded as just polymorphic (so-called "anonymous" polymorphisms) until proven otherwise, but this view is changing. Many of them have now been shown to have consequences for the level and/or activity of the protein encoded, and are termed functional polymorphisms. These can include, for example, sequence variations leading to alterations in the amino acid composition of the protein, changes in the 5′ promoter region leading to differences in mRNA expression, and/or polymorphisms in the 3′ region leading to differences in mRNA degradation. In particular, the GWAS (see below) have identified polymorphisms that can be very far away from an actual gene and most likely are involved in fine regulation of the gene of interest. As a result of this large amount of evidence that is being accumulated for DNA polymorphisms, we are now regarding all of them as potentially functional, until proven otherwise.

Polymorphisms of interest are usually first tested in population-based and/or case-control "association studies," to evaluate their contribution to the phenotype of interest at the population level. However, association studies do not establish cause and effect; they just show correlation or cooccurrence of one with the other. Cause and effect have to be established in truly functional cellular and molecular biological experiments involving, for example, transfection of cell lines with allelic constructs and testing activities of the different alleles. This can occur at different levels of organization and depends on the type of protein analyzed, for example, enzymes versus matrix molecules versus transcription factors. Acknowledging these complexities, it will remain a challenge, once an association has been observed, to identify the correct test of functionality, and once functionality has been established, to identify the correct endpoint in an epidemiologic study.

Functional polymorphisms lead to meaningful biological differences in function of the encoded "osteoporosis" protein, thus making the interpretation of association analyses using these variants quite straightforward. For example, for functional polymorphisms, it is expected that the same allele will be associated with the same phenotype in different populations. This can even be extended to similar associations being present in different ethnic groups, although allele frequencies can of course differ by ethnicity.

Out of the lines of evidence mentioned above, numerous candidate genes for risk of osteoporosis have emerged. These include "classical" candidate genes for osteoporosis such as collagen type I, the vitamin D receptor, and the estrogen receptors alpha and beta. Yet, recently identified "bone" genes, such as *LRP5*, also are candidate genes because their involvement in bone biology has now been established. These studies on monogenetic pedigrees in which an *LRP5* mutation was segregating (such as in the High Bone Mass phenotype pedigrees or in osteoporosis pseudoglioma pedigrees) have identified *LRP5* as a candidate gene for osteoporosis, while work from the GENOMOS consortium as well as the recent GWAS have also identified *LRP5* as a risk gene for osteoporosis (see below).

Genetic Effects: Large versus Small and Common versus Rare

From the analysis of the successfully identified genetic risk factors for complex disorders, it is now clear that for complex disorders in general, the risks associated with each individual common genetic variant are generally modest in terms of effect size. For polymorphisms involved in several complex disorders a trend can be discerned whereby the more common variants are associated with smaller risks (such as *PPARG Pro12Ala* in type 2 diabetes) than the more rare variants (such as Factor V Leiden and thrombosis).

While the risk of disease is indeed small for such individual genetic risk variants, because there are millions of these common variants in the human genome, the combined effect—or genetic load—of these risk variants can be substantial, both for the individual as well as at the population level. One can speculate that evolution has allowed these common variants to float around in the human population because they do not compromise reproductive success (or might even enhance it), and only start to affect fitness of the individual carrying such variants late in life, far after the reproductive period. On the other end of the spectrum, more rare variants might be selected out in evolution because they do affect reproductive success and/or will be private to individuals as newly arisen mutations.

Overall, the current thought about underlying genetic risk variants of complex diseases such as osteoporosis is that there may be hundreds of common variants conferring risk, but any given individual will also carry several genetic variants that are (very) rare in the population and might have bigger associated genetic risks. As discussed below, we now are successfully identifying these more common effects with the smaller effect sizes. We will have to wait until cost-effective total human genome sequencing techniques become available to identify in individuals the collections of the much rarer sequence variants that perhaps confer larger effects.

These small effect sizes of common variants also explain why it has been difficult to identify such risks convincingly, in spite of these genetic variants being so common. Common in this respect means allele frequencies of a genetic risk factor of 5% to 50%, and modest effect sizes means odds ratios of 1.1–2.0. Statistical power calculations show that indeed very large study populations of 1,000–10,000 subjects of case-control collections and/or population-based cohorts need to be studied in order to demonstrate convincingly such small effects by association analysis. Only recently have such large study populations become available and consortia been assembled to address these challenges in a robust manner using meta-analysis to estimate true effect sizes of individual variants.

Meta-Analysis

Since more and more association analyses are performed from an ever-increasing list of candidate gene polymorphisms, it is necessary to put all these data in perspective by performing meta-analyses of the individual association analyses. Meta-analysis can quantify the results of various studies on the same topic, and estimate and explain their diversity. Recent evidence indicates that a systematic meta-analysis approach can estimate population-wide effects of genetic risk factors for human disease (8), and that large studies are more conservative in these estimates and should preferably be used (9). An analysis of 301 studies on genetic associations (on many different diseases) concluded that there are many common variants in the human genome with modest, but real, effects on common disease risk, and that studies using large samples will be able to convincingly identify such variants (10). This notion in the field of complex genetics has led to the creation of consortia of investigators working on the same disease, and then in particular on the genetics of complex diseases and traits. While these consortia first operated in isolation, they are now collaborating through the HuGENet™ (http://www.cdc.gov/genomics/hugenet) instigated network of networks (11,12). Among such consortia, GENOMOS (http://www.genomos.eu), as the network of investigators working on genetics of osteoporosis, was one of the first (starting in 2003) and was involved in the first Network of Networks meetings.

Meta-analysis initially had some drawbacks because it was mostly based on combining sets of existing data resulting in, at times, substantial bias in the outcome. This is mainly because there is publication bias in the literature (positive studies reporting exaggerated effects) and there was virtually no standardization among investigators in methods of genotyping or phenotyping and data analysis. Yet, with the advent of growing consortia of investigators working on the subtle effects in complex genetics, the concept of meta-analysis has developed into one of prospective meta-analysis. Here, the investigators collectively perform genotyping under standardized conditions and agree on the outcomes, well before the outcome of individual studies is known. This approach will therefore include positive as well as negative studies on the polymorphism of interest. The GENOMOS consortium was one of the first networks to use such a prospective meta-analytic approach to start a systematic test of candidate gene polymorphisms in the field of osteoporosis.

The GENOMOS Consortium

The EU-sponsored GENOMOS (Genetic Markers for Osteoporosis) consortium attempts to perform such studies using standardized methods of genotyping and phenotyping. The GENOMOS project involves the large-scale study of several candidate gene polymorphisms in relation to osteoporosis-related outcomes in subjects drawn from several European centers. Its main outcomes are fractures and femoral neck and lumbar spine BMD. An overview of the participating centers and groups at the start of the project is given in Figure 17.3. Design details are further described

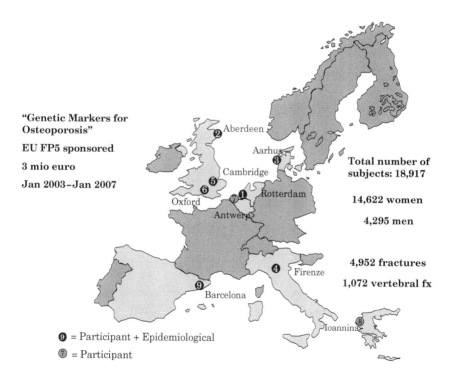

Figure 17.3 A geographical overview of the initial participating centers in the GENOMOS consortium at the start in 2003. These include the centers with study populations used for genotyping and association analysis (in black dots), and a center specializing in finding causative genes in monogenetic bone disorders (Antwerp, Belgium), and the statistical center for meta-analysis (Ioannina, Greece).

in the first meta-analysis of individual-level data on the *ESR1* gene (13) and can be found on the website (http://www.genomos.eu).

Apart from being a very large study of genetics of osteoporosis, an important aspect of this study is its prospective multicenter design. This means that the genotype data are generated for all centers first, and only AFTER that is completed is the association analysis done, thereby rendering it immune to possible publication bias. The targets of the study were initially polymorphisms for which some *a priori* evidence for involvement in osteoporosis was present already; it was not designed to be a risk gene-discovery tool and currently therefore could not, for example, assess all genetic diversity across a candidate gene. While fracture has been debated as an endpoint in genetics of osteoporosis studies, this was chosen in the GENOMOS study because it is clinically the most relevant endpoint. Statistical power of the GENOMOS study to detect genetic effects on fracture risk is high, with >5,000 fractures, while this number is still growing due to popularity of the symposium as well as the incidence of fracture with the passage of time in several of the longitudinal cohorts.

An overview of all the meta-analyses published by the GENOMOS consortium so far is presented in Table 17.2. The very first GENOMOS meta-analysis of three polymorphisms in the *ESR1* gene (intron 1 polymorphisms XbaI and PvuII and the promoter (TA) variable number of tandem repeats microsatellite) and haplotypes thereof, among 18,917 individuals in eight European centers, demonstrated no effects on BMD, but a modest effect on fracture risk (19–35% risk reduction for XbaI homozygotes), independent of BMD (13). Subsequent usual suspects in the genetics of osteoporosis scrutinized by GENOMOS were the Sp1 *COL1A1* gene polymorphism (14), five polymorphisms in the vitamin D receptor gene including the Cdx2 promoter variant, the FokI variant, and the BsmI, ApaI, and the TaqI variants (15), five polymorphisms in the *TGFbeta* gene (16), and the exon 9 and exon 13 variants in *LRP5* and the exon 9 variant in *LRP6* (17).

Overall, the major results of the GENOMOS study included the identification of the *LRP5* variants as true osteoporosis risk variants, but with modest effects size. The *LRP5* effects were very consistent across different populations, rendering very low *p*-values for the overall effect (although it was small), probably indicating that this is a universal genetic effect for osteoporosis, which can be expected to appear in nearly every population studied. In addition, we identified the *ESR1* SNPs as fracture risk factors and not so much as BMD associated variants, and also showed that the Sp1 *COL1A1* variant was associated with a modest increase in vertebral fracture risk, as we did for the Cdx2 variant in the *VDR* gene. These results show that the candidate gene approach is fruitful in identification of osteoporosis risk alleles, but only when applied as rigorously as in GENOMOS. In addition, it showed that the effect size of the common risk alleles in osteoporosis is modest. This might reflect our poor choice of candidate genes (not being able to select the most important risk genes for osteoporosis), but also illustrates the general allelic architecture of BMD. In view of the recent GWAS results, the latter scenario has proven to be correct.

Table 17.2 Large-scale evidence for candidate gene associations from the GENOMOS study

| | | | ASSOCIATIONS WITH OP PHENOTYPES | | | | |
| | | | BMD (SD) | | Fracture (Odds Ratio) | | |
Gene (n = 6)	SNPs (n = 17)	Sample n	Femoral Neck	Lumbar Spine	Vertebral	Non-Vertebral	Publication
ESR1	3	18,917	—	—	1.2–1.3	1.1–1.2	Ioannidis et al., *JAMA* 2004 (13)
COLIA1	1	20,786	0.15	0.15	1.1 (Sp1)	—	Ralston et al., *PLoS Med* 2006 (14)
VDR	5	26,242	—	—	1.1 (Cdx2)	—	Uitterlinden et al., *Ann Int Med* 2006 (15)
TGFbeta	5	28,924	—	—	—	—	Langdahl et al., *Bone* 2008 (16)
LRP5	2	37,760	0.15	0.15	1.12–1.26	1.06–1.14	Van Meurs et al., *JAMA* 2008 (17)
LRP6	1	37,760	—	—	—	—	*Ibid.* (17)

Importantly, we also excluded 5 *TGFbeta* variants to contribute to osteoporosis and most likely also other variants in the coding region of this prominent candidate gene for osteoporosis. This is equally important to the field of osteoporosis genetics as is finding risk alleles, as it signals to the scientific research community not to spend scarce resources studying *TGFbeta* variants further in relation to osteoporosis.

In the course of the GENOMOS project we have also evaluated several different approaches to find new potential genetic markers for osteoporosis. Of these, the work package on analyzing monogenetic families has been very successful in identifying new candidate genes, including *LRP5*, which was also identified in our consortium as a prominent risk gene for osteoporosis. Other approaches, such as linkage analysis in families or TDT testing in sib pairs selected on (mild) osteoporosis, were found to be not successful. In addition, we tested some techniques for genetic association studies, which were found to be helpful (haplotyping in population data using estimation algorithms) or not so helpful (LD mapping in pooled samples). These are all equally relevant messages to the scientific community on how to progress in the most efficient way in complex osteoporosis genetics.

While there were attempts in the original project to study gene–environment interactions relating to use of HRT medication in relation to *ESR1* genotypes, and dietary calcium intake in relation to *VDR* genotype, these were less successful. No major effect of HRT use was seen for the effect of the *ESR1* genotype on BMD or fracture risk, but the study was hampered by lack of standardized methods to assess HRT use and quality of the data sets. No major effect of dietary Ca intake was seen for the effect of the *VDR* genotype on BMD or fracture risk, but again, the study was hampered by lack of standardized methods and quality of the data sets.

In conclusion we can now say that

(a) GENOMOS has been established as the leading consortium of research groups working on the genetics of osteoporosis.
(b) GENOMOS has identified and refuted genetic risk factors for osteoporosis.
(c) The effects sizes of the identified genetic risk factors for osteoporosis is modest at best, with effects of 0.1 SD in BMD and 20–30% increases in risk for osteoporotic fracture.
(d) The results of GENOMOS activities have not yet led to clinically useful genetic markers and/or commercially interesting activities with any economic impact. This is due to the candidate gene approach taken so far, and the small effect sizes of individual genetic markers.

Although successful, drawbacks of the GENOMOS consortium include the fact that only well-known candidate genes were analyzed so far, and so we could not expect to generate much new biology, with the exception of studies on monogenetic diseases. In addition, GENOMOS only studied Caucasians, so the generalizability

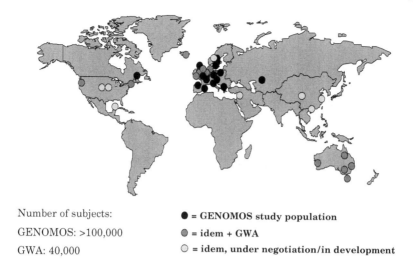

Number of subjects:

GENOMOS: >100,000

GWA: 40,000

● = GENOMOS study population

◉ = idem + GWA

○ = idem, under negotiation/in development

Figure 17.4   A geographical overview of the participating centers in the GEFOS consortium at the start in 2008. These include the centers with GWAS data in their study populations (dark gray dots) and the GENOMOS centers (black dots), and centers that have expressed interest in joining the GEFOS/GENOMOS effort (light gray dots).

of the findings is unknown for other ethnicities. The endpoints were limited to the classical osteoporosis endpoints BMD and fracture risk. Both of these are cumbersome to interpret in biological and clinical ways, and do not tell the complete story about osteoporosis. Finally, no risk modeling was performed to assess the contribution of the genetic risk factors we identified in GENOMOS in relation to well-established osteoporosis risk factors such as age, gender, BMI, use of a walking aid, and so on.

To address these shortcomings of the GENOMOS project, a follow-up project was sponsored under the FP7 program of the European Commission: GEFOS, the son of GENOMOS, was born. The GEFOS project (Figure 17.4; http://www.gefos. org) was started in March 2008, and uses the several GWAS on osteoporosis that are available or ongoing as its starting point. Under GEFOS, the sample size of the GENOMOS consortium has also increased further to ~100,000 samples, and is used to replicate hits coming from the GWAS. GEFOS will also include additional bone phenotypes (such as CT and ultrasound) to study as endpoints in the meta-analysis and/or GWAS, and will introduce risk modeling of the identified genetic risk factors in relation to other osteoporosis risk factors.

Genome-Wide Association Studies

Due to technological developments, the association study design has regained popularity, but now on a genome-wide scale, with an unprecedented density of genetic

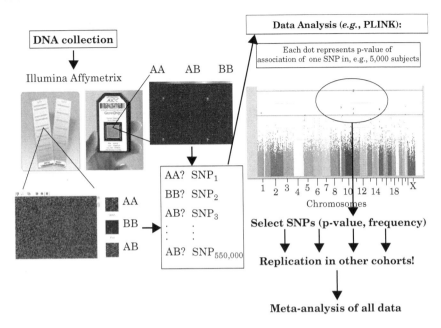

Figure 17.5   A schematic overview of the process of performing a GWA study. Each of the DNA samples from, for example, a typical case-control collection for a disease consisting of 5,000 DNA samples, are subjected to genome-wide SNP genotyping using any of two platforms (Illumina and Affymetrix). These will generate ~0.5 million genotypes per DNA sample, which combine to 2.5 billion genotypes across the 5,000 samples, which are then analyzed for association to the disease by standard chi-square tests in programs such as PLINK. The output of such programs is usually depicted as so-called "Manhattan plots," whereby each dot represents the p-value for association of one SNP (out of the 0.5 million). Selected SNPs are then identified ("the low-hanging fruit") to be subjected to replication efforts in additional DNA collections with the phenotype of interest. A meta-analysis on the combined evidence will establish consistency of the association, effect-size, and statistical significance.

markers: the GWAS (18). This renaissance has mostly been driven by the discovery of millions of SNPs throughout the human genome and the development of so-called microarray technology to type such SNPs accurately on a massive parallel scale.

   Genome-wide association studies (see Figure 17.5) have had considerable success in identifying common genetic susceptibility alleles (18). GWAS consist of screening the genome of many hundreds to thousands of subjects in a case-control study or population-based cohort study, with >300,000 SNPs, followed by a simple association analysis between a phenotype and all the genetic markers. This identifies genetic markers associated to the phenotype of interest with a certain statistical significance. Because of the multiplicity of testing with so many markers, thresholds have been considered to declare an association "genome-wide significant" (gws). For example, when analyzing 500,000 markers, this threshold is 1.10^{-7} (0.05/500,000), but given more recent approaches to exploit the linkage relationships between the millions of SNPs in the HapMap database (by imputation), 5.10^{-8} is now a more widely used gws level in GWAS. Seeing gws associations is dependent on factors such as the effect size of the genetic variants on the phenotype and the size of the study sample. Usually, a typical GWAS consists of a discovery sample with GWA data and a replication sample with GWA data. From the discovery sample of GWAS, the "top-hits" (e.g., all genetic markers that reach a significance of 1.10^{-4} or less) will be analyzed in the replication GWA data set(s) to see which markers replicate at nominal significance level, and which will reach the gws level after combining the data sets in a meta-analysis. Top hits can also be further analyzed in subsequent replication cohorts that do not necessarily have GWA data, but can be genotyped for the particular genetic markers identified. Such efforts now routinely include several thousands, if not tens of thousands, of individuals, and so the power is substantial to discover smaller and smaller effect sizes.

The current GWA genotyping platforms are optimized to discover common risk alleles rather than rare variants and thus, GWAS have their limitations in explaining all genetic variance of a disease or trait. For example, the explained genetic variance in type 2 diabetes mellitus by the recently discovered common variants in risk genes by GWAS is still limited to—at most—10% (18), and similar figures are observed for typical quantitative traits such as height (19–21). Yet, we must realize these are still early days in complex genetics, because we have only uncovered the "low-hanging fruit" in this first round of GWAS. Below the gws loci, there are many less significant signals with a smaller effects size, which will be identified by further increasing the sample size of either GWAS cohorts or replication cohorts. The complex genetics research community has now organized itself into a still-growing consortium of research groups who join GWAS data sets and are providing excellent forums for harmonizing phenotype definitions, such as GENOMOS. GWAS of osteoporosis phenotypes have only just been performed, and so progress in genetics of osteoporosis is lagging a bit behind in comparison to areas such as diabetes or traits such as height.

GWAS of Osteoporosis

The very first attempt to identify BMD loci through GWAS is presented by investigators from the Framingham study using the 100K Affymetrix platform and a limited sample size of $n = 1,141$ men and women (22). This effort did not result in BMD loci that reached the so-called gws, and made it clear that larger samples sizes were to be used, as well as genotyping platforms with a higher genome coverage such as the Illumina 317K or 550K platforms. Recently, the first three GWAS on BMD have been published, which identified several loci contributing to BMD that reached gws. One study was coming from analysis of the TwinsUK cohort and the Rotterdam Study, both looking at Caucasian women from the United Kingdom and the Netherlands, respectively (23), and the other studies were from deCODE and based on Icelandic subjects (24,25) (see Table 17.3 for an overview of the three studies). These three studies represent the first large-scale high-density GWAS efforts reporting BMD loci from a hypothesis-free approach. One locus was overlapping

Table 17.3 Comparison of three GWAS on bone mineral density

	Twins UK/ ERGO NL	*deCODE/DK/AUS*	*deCODE/DK/AUS*
Author	Richards B, Rivadeneira F, et al. (23)	Styrkarsdottir U, et al. (24)	Styrkarsdottir U, et al. (25)
Journal	*Lancet*, April 29, 2008	*NEJM*, April 30, 2008	*Nature Genetics*, December 14, 2008
GWA discovery	Twins UK ($n = 1,586$)	deCODE ($n = 5,861$)	deCODE ($n = 6,865$)
Platform	Illumina 317K	Illumina 317K	Illumina 317K
Replication cohorts	Rotterdam Study NL ($n = 4,877$) Chingford UK ($n = 718$)	Iceland ($n = 4,165$) Danish ($n = 2,269$) Australian ($n = 1,491$)	Iceland ($n = 3,135$) Danish ($n = 3,884$) Australian ($n = 1,491$)
Total *n*	8,557	13,786	15,375
gws hits: # BMD loci	2: *LRP5, OPG*	5: *OPG, RANKL, ESR1, ZFBTB40, MHC*	4: *SOST, MARK3, SP7, RANK*
Also fracture risk?	1 *(LRP5)*	3 (+3 post hoc)	1 *(SOST)*
Explained variance BMD	~1%	~3%	~4% (including previous SNPs)

between the efforts, that is, the OPG locus on chromosome 8, while the TwinsUK/ ERGO effort reported on an additional locus, that is, LRP5, and the deCODE GWAS reported eight additional loci, bringing the total now to ten BMD loci identified through GWAS. LRP5 was interesting because this gene and indeed this particular SNP (the exon 13 SNP) was reported just 1 month earlier by the GENOMOS consortium to be associated with very high confidence to BMD in the study by van Meurs et al. (17). The explained variance of the genetic factors for BMD that was reached by these studies was low (1–4%). This indicates that, as with the GWAS results for height (19–21), BMD is a truly complex trait with many loci (hundreds?) of small effect. This also indicates that even larger sample sizes than the one used by the deCODE study ($n = 15,375$) are necessary to identify these additional common factors. Taken together, this puts the GEFOS effort in the spotlight, because this consortium was able to eventually accumulate >40,000 samples with GWAS data (Figure 17.4) and therefore was well powered to identify the second wave of BMD loci in combination with the expanded GENOMOS consortium to include >100,000 replication samples. In addition, the range of subjects is now enlarged to include also younger subjects and subjects of different ethnic background such as Asians and African-Americans. The GWAS on osteoporosis in some of the GEFOS cohorts is still underway, and meta-analysis of combined data is planned soon to identify additional BMD loci beyond what the deCODE and TwinsUK/Rotterdam Study GWAS have identified. Initially, the GWAS in osteoporosis will focus on BMD as a normally distributed quantitative trait, a risk parameter for osteoporosis. In addition, it will be possible, across the several GWAS, to identify risk alleles for fracture risk (all types of fracture, hip fracture, vertebral fracture, etc.) and other phenotypes in osteoporosis such as bone geometry parameters and CT and QUS parameters. Yet, as we noted in the introduction, bone strength is only one of the risk factors for osteoporotic fracture. Together with loci coming from GWAS on cognitive function, muscle mass, and obesity/fat distribution, the bone strength loci will help to explain the variance in fracture risk, that is to say, for the common risk alleles involved in osteoporosis.

Rare Variants

The current round of GWAS tend to focus on this low-hanging fruit, while we know that there are many more such common, especially less common, variants to be discovered with less impressive *p*-values in the discovery phase, due to even smaller effect size and/or even smaller population frequency. Identifying such small effects is possible, but will require even larger sample sizes to detect them in a statistically robust and convincing way. All current GWAS focus on common variants with, say, >5% population frequency, but we have seen already that there are less common variants (0.5–5% population frequency) and even rare variants (<0.5% population frequency) that will help to explain risk of disease or the variance of a trait of interest.

Examples highlighting the existence of such less common variants involved in complex traits were demonstrated for sequence variations in genes related to cholesterol levels. Cohen et al. (26) tested whether rare DNA sequence variants collectively contributed to variation in plasma levels of high-density lipoprotein cholesterol (HDL-C). They sequenced three candidate genes (*ABCA1*, *APOA1*, and *LCAT*) that caused Mendelian forms of low HDL-C levels in individuals from a population-based study on cholesterol levels. Nonsynonymous sequence variants were significantly more common (16% vs 2%) in individuals with low HDL-C (<fifth percentile) than in those with high HDL-C (>95th percentile). Similar findings were obtained in an independent population, and biochemical studies indicated that most sequence variants in the low HDL-C group were functionally important and had substantial effect sizes. Thus, rare alleles with major phenotypic effects contribute significantly to low plasma HDL-C levels in the general population.

Similarly, such rare alleles of bone genes might contribute to variation in BMD and other bone parameters, and even fracture risk in the general population. Figure 17.6 highlights how such different genetic variants together constitute the genetic architecture of a trait like BMD in osteoporosis. At the extremes, with either very low or very high BMD, we have already identified bone genes mutations that lead to these rare and severe phenotypes, and become apparent as Mendelian bone diseases such as osteogenesis imperfecta and the High Bone Mass phenotype. In the normal range of the BMD distribution, efforts such as testing of candidate genes in GENOMOS and GWAS are now identifying genetic variants that are common and have modest effect size. Soon, we will embark on deep-sequencing projects, which will identify less common genetic variants (<5%), and which might have modest

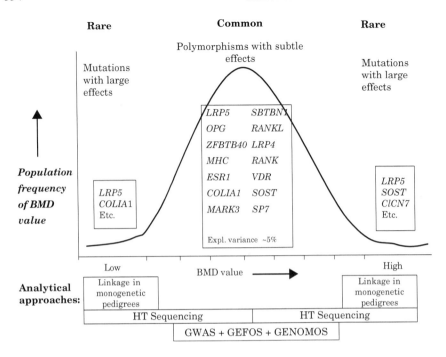

Figure 17.6 A schematic overview of the genetic architecture of BMD, as one of the risk parameters in osteoporosis, resulting from recent gene identification efforts. BMD is plotted as a normally distributed phenotype in any random population; indicated are some of the genetic variants that have been described explaining extreme values of BMD, mainly in monogenetic diseases, and the BMD loci that have now been identified through GENOMOS and two GWAS. Below, the category of analytical approaches is presented in relation to which genetic variants can be identified with them.

to substantial effect sizes. Again, these might include SNPs but also other types of genetic markers such as CNVs.

The future challenge, beyond the GWAS era, will therefore be to identify more rare variants through deep-sequencing approaches, for example, of the several loci/genes identified through GWAS on BMD and related phenotypes. Combinations of such rare and the more common genetic variants in these particular genes can then be scrutinized for their diagnostic potential in large, well-phenotyped cohorts, also in relation to the more classical risk factors such as age, BMI, and previous fracture. Such panels of combinations of genetic risk factors are expected to explain more of the genetic risk for osteoporosis than just the common variants or just the (very) rare variants.

Acknowledgments

The work described was sponsored by the European Commission under contract number QLK6-CT-2002–02629 (GENOMOS) and FP7-HEALTH-2007–201865 (GEFOS).

We would like to thank our colleagues in the GEFOS and GENOMOS consortia for their invaluable help with the projects described here and their inspiring discussions and criticism. We also thank Pascal Arp, Mila Jhamai, Lisette Stolk, Yue Fang, and Michael Moorhouse at Erasmus MC, who have all provided their help and expertise in the course of the GENOMOS and GEFOS projects.

References

1. Cummings SR, Nevitt MC, Browner WS, et al. Risk factors for hip fracture in white women. *N Engl J Med.* 1995;332:767–773.
2. Smith DM, Nance WE, Kang KW, Christian JC, Johnston CC. Genetic factors in determining bone mass. *J Clin Invest.* 1973;52:2800–2808.
3. Pocock NA, Eisman JA, Hopper JL, Yeates GM, Sambrook PN, Ebert S. Genetic determinants of bone mass in adults: a twin study. *J Clin Invest.* 1987;80:706–710.
4. Flicker L, Hopper JL, Rodgers L, Kaymakci B, Green RM, Wark JD. Bone density determinants in elderly women: a twin study. *J Bone Miner Res.* 1995;10:1607–1613.
5. Andrew T, Antioniades L, Scurrah KJ, Macgregor AJ, Spector TD. Risk of wrist fracture in women is heritable and is influenced by genes that are largely independent of those influencing BMD. *J Bone Miner Res.* 2005;20(1):67–74.
6. Michaelsson K, Melhus H, Ferm H, Ahlbom A, Pedersen NL. Genetic liability to fractures in the elderly. *Arch Intern Med.* 2005;165:1825–1830.
7. Kannus P, Palvanen M, Kaprio J, Parkkari J, Koskenvuo M. Genetic factors and osteoporotic fractures in elderly people: prospective 25 year follow up of a nationwide cohort of elderly Finnish twins. *BMJ.* 1999;319:1334–1337.
8. Ioannidis JP, Ntzani EE, Trikalinos TA, Contopoulos-Ioannidis DG. Replication validity of genetic association studies. *Nat Genet.* 2001;29(3):306–309.
9. Ioannidis JP, Trikalinos TA, Ntzani EE, Contopoulos-Ioannidis DG. Genetic associations in large versus small studies: an empirical assessment. *Lancet.* 2003;361(9357):567–571.
10. Lohmueller KE, Pearce CL, Pike M, Lander ES, Hirschhorn JN. Meta-analysis of genetic association studies supports a contribution of common variants to susceptibility to common disease. *Nat Genet.* 2003;33(2):177–182.
11. Ioannidis JP, Bernstein J, Boffetta P, et al. A network of investigator networks in human genome epidemiology. *Am J Epidemiol.* 2005;162(4):302–304.
12. Ioannidis JP, Gwinn M, Little J, et al. Human Genome Epidemiology Network and the Network of Investigator Networks. A roadmap for efficient and reliable human genome epidemiology. *Nat Genet.* 2006;38(1):3–5.
13. Ioannidis JPA, Ralston SH, Bennett ST, et al. Large-scale evidence for differential genetic effects of *ESR1* polymorphisms on osteoporosis outcomes: the GENOMOS Study. *JAMA.* 2004;292(17):2105–2114.
14. Ralston SH, Uitterlinden AG, Brandi ML, et al. Large-scale evidence for the effect of the COLIA1 Sp1 polymorphism on osteoporosis outcomes: the GENOMOS study. *PLoS Med.* 2006;3(4):e90 (EPub).
15. Uitterlinden AG, Ralston SH, Brandi ML, et al. Large-scale analysis of association between common vitamin D receptor gene variations and osteoporosis: the GENOMOS study. *Ann Int Med.* 2006;145(4):255–264.
16. Langdahl BL, Uitterlinden AG, Ralston SH, et al. Large-scale analysis of association between polymorphisms in the transforming growth factor beta 1 gene (TGFB1) and osteoporosis: the GENOMOS study. *Bone.* May 2008;42(5):969–981. Epub December 3, 2007.

17. van Meurs JBJ, Trikalinos T, Ralston SH, et al. Large-scale analysis of association between polymorphisms in the LRP-5 and -6 genes and osteoporosis: the GENOMOS Study. *JAMA.* 2008;299(11):1277–1290.

18. McCarthy MI, Abecasis GR, Cardon LR, et al. Genome-wide association studies for complex traits: consensus, uncertainty and challenges. *Nat Rev Genet.* 2008;9:356–369.

19. Weedon MN, Lango H, Lindgren CM, et al. Genome-wide association analysis identifies 20 loci that influence adult height. *Nat Genet.* 2008;40:575–583.

20. Lettre G, Jackson AU, Gieger C, et al. Identification of ten loci associated with height highlights new biological pathways in human growth. *Nat Genet.* 2008;40:584–591.

21. Gudbjartsson DF, Walters GB, Thorleifsson G, et al. Many sequence variants affecting diversity of adult human height. *Nat Genet.* 2008;40:609–615.

22. Kiel DP, Demissie S, Dupuis J, Lunetta KL, Murabito JM, Karasik D. Genome-wide association with bone mass and geometry in the Framingham Heart Study. *BMC Med Genet.* September 19, 2007;8(Suppl 1):S14.

23. Richards JB, Rivadeneira F, Inouye M, et al. Bone mineral density, osteoporosis, and osteoporotic fractures: a genome-wide association study. *Lancet.* May 3, 2008;371(9623):1505–1512.

24. Styrkarsdottir U, Halldorsson BV, Gretarsdottir S, et al. Multiple genetic loci for bone mineral density and fractures. *N Engl J Med.* 2008;358:2355–2365.

25. Styrkarsdottir U, Halldorsson BV, Gretarsdottir S, et al. New sequence variants associated with bone mineral density. *Nat Genet.* 2008;41:15–17.

26. Cohen JC, Kiss RS, Pertsemlidis A, et al. Multiple rare alleles contribute to low plasma levels of HDL cholesterol. *Science.* 2004;305:869–872.

18

Preterm birth

Siobhan M. Dolan

Preterm birth (PTB) is a perplexing clinical condition and major public health challenge. In 2006, 12.8% of all births in the United States were preterm, defined as occurring before 37 completed weeks of gestation (1). Preterm birth is the second leading cause of infant mortality and the leading cause of infant mortality among black infants in the United States, as well as the major contributor to worldwide infant mortality and morbidity (2). Children born preterm may suffer lifelong morbidities including lung disease, vision and hearing deficits, and other neurosensory impairments (3), and PTB can predispose children to adult diseases such as hypertension and diabetes (4).

Despite the significant public health burden of PTB, there are few effective strategies to reliably predict or prevent PTB (5,6). The etiology of this common complex condition remains elusive. Efforts to identify environmental contributors suggest that smoking, stress, black race, nutritional deficits, and infection contribute to, but do not explain, the majority of PTBs (7). Therefore, the discovery of predisposing genetic variants and relevant gene–environment interactions (see Figure 18.1) will likely be of great value in unraveling the mystery of PTB, by identifying women at risk and setting the stage for research and enhanced clinical and public health prevention strategies.

Systematic Review of the Literature

To summarize current knowledge of gene–disease associations in PTB—and to identify knowledge gaps—a team of researchers from the Preterm Birth International Collaborative (PREBIC), Human Genome Epidemiology Network (HuGENet), World Health Organization (WHO), Albert Einstein College of Medicine (AECOM), Massachusetts General Hospital (MGH), and March of Dimes (MOD) (see acknowledgments for complete list of participants) recently performed a systematic review of the literature on genetic associations with PTB (8), modeled after an approach developed at MGH (9,10). Using a comprehensive search strategy in PubMed and EMBASE, our team identified almost 6,000 relevant abstracts and screened them by hand according to inclusion and exclusion criteria. To be included, articles had to (1) describe human maternal, newborn, or paternal DNA variants in

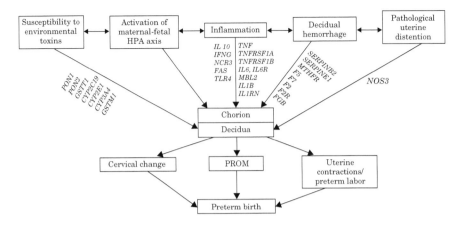

Figure 18.1 Pathways to preterm birth with select gene variants that have been studied. Source: Adapted from Lockwood CJ, Kuczynski E, Paediatr Perinat Epidemiol. *2001;15:78. With permission of Wiley-Blackwell Publishing.*

relation to preterm birth, (2) provide the case definition of preterm birth in gestational weeks at delivery, and (3) report the genotypes for cases and controls. Review articles, family-based studies, case reports, case-only studies, and studies exclusively of twins were excluded. Data were extracted for meta-analysis from the 48 articles that met the inclusion and exclusion criteria.

We compared the 48 articles identified by our search strategy with a search of the HuGE published literature (11) using the HuGE Navigator website (12,13), which identified 47 articles, and the Genetic Association Database (GAD) (14), which identified 3 articles. All articles found by HuGE Navigator and GAD had already been identified by our search strategy.

Overall, these 48 articles provided data on 144 polymorphisms in 76 genes. Thirty-four articles reported data on maternal DNA (15–48), describing 88 polymorphisms in 40 genes, while 26 articles reported on newborn DNA (18,23,27,31,34,35,39–41, 43,44,47,49–62), describing 114 polymorphisms in 63 genes; only 2 articles reported on paternal DNA (40,41), describing 4 polymorphisms in 3 genes.

Our meta-analysis found modest associations of preterm birth with three single nucleotide polymorphisms (SNPs), two in maternal DNA and one in neonatal DNA, which are described under Cumulative Evidence below. The complete field synopsis is available online at http://bioinformatics.aecom.yu.edu/ptbgene/index.html. In this analysis, many lessons were learned that might be valuable for researchers developing field synopses for other health outcomes. The principal challenges related to defining the phenotype, analyzing multiple genomes, capturing high-quality environmental data, reporting genotype data, and grading the evidence, all of which will be further addressed in this chapter.

Defining the Phenotype

Defining the phenotype for PTB is extremely challenging. It might seem straight-forward to determine which infants are born before 37 completed weeks gestation, which is the formal definition of PTB (63), because gestational ages are listed on birth certificates. However, because a multitude of factors contribute to PTB, defining a biologically homogeneous group, in which one might realistically expect to identify an underlying genetic predisposition, is much more difficult.

Approximately 40–45% of PTBs are estimated to follow spontaneous preterm labor, 30–35% are indicated due to maternal or fetal medical complications, and 25–30% follow preterm premature rupture of the membranes (PPROM, which is defined as spontaneous rupture of the membranes at less than 37 weeks gestation at least 1 hour before the onset of contractions) (7). Should we expect to find a genetic variant that contributes to all three types of PTB? For example, if we were to compare the DNA of a woman whose labor was induced at 36 weeks due to preeclampsia with another who underwent a cesarean section at 34 weeks for placenta previa and bleeding, is it plausible that we might identify genetic variants that contribute to both clinical scenarios? Could a spontaneous PTB at 26 weeks secondary to chorioamnionitis be related to the same genetic variants that predispose to delivery of a 35 week newborn whose mother had HELLP (hemolytic anemia, elevated liver enzymes, and low platelet count) syndrome? When etiology creeps into the phenotypic description, it is not clear how subgroups of the PTB phenotype should be defined. Thus, while gestational age dating seems the simplest of measures, the phenotype is much more nuanced. Stratifying the complex phenotype of PTB into sub-phenotypes likely to share underlying predisposing factors is an important step in designing studies to examine genetic associations with PTB.

For the purposes of our systematic review and field synopsis, we applied extremely liberal search criteria in PubMed and EMBASE and included all abstracts that had anything to do with preterm labor or PTB. As a result, we had to screen almost 6,000 abstracts to identify 48 articles that met our inclusion and exclusion criteria. We then read the articles and attempted to classify the PTB phenotype as (1) PTB following preterm labor; (2) PTB following PPROM; (3) PTB following maternal medical complications such as preeclampsia or diabetes; (4) PTB following fetal complications such as small for gestational age (SGA) or intrauterine growth restriction (IUGR); or (5) PTB, not otherwise specified. Our goal for the field synopsis was to identify genetic variants associated with *spontaneous singleton preterm birth*, as this phenotype may be most likely to have a genetic basis; however, in the end this was not possible because in many studies, it was difficult to determine exactly how the phenotype had been defined. Many studies did not differentiate between the five general types of PTB, or grouped all these types together. In the articles that reported maternal data, 18 defined the phenotype as PTB following spontaneous preterm labor, 7 defined the phenotype as spontaneous PTB or PTB following PPROM, and 9 defined the phenotype simply as PTB, without further specification. In the articles that reported newborn data, 6 defined the phenotype as PTB following spontaneous preterm labor, 1 defined it as PTB following PPROM, 3 combined spontaneous and PPROM cases, 1 defined the phenotype as PTB including maternal and fetal indications as well as spontaneous PTB, and 15 defined the phenotype simply as PTB. Neither of the two studies that reported paternal DNA defined the specific PTB phenotype.

Even studies that defined PTB as spontaneous varied in their choice of a gestational age threshold. Many investigators defined PTB, as the National Center for Health Statistics does, as birth before 37 completed weeks gestation (64), but others chose to define PTB as birth before 36 weeks, 35 weeks, 34 weeks, 32 weeks, and so on. Specifically, of the 34 articles that reported maternal genotypes, 24 defined preterm birth as birth before 37 completed weeks gestation, 2 articles used a definition of 36 weeks, 4 used 35 weeks, 2 used 34 weeks, and 2 used 32 weeks. Of the 26 articles reporting on newborn genotypes, 13 defined preterm birth as birth before 37 completed weeks gestation, but 4 used a definition of 36 weeks, 6 used 35 weeks, 1 used 34 weeks, 1 used 30 weeks, and 1 used 27 weeks. The 2 articles that reported paternal genotypes used 37 weeks as the case definition.

Gestational age dating is itself subject to much error and some methods of dating can lead to biased estimates. Methods commonly used for pregnancy dating—including calculation based on last menstrual period, second trimester ultrasound examination, and (more recently and most accurately) first trimester ultrasound examination—produce varying estimates of gestational age. One study in California demonstrated that early ultrasound (<20 weeks gestation) tends to underestimate gestational age and leads to a higher reported incidence of PTB (65). The articles we reviewed generally provided little or no data on the method of pregnancy dating.

Converting the continuous variable of gestational age into a dichotomous outcome—PTB versus term birth—might arbitrarily distort the analysis of biological relationships. Using a cutoff of 37 weeks to define PTB for health statistics serves a purpose by allowing for comparisons and trend analysis; however, it may not be biologically meaningful. Recent trends suggest that some late PTBs (34 0/7 weeks to 36 6/7 weeks) may be due to social factors, such as facility scheduling and patient preference (66); including these births as cases could hinder the analysis of underlying biological and genetic factors. Defining an earlier gestational age threshold (such as very preterm birth, which is defined as <32 weeks) or analyzing gestational age as a continuous variable might be useful to gain a better understanding of underlying genetic associations.

A final concern about phenotype is the relationship between PTB and low birth weight. Preterm birth and low birth weight are related but distinct conditions. Low birth weight is defined as birth weight less than 2,500 g at birth. Historically, PTB and low birth weight have sometimes been used interchangeably in reports of research studies; however, this further confuses accurate description of the PTB phenotype because low birth weight represents two different outcomes: (1) a neonate whose size is appropriate for gestational age but who is born preterm or (2) a neonate who is small for gestational age (SGA), and thus may be >37 weeks gestation but weighs <2,500 g. These two outcomes may derive from quite distinct physiologic processes that may or may not share underlying etiologies. Even now, some studies combine preterm birth with low birth weight to define a single phenotype, blurring the actual entity under study.

Multiple Genomes

Studying the genetic contribution to PTB requires the special consideration of potential interactions among three genomes: the maternal, the fetal, and the paternal. While studies have shown that the greatest contribution is from the maternal genome (67), followed by the fetal and the paternal (68), precise characterization of parental versus fetal genetic contribution to PTB is lacking. Many studies have utilized a case-control study design and compared genotypes of case mothers versus control mothers or case neonates versus control neonates. Another set of studies has used family-based approaches, looking at dyads (mother–newborn) or triads (mother–father–newborn), but these studies are not easily pooled with case-control studies for meta-analysis. Multifactor dimensionality reduction has been used as a nonparametric and genetic model-free alternative to logistic regression for the detection and characterization of nonlinear interactions among discrete genetic and environmental factors (69). Additional methods are needed to sort out the perplexing interplay of genetic variation in three genomes that contributes to PTB. Methods in human genome epidemiology that would allow us to understand the interactions of environmental factors with three genomes would be of great value in better understanding the etiology of PTB.

Further complicating the conduct of studies addressing the relative contributions to PTB of maternal and fetal genetic variation is the fact that the obstetrical research community studies PTB as an outcome, whereas the pediatric community sees PTB as a starting point. For example, many studies that examine genetic factors contributing to pediatric outcomes such as retinopathy of prematurity (70) or bronchopulmonary dysplasia (71) enroll PTBs as the entry cohort, genotype the babies, and follow them for the occurrence of these common outcomes. A large longitudinal study that enrolled mother–infant cohorts prenatally and followed them through the newborn period would have the added value of contributing to our understanding of not only the etiology of PTB but of its varied consequences. Collaborative studies that integrate both the obstetric and pediatric perspective and follow pregnancies and babies longitudinally, such as the National Children's Study (72), promise to add tremendously to our understanding of genetic associations with a host of aspects of pregnancy outcome as well as pediatric well-being.

Environmental Data

A few studies of PTB have examined relevant gene–environment interactions. These include studies of the relationship between *TNF*-α variants and bacterial vaginosis (73) and the interaction of genetic variation in the xenobiotic enzymes *GSTT1* and *CYP1A1* with smoking (32). Many genetic association studies of PTB do not report

any environmental data at all. The detailed description and classification of phenotype serves as a model for the detailed description and classification of environmental exposures that must be collected to study relevant gene–environment interactions
in PTB. Many traditional etiologic studies of PTB have collected detailed environmental data; such data should also be collected in studies of genetic associations
with PTB.

Genotype Data

One of the most surprising findings of our review was the variety of complex ways
in which genotypes were reported. In many analyses, subjects with the homozygous
minor allele and heterozygotes were combined into one category, presumably due to
small sample sizes. In addition, many studies only reported allele frequencies and
did not report genotypes. Sometimes allele frequency data or genotype data were
reported for mothers, sometimes for newborns, and sometimes for both. Paternal
data were reported in only a handful of studies.

A basic recommendation for future studies is to present the numbers of cases and
controls with each genotype in all groups studied. The following 2×3 table can be
used to present maternal genotype data in straightforward fashion:

Table 18.1 Mothers

	# Cases	# Controls
AA genotype		
Aa genotype		
aa genotype		

Genotype data for newborns and fathers should be represented in the same way.
If this simple presentation of the data were required for all publications, as it is by
some journals (74), readers would gain a better understanding of the study population and the process of pooling data for meta-analysis would be greatly enhanced.
Further stratifying such tables, for example, by detailed phenotype or by racial or
ethnic group, would also be useful.

Systematic review of gene–disease associations requires specific data at the level
of genetic variants. Although consistent reporting of SNPs and other variants in
the PTB literature has improved over time, identifying SNPs in older articles can
be challenging. Consistent identification of genetic variants according to a standard
classification scheme, such as dbSNP (75), will facilitate systematic data review and
synthesis. Even when a SNP is identified, deciphering which allele is reported as the
major versus minor allele is often difficult. Using references such as the ancestral
allele in dbSNP (75) can serve as a useful guidepost in the process of standardizing
the reporting of genetic variants.

Cumulative Evidence and Grading the Evidence

Our meta-analysis of ten *maternal* polymorphisms in nine genes found that SNPs in two genes—beta-2 adrenergic receptor (*ADRB2*, rs1042713) and interferon gamma (*IFNG*, rs2430561)—had nominally significant associations with PTB (p-values in the main, allele-based analyses were $p = 0.0096$ and $p = 0.014$, respectively). Meta-analysis of seven *neonatal* polymorphisms in seven genes found one SNP in coagulation factor 2 (*F2*, rs1799963) with a nominal association with PTB ($p = 0.03$). Updated data are available online at http://bioinformatics.aecom.yu.edu/ptbgene/index.html.

Cumulative evidence for genetic associations can be assessed by using three criteria (the "Venice criteria") proposed by the Network of Networks and HuGENet: (1) the amount of evidence; (2) the extent of replication; and (3) the degree of protection from bias (76). No gene–disease association in our field synopsis warranted an A grade in any of these three categories.

Amount of evidence. Many of the studies we reviewed were case reports (which we excluded) or small case-control studies, with an average size of 35–600 cases and usually a somewhat larger number of controls. Only 9 of the 34 reported analyses of maternal DNA and 10 of the 26 analyses of neonatal DNA included more than 100 cases; thus, even when 3 studies had evaluated a particular SNP, the total number of cases studied was usually well under 1,000.

Extent of replication. Many SNPs were evaluated in only one or two studies. Sufficient data for meta-analysis, reported from three or more studies, were available for ten polymorphisms in nine genes for maternal DNA and seven polymorphisms in seven genes for newborn DNA. Nearly all observed associations were statistically nonsignificant when the first study was excluded from analysis. The lack of replication we observed suggests that larger cohorts are needed for both gene discovery and replication.

Degree of protection from bias. Genetic association studies of PTB are also subject to many biases, beginning with those arising from inconsistencies in defining the phenotype.

Conclusion

The public health burden of PTB continues to mount and the clinical management remains challenging. Research attempting to understand the genetic contribution to PTB has produced a modest amount of literature, consisting mostly of candidate gene studies, which have thus far not revealed robust and replicated gene–disease associations. A better understanding of the genetic contribution to PTB and what it might reveal about the underlying biology and etiology of this common complex condition will likely be enhanced by genome-wide association studies (GWAS).

GWAS allow hypothesis-free interrogation of the genome and will likely uncover novel contributions to PTB. Although the technology for GWAS is becoming more accessible and affordable (77), our experience points out that the success of such studies is contingent upon (i) good clinical phenotyping; (ii) detailed data collection regarding environmental exposures; (iii) enhanced methods to look at the interaction of multiple genomes; and (iv) continued use of standardized genotyping and reporting methods using common nomenclature. Dissecting the complex, heterogeneous phenotype of PTB remains a huge research and clinical challenge. Human genome epidemiology holds promise for helping to address this public health challenge.

Acknowledgments

The systematic review and meta-analysis was performed by Mads V. Hollegaard, Mario Merialdi, Ana Pilar Betran, Tomas Allen, Chaya Abelow, Judith Nace, Bruce K. Lin, Muin J. Khoury, John P.A. Ioannidis, Sachin Bagade, Xin Zheng, Robert A. Dubin, Lars Bertram, Digna R. Velez, Ramkumar Menon, and Siobhan M. Dolan.

Thanks to Drs. Irwin Merkatz, Michael Katz, Calvin Hobel, Charles Lockwood, Alan Fleischman and the HuGENet and PREBIC memberships, June Kinoshita and the Alzheimer Research Forum, the Genetics and Aging Research Unit at Massachusetts General Hospital, Marta Gwinn, Wei Yu and the Office of Public Health Genomics at CDC, Vishwa Niranjan at Albert Einstein College of Medicine, and Motoko Oinuma at March of Dimes for technical assistance.

Funding has been provided by the World Health Organization, Preterm Birth International Collaborative, Albert Einstein College of Medicine, March of Dimes, and the Cure Alzheimer's Fund.

References

1. Martin JA, Hamilton BE, Sutton PD, et al. Births: final data for 2006. *Natl Vital Stat Rep.* 2009;57:1–101.
2. Merialdi M, Murray JC. The changing face of preterm birth. *Pediatrics.* 2007;120(5):1133–1134.
3. Fawke J. Neurological outcomes following preterm birth. *Semin Fetal Neonatal Med.* 2007;12(5):374–382.
4. Eriksson JG. The fetal origins hypothesis—10 years on. *BMJ.* 2005;330(7500):1096–1097.
5. Iams JD. Prediction and early detection of preterm labor. *Obstet Gynecol.* 2003;101(2):402–412.
6. Iams JD, Romero R, Culhane JF, Goldenberg RL. Primary, secondary, and tertiary interventions to reduce the morbidity and mortality of preterm birth. *Lancet.* 2008;371(9607):164–175.
7. Goldenberg RL, Culhane JF, Iams JD, Romero R. Epidemiology and causes of preterm birth. *Lancet.* 2008;371(9606):75–84.
8. PTBGene the preterm birth genetics knowledge base. Available at http://bioinformatics. aecom.yu.edu/ptbgene/index.html. Accessed September 4, 2009.
9. Bertram L, McQueen MB, Mullin K, Blacker D, Tanzi RE. Systematic meta-analyses of Alzheimer disease genetic association studies: the AlzGene database. *Nat Genet.* 2007;39(1):17–23.

10. Allen NC, Bagade S, McQueen MB, et al. Systematic meta-analyses and field synopsis of genetic association studies in schizophrenia: the SzGene database. *Nat Genet.* 2008;40(7):827–834.

11. Lin BK, Clyne M, Walsh M, et al. Tracking the epidemiology of human genes in the literature: the HuGE Published Literature database. *Am J Epidemiol.* 2006;164(1):1–4.

12. HuGE Navigator at http://www.hugenavigator.net. Accessed January 28, 2009.

13. Yu W, Gwinn M, Clyne M, Yesupriya A, Khoury MJ. A navigator for human genome epidemiology. *Nat Genet.* 2008;40(2):124–125.

14. Genetic Association Database at http://geneticassociationdb.nih.gov/. Accessed January 28, 2009.

15. Amory JH, Adams KM, Lin MT, Hansen JA, Eschenbach DA, Hitti J. Adverse outcomes after preterm labor are associated with tumor necrosis factor-(alpha) polymorphism -863, but not -308, in mother-infant pairs. *Am J Obstet Gynecol.* 2004;191(4):1362–1367.

16. Edwards RK, Ferguson RJ, Duff P. The interleukin-1(beta) +3953 single nucleotide polymorphism: Cervical protein concentration and preterm delivery risk. *Am J Reprod Immunol.* 2006;55(4):259–264.

17. Engel SM, Olshan AF, Siega-Riz AM, Savitz DA, Chanock SJ. Polymorphisms in folate metabolizing genes and risk for spontaneous preterm and small-for-gestational age birth. *Am J Obstet Gynecol.* 2006;195(5):1231.

18. Genc MR, Gerber S, Nesin M, Witkin SS. Polymorphism in the interleukin-1 gene complex and spontaneous preterm delivery. *Am J Obstet Gynecol.* 2002;187(1):157–163.

19. Jamie WE, Edwards RK, Ferguson RJ, Duff P. The interleukin-6 -174 single nucleotide polymorphism: cervical protein production and the risk of preterm delivery. *Am J Obstet Gynecol.* 2005;192(4):1023–1027.

20. Landau R, Xie HG, Dishy V, et al. (beta)(2)-adrenergic receptor genotype and preterm delivery. *Am J Obstet Gynecol.* 2002;187(5):1294–1298.

21. Lawlor DA, Gaunt TR, Hinks LJ, et al. The association of the PON1 Q192R polymorphism with complications and outcomes of pregnancy: findings from the British Women's Heart and Health cohort study. *Paediatr Perinat Epidemiol.* 2006;20(3): 244–250.

22. Mattar R, De Souza E, Daher S. Preterm delivery and cytokine gene polymorphisms. *Journal of Reproductive Medicine for the Obstetrician and Gynecologist.* 2006;51(4 SUPPL.):317–320.

23. Menon R, Velez DR, Thorsen P, et al. Ethnic differences in key candidate genes for spontaneous preterm birth: TNF-(alpha) and its receptors. *Hum Hered.* 2006;62(2):107–118.

24. Murtha AP, Nieves A, Hauser ER, et al. Association of maternal IL-1 receptor antagonist intron 2 gene polymorphism and preterm birth. *Am J Obstet Gynecol.* 2006;195(5):1249–1253.

25. Ozkur M, Dogulu F, Ozkur A, Gokmen B, Inaloz SS, Aynacioglu AS. Association of the Gln27Glu polymorphism of the beta-2-adrenergic receptor with preterm labor. *Int J Gynecol Obstet.* 2002;77(3):209–215.

26. Papazoglou D, Galazios G, Koukourakis MI, Kontomanolis EN, Maltezos E. Association of -634G/C and 936C/T polymorphisms of the vascular endothelial growth factor with spontaneous preterm delivery. *Acta Obstet Gynecol Scand.* 2004;83(5):461–465.

27. Resch B, Gallistl S, Kutschera J, Mannhalter C, Muntean W, Mueller WD. Thrombophilic polymorphisms—factor V Leiden, prothrombin G20210A, and methylenetetrahydrofolate reductase C677T mutations—and preterm birth. *Wien Klin Wochenschr.* 2004;116 (17 18):622–626.

28. Simhan HN, Krohn MA, Roberts JM, Zeevi A, Caritis SN. Interleukin-6 promoter—174 polymorphism and spontaneous preterm birth. *Am J Obstetr Gynecol.* 2003;189(4):915–918.

29. Stonek F, Hafner E, Philipp K, Hefler LA, Bentz EK, Tempfer CB. Methylenetetrahydrofolate reductase C677T polymorphism and pregnancy complications. *Obstet Gynecol.* 2007; 110(2 Pt 1):363–368.

30. Valdez LL, Quintero A, Garcio E, et al. Thrombophilic polymorphisms in preterm delivery. *Blood Cells Mol Dis.* 2004;33(1):51–56.

31. Velez DR, Menon R, Thorsen P, et al. Ethnic differences in interleukin 6 (IL-6) and IL6 receptor genes in spontaneous preterm birth and effects on amniotic fluid protein levels. *Ann Hum Genet.* 2007;71(Pt 5):586–600.

32. Wang X, Zuckerman B, Pearson C, et al. Maternal cigarette smoking, metabolic gene polymorphism, and infant birth weight. *JAMA.* 2002;287(2):195–202.

33. Annells MF, Hart PH, Mulligan CG, et al. Interleukins-1, -4, -6, -10, tumor necrosis factor, transforming growth factor-(beta), FAS, and mannose-binding protein C gene polymorphisms in Australian women: risk of preterm birth. *Am J Obstetr Gynecol.* 2004;191(6):2056–2067.

34. Doh K, Sziller I, Vardhana S, Kovacs E, Papp Z, Witkin SS. (beta)2-adrenergic receptor gene polymorphisms and pregnancy outcome. *J Perinat Med.* 2004;32(5):413–417.

35. Grisaru-Granovsky S, Tevet A, Bar-Shavit R, et al. Association study of protease activated receptor 1 gene polymorphisms and adverse pregnancy outcomes: results of a pilot study in Israel. *Am J Med Genet A.* 2007;143(21):2557–2563.

36. Moore S, Ide M, Randhawa M, Walker JJ, Reid JG, Simpson NA. An investigation into the association among preterm birth, cytokine gene polymorphisms and periodontal disease. *BJOG.* 2004;111(2):125–132.

37. Roberts AK, Monzon-Bordonaba F, Van Deerlin PG, et al. Association of polymorphism within the promoter of the tumor necrosis factor (alpha) gene with increased risk of preterm premature rupture of the fetal membranes. *Am J Obstetr Gynecol.* 1999;180(5):1297–1302.

38. Erichsen HC, Engel SA, Eck PK, et al. Genetic variation in the sodium-dependent vitamin C transporters, SLC23A1, and SLC23A2 and risk for preterm delivery. *Am J Epidemiol.* 2006;163(3):245–254.

39. Speer EM, Gentile DA, Zeevi A, Pillage G, Huo D, Skoner DP. Role of single nucleotide polymorphisms of cytokine genes in spontaneous preterm delivery. *Hum Immunol.* 2006;67(11):915–923.

40. Chen D, Hu Y, Chen C, et al. Polymorphisms of the paraoxonase gene and risk of preterm delivery. *Epidemiology.* 2004;15(4):466–470.

41. Chen DF, Hu Y, Yang F, et al. Mother's and child's methylenetetrahydrofolate reductase C677T polymorphism is associated with preterm delivery and low birth weight. *Beijing Da Xue Xue Bao.* 2004;36(3):248–253.

42. Erhardt E, Stankovics J, Molnár D, Adamovich K, Melegh B. High prevalence of factor V Leiden mutation in mothers of premature neonates. *Biol Neonate.* 2000; 78(2):145–146.

43. Hartel C, Finas D, Ahrens P, et al. Polymorphisms of genes involved in innate immunity: association with preterm delivery. *Mol Hum Reprod.* 2004;10(12):911–915.

44. Hartel C, von Otte S, Koch J, et al. Polymorphisms of haemostasis genes as risk factors for preterm delivery. *Thromb Haemost.* 2005;94(1):88–92.

45. Johnson WG, Scholl TO, Spychala JR, Buyske S, Stenroos ES, Chen X. Common dihydrofolate reductase 19-base pair deletion allele: a novel risk factor for preterm delivery. *Am J Clin Nutr.* 2005;81(3):664–668.

46. Kocher O, Cirovic C, Malynn E, et al. Obstetric complications in patients with hereditary thrombophilia identified using the LCx microparticle enzyme immunoassay: a controlled study of 5,000 patients. *Am J Clin Pathol.* 2007;127(1):68–75.

47. Nukui T, Day RD, Sims CS, Ness RB, Romkes M. Maternal/newborn GSTT1 null genotype contributes to risk of preterm, low birthweight infants. *Pharmacogenetics.* 2004;14(9):569–576.

48. Nurk E, Tell GS, Refsum H, Ueland PM, Vollset SE. Factor V Leiden, pregnancy complications and adverse outcomes: The Hordaland Homocysteine Study. *QJM.* 2006;99(5):289–298.

49. Aidoo M, McElroy PD, Kolczak MS, et al. Tumor necrosis factor-(alpha) promoter variant 2 (TNF2) is associated with pre-term delivery, infant mortality, and malaria morbidity in western Kenya: Asembo bay cohort project IX. *Genet Epidemiol.* 2001;21(3):201–211.

50. Ameglio F, Vento G, Romagnoli C, Giardina B, Capoluongo E. Association of MBL2 variants with early preterm delivery [1]. *Genet Med.* 2007;9(2):136–137.

51. Bessler H, Osovsky M, Sirota L. Association between IL-1ra gene polymorphism and premature delivery. *Biol Neonate.* 2004;85(3):179–183.

52. Bodamer OA, Mitterer G, Maurer W, Pollak A, Mueller MW, Schmidt WM. Evidence for an association between mannose-binding lectin 2 (MBL2) gene polymorphisms and pre-term birth. *Genet Med.* 2006;8(8):518–524.

53. Capasso M, Avvisati RA, Piscopo C, et al. Cytokine gene polymorphisms in Italian pre-term infants: association between interleukin-10 -1082 G/A polymorphism and respiratory distress syndrome. *Pediatr Res.* 2007;61(3):313–317.

54. Chen BH, Carmichael SL, Shaw GM, Iovannisci DM, Lammer EJ. Association between 49 infant gene polymorphisms and preterm delivery. *Am J Med Genet A.* 2007;143(17):1990–1996.

55. Fuks A, Parton LA, Polavarapu S, et al. Polymorphism of Fas and Fas ligand in pre-term premature rupture of membranes in singleton pregnancies. *Am J Obstet Gynecol.* 2005;193(3 Pt 2):1132–1136.

56. Gibson CS, MacLennan AH, Dekker GA, et al. Genetic polymorphisms and spontaneous preterm birth. *Obstet Gynecol.* 2007;109(2 PART 1):384–391.

57. Gopel W, Kim D, Gortner L. Prothrombotic mutations as a risk factor for preterm birth. *Lancet.* 1999;353(9162):1411–1412.

58. Liang HY, Wu BY, Chen DF, et al. Association of CYP2E1 and PON2311 polymorphisms in neonates with preterm. *Acta Genetica Sinica.* 2002;29(10):847–853.

59. Lorenz E, Hallman M, Marttila R, Haataja R, Schwartz DA. Association between the Asp299Gly polymorphisms in the toll-like receptor 4 and premature births in the Finnish population. *Pediatr Res.* 2002;52(3):373–376.

60. Meirhaeghe A, Boreham CA, Murray LJ, et al. A possible role for the PPARG Pro12Ala polymorphism in preterm birth. *Diabetes.* 2007;56(2):494–498.

61. Moonen RM, Paulussen AD, Souren NY, Kessels AG, Rubio-Gozalbo ME, Villamor E. Carbamoyl phosphate synthetase polymorphisms as a risk factor for necrotizing entero-colitis. *Pediatr Res.* 2007;62(2):188–190.

62. Wu BY, Liang HY, Chen DF, et al. Associations of Rsa I polymorphism at the 5' flanking region of CYP2E1 and PON2 148 polymorphism in neonates with preterm delivery. *Acta Genetica Sinica.* 2003;30(6):577–583.

63. Engle WA, Tomashek KM, Wallman C. "Late-preterm" infants: a population at risk. *Pediatrics.* 2007;120(6):1390–1401.

64. National Center for Health Statistics at http://www.cdc.gov/nchs/fastats/births.htm. Accessed January 28, 2009.

65. Dietz PM, England LJ, Callaghan WM, Pearl M, Wier ML, Kharrazi M. A comparison of LMP-based and ultrasound-based estimates of gestational age using linked California livebirth and prenatal screening records. *Paediatr Perinat Epidemiol.* 2007;21 (Suppl 2):62–71.

66. Raju TN. Late-preterm births: challenges and opportunities. *Pediatrics.* 2008;121(2): 402–403.

67. Wilcox AJ, Skaerven R, Lie RT. Familial patterns of preterm delivery: maternal and fetal contributions. *Am J Epidemiol.* 2008;167(4):474–479.

68. Lie RT, Wilcox AJ, Skjaerven R. Maternal and paternal influences on length of pregnancy. *Obstet Gynecol.* 2006;107(4):880–885.

69. Menon R, Velez DR, Simhan H, et al. Multilocus interactions at maternal tumor necrosis factor-(alpha), tumor necrosis factor receptors, interleukin-6 and interleukin-6 receptor genes predict spontaneous preterm labor in European-American women. *Am J Obstet Gynecol.* 2006;194(6):1616–1624.

70. Banyasz I, Bokodi G, Vannay A, et al. Genetic polymorphisms of vascular endothelial growth factor and angiopoietin 2 in retinopathy of prematurity. *Curr Eye Res.* 2006;31(7–8):685–690.

71. Hilgendorff A, Heidinger K, Pfeiffer A, et al. Association of polymorphisms in the mannose-binding lectin gene and pulmonary morbidity in preterm infants. *Genes Immun.* 2007;8(8):671–677.

72. The National Children's Study. Available at http://www.nationalchildrensstudy.gov/Pages/default.aspx. Accessed January 28, 2009.

73. Macones GA, Parry S, Elkousy M, Clothier B, Ural SH, Strauss JF. A polymorphism in the promoter region of TNF and bacterial vaginosis: Preliminary evidence of gene-environment interaction in the etiology of spontaneous preterm birth. *Am J Obstet Gynecol.* 2004;190(6):1504–1508.

74. Framework for a fully powered risk engine. *Nat Genet.* 2005;37(11):1153.

75. dbSNP at http://www.ncbi.nlm.nih.gov/projects/SNP/. Accessed January 28, 2009.

76. Ioannidis JP, Boffetta P, Little J, et al. Assessment of cumulative evidence on genetic associations: interim guidelines. *Int J Epidemiol.* 2008;37(1):120–132.

77. Chanock SJ, Manolio T, Boehnke M, et al. Replicating genotype-phenotype associations. *Nature.* 2007;447(7145):655–660.

19

Coronary heart disease

Adam S. Butterworth, Julian P. T. Higgins, Nadeem Sarwar, and John Danesh

Introduction

Coronary heart disease (CHD)—which includes myocardial infarction, angina pectoris, and stenosis of the coronary arteries—is a public health problem of substantial international importance. It is the leading cause of death worldwide, with over 7 million deaths per year (1), a major source of disability and a considerable economic burden (2). Over the past half-century, several major modifiable risk factors have been identified, such as smoking, diabetes, elevated levels of blood pressure, and circulating lipids. The tendency for CHD to cluster in families (coefficient of familial clustering [λs] estimated to be between two and seven) suggests that genetic variation, either directly or through modulation of known or as yet unidentified risk factors, importantly influences CHD risk (3). Identification of CHD susceptibility variants is of potential interest because it should contribute to insights into disease pathophysiology that may translate into clinical benefits through (i) identification of novel therapeutics; (ii) improved stratification of disease risk in vulnerable populations; (iii) more cost-effective targeting of existing interventions; and (iv) identification and understanding of joint gene–environment effects. The realization of these potential benefits is, however, predicated on reliable genetic discovery and validation.

Progress in identifying the genome sequence variants underlying the inherited effects has been slow. Until recently, studies have typically involved biological approaches to candidate identification, leading to specific explorations of candidate genes in lipid, inflammatory, hemostatic, and other pathways suggested by prevailing mechanistic understanding. Many of the early reports of promising findings using this approach have, however, not been confirmed by later and larger studies. More recently, genome-wide association studies (GWAS) have examined CHD associations with large numbers of variants distributed across the genome, entailing hypothesis-free global-testing methods. This approach is starting to uncover novel loci with strong evidence of association with CHD, but with as-yet unknown biological relevance.

This chapter provides a critical and quantitative review of the current state of evidence regarding potential genetic susceptibility loci and CHD. We review published quantitative reviews of candidate gene polymorphisms and published GWAS addressing CHD.

Methods

Candidate Gene Association Studies

We sought all published quantitative reviews of association studies of genetic variants and CHD outcomes. Quantitative reviews were defined as reviews of at least three gene–disease association studies in which numerical data from each study were presented systematically. CHD endpoints were defined as myocardial infarction (MI), angina pectoris (stable or unstable), coronary stenosis, or coronary death. Search strategies included coronary disease terms, genetic terms, and phrases to identify reviews or meta-analyses and were applied to electronic databases including PubMed, Embase, BIOSIS, and Web of Science. We scanned titles and abstracts of identified articles to exclude papers that were obviously irrelevant. Full text copies of remaining articles were collected and examined against prespecified inclusion criteria.

For each polymorphism that had been reviewed, we selected the single most informative review based on the number of studies included, total number of participants across studies, and the date of publication. We collected details of the polymorphisms studied, the methods used to find and assess studies, and summary results, and collated the information into a highly structured database. In addition, we collected details of participants and design of all association studies in each review, referring back to the original articles where necessary. We conducted rigorous meta-analyses based on the studies included in the original quantitative reviews, and made adjustments to results where investigators appeared to have extracted data incorrectly or used inappropriate methods to pool studies (e.g., double counting of cases or controls).

Analysis

We conducted meta-analyses using standard fixed-effect and random-effects methods, assuming a per-allele genetic model when data were available by genotype. For variants where some studies reported only partial genotype data (i.e., numbers of carriers and noncarriers), prohibiting a per-allele model, we used the genetic model adopted by authors of the original review. We also conducted fixed-effect meta-analyses to contrast results from larger studies (at least 500 cases or 1,000 total participants) with those from smaller studies, and to contrast studies conducted in exclusively white populations with those in exclusively East Asian populations. The fixed-effect model was chosen for these subsidiary analyses, recognizing that this does not account for heterogeneity, in order to avoid placing excess weight on smaller studies that may be more prone to selective reporting bias and inflated effect sizes. Formal tests for differences between subgroups were performed using a chi-squared test, with Harbord's modified regression test used to assess funnel plot asymmetry (4).

For presentation in the main table of findings, we undertook a more complex meta-analysis for each variant that enabled us to (i) present a per-allele odds ratio in every case, irrespective of how data were reported and (ii) address to some extent the dependence of association magnitudes on study size. For this we implemented a model that exploits a Hardy–Weinberg equilibrium (HWE) assumption to "recreate" genotype data from incompletely reported results (5). We further extended this to a random-effects meta-regression of (log) odds ratio on inverse sample size, and calculated the predicted magnitude corresponding to the largest observed study within each meta-analysis, along with its confidence interval (6). The model was implemented in a Bayesian framework using WinBUGS (7), assuming noninformative prior distributions.

We describe the amount of evidence available for each variant using the number of included association studies, the numbers of participants (cases and controls), and the amount of information in each review, defined by the sum of the weights from an inverse variance meta-analysis model. We describe the consistency of evidence using the I^2 statistic, since it can be compared across different effect measures and across different numbers of studies (8). Allele frequencies for the allele of interest were calculated by pooling genotype counts in the control groups across studies, assuming HWE in studies for which complete genotype information was not available.

Concerns about Bias

Bias in a genetic association study can arise at several different stages of investigation: definition of outcomes, ascertainment of participants, assessment of genotypes, and reporting of results (9). Further biases may occur at the quantitative review stage if reporting of studies is related to the magnitude of association (publication bias). Characteristics of studies and reviews that could suggest presence of such biases were collected with emphasis on the numbers of studies for which the control group deviated from HWE, the number of studies in which it was known that investigators were blinded to case-control status when calling genotypes, the design of studies (retrospective or prospective), source of study controls (general population or other, for example, hospital or clinic controls), use of formal systematic review methods to ascertain association studies, and attempts to correspond with study authors to confirm, collect, or ascertain data. Insufficient information was generally provided by individual reports to enable assessment of the possibility of genotyping errors. We provide comments on concerns about potential biases in each review in preference to using quality assessment scales.

For presentation in the main summary table, we classified each meta-analysis using the following criteria. A nonsystematic review indicated that a thorough attempt to find all published literature had not been described in the review methods. Funnel plot asymmetry (FPA) was considered to be present when there were at least ten studies and either the Harbord test or a test comparing larger and smaller studies was statistically significant at the 5% level. Concerns over ethnicity arose when a test of difference between whites and East Asians was statistically significant at a 5% level and there were at least two studies in each category. We expressed concern over HWE if exclusion of studies that could be determined to have statistically significant departure from HWE changed the summary odds ratio by more than 5%. Heterogeneity was considered to be present when there were at least five studies and either I^2 was greater than 50% or a lower 95% confidence interval for I^2 exceeded 20%.

GWA Studies

We sought GWAS involving more than 10,000 variants by searching the recent literature for terms such as "genome-wide" and "whole-genome." We extracted summary information from each GWA study with details of most significant loci identified and significance thresholds required for replication. We also examined whether these findings had been replicated in independent samples, and collected per-allele odds ratios for the strongest signals. For the locus at 9p21.3, these odds ratios and their confidence intervals were pooled across samples using a random-effects meta-analysis model with inverse variance weighting.

Results

Candidate Gene Reviews

We identified quantitative reviews of 48 variants in 33 candidate genes, reported in 24 articles (10–33) (Table 19.1). Numbers of studies included in each review ranged from 3 to 108 studies per variant, with a median of 19. Most variants had been studied in a total of between 10,000 and 100,000 participants, although only 15 variants had been studied in more than 10,000 cases.

Despite the existence of considerable evidence on several polymorphisms, few appeared to have strong, consistent associations with CHD. Only one polymorphism—the *e4* variant of the apolipoprotein E (*APOE*) gene—had a 95% confidence interval that excludes the null, once size effects were taken into account. Excluding variants with so much uncertainty that 95% confidence intervals extend beyond the scale in Table 19.1, per-allele odds ratio estimates ranged from 0.88 to 1.24. Considerable heterogeneity was seen for half of the variants with I^2 values greater than 50% in 24 of the meta-analyses and a lower 95% confidence interval exceeding 20% in two further meta-analyses. Study size effects, which may be indicative of publication bias, were also commonly seen with 18 variants showing funnel plot asymmetry or having significantly different summary results in larger and smaller studies (Table 19.2). Despite the heterogeneity present in the data on many variants, the results calculated using random-effects models were generally similar to those using fixed-effect models. For five variants, the statistical significance of the meta-analytic mean depended on the meta-analysis model used, and for *e4* carriers of the *APOE* gene the confidence intervals for fixed-effect and random-effects meta-analyses do not overlap (see Section "Discussion").

A number of polymorphisms appeared to exhibit different effects in populations of different ethnicity. Summary estimates differed significantly ($p < 0.05$) between whites and East Asians in 9 of the 32 meta-analyses in which participants from each group were included. In some cases, allele frequencies also differed importantly between the two groups. For example, the *XbaI* polymorphism of the apolipoprotein B gene has a frequency of 0.52 in white controls, but a frequency of 0.95 in East Asian controls, with apparently opposing associations (although the estimate in East Asian populations was not significantly different from the null).

We summarized study characteristics that might be associated with biases in Table 19.3. Nearly half of the meta-analyses (23/48) contained at least 10% of studies with a statistically significant ($p < 0.05$) deviation from HWE in controls, suggestive of potential genotyping error in these studies; however, exclusion of these studies from meta-analyses only altered the summary odds ratio by more than 5% for four of the variants. Genotyping call rates were rarely reported, so we could not assess this important feature. A third of studies (374/1126, or 34%) reported that laboratory technicians were blinded to case-control status when genotyping. The majority of studies (89%) were case-control or cross-sectional in design, with a small proportion of prospective cohort studies or nested case-control studies based in prospective cohorts (and, therefore, using "internal" population controls). Overall, controls in available studies were drawn approximately evenly from essentially general population sources and other sources such as clinics or hospitals where disease-free status was not guaranteed.

Genome-Wide Studies

By January 2009, seven GWAS assessing associations with CHD had been published that included at least 10,000 variants (34–40) (Table 19.4). One particular locus (9p21.3) has been consistently replicated in the four densest studies, indicating the presence of a potentially "true" association with a single nucleotide polymorphism (SNP) at this locus, although the exact causal SNP has not yet been identified. A meta-analysis of SNPs from GWAS and replication studies that have genotyped SNPs in this region (35,37,39,41–50) showed a highly significant association with an increase in risk of about 30% for each copy of the risk allele carried (Figure 19.1). Other loci that warrant further investigation are those that have been replicated in large studies, such as 6q25.1 and 2q36.3 replicated in the German MI study (39). Significant SNPs at 16q23 have also been identified in two initial GWAS (WTCCC and Framingham Heart Study), although the *p*-values in each study did not reach genome-wide statistical significance and the region was not replicated in other samples. Focused genotyping in large numbers of cases will be required to confirm or refute these weaker findings, as seen when apparent associations with the rs909253 SNP in the lymphotoxin alpha gene at 6p21.3 discovered by the OACIS GWA study (38) were not replicated in a number of follow-up studies, including the ISIS study of over 6,000 cases (14).

Table 19.1 Summary details of 48 reviews of polymorphisms with CHD outcomes

Biological pathway	REPORT		First study	Reviews*	GENETIC VARIANT					Freq†	Outcome
	Author	Year			Gene	Variant	Allele	Posn	rs		
Lipids											
	Bennet	2007	1983	5	APOE	e4	e4	exon4	7412/429358	0.15	CHD
	Bennet	2007	1983	5	APOE	e2	e2	exon4	7412/429358	0.09	CHD
	Sagoo	2008	1995	5	LPL	N291S	S	exon 6	268	0.03	CHD
	Sagoo	2008	1992	6	LPL	S447X	X	exon 9	328	0.10	CHD
	Sagoo	2008	1995	4	LPL	D9N	N	exon2	1801177	0.02	CHD
	Sagoo	2008	1990	3	LPL	PvuII	P2	intron 6	285	0.46	CHD
	Sagoo	2008	1996	2	LPL	T-93G	G	promoter	1800590	0.02	CHD
	Sagoo	2008	1989	2	LPL	HindIII	H1	intron 8	320	0.29	CHD
	Sagoo	2008	1997	3	LPL	G188E	E	exon 5	–	<0.01	CHD
	Lawlor	2004	1995	3	PON1	Q192R	R	exon 6	662	0.32	CHD
	Wheeler	2004	1997	2	PON1	L55M	M	exon 3	854560	0.27	CHD
	Wheeler	2004	2000	1	PON1	T-107C	C	promoter	705379	0.47	CHD
	Wheeler	2004	1998	1	PON2	S311C	C	exon 9	7493	0.22	CHD
	Boekholdt	2005	1995	1	CETP	TaqIB	B2	intron 1	708272	0.44	CHD
	Chiodini	2003	1990	2	APOB	SpIns/Del	Del	exon 1	11279109	0.31	CHD
	Chiodini	2003	1986	2	APOB	XBal	X-	exon 26	693	0.63	CHD
	Chiodini	2003	1986	2	APOB	EcoRI	E-	exon 29	1042031	0.14	CHD
Inflammation											
	Sie	2006	2001	1	IL6	G-174C	C	promoter	1800795	0.42	CHD
	Clarke	2006	2002	1	LTA	rs909253	C	intron 1	909253	0.37	MI
	Koch	2008	2001	1	THBS4	A387P	P	exon 10	1866389	0.22	MI
	Koch	2008	2001	1	THBS1	N700S	S	exon 13	2228262	0.10	MI
	Koch	2008	2001	1	THBS2	T3949G	G	3'UTR	8089	0.24	MI
	Pereira	2007	1998	2	TNF-alpha	G-308A	A	promoter	1800629	0.15	CHD
	Koch	2006	2003	1	TLR4	D299G	G	exon 3	4986790	0.07	MI
	Abilleira	2006	1999	1	MMP3	5A/6A	5A	promoter	3025058	0.31	MI
	Abilleira	2006	2001	1	MMP9	C-1562T	T	promoter	3918242	0.12	Stenosis
Renin-angiotensin											
	Morgan	2003	1992	9	ACE	I/D	Del	intron 16	1799752	0.52	MI
	Xu	2007	1995	2	AGT	M235T	T	exon 2	699	0.48	CHD
	Xu	2007	1995	2	AGT	T174M	M	exon 2	4762	0.12	CHD
	Casas	2006	1998	2	NOS3	E298D	D	exon 8	1799983	0.26	CHD
	Casas	2006	1998	2	NOS3	T-786C	C	promoter	2070744	0.23	CHD
	Casas	2006	1996	2	NOS3	intron 4	a	intron 4	–	0.14	CHD
	Ntzani	2007	1994	1	AGTR1	A1166C	C	3'UTR	5186	0.27	MI
Hemostasis											
	Ye	2006	1995	8	Factor V	R506Q	Q	exon 10	6025	0.03	CHD
	Ye	2006	1996	9	ITGB3/GPIIIa	P1A1/A2	A2	exon 2	5918	0.15	CHD
	Ye	2006	1997	5	Factor II	G20210A	A	3'UTR	1799963	0.01	CHD
	Ye	2006	1991	4	PAI-1	4G/5G	4G	promoter	1799889	0.52	CHD
	Ye	2006	1995	2	Factor VII	R353Q	Q	exon 8	6046	0.12	CHD
	Ye	2006	1999	1	GPIa	C807T	T	exon 7	1126643	0.38	CHD
	Ye	2006	1997	1	GPIba	T-5C	C	promoter	2243093	0.13	CHD
	Keavney	2006	1993	3	FGB	G-455A	A	promoter	1800790	0.20	CHD
	Voko	2007	1998	2	Factor XIII	V34L	L	exon 2	5985	0.24	CHD

Cases	Controls	Total	n‡	Info§	Per-allele OR & 95% CI	I² & 95% CI		Non	FPA	Ethn	HWE	Het
31816	69017	100833	108	3227	1.15 (1.03, 1.28)	70	(64, 75)	○	●	●	○	●
26469	59724	86193	108	1733	0.90 (0.80, 1.02)	57	(46, 65)	○	○	●	○	●
13883	24145	38028	21	371	1.02 (0.88, 1.21)	5	(0, 49)	○	○	◐	○	○
11050	20221	31271	26	878	0.88 (0.74, 1.00)	50	(21, 68)	○	○	●	○	●
9812	18519	28331	21	272	1.24 (1.00, 1.56)	17	(0, 51)	○	○	◐	○	○
8440	8774	17214	18	1985	0.99 (0.86, 1.16)	32	(0, 61)	○	○	○	○	○
5045	10395	15440	7	107	1.11 (0.72, 1.52)	10	(0, 74)	○	◐	◐	○	○
6226	5244	11470	23	635	0.94 (0.84, 1.07)	16	(0, 49)	○	○	○	○	○
2524	8595	11119	3	3	1.41 (0.26, 6.99)	0	–	○	◐	◐	○	◐
10816	16706	27522	38	2244	1.07 (0.96, 1.21)	61	(0, 64)	○	●	●	○	●
5989	6427	12416	20	944	1.00 (0.91, 1.10)	0	(0, 49)	○	○	○	○	○
1366	1332	2698	4	334	1.01 (0.79, 1.44)	43	(0, 81)	○	◐	●	●	◐
1498	2100	3598	7	288	1.01 (0.72, 1.39)	67	(26, 85)	○	◐	○	●	●
2857	5938	8795	7	767	0.88 (0.78, 1.03)	0	(0, 71)	○	◐	◐	○	○
3777	4834	8611	19	859	1.10 (0.89, 1.45)	57	(28, 74)	○	○	○	○	●
2503	3071	5574	19	467	1.01 (0.79, 1.34)	59	(31, 75)	○	○	●	○	●
1677	1900	3577	14	160	1.16 (0.89, 1.49)	19	(0, 56)	○	○	○	○	○
6927	13374	20301	8	1509	1.00 (0.92, 1.09)	54	(0, 79)	○	◐	◐	○	●
9772	5356	15128	5	1534	1.04 (0.92, 1.28)	62	(0, 86)	●	◐	◐	○	●
6978	5745	12723	8	949	0.99 (0.84, 1.20)	63	(21, 83)	○	◐	◐	○	●
6388	4736	11124	5	440	1.06 (0.81, 1.36)	35	(0, 76)	○	◐	◐	○	○
4930	3277	8207	4	592	1.00 (0.67, 1.40)	70	(14, 90)	○	◐	◐	○	◐
6740	5678	12418	17	560	0.93 (0.80, 1.08)	49	(11, 71)	○	○	◐	○	○
6143	4158	10301	7	213	0.91 (0.55, 1.36)	64	(18, 84)	●	◐	◐	○	●
2549	3202	5751	7	269	1.23 (0.87, 1.80)	87	(76, 93)	○	◐	◐	○	●
3909	1251	5160	5	211	1.05 (0.67, 1.78)	67	(15, 87)	○	◐	○	●	●
13506	27508	41014	40	1530	1.02 (0.96, 1.09)	60	(44, 72)	○	●	●	○	●
13279	16701	29980	41	2714	1.00 (0.88, 1.12)	56	(37, 69)	○	●	○	○	●
8605	11967	20572	16	785	0.93 (0.81, 1.24)	54	(19, 74)	○	●	○	○	●
13298	12197	25495	40	1837	0.95 (0.85, 1.08)	69	(57, 77)	○	●	○	○	●
10004	12829	22833	21	1414	1.09 (0.94, 1.28)	64	(42, 77)	○	●	○	○	●
9704	9324	19028	30	945	1.04 (0.89, 1.20)	57	(35, 71)	○	○	○	○	●
9663	15484	25147	25	2232	1.05 (0.92, 1.24)	62	(41, 75)	○	●	○	○	●
15121	26909	42030	57	437	1.02 (0.90, 1.16)	15	(0, 40)	○	●	◐	○	○
12524	21616	34140	44	1440	0.94 (0.81, 1.09)	60	(45, 72)	○	○	◐	○	●
11309	14015	25324	32	134	1.00 (0.80, 1.24)	28	(0, 53)	○	●	◐	○	○
10770	12388	23158	35	2658	0.99 (0.90, 1.07)	57	(37, 71)	○	●	○	○	●
6875	11217	18092	24	756	1.02 (0.92, 1.14)	0	(0, 45)	○	○	○	○	○
5853	5998	11851	15	1311	1.01 (0.89, 1.16)	47	(2, 71)	○	○	○	○	○
4898	5185	10083	13	474	1.07 (0.87, 1.27)	39	(0, 68)	○	○	○	●	○
12220	18715	30935	20	1915	0.96 (0.87, 1.03)	25	(0, 57)	○	○	○	○	○
5751	6526	12277	16	990	1.02 (0.89, 1.14)	65	(40, 79)	○	●	◐	○	●

.5   1   2

Table 19.1 Continued

Biological pathway	REPORT Author	Year	First study	Reviews*	GENETIC VARIANT Gene	Variant	Allele	Posn	rs	Freq†	Outcome
Others											
	van der A	2006	1998	1	HFE	C282Y	Y	exon 4	1800562	0.06	CHD
	van der A	2006	1998	1	HFE	H63D	D	exon 2	1799945	0.15	CHD
	Lewis	2005	1996	8	MTHFR	C677T	T	exon 5	1801133	0.34	CHD
	Kjaergaard	2007	2000	1	ESR1	T-397C	C	intron 1	2234693	0.45	MI
	Di Castelnuovo	2008	1998	1	CYBA	C242T	T	exon 4	4673	0.24	CHD
	Zafarmand	2008	1997	1	ADRB3	W64R	R	exon 1	4994	0.08	CHD

Ordered by biological category, review, then variant in descending order of total number of participants.
Abbreviations: CHD = coronary heart disease, defined as myocardial infarction (MI), coronary stenosis, angina or fatal
Reviews* - Total number of reviews for each variant including the one listed; Freq† - Frequency of allele of interest, not necessarily
information in each meta-analysis defined as the sum of the weights from an inverse-variance weighted analysis; Summary estimates§ - Pooled
Comments on potential concerns about bias (Non-sys, no evidence of systematic review methods; FPA, funnel plot asymmetry/study size
high proportion of studies deviating from Hardy-Weinberg equilibrium)—see Tables 19.2 and 19.3.
○ = no concerns; ● = concerns; ◑ = insufficient evidence to judge.

Table 19.2 Subsidiary analyses of reviews

Biological pathway	REPORT Author	Year	GENETIC VARIANT Gene	Variant	n	Model*	FIXED† OR	95% CI	RANDOM OR	95% CI	CONSISTENCY I²	95% CI
Lipids												
	Bennet	2007	APOE	e4	108	Dominant	1.19	(1.15, 1.24)	1.39	(1.29, 1.50)	70	(64, 75)
	Bennet	2007	APOE	e2	108	Dominant	0.91	(0.86, 0.95)	0.93	(0.86, 1.02)	57	(46, 65)
	Sagoo	2008	LPL	N291S	21	Dominant	1.06	(0.96, 1.17)	1.07	(0.96, 1.20)	5	(0, 49)
	Sagoo	2008	LPL	S447X	26	Dominant	0.88	(0.82, 0.94)	0.84	(0.75, 0.94)	50	(21, 68)
	Sagoo	2008	LPL	D9N	21	Dominant	1.26	(1.12, 1.42)	1.33	(1.14, 1.56)	17	(0, 51)
	Sagoo	2008	LPL	PvuII	18	Per-allele	0.97	(0.93, 1.01)	0.97	(0.89, 1.05)	32	(0, 61)
	Sagoo	2008	LPL	T-93G	7	Dominant	1.24	(1.03, 1.50)	1.22	(0.98, 1.52)	10	(0, 74)
	Sagoo	2008	LPL	HindIII	23	Dominant	0.89	(0.83, 0.96)	0.89	(0.81, 0.98)	16	(0, 49)
	Sagoo	2008	LPL	G188E	3	Dominant	2.80	(0.88, 8.87)	2.80	(0.88, 8.87)	0	–
	Lawlor	2004	PON1	Q192R	38	Per-allele	1.12	(1.07, 1.16)	1.16	(1.08, 1.25)	61	(0, 64)
	Wheeler	2004	PON1	L55M	20	Dominant	0.97	(0.89, 1.05)	0.96	(0.88, 1.06)	0	(0, 49)
	Wheeler	2004	PON1	T-107C	4	Per-allele	1.02	(0.92, 1.14)	1.05	(0.90, 1.22)	43	(0, 81)
	Wheeler	2004	PON2	S311C	7	Per-allele	1.04	(0.93, 1.17)	1.02	(0.83, 1.26)	67	(26, 85)
	Boekholdt	2005	CETP	TaqIB	7	Per-allele	0.88	(0.82, 0.95)	0.88	(0.82, 0.95)	0	(0, 71)
	Chiodini	2003	APOB	SpIns/Del	19	Per-allele	1.10	(1.03, 1.81)	1.09	(0.98, 1.22)	57	(28, 74)
	Chiodini	2003	APOB	XBaI	19	Per-allele	1.09	(1.00, 1.19)	1.13	(0.97, 1.32)	59	(31, 75)
	Chiodini	2003	APOB	EcoRI	14	Dominant	1.33	(1.14, 1.55)	1.36	(1.14, 1.63)	19	(0, 56)
Inflammation												
	Sie	2006	IL6	G-174C	8	Per-allele	1.03	(0.98, 1.08)	1.05	(0.97, 1.14)	54	(0, 79)
	Clarke	2006	LTA	909253	5	Per-allele	1.05	(1.00, 1.11)	1.10	(1.00, 1.21)	62	(0, 86)
	Koch	2008	THBS4	A387P	8	Per-allele	1.03	(0.97, 1.10)	1.05	(0.93, 1.17)	63	(21, 83)
	Koch	2008	THBS1	N700S	5	Per-allele	1.08	(0.98, 1.19)	1.07	(0.93, 1.24)	35	(0, 76)
	Koch	2008	THBS2	T3949G	4	Per-allele	1.04	(0.96, 1.13)	0.98	(0.83, 1.16)	70	(14, 90)
	Pereira	2007	TNF-alpha	G-308A	17	Dominant	1.04	(0.96, 1.13)	1.07	(0.94, 1.21)	49	(11, 71)
	Koch	2006	TLR4	D299G	7	Dominant	0.93	(0.82, 1.07)	0.90	(0.69, 1.17)	64	(18, 84)
	Abilleira	2006	MMP3	5A/6A	7	Dominant	1.24	(1.10, 1.39)	1.38	(0.98, 1.95)	87	(76, 93)
	Abilleira	2006	MMP9	C-1562T	5	Per-allele	1.08	(0.94, 1.24)	1.18	(0.89, 1.56)	67	(15, 87)

376

AMOUNT OF INFORMATION					SUMMARY ESTIMATES[¶]		CONSISTENCY		CONCERNS ABOUT VALIDITY[#]				
Cases	Controls	Total	n[‡]	Info[§]	Per-allele OR & 95% CI		I² & 95% CI		Non	FPA	Ethn	HWE	Het
8839	51105	59944	23	709	+	1.02 (0.91, 1.15)	22	(0, 53)	○	○	◑	○	○
7239	47129	54368	13	1109	+	1.05 (0.96, 1.12)	14	(0, 53)	○	●	◑	○	○
25428	33041	58469	79	1033	+	1.02 (0.96, 1.08)	41	(23, 55)	○	○	●	○	●
4516	12190	16706	8	888	—+—	1.02 (0.91, 1.22)	47	(0, 76)	○	◑	◑	○	○
5406	2991	8397	8	630	—+—	0.93 (0.69, 1.22)	63	(20, 83)	○	◑	●	○	●
4062	4962	9024	10	244	—+—	1.04 (0.82, 1.31)	42	(0, 72)	○	○	○	○	○

5   1   2

coronary event.
the rare allele, calculated under HWE where 3 × 2 data unavailable; n[‡] - Number of studies included in meta-analysis; Info[§] - Amount of
additive (per-allele) odds ratios from a random-effects meta-regression accounting for study sample size (see Methods); Validity[#] -
effects, Het, moderate/high between-study heterogeneity, Ethn, difference in results between White/East Asian studies, HWE,

STUDY SIZE								X²	HARBORD	PARTICIPANT ETHNICITY							X²
LARGER[‡]				SMALLER						WHITE				EAST ASIAN			
n	OR	95% CI	I²	n	OR	95% CI	I²	p[#]	p	n	OR	95% CI	Freq	n	OR	95% CI	Freq	p[§]
23	1.09	(1.04, 1.13)	51	85	1.51	(1.42, 1.61)	65	<0.001	<0.001	33	1.12	(1.05, 1.18)	0.16	36	1.73	(1.56, 1.92)	0.09	<0.001
21	0.88	(0.83, 0.94)	59	87	0.95	(0.88, 1.03)	56	0.133	0.33	33	0.86	(0.80, 0.93)	0.10	36	1.10	(0.96, 1.24)	0.06	0.001
8	1.05	(0.94, 1.17)	40	13	1.10	(0.83, 1.46)	0	0.785	0.39	11	1.13	(0.85, 1.49)	0.02	0	–	–	–	–
9	0.91	(0.85, 0.98)	19	17	0.79	(0.69, 0.90)	56	0.069	0.19	13	0.90	(0.81, 1.01)	0.12	3	0.60	(0.42, 0.85)	0.12	0.030
9	1.22	(1.06, 1.40)	54	11	1.39	(1.10, 1.77)	0	0.339	0.10	11	1.36	(1.04, 1.79)	0.02	0	–	–	–	–
3	0.96	(0.91, 1.01)	44	15	1.00	(0.92, 1.10)	32	0.422	0.82	10	0.94	(0.86, 1.03)	0.48	3	1.13	(0.90, 1.41)	0.38	0.142
4	1.28	(1.04, 1.57)	0	3	1.03	(0.62, 1.70)	46	0.435	0.90	4	1.13	(0.74, 1.71)	0.02	0	–	–	–	–
5	0.91	(0.82, 1.01)	0	18	0.87	(0.77, 0.98)	30	0.578	0.69	14	0.90	(0.82, 0.99)	0.29	4	0.73	(0.56, 0.95)	0.29	0.139
1	3.20	(0.86, 11.9)	–	1	1.78	(0.16, 19.7)	–	0.674	–	2	2.80	(0.88, 8.87)	<0.01	0	–	–	–	–
7	1.05	(0.99, 1.11)	0	31	1.18	(1.12, 1.25)	64	0.004	0.07	23	1.08	(1.03, 1.14)	0.28	11	1.19	(1.10, 1.29)	0.43	0.038
3	1.02	(0.93, 1.11)	0	16	0.99	(0.90, 1.08)	0	0.649	0.09	12	1.02	(0.95, 1.09)	0.35	4	0.87	(0.67, 1.13)	0.07	0.267
0	–	–	–	4	1.02	(0.92, 1.14)	43	–	0.06	2	1.26	(1.01, 1.56)	0.49	2	0.95	(0.84, 1.08)	0.47	0.030
0	–	–	–	7	1.04	(0.93, 1.17)	67	–	0.77	2	1.06	(0.82, 1.38)	0.23	4	1.12	(0.97, 1.28)	0.19	0.743
4	0.88	(0.82, 0.95)	22	3	0.92	(0.80, 1.07)	0	0.520	0.08	6	0.88	(0.82, 0.95)	0.44	0	–	–	–	–
1	1.15	(1.01, 1.30)	–	18	1.09	(1.01, 1.18)	59	0.485	0.79	12	1.14	(1.06, 1.23)	0.34	5	0.98	(0.82, 1.16)	0.23	0.104
0	–	–	–	19	1.09	(1.00, 1.19)	59	–	0.62	12	1.13	(1.02, 1.25)	0.52	3	0.81	(0.56, 1.18)	0.95	0.048
0	–	–	–	14	1.33	(1.14, 1.55)	19	–	0.17	9	1.31	(1.10, 1.56)	0.18	3	1.43	(0.93, 2.18)	0.05	0.708
7	1.02	(0.97, 1.07)	1	1	2.04	(1.30, 3.20)	–	0.002	0.007	6	1.03	(0.97, 1.10)	0.42	0	–	–	–	–
4	1.03	(0.98, 1.09)	0	1	1.39	(1.14, 1.69)	–	0.005	0.07	1	1.08	(0.90, 1.29)	0.34	3	1.14	(1.05, 1.25)	0.39	0.549
4	0.98	(0.91, 1.05)	52	4	1.19	(1.05, 1.35)	49	0.009	0.35	7	1.03	(0.97, 1.10)	0.22	0	–	–	–	–
4	1.08	(0.98, 1.19)	65	1	1.15	(0.77, 1.70)	–	0.756	0.82	5	1.08	(0.98, 1.19)	0.10	0	–	–	–	–
3	1.05	(0.96, 1.14)	79	1	0.95	(0.72, 1.27)	–	0.544	0.25	4	1.04	(0.96, 1.13)	0.25	0	–	–	–	–
4	1.02	(0.91, 1.14)	0	13	1.06	(0.94, 1.20)	61	0.636	0.15	7	1.09	(0.96, 1.25)	0.16	0	–	–	–	–
3	0.95	(0.82, 1.11)	69	4	0.85	(0.62, 1.17)	69	0.515	0.63	4	0.80	(0.67, 0.95)	0.07	0	–	–	–	–
2	1.00	(0.84, 1.19)	95	5	1.48	(1.26, 1.74)	78	0.001	0.14	1	1.85	(1.12, 3.06)	0.50	4	1.17	(1.01, 1.36)	0.20	0.086
3	1.08	(0.93, 1.25)	63	2	1.09	(0.80, 1.50)	86	0.924	0.15	3	1.08	(0.93, 1.25)	0.12	2	1.09	(0.80, 1.50)	0.15	0.924

Table 19.2 Continued

Biological pathway					Model*	FIXED†		RANDOM		CONSISTENCY	
	REPORT		GENETIC VARIANT								META-ANALYSIS MODEL
	Author	Year	Gene	Variant	n		OR	95% CI	OR	95% CI	I² 95% CI

Biological pathway	Author	Year	Gene	Variant	n	Model*	OR	95% CI	OR	95% CI	I²	95% CI
Renin-angiotensin												
	Morgan	2003	ACE	I/D	40	Recessive	1.15	(1.09, 1.21)	1.24	(1.13, 1.37)	60	(44, 72)
	Xu	2007	AGT	M235T	41	Per-allele	1.05	(1.01, 1.09)	1.10	(1.03, 1.17)	56	(37, 69)
	Xu	2007	AGT	T174M	16	Per-allele	1.03	(0.96, 1.10)	1.09	(0.96, 1.24)	54	(19, 74)
	Casas	2006	NOS3	E298D	40	Per-allele	1.10	(1.05, 1.15)	1.17	(1.07, 1.28)	69	(57, 77)
	Casas	2006	NOS3	T-786C	21	Per-allele	1.13	(1.07, 1.19)	1.16	(1.06, 1.28)	64	(42, 77)
	Casas	2006	NOS3	Intron 4	30	Per-allele	1.10	(1.03, 1.17)	1.13	(1.02, 1.25)	57	(35, 71)
	Ntzani	2007	AGT1R	A1166C	25	Per-allele	1.04	(1.00, 1.08)	1.12	(1.03, 1.22)	62	(41, 75)
Hemostasis												
	Ye	2006	Factor V	R506Q	57	Per-allele	1.17	(1.06, 1.28)	1.21	(1.08, 1.36)	15	(0, 40)
	Ye	2006	ITGB3/ GPIIIa	P1A1/A2	44	Per-allele	0.99	(0.94, 1.04)	1.02	(0.93, 1.12)	60	(45, 72)
	Ye	2006	Factor II	G20210A	32	Per-allele	1.28	(1.08, 1.51)	1.36	(1.10, 1.69)	28	(0, 53)
	Ye	2006	PAI-1	4G/5G	35	Per-allele	1.05	(1.01, 1.09)	1.08	(1.01, 1.15)	57	(37, 71)
	Ye	2006	Factor VII	R353Q	24	Per-allele	0.98	(0.91, 1.05)	0.98	(0.91, 1.05)	0	(0, 45)
	Ye	2006	GPIa	C807T	15	Per-allele	1.03	(0.97, 1.08)	1.04	(0.96, 1.13)	47	(2, 71)
	Ye	2006	GPIba	T-5C	13	Per-allele	1.05	(0.96, 1.15)	1.03	(0.90, 1.17)	39	(0, 68)
	Keavney	2006	FGB	G-455A	20	Per-allele	1.00	(0.95, 1.04)	0.99	(0.93, 1.05)	25	(0, 57)
	Voko	2007	Factor XIII	V34L	16	Per-allele	0.93	(0.87, 0.99)	0.86	(0.76, 0.96)	65	(40, 79)
Others												
	van der A	2006	HFE	C282Y	23	Dominant	1.02	(0.95, 1.10)	1.02	(0.93, 1.13)	22	(0, 53)
	van der A	2006	HFE	H63D	13	Dominant	1.04	(0.98, 1.11)	1.03	(0.96, 1.10)	14	(0, 53)
	Lewis	2005	MTHFR	C677T	79	Homozygote	1.11	(1.05, 1.18)	1.15	(1.05, 1.27)	41	(23, 55)
	Kjaergaard	2007	ESR1	T-397C	8	Per-allele	1.01	(0.95, 1.08)	1.06	(0.95, 1.17)	47	(0, 76)
	Di Castelnuovo	2008	CYBA	C242T	8	Per-allele	0.97	(0.90, 1.05)	0.98	(0.85, 1.13)	63	(20, 83)
	Zafarmand	2008	ADRB3	W64R	10	Dominant	1.08	(0.95, 1.22)	1.10	(0.92, 1.31)	42	(0, 72)

Fixed-effect meta-analysis used unless stated.

Model* - Genetic model used (per-allele where data allow); Fixed† - Summary odds ratio and 95% confidence interval from frequentist chi-squared test for significant between-subgroup heterogeneity.

Discussion

The HuGENet roadmap has encouraged preparation of cumulative overviews of genetic association studies of various complex disease outcomes in order to "identify gaps, avoid wasteful duplication, and promote translation" of emerging knowledge in genetic epidemiology (51). In this chapter, we have presented such a synopsis in relation to CHD, a condition that may involve one of the largest evidence bases in relation to both candidate genes and genome-wide studies of any complex outcome.

After making allowances for the potential impact of study size, the *e2/e3/e4* variant of the *APOE* gene was the only susceptibility locus among the several dozen candidate genes reviewed here that showed convincing evidence of associations with CHD. A recent systematic review of *APOE* genotypes involved tabular data from authors of available studies as well as from previously unreported studies. It reported approximately linear associations of *APOE* genotypes with low-density

| | STUDY SIZE | | | | | | PARTICIPANT ETHNICITY | | | | | | | |
| LARGER[‡] | | | | SMALLER | | | | χ² | HARBORD | WHITE | | | | EAST ASIAN | | | | χ² |
n	OR	95% CI	I²	n	OR	95% CI	I²	p*	p	n	OR	95% CI	Freq	n	OR	95% CI	Freq	p§
7	1.08	(1.01, 1.15)	0	33	1.27	(1.17, 1.38)	62	0.002	0.007	24	1.16	(1.08, 1.24)	0.52	7	1.52	(1.22, 1.89)	0.35	0.022
4	0.98	(0.93, 1.04)	0	37	1.12	(1.06, 1.18)	54	0.001	0.03	14	1.07	(1.02, 1.14)	0.42	12	1.17	(1.05, 1.29)	0.78	0.181
4	0.99	(0.91, 1.07)	0	12	1.19	(1.03, 1.38)	60	0.030	0.17	5	1.02	(0.92, 1.14)	0.13	6	1.02	(0.84, 1.24)	0.10	0.991
11	0.99	(0.93, 1.06)	65	29	1.24	(1.16, 1.33)	61	<0.001	0.008	21	1.06	(1.01, 1.12)	0.33	11	1.16	(1.01, 1.32)	0.08	0.229
9	1.07	(1.00, 1.14)	61	12	1.26	(1.15, 1.37)	58	0.004	0.15	10	1.10	(1.03, 1.18)	0.39	6	1.13	(1.03, 1.24)	0.10	0.678
9	1.08	(0.99, 1.17)	68	21	1.13	(1.02, 1.24)	52	0.494	0.20	14	1.09	(1.01, 1.18)	0.14	10	1.07	(0.94, 1.23)	0.12	0.870
5	0.98	(0.93, 1.03)	0	20	1.20	(1.11, 1.29)	56	<0.001	0.04	15	1.12	(1.05, 1.19)	0.28	2	1.47	(0.88, 2.44)	0.06	0.299
10	1.06	(0.93, 1.20)	28	43	1.31	(1.14, 1.50)	3	0.026	0.01	28	1.25	(1.09, 1.43)	0.02	1	2.82	(0.63, 12.7)	0.00	0.291
8	0.98	(0.92, 1.05)	0	34	1.00	(0.93, 1.09)	67	0.644	0.39	31	0.98	(0.92, 1.04)	0.15	1	3.09	(0.32, 29.9)	0.01	0.320
9	1.02	(0.81, 1.28)	6	23	1.69	(1.31, 2.18)	15	0.004	0.03	17	1.19	(0.96, 1.47)	0.01	0	–	–	–	–
8	1.02	(0.97, 1.07)	17	27	1.10	(1.04, 1.17)	61	0.049	0.05	22	1.05	(1.00, 1.10)	0.49	7	1.04	(0.94, 1.15)	0.61	0.873
6	1.02	(0.93, 1.11)	0	18	0.92	(0.82, 1.03)	0	0.171	0.18	16	1.00	(0.92, 1.08)	0.13	5	0.90	(0.72, 1.14)	0.07	0.434
4	0.99	(0.92, 1.07)	10	11	1.07	(0.99, 1.16)	52	0.167	0.35	9	1.01	(0.95, 1.08)	0.38	4	1.05	(0.94, 1.18)	0.37	0.578
4	1.08	(0.97, 1.22)	0	9	1.00	(0.86, 1.15)	54	0.375	0.29	7	1.08	(0.97, 1.19)	0.12	3	1.08	(0.86, 1.35)	0.15	0.996
8	1.00	(0.95, 1.05)	0	12	0.99	(0.90, 1.09)	47	0.916	0.79	8	0.96	(0.90, 1.04)	0.20	3	1.07	(0.87, 1.31)	0.14	0.369
4	1.03	(0.95, 1.12)	0	12	0.81	(0.73, 0.89)	61	<0.001	0.002	10	0.98	(0.92, 1.06)	0.23	0	–	–	–	–
12	1.02	(0.95, 1.10)	7	11	1.01	(0.80, 1.28)	39	0.933	0.63	14	1.03	(0.95, 1.12)	0.06	0	–	–	–	–
8	1.06	(1.00, 1.13)	0	5	0.85	(0.69, 1.05)	0	0.048	0.008	8	1.06	(1.00, 1.14)	0.14	0	–	–	–	–
17	1.07	(0.98, 1.16)	37	62	1.17	(1.07, 1.28)	42	0.128	0.10	29	1.01	(0.92, 1.11)	0.36	16	1.25	(1.07, 1.46)	0.35	0.024
5	0.98	(0.91, 1.06)	18	3	1.16	(1.00, 1.34)	55	0.050	0.007	6	1.01	(0.94, 1.09)	0.45	0	–	–	–	–
4	0.97	(0.89, 1.04)	64	4	1.01	(0.82, 1.24)	71	0.693	0.99	3	1.04	(0.94, 1.15)	0.34	3	0.78	(0.67, 0.90)	0.12	0.001
4	1.05	(0.90, 1.23)	53	6	1.11	(0.90, 1.37)	43	0.686	0.44	3	0.92	(0.76, 1.11)	0.08	4	1.06	(0.81, 1.37)	0.12	0.411

fixed-effect meta-analysis using original model; Larger[‡] - Results from larger studies defined as ≥500 cases or ≥1,000 participants; p§ - p value from a

lipoprotein cholesterol levels and with coronary risk (11). This meta-analysis also reported striking discrepancies in odds ratios for CHD between the larger studies of *APOE* genotypes (at least 500 cases) and the smaller studies (fewer than 500 cases), with inclusion of the smaller studies resulting in overestimation of the relevance of the *e4* variant and obscuring the relevance of the *e2* variant. Interim guidelines for assessing the strength of evidence from association studies have been published recently, proposing a "semi-quantitative index" to class epidemiologic evidence into strong, moderate, or weak categories (9). Despite the large amounts of evidence compiled for many variants with CHD, heterogeneity between studies, a lack of replication, and concerns about biases—particularly about publication bias—would give all candidate genes other than *APOE* a "weak" grading.

Several conclusions can be derived from this analysis of data on candidate variants in CHD. The size of any realistic effects of any particular variant in CHD is likely to be much more moderate than initially anticipated, as demonstrated by the

Table 19.3 Characteristics of studies allowing assessment of susceptibility to bias

Biological pathway				GENOTYPING							STUDY POPULATION				REVIEW METHODS	
REPORT		Gene	Variant			HWE			BLINDED		STUDY DESIGN		CONTROL SOURCE		Review	
Author	Year			Dev*	n†	OR	OR	%	Yes‡	No§	Retro¶	Prosp#	Popn**	Other††	Corr‡‡	Sys§§
Lipids																
Bennet	2007	APOE	e4	12	103	1.18	1.19	−0.8	37	63	87	21	51	32	Y	Y
Bennet	2007	APOE	e2	7	103	0.90	0.91	1	37	63	87	21	51	32	Y	Y
Sagoo	2008	LPL	N291S	1	15	1.07	1.11	3.7	10	11	16	5	16	5	Y	Y
Sagoo	2008	LPL	S447X	1	21	0.84	0.83	1	10	16	22	4	17	9	Y	Y
Sagoo	2008	LPL	D9N	2	17	1.33	1.36	2.3	10	11	17	4	14	7	Y	Y
Sagoo	2008	LPL	PvuII	1	18	0.97	0.98	1.0	6	12	18	0	6	11	Y	Y
Sagoo	2008	LPL	T-93G	1	6	1.22	1.21	0.8	1	6	7	0	3	4	Y	Y
Sagoo	2008	LPL	HindIII	1	22	0.89	0.89	0	6	17	22	1	13	8	Y	Y
Sagoo	2008	LPL	G188E	0	1	2.80	–	–	0	3	3	0	3	0	Y	Y
Lawlor	2004	PON1	Q192R	4	38	1.16	1.14	1.7	10	28	33	5	12	26	N	Y
Wheeler	2004	PON1	L55M	2	19	0.96	0.97	1.0	2	18	18	2	5	15	Y	Y
Wheeler	2004	PON1	T-107C	1	4	1.05	1.11	5.7	1	3	4	0	1	3	Y	Y
Wheeler	2004	PON2	S311C	1	7	1.02	1.08	5.9	0	7	7	0	3	4	Y	Y
Boekholdt	2005	CETP	TaqIB	1	7	0.88	0.88	0	3	4	3	4	6	1	Y	Y¶¶
Chiodini	2003	APOB	SpIns/Del	1	19	1.09	1.11	1.8	5	14	19	0	11	8	N	Y##
Chiodini	2003	APOB	XbaI	1	19	1.13	1.14	0.9	2	17	19	0	11	8	N	Y##
Chiodini	2003	APOB	EcoRI	1	13	1.36	1.31	3.7	2	12	14	0	8	6	N	Y##

Inflammation

Sie	2006	IL6	G-174C	0	8	1.05	—	—	3	5	5	3	6	2	N	Y¶¶
Clarke	2006	LTA	909253	0	5	1.10	—	—	3	2	5	0	2	3	N	N
Koch	2008	THBS4	A387P	0	8	1.05	—	—	3	5	6	2	6	2	N	Y¶¶
Koch	2008	THBS1	N700S	0	5	1.07	—	—	3	2	5	0	4	1	N	Y¶¶
Koch	2008	THBS2	T3949G	0	4	0.98	—	—	2	2	4	0	3	1	N	Y¶¶
Pereira	2007	TNF-alpha	G-308A	0	14	1.07	—	—	5	12	16	0	10	7	Y	Y¶#
Koch	2006	TLR4	D299G	1	4	0.90	0.94	4.4	1	6	6	1	4	3	N	N¶¶
Abilleira	2006	MMP3	5A/6A	2	6	1.38	1.41	2.2	2	5	7	0	2	5	N	Y
Abilleira	2006	MMP9	C-1562T	1	5	1.18	1.29	9.3	1	4	5	0	0	5	N	Y

Renin-angiotensin

Morgan	2003	ACE	I/D	7	36	1.24	1.22	1.6	15	25	39	1	21	19	N	Y
Xu	2007	AGT	M235T	6	41	1.10	1.07	2.7	8	33	38	3	18	23	N	Y
Xu	2007	AGT	T174M	0	16	1.09	—	—	2	14	16	0	7	9	N	Y
Casas	2006	NOS3	E298D	2	40	1.17	1.19	1.7	20	20	36	2	18	22	Y	Y
Casas	2006	NOS3	T-786C	0	21	1.16	—	—	12	9	20	1	13	8	Y	Y
Casas	2006	NOS3	Intron 4	2	30	1.13	1.15	1.8	12	18	28	1	13	17	Y	Y
Ntzani	2007	AGT1R	A1166C	3	25	1.12	1.12	0	13	12	22	3	16	9	Y	Y

Hemostasis

Ye	2006	Factor V	R506Q	1	57	1.21	1.21	0	26	31	51	4	34	23	Y	Y
Ye	2006	ITGB3/GPIIIa	PIA1/A2	5	44	1.02	1.06	3.9	18	26	42	2	18	26	Y	Y
Ye	2006	Factor II	G20210A	2	32	1.36	1.41	3.7	16	16	34	2	22	16	Y	Y
Ye	2006	PAI-1	4G/5G	7	35	1.08	1.06	1.9	13	22	30	3	18	17	Y	Y
Ye	2006	Factor VII	R353Q	3	24	0.98	0.97	1.0	12	12	22	2	11	13	Y	Y

(Continued)

Table 19.3 Continued

| Biological pathway | REPORT | | Gene | Variant | GENOTYPING | | | | | | | | | STUDY POPULATION | | REVIEW METHODS | |
| | | | | | HWE | | | | | BLINDED | | STUDY DESIGN | | CONTROL SOURCE | | Review | |
	Author	Year			Dev*	n†	OR	OR	%	Yes‡	No§	Retro¶	Prosp#	Popn**	Other††	Corr‡‡	Sys§§
	Ye	2006	GPIa	C807T	4	15	1.04	0.99	4.8	5	10	14	1	6	9	Y	Y
	Ye	2006	GPIba	T-5C	2	13	1.03	1.09	5.8	6	7	13	0	3	10	Y	Y
	Keavney	2006	FGB	G-455A	2	20	0.99	1.01	2.0	6	14	15	3	13	7	Y	Y
	Voko	2007	Factor XIII	V34L	0	16	0.86	–	–	6	10	15	0	9	7	N	Y
Others																	
	van der A	2006	HFE	C282Y	1	14	1.02	1.03	1.0	7	16	15	6	13	10	N	Y¶¶
	van der A	2006	HFE	H63D	1	9	1.03	1.05	1.9	2	11	10	2	7	6	N	Y¶¶
	Lewis	2005	MTHFR	C677T	5	73	1.16	1.17	0.9	19	61	74	4	37	43	Y	Y
	Kjaergaard	2007	ESR1	T-397C	0	8	1.06	–	–	1	9	4	4	4	4	Y	Y
	Di Castelnuovo	2008	CYBA	C242T	1	8	0.97	0.99	2.1	2	6	8	0	3	5	N	Y
	Zafarmand	2008	ADRB3	W64R	1	9	1.10	1.05	4.5	8	9	8	2	3	7	N	Y

Dev* - Number of studies where controls deviate ($p < 0.05$) from Hardy-Weinberg equilibrium; n† - Number of studies in which deviation from HWE could be assessed; OR - Summary odds ratio with HWE-deviating studies excluded; % - Percentage change in odds ratio once HWE-deviating studies are excluded; Yes‡ - Number of studies which reported blinded genotyping; No§ - Number of studies where blinding was not used or not reported; Retro¶ - Studies using a retrospective (case-control/cross-sectional) design; Prosp# - Studies using a prospective cohort (or nested case-control) design; Popn** - Studies where controls were drawn from disease-free population samples; Other†† - Other control sources, for example, hospital or angiography clinic; Corr‡‡ - Review where correspondence with authors was used to obtain data; Sys§§ - Reviews where a systematic review approach was reportedly taken; Y/N¶¶ - Restricted to White/European studies only; Y## - Restricted to retrospective studies only.

per-allele odds ratio in this review, which for most variants ranged from about 0.9 to 1.2. It may be that some of these inconclusively studied variants have real but only modest associations with CHD. This residual uncertainty, despite years of investigation in small-to-moderate sized studies, implies the need for research strategies that enable the reliable assessment of moderate effects. There is, in particular, the need for studies that can minimize random error (by inclusion of much larger number of CHD cases and controls than hitherto), reporting biases (by conduct of very large individual studies or by analyses in prespecified consortia of smaller studies), and genotyping errors (by application of rigorous assay methods and laboratory approaches, such as mixing samples from cases and controls in assay plates, masking laboratory technicians to the samples' case-control status and reporting genotyping call rates).

The seven GWAS of clinical coronary outcomes published by January 2009 have generally been conducted in populations of Northern European ancestry (Table 19.4). These studies have involved between 94 and 1,926 coronary cases, some providing adequate power to detect odds ratios of 1.5 or larger but not to detect more moderate odds ratios. As initial GWAS in CHD reported on loci with odds ratios less than 1.5 (notably the 9p21.3 locus: Figure 19.1), it suggests that several (perhaps many) additional loci with effects of similar magnitude remain undetected and await discovery. Similar considerations apply to the evaluation of less common genetic variants, as acknowledged in the WTCCC report: "even with 2,000 cases and 3,000 controls, adequate power is restricted to common variants of relatively large effect" and "given the likely distribution of effect sizes for most complex traits, there are strong grounds for prosecution of GWA studies on an even larger scale than ours" (34). Combined analysis of data from the WTCCC and the German MI Family studies (involving a total of 2,801 coronary cases) suggested possible associations with a further four loci not detected in either study separately, reinforcing how greater power can enhance discovery (39). Other variants, such as those seen at 16q23 and 6q25.1, have been replicated in at least one independent sample and require further investigation. As the numbers of SNPs assessed continues to increase, the sharing of findings and datasets by investigators will enable more rapid validation. For example, the lack of association at the 9p21.3 locus in the Japanese OACIS study (38) may be an indication that the association varies between populations, although without access to full details of the SNPs genotyped it is not possible to determine if this region was adequately covered in the study.

The current review was limited by inclusion of only candidate variants that had already been studied in a meta-analysis, although our database searches identified fewer than 20 further candidate variants in CHD that had been investigated in at least five individual studies. As the genetic and genomic epidemiology of CHD is a particularly rapidly moving field, bespoke field synopses can become quickly outdated, arguing for the creation of publicly accessible electronic systems that enable rapid (and, to some extent, automated) updating and searching methods to provide summaries of the available evidence. An early exemplar of such an approach

Table 19.4 Summary of genome-wide association studies of over 10,000 SNPs in CHD

	INITIAL GENOME-WIDE STUDIES									
Study	*Location*	*Cases*	*Controls*	*Outcome*	*SNPs**	*Threshold†*	*Hits‡*	*Locus*	*p*	*Study*
WTCCC (34,39)	UK	1,926	2,938	CHD	392,975	$p < 0.001$ & FPRP<0.5	9			WTCCC hits replicated with German MI study
German MI Family Study (39)	Germany	875	1,644	MI with FH	272,602	–	–			Combined analysis of both GWAS
deCODE (35)	Iceland	1,607	6,728	MI	305,593	None Top hit only	1			Icelandic B Atlanta Philadelphia Durham
Ottawa Heart Study (37)	Canada	322	312	Severe CHD	72,864	$P < 0.025$	2,586			Ottawa Heart Study 2 ARIC CCHS Dallas Heart Study Ottawa Heart Study 3
Framingham (36)	USA	118	1,227	Major CHD	70,987	$P < 10^{-5}$	1	16q23 (9p21.3	9.7×10^{-6} 2.5×10^{-4})	–
OACIS (38)	Japan	94	658	MI	65,671	$P < 0.01$	≥773			OACIS replication
Celera (40)	USA	340	346	MI	11,053	$P < 0.05$	637			Celera 2 Celera 3

Abbreviations: WTCCC - Wellcome Trust Case-Control Consortium; OACIS - Osaka Acute Coronary Insufficiency Study; history; CAD, coronary artery disease; IHD - ischemic heart disease; FDR - false-discovery rate; SNP - single nucleotide SNPs* - Number of SNPs that passed error-checking stages; Threshold† - Significance threshold for genotyping in replication

Location	Cases	Controls	Outcome	SNPs*	Threshold†	Hits‡	Locus	p	Per-allele OR§
					$p < 0.05$	3	9p21.3	6.8×10^{-6}	1.33 (1.18, 1.51)
							6q25.1	1×10^{-3}	1.24 (1.09, 1.41)
							2q36.3	4×10^{-3}	1.20 (1.06, 1.35)
					Joint $p < 1.3 \times 10^{-6}$ & FPRP<0.2	4	1p13.3	4.1×10^{-9}	1.29 (1.18, 1.40)
							1q41	1.3×10^{-6}	1.20 (1.12, 1.30)
							10q11.21	9.5×10^{-8}	1.33 (1.20, 1.48)
							15q22.33	1.2×10^{-7}	1.21 (1.13, 1.30)
Iceland	665	3,533	MI	3–		1	9p21.3	1.4×10^{-5}	1.31 (1.16, 1.47)
USA	596	1,284	MI	MI			9p21.3	1.5×10^{-4}	1.31 (1.14, 1.50)
USA	582	504	MI	3			9p21.3	1.9×10^{-4}	1.38 (1.17, 1.64)
USA	1,137	718	MI	3			9p21.3	2.7×10^{-4}	1.28 (1.12, 1.46)
Canada	311	326	Severe CHD	2,586	$p < 0.025$	50			
USA	1,347	9,054	Incident CHD	50	$p < 0.025$	1	9p21.3	4×10^{-3}	1.16 (1.06, 1.28)
Denmark	1,525	9,053	Incident IHD	2	–		9p21.3	4×10^{-4}	1.17 (1.08, 1.26)
USA	154	527	CAD	2	–		9p21.3	2.5×10^{-2}	1.34 (1.04, 1.74)
Canada	647	847	CHD	2	–		9p21.3	3×10^{-4}	1.41 (1.21, 1.64)
Japan	1,133	1,878	MI	>773	Unknown	1	6p21	3.3×10^{-6}	1.21 (1.09, 1.35)
USA	445	606	MI	637	$p < 0.05$	30			
USA	560	891	MI	31	$p < 0.05$ & FDR < 0.1	5	4q32	2.8×10^{-3}	1.25 (1.10, 1.43)
							6q22	6.7×10^{-3}	1.23 (1.06, 1.42)
							12p13	1.8×10^{-3}	1.28 (1.11, 1.46)
							1q44	1.3×10^{-2}	1.19 (1.05, 1.36)
							19p13.2	3.4×10^{-3}	1.25 (1.09, 1.44)

ARIC - Atherosclerosis Risk in Communities; CCHS - Copenhagen City Heart Study; MI - myocardial infarction; FH - family polymorphism; FPRP, false positive report probability.
study; Hits‡ - Number of loci reaching threshold; Per-allele OR§ - Per-allele odds ratio with 95% confidence interval.

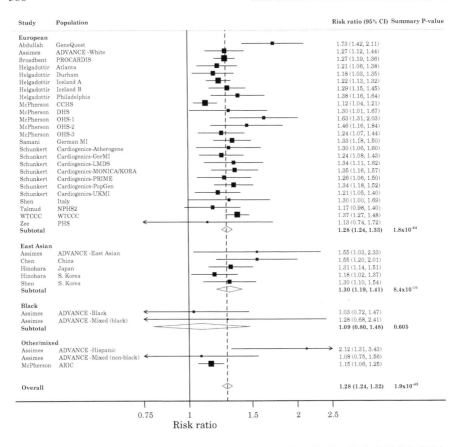

Study	Population	Risk ratio (95% CI)	Summary P-value
European			
Abdullah	GeneQuest	1.73 (1.42, 2.11)	
Assimes	ADVANCE -White	1.27 (1.12, 1.44)	
Broadbent	PROCARDIS	1.27 (1.19, 1.36)	
Helgadottir	Atlanta	1.21 (1.06, 1.38)	
Helgadottir	Durham	1.18 (1.03, 1.35)	
Helgadottir	Iceland A	1.22 (1.13, 1.32)	
Helgadottir	Iceland B	1.29 (1.15, 1.45)	
Helgadottir	Philadelphia	1.38 (1.16, 1.64)	
McPherson	CCHS	1.12 (1.04, 1.21)	
McPherson	DHS	1.30 (1.01, 1.67)	
McPherson	OHS-1	1.63 (1.31, 2.03)	
McPherson	OHS-2	1.46 (1.16, 1.84)	
McPherson	OHS-3	1.24 (1.07, 1.44)	
Samani	German MI	1.33 (1.18, 1.50)	
Schunkert	Cardiogenics-Atherogene	1.30 (1.06, 1.60)	
Schunkert	Cardiogenics-GerMI	1.24 (1.08, 1.43)	
Schunkert	Cardiogenics-LMDS	1.34 (1.11, 1.62)	
Schunkert	Cardiogenics-MONICA/KORA	1.35 (1.16, 1.57)	
Schunkert	Cardiogenics-PRIME	1.26 (1.06, 1.50)	
Schunkert	Cardiogenics-PopGen	1.34 (1.18, 1.52)	
Schunkert	Cardiogenics-UKMI	1.21 (1.05, 1.40)	
Shen	Italy	1.30 (1.00, 1.69)	
Talmud	NPHS2	1.17 (0.98, 1.40)	
WTCCC	WTCCC	1.37 (1.27, 1.48)	
Zee	PHS	1.13 (0.74, 1.72)	
Subtotal		**1.28 (1.24, 1.33)**	1.8×10^{-44}
East Asian			
Assimes	ADVANCE -East Asian	1.55 (1.03, 2.33)	
Chen	China	1.55 (1.20, 2.01)	
Hinohara	Japan	1.31 (1.14, 1.51)	
Hinohara	S. Korea	1.18 (1.02, 1.37)	
Shen	S. Korea	1.30 (1.10, 1.54)	
Subtotal		**1.30 (1.19, 1.41)**	8.4×10^{-10}
Black			
Assimes	ADVANCE -Black	1.03 (0.72, 1.47)	
Assimes	ADVANCE -Mixed (black)	1.28 (0.68, 2.41)	
Subtotal		**1.09 (0.80, 1.48)**	0.605
Other/mixed			
Assimes	ADVANCE -Hispanic	2.12 (1.31, 3.43)	
Assimes	ADVANCE -Mixed (non-black)	1.08 (0.75, 1.56)	
McPherson	ARIC	1.15 (1.06, 1.25)	
Overall		**1.28 (1.24, 1.32)**	1.9×10^{-49}

0.75   1   1.5   2   2.5

Risk ratio

CCHS - Copenhagen City Heart Study; OHS - Ottawa Heart Study; DHS - Dallas Heart Study; LMDS - Left Main Disease Study; NPHS2 - Northwick Park Heart Study 2; WTCCC - Wellcome Trust Case-Control Consortium; PHS - Physicians' Health Study; ARIC - Atherosclerosis Risk In Communities.

Figure 19.1 Random-effects meta-analysis of per-allele odds ratios from SNPs at locus 9p21.3.

has been the AlzGene database (52), which collects data on all genetic association studies with Alzheimer disease outcomes and produces crude, up-to-date meta-analyses, enabling cumulative assessment of the state of the evidence of variants investigated in at least four separate studies. A number of other examples of such synopses have also been created, including SzGene for schizophrenia (www.szgene. org) (53), PDGene for Parkinson disease (www.pdgene.org), and Episat for DNA repair gene variants and cancer (www.episat.org) (54). Such resources may be useful for researchers (e.g., to prioritize hypotheses for new genotyping and to help control publication bias) and funding agencies (e.g., to optimize the use of resources). Following this successful example, we are in the process of developing "CHDGene" as such a resource for those interested in the genetic epidemiology of cardiovascular disease.

References

1. Mathers CD, Loncar D. Projections of global mortality and burden of disease from 2002 to 2030. *PLoS Med.* 2006;3(11):e442.
2. Rosamond W, Flegal K, Friday G, et al. Heart disease and stroke statistics—2007 update: a report from the American Heart Association Statistics Committee and Stroke Statistics Subcommittee. *Circulation.* 2007;115(5):e69–e171.
3. Lusis AJ, Mar R, Pajukanta P. Genetics of atherosclerosis. *Annu Rev Genomics Hum Genet.* 2004;5:189–218.
4. Harbord RM, Egger M, Sterne JA. A modified test for small-study effects in meta-analyses of controlled trials with binary endpoints. *Stat Med.* 2006;25(20):3443–3457.
5. Salanti G, Higgins JP. Meta-analysis of genetic association studies under different inheritance models using data reported as merged genotypes. *Stat Med.* 2008;27(5):764–777.
6. Shang A, Huwiler-Müntener K, Nartey L, et al. Are the clinical effects of homoeopathy placebo effects? Comparative study of placebo-controlled trials of homoeopathy and allopathy. *Lancet.* 2005;366(9487):726–732.
7. Lunn DJ, Thomas A, Best N, Spiegelhalter D. WinBUGS—a Bayesian modelling framework: concepts, structure, and extensibility. *Stat Comput.* 2000;10:325–337.
8. Higgins JP, Thompson SG. Quantifying heterogeneity in a meta-analysis. *Stat Med.* 2002;21(11):1539–1558.
9. Ioannidis JP, Boffetta P, Little J, et al. Assessment of cumulative evidence on genetic associations: interim guidelines. *Int J Epidemiol.* 2007;37(1):120–132.
10. Abilleira S, Bevan S, Markus HS. The role of genetic variants of matrix metalloproteinases in coronary and carotid atherosclerosis. *J Med Genet.* 2006;43(12):897–901.
11. Bennet AM, Di Angelantonio E, Ye Z, et al. Association of apolipoprotein E genotypes with lipid levels and coronary risk. *JAMA.* 2007;298(11):1300–1311.
12. Casas JP, Cavalleri GL, Bautista LE, Smeeth L, Humphries SE, Hingorani AD. Endothelial nitric oxide synthase gene polymorphisms and cardiovascular disease: a HuGE review. *Am J Epidemiol.* 2006;164(10):921–935.
13. Chiodini BD, Barlera S, Franzosi MG, Beceiro VL, Introna M, Tognoni G. APO B gene polymorphisms and coronary artery disease: a meta-analysis. *Atherosclerosis.* 2003;167(2):355–366.
14. Clarke R, Xu P, Bennett D, et al. Lymphotoxin-alpha gene and risk of myocardial infarction in 6,928 cases and 2,712 controls in the ISIS case-control study. *PLoS Genet.* 2006;2(7):e107.
15. Di Castelnuovo A, Soccio M, Iacoviello L, et al. The C242T polymorphism of the p22phox component of NAD(P)H oxidase and vascular risk. Two case-control studies and a meta-analysis. *Thromb Haemost.* 2008;99(3):594–601.
16. Keavney B, Danesh J, Parish S, et al. Fibrinogen and coronary heart disease: test of causality by "Mendelian randomization." *Int J Epidemiol.* 2006;35(4):935–943.
17. Kjaergaard AD, Ellervik C, Tybjærg-Hansen A, et al. Estrogen receptor alpha polymorphism and risk of cardiovascular disease, cancer, and hip fracture: cross-sectional, cohort, and case-control studies and a meta-analysis. *Circulation.* 2007;115(7):861–871.
18. Koch W, Hoppmann P, Pfeufer A, Schomig A, Kastrati A. Toll-like receptor 4 gene polymorphisms and myocardial infarction: no association in a Caucasian population. *Eur Heart J.* 2006;27(21):2524–2529.
19. Koch W, Hoppmann P, Pfeufer A, Schomig A, Kastrati A. Polymorphisms in thrombospondin genes and myocardial infarction: a case-control study and a meta-analysis of available evidence. *Hum Mol Genet.* 2008;17(8):1120–1126.

20. Lawlor DA, Day INM, Gaunt TR, et al. The association of the PON1 Q192R polymorphism with coronary heart disease: findings from the British Women's Heart and Health cohort study and a meta-analysis. *BMC Genet.* 2004;5:17.

21. Lewis SJ, Ebrahim S, Davey Smith G. Meta-analysis of MTHFR 677C->T polymorphism and coronary heart disease: does totality of evidence support causal role for homocysteine and preventive potential of folate? *BMJ.* 2005;331(7524):1053.

22. Morgan TM, Coffey CS, Krumholz HM. Overestimation of genetic risks owing to small sample sizes in cardiovascular studies. *Clin Genet.* 2003;64(1):7–17.

23. Ntzani EE, Rizos EC, Ioannidis JP. Genetic effects versus bias for candidate polymorphisms in myocardial infarction: case study and overview of large-scale evidence. *Am J Epidemiol.* 2007;165(9):973–984.

24. Pereira TV, Rudnicki M, Franco RF, Pereira AC, Krieger JE. Effect of the G-308A polymorphism of the tumor necrosis factor alpha gene on the risk of ischemic heart disease and ischemic stroke: a meta-analysis. *Am Heart J.* 2007;153(5):821–830.

25. Qi L, Doria A, Manson JE, et al. Adiponectin genetic variability, plasma adiponectin, and cardiovascular risk in patients with type 2 diabetes. *Diabetes.* 2006;55(5):1512–1516.

26. Sagoo GS, Tatt I, Salanti G, et al. Seven lipoprotein lipase gene polymorphisms, lipid fractions, and coronary disease: a HuGE association review and meta-analysis. *Am J Epidemiol.* 2008;168(11):1233–1246.

27. Sie MP, Sayed-Tabatabaei FA, Oei HHS, et al. Interleukin 6 -174 g/c promoter polymorphism and risk of coronary heart disease: results from the Rotterdam study and a meta-analysis. *Arterioscler Thromb Vasc Biol.* 2006;26(1):212–217.

28. van der A DL, Peeters PHM, Grobbee DE, et al. HFE mutations and risk of coronary heart disease in middle-aged women. *Eur J Clin Invest.* 2006;36(10):682–690.

29. Vokó Z, Bereczky Z, Katona E, Adány R, Muszbek L. Factor XIII Val34Leu variant protects against coronary artery disease. A meta-analysis. *Thromb Haemost.* 2007; 97(3):458–463.

30. Wheeler JG, Keavney BD, Watkins H, Collins R, Danish J. Four paraoxonase gene polymorphisms in 11212 cases of coronary heart disease and 12786 controls: meta-analysis of 43 studies. *Lancet.* 2004;363(9410):689–695.

31. Xu MQ, Ye Z, Hu FB, He L. Quantitative assessment of the effect of angiotensinogen gene polymorphisms on the risk of coronary heart disease. *Circulation.* 2007; 116(12):1356–1366.

32. Ye Z, Liu EH, Higgins JP, et al. Seven haemostatic gene polymorphisms in coronary disease: meta-analysis of 66,155 cases and 91,307 controls. *Lancet.* 2006; 367(9511):651–658.

33. Zafarmand MH, van der Schouw YT, Grobbee DE, de Leeuw PW, Bots ML. T64A polymorphism in beta3-adrenergic receptor gene (ADRB3) and coronary heart disease: a case-cohort study and meta-analysis. *J Intern Med.* 2008;263(1):79–89.

34. Wellcome Trust Case Control Consortium. Genome-wide association study of 14,000 cases of seven common diseases and 3,000 shared controls. *Nature.* 2007;447(7145):661–678.

35. Helgadottir A, Thorleifsson G, Manolescu A, et al. A common variant on chromosome 9p21 affects the risk of myocardial infarction. *Science.* 2007;316(5830):1491–1493.

36. Larson MG, Atwood LD, Benjamin EJ, et al. Framingham Heart Study 100K project: genome-wide associations for cardiovascular disease outcomes. *BMC Med Genet.* 2007;8(Suppl 1): S5.

37. McPherson R, Pertsemlidis A, Kavaslar N, et al. A common allele on chromosome 9 associated with coronary heart disease. *Science.* 2007;316(5830):1488–1491.

38. Ozaki K, Ohnishi Y, Iida A, et al. Functional SNPs in the lymphotoxin-alpha gene that are associated with susceptibility to myocardial infarction. *Nat Genet.* 2002;32(4):650–654.

39. Samani NJ, Erdmann J, Hall AS, et al. Genomewide association analysis of coronary artery disease. *N Engl J Med.* 2007;357(5):443–453.

40. Shiffman D, Ellis SG, Rowland CM, et al. Identification of four gene variants associated with myocardial infarction. *Am J Hum Genet.* 2005;77(4):596–605.

41. Abdullah KG, Li L, Shen GQ, et al. Four SNPS on chromosome 9p21 confer risk to premature, familial CAD and MI in an American Caucasian population (GeneQuest). *Ann Hum Genet.* 2008;72(5):654–657.

42. Assimes TL, Knowles JW, Basu A, et al. Susceptibility locus for clinical and subclinical coronary artery disease at chromosome 9p21 in the multi-ethnic ADVANCE Study. *Hum Mol Genet.* 2008;17(15):2320–2328.

43. Broadbent HM, Peden JF, Lorkowski S, et al. Susceptibility to coronary artery disease and diabetes is encoded by distinct, tightly linked SNPs in the ANRIL locus on chromosome 9p. *Hum Mol Genet.* 2008;17(6):806–814.

44. Chen Z, Qian Q, Ma G, et al. A common variant on chromosome 9p21 affects the risk of early-onset coronary artery disease. *Mol Biol Rep.* 2008;36(5):889–893.

45. Hinohara K, Nakajima T, Takahashi M, et al. Replication of the association between a chromosome 9p21 polymorphism and coronary artery disease in Japanese and Korean populations. *J Hum Genet.* 2008;53(4):357–359.

46. Schunkert H, Götz A, Braund P, et al. Repeated replication and a prospective meta-analysis of the association between chromosome 9p21.3 and coronary artery disease. *Circulation.* 2008;117(13):1675–1684.

47. Shen GQ, Li L, Rao S, et al. Four SNPs on chromosome 9p21 in a South Korean population implicate a genetic locus that confers high cross-race risk for development of coronary artery disease. *Arterioscler Thromb Vasc Biol.* 2008;28(2):360–365.

48. Shen GQ, Rao S, Martinelli N, et al. Association between four SNPs on chromosome 9p21 and myocardial infarction is replicated in an Italian population. *J Hum Genet.* 2008;53(2):144–150.

49. Talmud PJ, Cooper JA, Palmen J, et al. Chromosome 9p21.3 coronary heart disease locus genotype and prospective risk of CHD in healthy middle-aged men. *Clin Chem.* 2008;54(3):467–474.

50. Zee RY, Ridker PM. Two common gene variants on chromosome 9 and risk of atherothrombosis. *Stroke.* 2007;38(10):e111.

51. Ioannidis JP, Gwinn M, Little J, et al. A road map for efficient and reliable human genome epidemiology. *Nat Genet.* 2006;38(1):3–5.

52. Bertram L, McQueen MB, Mullin K, Blacker D, Tanzi RE. Systematic meta-analyses of Alzheimer disease genetic association studies: the AlzGene database. *Nat Genet.* 2007;39(1):17–23.

53. Allen NC, Bagade S, McQueen MB, et al. Systematic meta-analyses and field synopsis of genetic association studies in schizophrenia: the SzGene database. *Nat Genet.* 2008;40(7):827–834.

54. Vineis P, Manuguerra M, Kavvoura FK, et al. A field synopsis on low-penetrance variants in DNA repair genes and cancer susceptibility. *J Natl Cancer Inst.* 2009;101(1):24–36.

20

Schizophrenia

Lars Bertram

Introduction

As is the case for most of the other phenotypes described in this part of the book, efforts to identify the genes that modulate the risk for schizophrenia (SZ) have met with only limited success. This is at least in part due to problems that aggravate epidemiologic research in many psychiatric diseases, for example, a considerable degree of phenotypic variability and diagnostic uncertainty, the lack of extended pedigrees with Mendelian inheritance, and the absence of definitive disease-specific neuropathological features or biomarkers (1). The identification of susceptibility genes is further complicated by gene–gene interactions that are difficult to predict and model, and a likely substantial but difficult to detect, environmental component. Notwithstanding these challenges, several chromosomal regions thought to harbor SZ genes have been identified via whole genome linkage analyses, a few overlapping across different samples (2,3). In the search for the genes putatively underlying these and other chromosomal regions, over 1,300 SZ "candidate gene" studies have been published over the past two decades claiming or refuting genetic association between certain alleles and affection status and/or certain endophenotypes (4). Currently, more than 150 SZ genetic association papers are published each year, at an ever-increasing pace (5). Despite these tremendous efforts, no single gene or genetic variant has yet been established as a bona fide SZ gene, at least not with the confidence attributed to other complex disease genes, such as *APOE* in Alzheimer disease (6) or *CFH* in macular degeneration (7). For geneticists as well as clinicians, the growing number of (mostly conflicting) genetic findings has become increasingly difficult to follow, evaluate, and interpret, calling for a systematic field synopsis and online encyclopedia as proposed by the HuGE investigators in 2006 (8).

Field Synopsis and Online Encyclopedia: The SzGene Database

In 2006 our group in collaboration with the Schizophrenia Research Forum started building a publicly available database, "SzGene" (http://www.szgene.org), which systematically collects, summarizes, and meta-analyzes all genetic association studies published in the field of SZ, including genome-wide association studies (GWAS) (4). After thorough and still ongoing searches of the available scientific literature, key variables are extracted from original publications and summarized on the SzGene web site. Furthermore, if published genotype data are available from at least four independent case-control studies, they are subjected to random effects meta-analyses of study-level allelic odds ratios (ORs). As of October 1, 2008, SzGene includes over 1,300 individual studies, and showcases the results of over 150 meta-analyses. In these, 27 genes show nominally significant risk effects in a recent freeze of the database content (Table 20.1). The average allelic summary ORs are generally very modest, that is ~1.2 (range: 1.06–1.63) for "risk" alleles, and ~0.8 (range: 0.69–0.94) for "protective" alleles, compared to an OR of ~3–4 for a single copy of the *APOE* ε4-allele in Alzheimer disease (6). These modest effect sizes are in good agreement with those found in other large-scale studies on the genetics of complex diseases (6,9,10), and have important (and well-known) implications for the design of future genetic association studies in SZ, as sample sizes will need to be vastly increased in order to detect or exclude ORs of 1.5 or below with sufficient confidence. For instance, to detect an allelic OR of 1.25 with 80% power at a p-value of 0.05, sample sizes between ~1,400 and 6,000 combined cases and controls are needed for disease allele frequencies ranging from 0.50 to 0.05, respectively (based on calculations using the tools described in References 11 and 12). Sample sizes need to be increased approximately fivefold to detect such modest effects with the same power at p-values below 5×10^{-8}, which is one threshold that has been proposed for declaring genome-wide significance (13,14).

Summary of SzGene Methods

SzGene was modeled after a database developed earlier by our research group for the systematic annotation and meta-analysis of genetic association studies in Alzheimer disease ("AlzGene") (6). AlzGene was the first systematic and continuously updated field synopsis of any genetically complex disease. The corresponding web site (http://www.alzgene.org) was first launched in July of 2004 and included detailed summaries of ~150 publications for approximately 20 genes. Current AlzGene statistics exceed 1,100 publications and 550 genes/loci. From these figures it becomes clear that the "engine" underlying AlzGene, SzGene, and related databases are the ongoing *literature searches* for publications eligible for inclusion. Studies are considered eligible if: (a) they represent genetic association studies, (b) they are published in a peer-reviewed journal, and (c) they are published in English. Clearly, these criteria are arbitrary and nonexhaustive and therefore may lead to bias in the resulting meta-analyses (e.g., because data presented at scientific meetings or published in a language other than English are ignored). However, to the degree that it can be detected, we found no evidence that this strategy, which could lead to the exclusion of a disproportionate amount of "negative" data, resulted in any significant bias, at least not in the majority of meta-analyses with a nominally significant

Table 20.1 SzGene "Top Results" (current on October 1, 2008)

Locus/Gene	Polymorphism	SzGene OR (95% CI)*	p-value*	# SZ Cases	# Controls	# Samples†	Ethnicity
AKT1	rs2494732	1.09 (1.00–1.18)	0.05	4,194	4,416	6	ALL
APOE	ε2/3/4‡	1.16 (1.01–1.33)	0.04	1,563	3,003	16	CAU
DAO	rs4623951	0.88 (0.79–0.98)	0.03	1,509	1,521	4	ALL
DAOA	rs3916971	0.84 (0.73–0.96)	0.01	844	922	4	ALL
DRD1	rs4532	1.18 (1.01–1.38)	0.04	725	1,075	5	ALL
DRD2	rs6277	1.34 (1.07–1.68)	0.01	2,653	3,262	5	CAU
DRD4	120-bp TR	0.81 (0.7–0.94)	0.005	1,236	1,199	4	ALL
DTNBP1	rs1011313	1.12 (1.01–1.25)	0.03	5,319	5,454	11	CAU
GABRB2	rs6556547	0.70 (0.52–0.95)	0.02	774	620	3	CAU
GRIN2B	rs1019385	0.69 (0.54–0.88)	0.003	502	466	4	ALL
HP	Hp1/2	0.88 (0.8–0.98)	0.02	1,346	2,018	6	ALL
GWA_11p14.1	rs1602565	1.19 (1.08–1.31)	0.0007	5,475	10,845	7	CAU
GWA_16p13.12	rs7192086	1.12 (1.06–1.18)	0.00003	7,179	12,623	9	ALL
HTR2A	rs6311	1.16 (1.01–1.33)	0.03	2,678	2,964	8	ALL
IL1B	rs16944	0.84 (0.74–0.96)	0.01	882	1,295	5	CAU
MTHFR	rs1801133	1.14 (1.03–1.25)	0.009	2,529	4,068	16	ALL
NRG1	rs10503929	0.87 (0.79–0.97)	0.009	2,524	2,797	4	ALL

PLXNA2	rs1327175	0.76 (0.58–0.99)	0.04	1,711	1,770	7	ALL
OPCML	rs3016384	0.93 (0.87–0.99)	0.02	7,187	12,675	9	ALL
PPP3CC	rs2461491	1.06 (1.01–1.12)	0.02	5,991	5,960	5	ALL
RELN	rs7341475	0.86 (0.79–0.95)	0.003	2,594	6,587	4	CAU
RGS4	rs2661319	0.94 (0.89–0.99)	0.01	7,765	8,629	12	ALL
TP53	rs1042522	1.13 (1.01–1.26)	0.03	1,418	1,410	5	ALL
RPGRIP1L	rs9922369	1.30 (1.04–1.63)	0.02	5,473	10,823	7	CAU
SLC18A1	rs2270641	1.63 (1.03–2.57)	0.04	759	885	4	ALL
TPH1	rs1800532	1.25 (1.08–1.44)	0.002	1,239	1,708	6	ALL
ZNF804A	rs1344706	0.89 (0.84–0.95)	0.0005	7,183	12,663	9	ALL

List of loci containing at least one polymorphism showing nominally significant (p-value ≤0.05) summary ORs in SzGene on October 1, 2008. To be considered as "Top Result," summary OR needs to be significant across samples from all ethnic backgrounds ("ALL") or in Caucasians only ("CAU"). Whenever nominally statistically significant results are observed for both, that is, ALL and CAU, only the analysis that has the largest genetic effect size (OR deviating the most from 1) is reported here. Note that SzGene is continuously updated, so results displayed online may differ from the results above; consult the SzGene web site for up-to-date numbers and additional meta-analyses in these and other loci (http://www.szgene.org). Shaded loci (DRD1, DTNBP1, MTHFR, and TPH1) showed "strong epidemiologic credibility" applying recently proposed (17) guidelines in our original SzGene publication (4). Loci prefixed with "GWA_" were originally identified in a GWAS and have not yet been assigned to a specific gene.

*Summary ORs, 95% confidence intervals (CI), and p-values are based on random-effects allelic contrasts comparing minor versus major alleles.

†Number of samples refers to the number of independent case-control samples used in the meta-analyses; multiple samples may be reported in the same publication and are considered separately if they are independent, that is, nonoverlapping. Samples overlapping across publications are only used once, usually by including the data sets with the largest number of available genotypes.

‡Results are based on comparing ε4- versus ε3-alleles at this locus.

outcome. For more details on the methods related to the literature searches, data management, and statistical procedures, please consult the original SzGene paper (4) and the database web site (http://www.szgene.org).

To allow for an unbiased and systematic extraction of demographic variables and genotype data from each study, several *data management* procedures were put into place. Full length copies of all papers eligible for inclusion in SzGene are obtained and stored offline. As a general rule, all applicable data are first entered into an offline version of the database, where they are double-checked against the original publications before any further processing (e.g., meta-analysis and posting on the SzGene web site). Each SzGene study entry consists of the name of the first author, year of publication, and PubMed ID number, along with key population-specific details extracted from each study, such as: ascertainment design (family-based or case-control), ethnic background and population (i.e., country) of origin, as well as sample source (clinic-, population-, or community-based), the number of cases with gender ratio, age at onset, age at examination, method of diagnosis, the number of controls with gender ratio and age at examination, and the reported study results. Whenever possible, NCBI's "dbSNP" identifiers ("rs numbers") were used to designate polymorphism identities throughout the database. Genotype distributions are listed for each polymorphism as provided in the original publication. Whenever genotype distributions are not presented in the publication, they are calculated from reported allele frequencies and sample sizes (assuming no deviations from HWE unless reported otherwise in the original paper). In many instances, authors reported genotype data in the same or largely overlapping samples in separately published articles. Where such overlap was specified by the authors or suspected overlap was confirmed by the authors, the overlap is indicated and only genotype data from the largest cohort is included in SzGene and its meta-analyses.

Statistical analyses in SzGene revolve mainly around the meta-analysis of study-specific ORs. For all variants with minor allele frequencies >0.01 in "healthy" controls and with case-control genotype data available from four or more samples, crude study-level ORs and 95% confidence intervals (CIs) are calculated for each study using allelic contrasts (generally, minor vs major allele). Summary ORs and 95% CIs are calculated using the DerSimonian and Laird random-effects model (15), which utilizes weights that incorporate both the within-study and between-study variance. This procedure is first performed on all studies regardless of ethnicity (denoted by "All Studies" on the meta-analysis graphs; Figure 20.1c). Summary ORs and 95% CIs are also calculated for studies of Caucasian ancestry if three or more such studies existed ("All Caucasian Studies"). Generally, too few samples of non-Caucasian ancestry exist to allow meaningful meta-analyses on non-Caucasian ancestry populations. Routine sensitivity analyses include the calculation of summary ORs and 95% CIs for all studies excluding the initial report ("All Excluding Initial") and after excluding studies violating HWE according to a chi-square test at $p \leq 0.05$ ("All Excl HWE Deviations"). We also routinely construct funnel plots that depict the ORs (on a logarithmic scale) against their standard error for each study (16), and these plots are available online for all variants. Finally, the online version of SzGene maintains a continuously updated list of associations that have been evaluated in meta-analyses and yield statistically significant results ($p < 0.05$) in the main analysis of all ethnicities or in studies of Caucasian descent ("Top Results").

To all "Top Results" we also applied a recently proposed grading scheme to assess the strength of the "epidemiologic credibility" of each meta-analysis. This interim grading scheme has recently been developed by investigators from HuGENet and details on its background are published elsewhere (see also Chapter 4) (17). Briefly, each meta-analyzed association is graded (using grades A to C, where A represents the "best" possible grade) based on the: (a) amount of evidence (i.e., sample size), (b) consistency of replication (i.e., degree of heterogeneity), and (c) protection from bias (e.g., publication bias, loss of significance after exclusion of the initial study). Overall epidemiologic credibility is then rated as A, (or "strong,") if associations receive three A grades; as B, (or "moderate,") if they received any B, but no C; and C, (or "weak,") if they received at least one C grade in any of the three assessment criteria (17). Future versions of SzGene will provide a list of "Top Results" rank-ordered based on the outcome of this (and possibly other) grading assessments.

After completing the data entry, processing, and analysis procedures described above, all study-specific variables, genotype data, and meta-analysis results are posted to the *online database* version of SzGene. This is written in a server-side scripting environment (using Microsoft Active Server Pages), and all data is stored and managed in Microsoft SQL Server, a relational database management system. The online database is hosted by the "Schizophrenia Research Forum," a nonprofit, internet-based community portal dedicated to furthering collaboration among researchers to help in the search for causes, treatments, and understanding of schizophrenia. The SzGene site can be accessed via its own designated URLs (http://www.szgene.org or http://www.schizophreniagene.org) or directly through the Schizophrenia Research Forum (http://www.schizophreniaforum.org/res/scz-gene/default.asp; see Figure 20.1a for a screenshot of the home page, including an expanded list of recent "Top Results").

The SzGene site is divided into three sections: (i) "Gene-specific summary" pages, which list all studies and study-specific descriptors for any gene included in SzGene (Figure 20.1b); (ii) "Polymorphism detail" pages, which list published genotype distributions for each polymorphism and sample analyzed per study (Figure 20.1c); (iii) "Meta-analysis" pages, which provide ethnicity-specific pooled genotype distributions (after summation of study-specific genotype counts; Figure 20.1d), and forest plots based on allele-specific random-effects analyses including summary ORs and 95% CIs for each polymorphism with data available in at least four independent samples. Each meta-analysis page also provides a link to a polymorphism-specific funnel plot to allow a visual assessment of publication bias. The SzGene web interface (Figure 20.1a) can be searched either by gene name or alias (with direct links to the appropriate entries in NCBI's "EntrezGene," by protein name or alias (with links to NCBI's "EntrezProtein"), by polymorphism name or alias (with links to NCBI's "dbSNP"), by

(a) SzGene homepage (http://www.szgene.org) with "Top Results" list expanded (current on October 1, 2008; for details on these results see Table 20.1).

SchizophreniaGene (SZGene)
Published Candidate Genes for Schizophrenia

◀ BACK   SEARCH   METHODS   DISCLAIMER   CREDITS

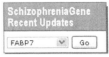

SchizophreniaGene Recent Updates

FABP7   ∨   Go

SZGene   Updated 1 October 2008

Chromosome: 1 2 3 4 5 6 7 8 9 10 11 12 13
            14 15 16 17 18 19 20 21 22 X Y MT

Gene: -- Select --   ∨   Go

Protein: -- Select --   ∨   Go

Polymorphism: -- Select --   ∨   Go

Study: -- Select --   ∨   Go

Keyword: [   ]   Go

GWAS and other large-scale association studies

Display, print, and download SZGene database content

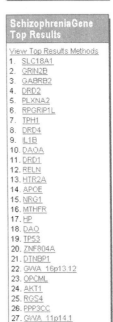

SchizophreniaGene Top Results

View Top Results Methods
1. SLC18A1
2. GRIN2B
3. GABRB2
4. DRD2
5. PLXNA2
6. RPGRIP1L
7. TPH1
8. DRD4
9. IL1B
10. DAOA
11. DRD1
12. RELN
13. HTR2A
14. APOE
15. NRG1
16. MTHFR
17. HP
18. DAO
19. TP53
20. ZNF804A
21. DTNBP1
22. GWA_16p13.12
23. OPCML
24. AKT1
25. RGS4
26. PPP3CC
27. GWA_11p14.1

The SchizophreniaGene database aims to provide a comprehensive, unbiased and regularly updated collection of genetic association studies performed on schizophrenia phenotypes. Eligible publications are identified following systematic searches of scientific literature databases, as well as the table of contents of journals in genetics and psychiatry.

The database can be searched either by a variety of dropdown menus or by specific keywords. For each gene, summary overviews are provided displaying key characteristics for each publication, including links to genotype distributions of the polymorphisms studied, random-effects allelic meta-analyses, and funnel plots for an assessment of publication bias.

For more details on the background and methods, see Methods, Disclaimer, and Credits. We encourage authors and readers to contact us to report errors in the presentation of study details, or to notify us of studies that have mistakenly been left out.

How to Cite Content on SchizophreniaGene:
Allen NC, Bagade S, McQueen MB, Ioannidis JPA, Kawoura FK, Khoury MJ, Tanzi RE, Bertram L (2008) "Systematic Meta-Analyses and Field Synopsis of Genetic Association Studies in Schizophrenia: The SzGene Database" Nat Genet 40(7): 827-34.

Figure 20.1 Example screenshots from SzGene.

(b) "Gene summary" page: summarizes key variables of each study published for DRD2 and eligible for inclusion in SzGene. Note that this screenshot only depicts the top section of this page which on June 7, 2008 listed a total of 65 individual publications.

Gene Overview of All Published Schizophrenia-Association Studies for DRD2

| ◀ BACK | SEARCH | METHODS | DISCLAIMER | CREDITS |

Gene: DRD2 (D2R, D2DR) Enter Gene   View on PDGene

Protein: dopamine receptor D2 (seven transmembrane helix receptor) [••••] Protein

Chromosome: 11 (View: 1 2 3 4 5 6 7 8 9 10 11 12 13 14 15 16 17 18 19 20 21 22 X Y)

Status: Updated 1 October 2008

| VIEW META-ANALYSIS |

1. CASE-CONTROL STUDIES (BY ETHNIC GROUP)

Study	Population	Source	# Polys	SZ Cases # Subjects (% women)	DX	Onset Age (range)	Age (range)	Normal Controls # Subjects (% women)	Age (range)	Result	Comment
CAUCASIAN											
Asherson, 1994	UK	CL	1 (detail)	112 (-)	BIP	-	-	64 (-)	-	Negative	SUBMIT COMMENT
Breen, 1999	UK	CL	1 (detail)	439 (-)	M	-	-	437 (-)	-	Positive	SUBMIT COMMENT
Campion, 1994	France	CL	1 (detail)	88 (-)	BIP	-	-	88 (-)	-	Negative	SUBMIT COMMENT
* Initial Study * Comings, 1991	USA	CL	1 (detail)	87 (-)	BI	-	-	314 (-)	-	Negative	SUBMIT COMMENT
Crawford, 1996	USA	CL	1 (detail)	84 (-)	BIP	-	-	84 (-)	-	Negative	SUBMIT COMMENT
Dollfus, 1996	France	CL	1 (detail)	62 (-)	M	-	-	161 (-)	-	Negative	SUBMIT COMMENT
Dubertret, 2001	France	CL	2 (detail)	58 (26%)	IV	20.6 + 3.1 (-)	-	58 (22%)	-	Positive	SUBMIT COMMENT

Figure 20.1 Continued.

name of the first author and year of publication (with links to NCBI's "PubMed"), or by a free-text search. Finally, users can search by chromosomal location, where gene symbols are listed according to their approximate location next to cytogenetic images of each chromosome. As an experimental addition to these chromosome overviews, we have highlighted potential SZ linkage regions as reported by Lewis et al. (3).

First SzGene Results

For the purpose of this summary, the database content was "frozen" on October 1, 2008, similar to what was done for the original SzGene paper (4). At that time, 1,374 individual publications reporting on 6,397 genetic variants (or polymorphisms) in 739 different genes were included, after screening approximately 16,000 titles and abstracts (note that the database continues to be regularly updated; therefore, the results presented below may differ from those found online).

Of the 6,397 included polymorphisms, 154 variants in 63 genes had sufficient data to warrant meta-analysis (i.e., genotype data available from at least four independent case-control samples) on October 1, 2008. On average, these meta-analyses were based on ~7,600 combined cases and controls, originating from seven

*(c) "Polymorphism details" page: summarizes the genotype distributions for each polymor-
phism and sample investigated by each study (using Dubertret, 2001 as an example).*

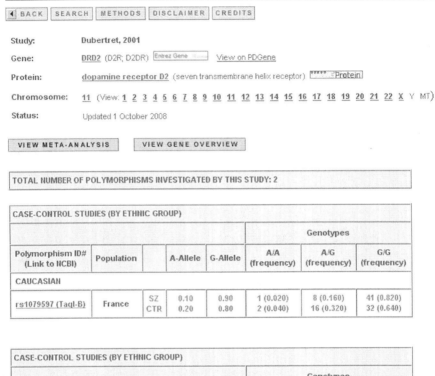

Figure 20.1 Continued.

independent data sets. While 37 of the meta-analyzed variants in 27 genes showed
nominally significant ($p \leq 0.05$) summary ORs (*AKT1, APOE, DAO, DAOA, DRD1,
DRD2, DRD4, DTNBP1, GABRB2, GRIN2B, HP, GWA_11p14.1, GWA_16p13.12,
HTR2A, IL1B, MTHFR, NRG1, PLXNA2, OPCML, PPP3CC, RELN, RGS4, TP53,
RPGRIP1L, SLC18A1, TPH1,* and *ZNF804A*; Table 20.1), the vast majority of polymorphisms yielded no significant association with SZ risk. However, in only about
half of all meta-analyses was the combined sample size sufficient to detect an allelic
OR of ~1.25 with 80% power (see above), which could have affected both positive
and negative results. Overall, our systematic approach applied to the SZ genetics literature nearly doubled the number of meta-analyses published in the field, including
the detection of significant effects in seven genes (*DAO, DRD1, DTNBP1, GABRB2,*

(d) "Meta-analysis" page: shows forest plots for all polymorphisms with sufficient geno-type data to warrant meta-analyses (note that for many loci, several polymorphisms had sufficient data and that meta-analyses can be chosen from a pull-down menu; here rs6277 [Pro319Pro] was chosen as an example).

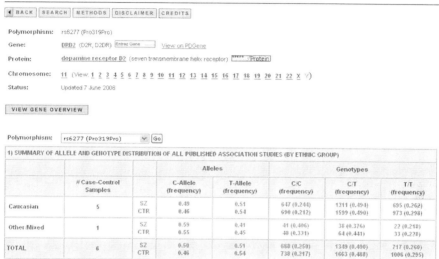

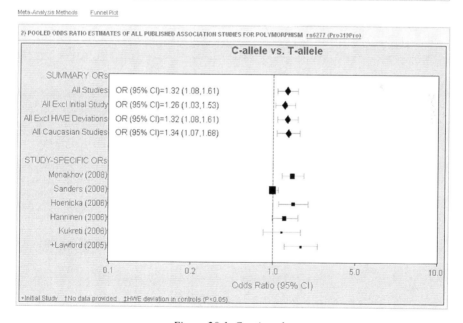

Figure 20.1 Continued.

HP, PLXNA2, and *TP53*) that were not meta-analyzed prior to the freeze data of the original SzGene publication (4). Finally, application of the HuGENet grading scheme (17) to all nominally significant associations of the initial data freeze sug-gested that variants in at least four genes obtained an overall "A grade," implying that their meta-analysis results showed a strong degree of "epidemiologic credibility" (i.e., *DRD1, DTNBP1, MTHFR, TPH1*; Table 20.1 and Reference 4). Thus, at least based on these interim criteria, these genes currently appear as the best contenders to harbor genuine susceptibility alleles within the whole domain of genetic epidemiology in SZ.

Inclusion of GWAS in SzGene

As described in more detail elsewhere in this book (Chapter 8), recent advances in large-scale genotyping technologies now enable researchers to perform comprehensive and largely hypothesis-free GWAS. As of July 2008, six groups had reported results using this approach in SZ (18–23) (Table 20.2), testing between ~25,000 and ~500,000 markers in the initial screening phase. The sheer scale of GWAS makes their systematic inclusion in SzGene a daunting and computationally demanding task. We have devised the following three-stage protocol to capture the most relevant genetic information from GWAS without the need to display each data point or result online.

Stage 1 focuses on the inclusion and display of genes and polymorphisms highlighted (or "featured") by the authors of a GWAS (Table 20.2). Usually, these loci are emphasized in the original publication because they show some degree of genetic association after completion of all analyses, for example, correction for multiple comparisons and/or replication in multiple independent data sets. Stage 1 data represent the core findings of each GWAS, and their inclusion is relatively straightforward as the distributions of these genes and polymorphisms are usually readily available from the original publication.

Stage 2 makes use of "non-featured" genotypes, that is, of polymorphisms not reported as associated with SZ in the original publications, provided the complete GWAS data are publicly available. Practically, this entails identifying all markers not addressed in Stage 1 for overlap with polymorphisms already included in SzGene and including data on their distribution to recalculate the meta-analyses. Note that the failure to identify previously proposed candidate gene effects within the setting of a GWAS does not necessarily preclude such effects from existing. Rather, this scenario could reflect insufficient power due to small sample size. For instance, the combined (cases and controls) sample sizes used for GWAS in the five currently published studies in SZ ranged from ~300 to ~3,500. Thus, none of these studies came even close to the minimum sample sizes needed (~7,000 combined cases and controls, see above) to detect ORs ~1.25 with 80% power at p-values $\leq 5 \times 10^{-8}$.

Stage 3 entails conducting systematic meta-analyses for all variants overlapping across independent samples, provided that at least four complete GWAS data sets have been made publicly available. Only variants showing genome-wide significant summary ORs in these meta-analyses will be displayed on the SzGene web site. The threshold for declaring statistical significance in this context will be more stringent than for meta-analyses of individual candidate polymorphisms, due to the large number of tests performed. Procedures for implementing this stage, and

Table 20.2 Overview of published GWAS in SZ (current on October 1, 2008)

GWAS	Design	Population	Platform	# SNPs	Data Available?	# SZ Cases* (Total)	# Controls* (Total)	"Featured" Genes
Mah, 2006 (18)	Case-control & Family-based	USA, Australia & Other	Customized cSNPs	25,494	No	320 (1,082)	325 (1,123)	PLXNA2[1]
Lencz, 2007 (19)	Case-control	USA	Affymetrix (500K)	439,511	No	178 (249)	144 (175)	CSF2RA[2], IL3RA[3]
Shifman, 2008 (21)	Case-control	Israel, USA, EU	Affymetrix (500k)	510,552	No	660 (3,015)	2,771 (7,183)	RELN[4]
Kirov, 2008 (20)	Family-based	Bulgaria	Illumina (550K)	43,680	No	574 (n.a.)	1,753 (n.a.)	CCDC60[5], RBP1[6]
Sullivan, 2008 (22)	Case-control	USA	Affymetrix (500K) & Perlegen	492,900	Yes†	738 (n.a.)	733 (n.a.)	none
O'Donovan, 2008 (23)	Case-control	Mixed	Affymetrix (500K)	362,532	No	479 (6829)	2,937 (9,897)	ZNF804A,[7] GWA_11p14.1,[8] GWA_16p13.12[9]

Modified after content on the SzGene web site (http://www.szgene.org) (5); current on October 1, 2008. Studies are listed in order of publication date. "Featured Genes" are those genes/loci that were declared as "associated" in the original publication; but criteria for declaring association may vary across studies. Note that the studies by Mah, 2006, Shifman, 2008, and Kirov, 2008 used pooled genotypes in their initial GWAS analyses.

*Numbers of "SZ Cases" and "Controls" refers to sample sizes used in initial GWAS, whereas "Total" refers to initial sample plus any follow-up samples (where applicable); please consult SzGene web site for more details on these studies.

†Original publication states that "individual phenotype and genotype data (has been) made available to the scientific community"; application from SzGene curatorial team for access to these data is currently pending.

The following URLs are to the respective gene summaries on the database's web site:
1. http://www.schizophreniaforum.org/res/sczgene/geneoverview.asp?geneID=259
2. http://www.schizophreniaforum.org/res/sczgene/geneoverview.asp?geneID=495
3. http://www.schizophreniaforum.org/res/sczgene/geneoverview.asp?geneID=204
4. http://www.schizophreniaforum.org/res/sczgene/geneoverview.asp?geneID=18
5. http://www.schizophreniaforum.org/res/sczgene/geneoverview.asp?geneID=692
6. http://www.schizophreniaforum.org/res/sczgene/geneoverview.asp?geneID=691
7. http://www.schizophreniaforum.org/res/sczgene/geneoverview.asp?geneID=739
8. http://www.schizophreniaforum.org/res/sczgene/geneoverview.asp?geneID=731
9. http://www.schizophreniaforum.org/res/sczgene/geneoverview.asp?geneID=733

the definition of appropriate threshold criteria are currently being developed by our group and by others (24).

Strengths and Limitations of the SzGene Approach

Assuming that the literature searches, inclusion criteria, data management, and data analysis procedures work reasonably well and actually provide a correct and exhaustive account of the available literature, SzGene is the single most comprehensive resource for the status of genetics research in SZ available to date (see below for important limitations to this and the following statements). In our original datafreeze (4) we could show that literature searches in SzGene outperformed those of several other literature/genetics databases, and that the results of our meta-analyses were in very good agreement with those published previously in nearly 80 individual papers. Published meta-analyses, however, have one important disadvantage: by nature of their design, they run the risk of becoming outdated quickly, possibly as soon as new data from one or two additional studies are published. Provided that sufficient funding remains available, SzGene does not have this caveat. Any meta-analysis in the database can be updated shortly after the publication of new data. Another strength of SzGene and related databases is that it is not limited to meta-analyses on certain genes or networks of genes (e.g., those that are in the same pathway or gene family), but considers all published loci simultaneously, making the comparison of results across studies, genes, pathways, chromosomal regions, and so on very easy. Furthermore, all loci containing at least one polymorphism nominally significant for meta-analysis are separately highlighted on the database homepage in a section called "Top Results." Thus, consulting this section of the SzGene web site will provide the user with a complete—and essentially real-time—snapshot of the "most promising" SZ candidate genes, based on the systematic evaluation of literally hundreds of individual studies and thousands of data points. As such, the "Top Results" list could help prioritize future genetic association studies (e.g., for further independent replication, or fine-mapping), and guide functional genomics and molecular studies investigating the potential pathogenetic mechanisms underlying the putative genetic associations.

While regularly updated online encyclopedias such as SzGene and related databases drastically facilitate the evaluation and interpretation of genetic association data in their respective fields, their overall approach, naturally, is not without caveats. First and foremost, despite the comprehensive and systematic searches of the scientific literature, we cannot exclude the possibility that some association studies were overlooked or entered erroneously. This can be partly alleviated with the help of database users who are explicitly encouraged to alert the curatorial team of any errors or omissions, which will be fixed as soon as possible. Other limitations include our restriction to allele contrasts in the meta-analyses (which allows no inference of the true mode of inheritance and is usually less powerful than genotype-based tests), the nonconsideration of haplotype-based genotype data or imputed single-locus genotypes (possibly missing important associations), the exclusive focus on "main effects" (and the inherent inability to account for gene–gene and gene–environment interactions), and the lack of adjustment for certain covariates such as age and gender (which is impossible to do systematically without access to study-level raw data). Furthermore, protection from bias is particularly difficult to ensure or assess, since latent bias is always possible and no test can have very high sensitivity and specificity for all types of possible biases. Finally, it needs to be stressed that the number of "true" associations is almost certainly going to be smaller than the number of nominally significant findings listed at any time on the SzGene web site (25,26). This has a number of reasons, including multiple testing, linkage disequilibrium among associated variants, undetected publication or other reporting biases, as well as study-level technical artifacts that may have gone unnoticed or may be impossible to detect. Moreover, most of the "positive" meta-analysis outcomes in SzGene currently do not reach very high levels of statistical significance (see Table 20.1), none even approaching the common thresholds used to establish genome-wide significance, for example, a p-value $\leq 5 \times 10^{-8}$ (note that this is different for the "Top Results" of AlzGene or PDGene [http://www.pdgene.org], where several meta-analyses show p-values below 5×10^{-8}).

Generally, the possibility of a false-positive meta-analysis finding always exists, even for the highest ranked "Top Result." Eventually, genuine risk effects can only be proven by the accumulation of sufficient unbiased genotype data in favor of the presumed association *in combination* with functional genomics and biological evidence suggesting a direct biochemical involvement of the associated variant (13). Notwithstanding these limitations, there is good reason to believe that the variants and loci highlighted in the "Top Results" section of SzGene and related databases currently represent the best bets as to which of the hundreds of putative candidate genes might genuinely contribute to disease susceptibility and pathogenesis. As such, they probably warrant follow-up with high priority.

Acknowledgments
Funding for SzGene is provided by the National Alliance on Research in Schizophrenia and Depression (to LB). The SzGene team would like to express their gratefulness to the Schizophrenia Research Forum for hosting SzGene on their web site.

References

1. Kennedy JL, FarrerLA, Andreasen NC, Mayeux R, St George-Hyslop P. The genetics of adult-onset neuropsychiatric disease: complexities and conundra? *Science.* 2003;302(5646):822–826.
2. Badner JA, Gershon ES. Meta-analysis of whole-genome linkage scans of bipolar disorder and schizophrenia. *Mol Psychiatry.* 2002;7(4):405–411.
3. Lewis CM, Levinson DF, Wise LH, et al. Genome scan meta-analysis of schizophrenia and bipolar disorder, part II: schizophrenia. *Am J Hum Genet.* 2003;73(1):34–48.
4. Allen NC, Bagade S, McQueen MB, et al. Systematic meta-analyses and field synopsis of genetic association studies in schizophrenia: the SzGene database. *Nat Genet.* 2008;40(7):827–834.

5. Bertram L. Genetic research in schizophrenia: new tools and future perspectives. *Schizophr Bull.* 2008;34(5):806–812.

6. Bertram L, McQueen MB, Mullin K, Blacker D, Tanzi RE. Systematic meta-analyses of Alzheimer disease genetic association studies: the AlzGene database. *Nat Genet.* 2007;39(1):17–23.

7. Thakkinstian A, Han P, McEvoy M, et al. Systematic review and meta-analysis of the association between complement factor H Y402H polymorphisms and age-related macular degeneration. *Hum Mol Genet.* 2006;15(18):2784–2790.

8. Ioannidis JP, Gwinn M, Little J, et al. A road map for efficient and reliable human genome epidemiology. *Nat Genet.* 2006;38(1):3–5.

9. Lohmueller KE, Pearce CL, Pike M, Lander ES, Hirschhorn JN. Meta-analysis of genetic association studies supports a contribution of common variants to susceptibility to common disease. *Nat Genet.* 2003;33(2):177–182.

10. Ioannidis JP, Ntzani EE, Trikalinos TA, Contopoulos-Ioannidis DG. Replication validity of genetic association studies. *Nat Genet.* 2001;29(3):306–309.

11. Purcell S, Cherny SS, Sham PC. Genetic Power Calculator: design of linkage and association genetic mapping studies of complex traits. *Bioinformatics.* 2003;19(1):149–150.

12. Lange C, DeMeo D, Silverman EK, Weiss ST, Laird NM. PBAT: tools for family-based association studies. *Am J Hum Genet.* 2004;74(2):367–369.

13. McCarthy MI, Abecasis GR, Cardon LR, et al. Genome-wide association studies for complex traits: consensus, uncertainty and challenges. *Nat Rev Genet.* 2008;9(5):356–369.

14. Hoggart CJ, Clark TG, De Iorio M, Whittaker JC, Balding DJ. Genome-wide significance for dense SNP and resequencing data. *Genet Epidemiol.* 2008;32(2):179–185.

15. DerSimonian R, Laird N. Meta-analysis in clinical trials. *Control Clin Trials.* 1986;7(3):177–188.

16. Egger M, Davey Smith G, Schneider M, Minder C. Bias in meta-analysis detected by a simple, graphical test. *BMJ.* 1997;315(7109):629–634.

17. Ioannidis JP, Boffetta P, Little J, et al. Assessment of cumulative evidence on genetic associations: interim guidelines. *Int J Epidemiol.* 2008;37(1):120–132.

18. Mah S, Nelson MR, Delisi LE, et al. Identification of the semaphorin receptor PLXNA2 as a candidate for susceptibility to schizophrenia. *Mol Psychiatry.* 2006;11(5):471–478.

19. Lencz T, Morgan TV, Athanasiou M, et al. Converging evidence for a pseudoautosomal cytokine receptor gene locus in schizophrenia. *Mol Psychiatry.* 2007;12(6):572–580.

20. Kirov G, Zaharieva I, Georgieva L, et al. A genome-wide association study in 574 schizophrenia trios using DNA pooling. *Mol Psychiatry.* 2008.

21. Shifman S, Johannesson M, Bronstein M, et al. Genome-wide association identifies a common variant in the reelin gene that increases the risk of schizophrenia only in women. *PLoS Genet.* 2008;4(2):e28.

22. Sullivan PF, Lin D, Tzeng JY, et al. Genomewide association for schizophrenia in the CATIE study: results of stage 1. *Mol Psychiatry.* 2008;13(6):570–584.

23. O'Donovan MC, Craddock N, Norton N, et al. Identification of loci associated with schizophrenia by genome-wide association and follow-up. *Nat Genet.* 2008;40(9):1053–1055.

24. Evangelou E, Maraganore DM, Ioannidis JP. Meta-analysis in genome-wide association datasets: strategies and application in Parkinson disease. *PLoS ONE.* 2007;2e196.

25. Wacholder S, Chanock S, Garcia-Closas M, El Ghormli L, Rothman N. Assessing the probability that a positive report is false: an approach for molecular epidemiology studies. *J Natl Cancer Inst.* 2004;96(6):434–442.

26. Ioannidis JP. Why most published research findings are false. *PLoS Med.* 2005;2(8):e124.

IV

APPLICATIONS OF EPIDEMIOLOGIC METHODS FOR USING GENETIC INFORMATION IN MEDICINE AND PUBLIC HEALTH

21

Mendelian randomization: the contribution of genetic epidemiology to elucidating environmentally modifiable causes of disease

George Davey Smith and Shah Ebrahim

Introduction

Conventional risk factor epidemiology—directly studying environmentally modifiable exposures that may influence disease risk—and genetic epidemiology have similarities and differences. The case-control design is, for example, more popular in genetic epidemiology than it currently is in conventional risk factor epidemiology, and while the importance of sample size is recognized in conventional epidemiology, the huge collaborative ventures currently being undertaken in genetic epidemiology have not been the norm, since special attention has, appropriately, been paid to detailed exposure and outcome measurement (1). In genetic epidemiology there has recently been much attention paid to false-positive findings generated by multiple hypothesis testing against a background of inadequate statistical power (2,3) whereas in risk factor epidemiology problems generated by confounding and bias have been to the forefront (4). In this chapter we deal with Mendelian randomization, a principle that underlies some of the differences between conventional risk factor and genetic epidemiology, and also renders genetic epidemiology a useful tool for improving the identification of environmentally modifiable risk factors that are causally related to disease outcomes, and therefore targets for therapeutic or preventative intervention.

Understanding Environmentally Modifiable Causes of Disease: Why We Need New Approaches

Conventional risk factor epidemiology approaches have had major successes in identifying modifiable causes of disease. However, in recent years there have been several high-profile cases in which such approaches have appeared to produce misleading findings.

Consider cardiovascular disease, where observational studies suggesting that beta-carotene (5), vitamin E supplements (6,7), vitamin C supplements (8), and hormone replacement therapy (9) were protective were followed by large randomized controlled trials (RCTs) showing no such protection (10–15). In each case, special pleading was advanced to explain the discrepancy; were the doses of vitamins given in the trials too high, too low, or of too short duration to be comparable to the observational studies (16,17)? Did hormone replacement therapy use start too late in the trials (18)? Were differences explained by duration of follow-up or other design aspects (19)? Were interactions with other factors such as smoking or alcohol consumption key? Rather than such specific—and post hoc—explanations being true (with the reassuring conclusion that both the observational studies and the trials had got the right answers, but to different questions), it is likely that a general problem of confounding—by lifestyle and socioeconomic factors, or by baseline health status and prescription policies—is responsible (20–23). Indeed, in the vitamin E supplements example, the observational studies and the trials tested precisely the same thing. Figures 21.1a and 21.1b show the findings from observational studies of taking vitamin E supplements (6,7) and a meta-analysis of trials of supplements (24). The point here is that the observational studies specifically investigated the effect of taking supplements for a short period (2–4 years) and found an apparent robust and large protective effect, even after adjustment for confounders. The trials tested randomization to essentially the same supplements for the same period, and found no protective effect.

The potentially misleading findings from observational studies have consequences, of course. For example, Figure 21.2 demonstrates that nearly half of U.S. adults are taking either vitamin E supplements or multivitamin/multimineral supplements that generally contain vitamin E (25). Figure 21.3 presents data from the three available time points, where it is seen that there appears to have been a particular increase in vitamin E use after 1992 (26), possibly consequent upon the publication of the two observational studies mentioned above, which have received nearly 3,000 citations between them since publication.

What underlies the discrepancy between these findings? One likely possibility is that there is considerable confounding between use of vitamin E supplements

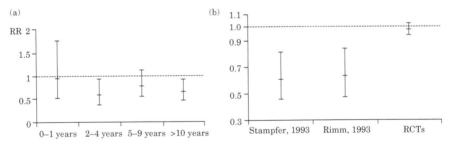

Figure 21.1 (a) Observed effect of duration of vitamin E supplement use compared to no use on coronary heart disease (CHD) events in the Health Professionals Follow-up Study (6). (b) Vitamin E supplement use and risk of CHD in that and another observational study (6,7) and in a meta-analysis of RCTs (24) (relative risks and 95% confidence intervals for taking and not taking vitamin E supplements).

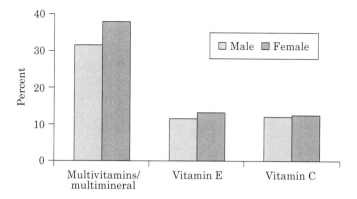

Figure 21.2 Use of vitamin supplements in past month among U.S. adults, 1999–2000 (25).
Source: *Radimer K, et al.,* Am J Epidemiol *2004;160:339–349.*

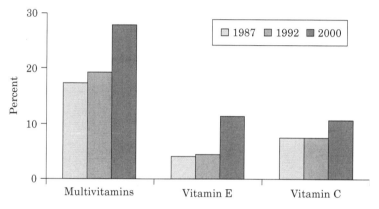

Figure 21.3 Use of vitamin supplements by U.S. adults, 1987–2000 (26). Source: *Millen AE, et al.,* Journal of American Dietetic Assoc *2004;104:942–950.*

and other exposures that could increase the risk of coronary heart disease (CHD). Such confounding is extensive, as has been demonstrated with respect to vitamin C (27), and can generate the magnitude of associations found in observational studies (27,28). Other processes in addition to confounding can generate robust, but non-causal, associations in observational studies. Reverse causation—where the disease influences the apparent exposure, rather than *vice versa*—may generate strong and replicable associations. For example, many studies have found that people with low circulating cholesterol levels are at increased risk of several cancers, including colon cancer. If causal, this is an important association as it might mean that efforts to lower cholesterol levels would increase the risk of cancer. However, it is possible that the early stages of cancer may, many years before diagnosis or death, lead to a lowering in cholesterol levels, rather than low cholesterol levels increasing the risk of cancer. Similarly, in studies of inflammatory markers such as C-reactive protein and cardiovascular disease risk, it is possible that early stages of atherosclerosis—which is an inflammatory process—lead to elevation in circulating inflammatory markers. Since people with atherosclerosis are more likely to experience cardiovascular events, a robust, but noncausal, association between levels of inflammatory markers and incident cardiovascular disease is generated. Reverse causation can also occur through behavioral processes—for example, people with early stages and symptoms of cardiovascular disease may reduce their consumption of alcohol, which would generate a situation in which alcohol intake appears to protect against cardiovascular disease. Finally, a form of reverse causation can occur through reporting bias, with the presence of disease influencing reporting disposition. In case-control studies, people with the disease under investigation may report on their prior exposure history in a different way than do controls—perhaps because the former will think harder about potential reasons that account for why they have developed the disease.

In observational studies, associations between an exposure and disease will generally be biased if there is selection according to an exposure–disease combination in case-control studies, or according to an exposure–disease risk combination in prospective studies. Such selection may arise through differential participation in research studies, for example, conducting studies in settings such as hospitals where cases and controls are not representative of the general population. If, for example, those people experiencing an exposure but at low risk of disease for other reasons were differentially excluded from a study, the exposure would appear to be positively related to disease outcome, even if there were no such association in the underlying population. This is a form of "Berkson's bias," well known to epidemiologists (29). A possible example of such associative selection bias relates to the finding in the large American Cancer Society volunteer cohort that high alcohol consumption (which would be expected to increase stroke risk through association with high blood pressure), was associated with a reduced risk of stroke (30). While ischemic stroke risk might be reduced by the HDL-cholesterol raising effects of alcohol, the outcome category included hemorrhagic stroke, for which there is no obvious mechanism through which alcohol would reduce risk. Population-based studies have found that heavy alcohol consumption tends to increase stroke risk, particularly hemorrhagic stroke (31,32). These discordant findings are likely explained by the small proportion of heavy drinkers who volunteer for a study about the health effects of their lifestyle being unrepresentative of all heavy drinkers in the population, the volunteers among heavy drinkers being healthier than those who do not volunteer. Moderate drinkers and nondrinkers who volunteer may be more representative of moderate drinkers and nondrinkers in the underlying population. Thus the low risk of stroke in the heavy drinkers who volunteer for the study could erroneously make it appear that alcohol reduces the risk of stroke.

The problems of confounding and bias discussed above relate to the production of associations in observational studies that are not reliable indicators of the true direction of causal associations. A separate issue is that the strength of associations between causal risk factors and disease in observational studies will generally be underestimated due to random measurement imprecision in indexing the exposure. A century ago, Charles Spearman demonstrated mathematically how such measurement imprecision would lead to what he termed the "attenuation by errors" of associations (33,34). This has lately been renamed "regression dilution bias."

Observational studies can and do produce findings that either spuriously enhance or downgrade estimates of causal associations between modifiable exposures and disease. This has serious consequences for the appropriateness of interventions that aim to reduce disease risk in populations. It is for these reasons that alternative approaches—including those within the Mendelian randomization framework—need to be applied.

Phenocopies, Genocopies, and the Causes of Disease

An approach that can strengthen inference from observational studies is to apply the concepts of phenocopy and genocopy to population-based research settings. The term phenocopy is attributed to Goldschmidt (35) and is used to describe the situation where an environmental exposure could produce the same outcome as was produced by a genetic mutation. As Goldschmidt explained, "different causes produce the same end effect, presumably by changing the same developmental processes in an identical way" (35). In human genetics the term phenocopy refers to an environmentally produced disease state that is similar to a clear genetic syndrome. For example, the niacin-deficiency disease pellagra is clinically similar to the autosomal recessive condition Hartnup disease (36), and pellagra has been referred to as a phenocopy of the genetic disorder (37,38). Hartnup disease is due to reduced neutral amino acid absorption from the intestine and reabsorption from the kidney, leading to low levels of blood tryptophan, which in turn leads to a biochemical anomaly that is similar to that seen when the diet is deficient in niacin (39,40). Genocopy is a less utilized term, attributed to Schmalhausen (Schmalhausen 1938 cited by Gause 1942) (41) but has generally been considered to be the reverse of phenocopy—that is, when genetic variation generates an outcome that could be produced by an environmental exposure (42). It is clear that, even when the term genocopy is used polemically, as, for example, in a critique of excessively reductionist uses of neurogenetics in explaining behavioral variation (43), phenocopy and genocopy are the converse of one another, reflecting differently motivated accounts of how both genetic and environmental factors influence physical state. Thus, for example, Hartnup disease can be called a genocopy of pellagra, while pellagra can be considered a phenocopy of Hartnup disease. Mendelian randomization can, therefore, be viewed as an application of the phenocopy–genocopy nexus that allows causation to be separated from association through the common outcome produced by different starting points.

Phenocopies of major genetic disorders are generally rarely encountered in clinical medicine, but as Lenz comments (44), "they are, however, most important as models which might help to elucidate the pathways of gene action." As we will discuss, Mendelian randomization is concerned with less major (and thus more common) disturbances, and reverses the direction of phenocopy $\rightarrow$ genocopy, to utilize genocopies, of known genetic mechanism, to inform us better about pathways through which the environment influences health.

The scope of phenocopy–genocopy has been discussed by Zuckerlandl and Villett (45), who advance mechanisms through which there can be equivalence between environmental and genotypic influences. Indeed, they state that there is "no doubt that all environmental effects can be mimicked by one or several mutations." The notion that genetic and environmental influences can be both equivalent and interchangeable has received considerable attention in developmental biology (46,47). Furthermore, population genetic analyses of correlations between different traits suggest that there are common pathways of genetic and environmental influences, with Cheverud concluding that "most environmentally caused phenotypic variants should have genetic counterparts and vice versa" (48).

Mendelian Randomization: What Is It and How Does It Work?

The basic principle utilized in the Mendelian randomization approach is that if genetic variants either alter the level of, or mirror the biological effects of, a modifiable environmental exposure that itself alters disease risk, then these genetic variants should be related to disease risk to the extent predicted by their influence on exposure to the risk factor. Common genetic polymorphisms that have a well-characterized biological function (or are markers for such variants) can therefore be utilized to study the effect of a suspected environmental exposure on disease risk (49–55).

It may seem illogical to study genetic variants as proxies for environmental exposures rather than measure the exposures themselves. However, there are several crucial advantages of utilizing functional genetic variants (or their markers) in this manner that relate to the problems with observational studies outlined above. First, unlike environmental exposures, genetic variants are not generally associated with the wide range of behavioral, social, and physiological factors that, for example, confound the association between vitamin E supplementation use and CHD. This means that if a genetic variant is used as a proxy for an environmentally modifiable exposure, it is unlikely to be confounded in the way that direct measures of the exposure will be. Further, aside from the effects of population structure (56), such variants will not be associated with other genetic variants, except through linkage disequilibrium.

Second, we have seen how inferences drawn from observational studies may be subject to bias due to reverse causation. Disease processes may influence exposure levels such as alcohol intake, or measures of intermediate phenotypes such as cholesterol levels and C-reactive protein. However, germline genetic variants associated with average alcohol intake or circulating levels of intermediate phenotypes will not be influenced by the onset of disease. This will be equally true with respect to reporting bias generated by knowledge of disease status in case-control studies, or to differential reporting bias in any study design.

Third, selection bias, whereby selection into a study is related to both exposure level and disease risk and can generate spurious associations (as illustrated above with respect to alcohol and hemorrhagic stroke), is unlikely to occur with respect to genetic variants. For example, in a series of cancer case-control studies, there was no association between a wide range of genetic variants and participation rates (57).

Finally, a genetic variant will indicate long-term levels of exposure, and, if the variant is considered to be a proxy for such exposure, it will not suffer from the measurement error inherent in phenotypes that have high levels of variability. For example, differences between groups defined by cholesterol level-related genotype will, over a long period, reflect the cumulative differences in absolute cholesterol levels between the groups. For individuals, blood cholesterol is variable over time, and the use of single measures of cholesterol will underestimate the true strength of association between cholesterol and, for instance, coronary heart disease. Indeed, use of the Mendelian randomization approach predicts a strength of association that is in line with randomized controlled trial findings of effects of cholesterol lowering, when the increasing benefits seen over the relatively short trial period are projected to the expectation for differences over a lifetime (50).

Mendelian Randomization: Is the Principle Sound?

The principle of Mendelian randomization relies on the basic (but approximate) laws of Mendelian genetics. If the probability that a postmeiotic germ cell that has received any particular allele at segregation contributes to a viable conceptus is independent of environment (following on from Mendel's first law), and if genetic variants sort independently (following on from Mendel's second law), then at a population level these variants will tend to be unassociated with the confounding factors that generally distort conventional observational studies. This particular strength of genetic studies was explicitly recognized by the pioneering geneticist and statistician R.A. Fisher from the 1920s onward. As Fisher said:

> Genetics is indeed in a peculiarly favored condition in that Providence has shielded the geneticist from many of the difficulties of a reliably controlled comparison. The different genotypes possible from the same mating have been beautifully randomized by the meiotic process...Generally speaking, the geneticist, even if he foolishly wanted to, could not introduce systematic errors into the comparison of genotypes, because for most of the relevant time he has not yet recognized them. (58)

The principle was explicitly utilized in observational studies from the 1960s (59–62), with the term Mendelian randomization being introduced by Richard Gray and Keith Wheatley in 1991 (63), in the context of an innovative genetically informed observational approach to asses the effects of bone marrow transplantation in the treatment of childhood acute myeloid leukaemia. More recently the term has been widely used in discussions of observational epidemiologic studies (49,64–67). Further discussion of the origin of this approach is given elsewhere (68).

Empirical evidence that there is lack of confounding of genetic variants with factors that confound exposures in conventional observational epidemiologic studies comes from several sources. For example, consider the virtually identical allele frequencies in the British 1958 birth cohort and British blood donors (69). Blood donors are clearly a very selected sample of the population, whereas the 1958 birth cohort comprised all births born in one week in Britain with relatively low selection bias. Blood donors and the general population sample would differ considerably with respect to the behavioral, socioeconomic, and physiological risk factors that are the confounding factors in observational epidemiologic studies. Figure 21.4 shows in its top panel the statistical evidence of differences in allele frequencies of 500,568 SNPs assayed using the Affymetrix 500K chip between subjects from the 1958 birth cohort and the U.K. blood donors, stratified by 12 broad regions of Britain. The bottom panel shows good agreement of the test statistics found with those expected on the basis of there being no actual differences in allele frequencies. The fact that very

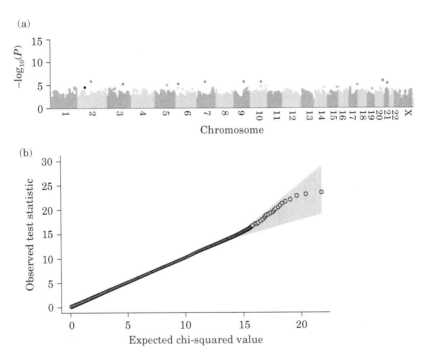

Figure 21.4 Comparisons of 500,568 SNP variants in the 1958 birth cohort and U.K. blood donors. Data from Wellcome Trust Case Control Consortium, Nature *(2007) (69) (a) Statistical significance of differences in allele frequencies; (b) agreement with null distribution of differences. Reprinted by permission from Macmillan Publishers Ltd:* Nature *(doi:10.1038/nature)*

few robust differences between these two groups were found despite the considerable differences there are between the groups with respect to many social, behavioral, and environmental factors is in line with expectations based on the Mendelian randomization principle. Similarly, we have recently demonstrated the lack of association between a range of SNPs of known phenotypic effects and nearly 100 sociocultural, behavioral, and biological risk factors for disease (70).

Mendelian Randomization in Practice

The term Mendelian randomization has now become widely used, with a variety of meanings. This partly reflects the fact that there are several categories of inference that can be drawn from studies utilizing the Mendelian randomization approach. In the most direct forms, genetic variants can be related to the probability or level of exposure ("exposure propensity") or to intermediate phenotypes believed to influence disease risk. Less direct evidence can come from genetic variant–disease associations that indicate that a particular biological pathway may be of importance, perhaps because the variants modify the effects of environmental exposures. Several examples of these categories have been given elsewhere (49,50,52,54,55); here a few illustrative cases are briefly outlined.

Exposure Propensity

Alcohol Intake and Health

The possible protective effect of moderate alcohol consumption on CHD risk remains controversial (71–73). Nondrinkers may be at a higher risk of CHD because health problems (perhaps induced by previous alcohol abuse) dissuade them from drinking (74). As well as this form of reverse causation, confounding could play a role, with nondrinkers being more likely to display an adverse profile of socioeconomic or other behavioral risk factors for CHD (31). Alternatively, alcohol may have a direct biological effect that lessens the risk of CHD—for example, by increasing the levels of protective high-density lipoprotein (HDL) cholesterol (75). It is, however, unlikely that an RCT of alcohol intake, able to test whether there is a protective effect of alcohol on CHD events, will be carried out.

Alcohol is oxidized to acetaldehyde, which in turn is oxidized by aldehyde dehydrogenases (ALDHs) to acetate. Half of Japanese people are heterozygotes or homozygotes for a null variant of *ALDH2* and peak blood acetaldehyde concentrations post alcohol challenge are 18 times and 5 times higher respectively among homozygous null variant and heterozygous individuals compared with homozygous wild type individuals (76). This renders the consumption of alcohol unpleasant through inducing facial flushing, palpitations, drowsiness, and other symptoms. As Figure 21.5 shows, there are very considerable differences in alcohol consumption according to genotype (77). The principles of Mendelian randomization are seen to apply—two factors that would be expected to be associated with alcohol

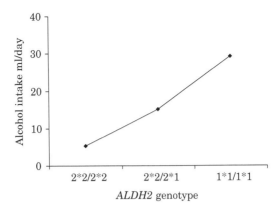

Figure 21.5 Relationship between alcohol intake and ALDH2 genotype (*1*1 homozygous wild variant, *1*2 heterozygous variant, *2*2 homozygous null variant). Data from Takagi et al. 2002 (77).

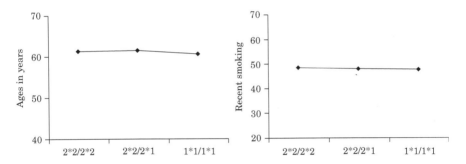

Figure 21.6 Relationship between characteristics and ALDH2 genotype (*1*1 homozygous wild variant, *1*2 heterozygous variant, *2*2 homozygous null variant). Data from Takagi et al. 2002 (77).

consumption, age, and cigarette smoking, which would confound conventional observational associations between alcohol and disease, are not related to genotype despite the strong association of genotype with alcohol consumption (Figure 21.6).

It would be expected that *ALDH2* genotype influences diseases known to be related to alcohol consumption, and as proof of principle it has been shown that *ALDH2* null variant homozygosity—associated with low alcohol consumption—is indeed related to a lower risk of liver cirrhosis (78). Considerable evidence, including data from randomized controlled trials, suggests that alcohol increases HDL cholesterol levels (79,80) (which should protect against CHD). In line with this, *ALDH2* genotype is strongly associated with HDL cholesterol in the expected direction (Figure 21.7). With respect to blood pressure, observational evidence suggests that long-term alcohol intake produces an increased risk of hypertension and higher prevailing blood pressure levels. A meta-analysis of studies of *ALDH2*

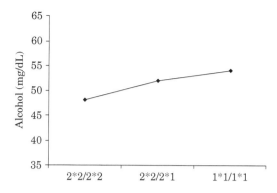

Figure 21.7 Relationship between HDL cholesterol and ALDH2 genotype (*1*1 homozygous wild variant, *1*2 heterozygous variant, *2*2 homozygous null variant). Data from Tagaki et al. 2002 (77).

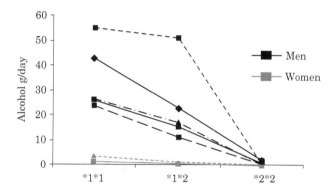

Figure 21.8 ALDH2 genotypes (*1*1 homozygous wild variant, *1*2 heterozygous variant, *2*2 homozygous null variant) by alcohol consumption, g/day: five studies, n = 6815. Data from chen et al.(81).

genotype and blood pressure suggests there is indeed a substantial effect in this direction (81). As shown in Figure 21.8, alcohol consumption is strongly related to genotype among men, and despite higher levels of overall alcohol consumption in some studies compared with others the shape of the association remains similar. Among women, however, there is no evidence of association between drinking and genotype with aelohol consumption being universely low in women in the populations studied. Figure 21.9 demonstrates that among men homozygous for the null variant, who drink considerably less alcohol than those homozygous for the common wild type, systolic blood pressures are considerably lower (Figure 21.10). By contrast, among women, for whom genotype is unrelated to alcohol intake, there is no association between genotype and systolic blood pressure. The differential genotype blood pressure associations in men and women indicate that there is no other mechanism linking genotype and blood pressure than that relating to alcohol intake. If alternative pathways existed, both men and women would be expected to have

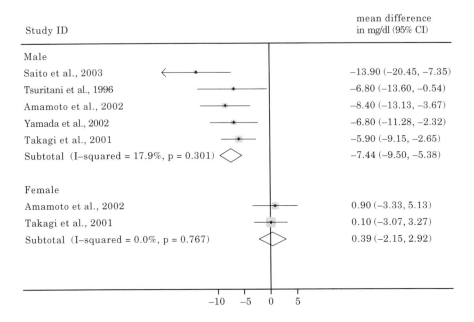

Figure 21.9 ALDH2 genotype and systolic blood pressure. Data from Chen et al. (81).

the same genotype-blood pressure association. Figure 21.11 demonstrates that men who are homozygous for the wild type have nearly two and a half times the risk of hypertension than men who are homozygous for the null variant. Heterozygous men who drink an intermediate amount of alcohol have a more modest elevated risk of hypertension compared to men with homozygous null variant. Thus, a dose–response association of hypertension and genotype is seen, in line with the dose–response association between genotype and alcohol intake.

Alcohol intake has also been postulated to increase the risk of esophageal cancer; however, some have questioned the importance of its role (82). Figure 21.12 presents findings from a meta-analysis of studies of *ALDH2* genotype and esophageal cancer risk (83), clearly showing that people who are homozygous for the null variant, who therefore consume considerably less alcohol, have a greatly reduced risk of esophageal cancer. The reduction in risk is close to that predicted from size of effect of genotype on alcohol consumption and the dose–response of alcohol on esophageal cancer risk (84). When the heterozygous individuals are compared with those homozygous for the functional variant, an interesting picture emerges—the risk of esophageal cancer is *higher* in the heterozygotes who drink rather *less* alcohol than those with the homozygous functional variant. If alcohol itself were the direct causal factor cancer risk would be intermediate in the heterozygotes compared with the other two groups. Acetaldehyde is the more likely direct causal factor, as heterozygotes drink some alcohol but metabolize it inefficiently, leading to accumulation of higher levels of acetaldehyde than would occur in homozygotes for the common

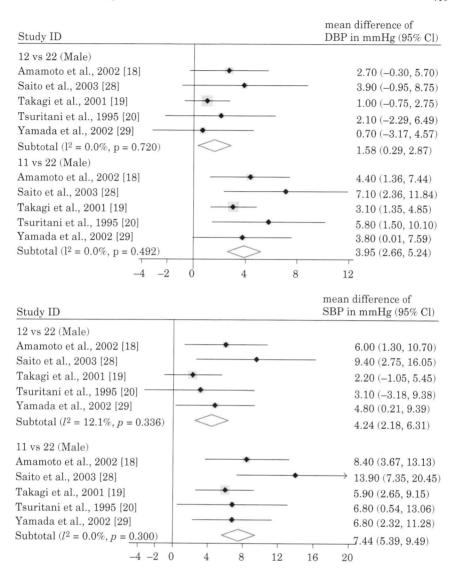

Figure 21.10 Mean difference in diastolic (top panel) and systolic (bottom panel) blood pressure in males by ALDH2 genotypes: heterozygous variant (12) versus homozygous null variant (22) and homozygous common variant (11) versus homozygous null variant (22). Data from Chen et al. (81).

variant, who metabolize alcohol efficiently, and homozygote null individuals, who drink insufficient alcohol to produce raised acetaldehyde levels.

Intermediate Phenotypes

Genetic variants can influence circulating biochemical factors such as cholesterol, homocysteine, or fibrinogen levels. This provides a method for assessing causality

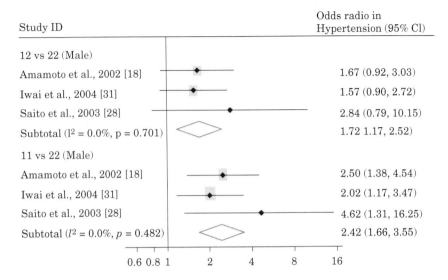

Figure 21.11 Odds ratios for association of hypertension in males with ALDH2 genotypes and hypertension: heterozygous variant (12) versus homozygous null variant (22) and homozygous common variant (11) versus homozygous null variant (22). Data from Chen et al. (81).

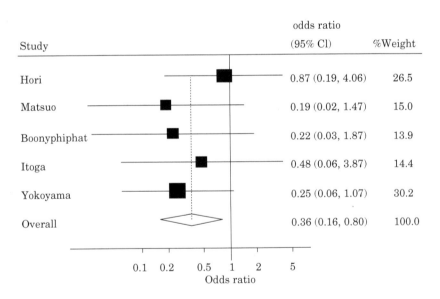

Figure 21.12 Risk of esophageal cancer in individuals with the ALDH2*2*2 versus ALDH2*1*1 genotype. Data from Lewis and Davey Smith (83).

in associations observed between these measures (*intermediate phenotypes*) and disease, and thus whether interventions to modify the intermediate phenotype could be expected to influence disease risk.

Cholesterol and Coronary Heart Disease

Familial hypercholesterolaemia is a dominantly inherited condition in which many rare mutations (over 700 DNA sequence variations (85)) of the low-density lipo-protein receptor gene (about 10 million people affected worldwide, a prevalence of around 0.2%) lead to high circulating cholesterol levels (86). The high risk of prema-ture CHD in people with this condition was readily appreciated, with an early U.K. report demonstrating that by age 50 half of men and 12% of women had suffered from CHD (87). Compared with the population of England and Wales (mean total cholesterol 6.0 mmol/L), people with familial hypercholesterolaemia (mean total cholesterol 9 mmol/l) suffered a 3.9-fold increased risk of CHD mortality, although very high relative risks among those aged less than 40 years have been observed (88). These observations, regarding genetically determined variation in risk, pro-vided strong evidence that the associations between blood cholesterol and CHD seen in general populations reflected a causal relationship. The causal nature of the association between blood cholesterol levels and CHD has historically been contro-versial (89). As both Daniel Steinberg (90) and Ole Færgeman (91) discuss, many clinicians and public health practitioners rejected the notion of a causal link for a range of reasons. However, from the late 1930s onward, evidence that people with genetically high levels of cholesterol had high risk for CHD should have been pow-erful and convincing evidence of the causal influence of elevated blood cholesterol in the general population.

With the advent of effective means of reducing blood cholesterol through statin treatment, there remains no serious doubt that the cholesterol-CHD relationship is causal. Among people without CHD, reducing total cholesterol levels with statin drugs by around 1–1.5 mmol/l reduces CHD mortality by around 25% over 5 years. Assuming a linear relationship between blood cholesterol and CHD risk, and given the difference in cholesterol of 3.0 mmol/l between people with familial hypercho-lesterolaemia and the general population, the randomized controlled trial evidence on the effect on CHD mortality of lowering total cholesterol would predict a rela-tive risk for CHD of around 2, as opposed to 3.9, for people with familial hyperc-holesterolaemia. However, the trials also demonstrate that the relative reduction in CHD mortality increases over time from randomization—and thus time with low-ered cholesterol—as would be expected if elevated levels of cholesterol operate over decades to influence the development of atherosclerosis. People with familial hyper-cholesterolaemia will have had high total cholesterol levels throughout their lives, and this would be expected to generate a greater risk than that predicted by the results of lowering cholesterol levels for only 5 years. Furthermore, ecological stud-ies relating cholesterol levels to CHD demonstrate that the strength of association increases as the lag period between cholesterol level assessment and CHD mortality increases (92), again suggesting that long-term differences in cholesterol level are the important etiological factor in CHD. As discussed above, Mendelian randomization is one method for assessing the effects of long-term differences in exposures on disease risk, free from the diluting problems of both measurement error and of only having short-term assessment of risk factor levels. This reasoning provides an indication that cholesterol-lowering efforts should be lifelong rather than limited to the period for which RCT evidence with respect to CHD outcomes is available. Recently, several common genetic variants that are related to cholesterol level and CHD risk have been identified, and these have also demonstrated effects on CHD risk consistent with lifelong differences in cholesterol level (55,93–95).

C-Reactive Protein (CRP) and Coronary Heart Disease

Strong associations of C-reactive protein (CRP), an acute phase inflammatory marker, with hypertension, insulin resistance, and CHD have been repeatedly observed (96–101), with the obvious inference that CRP is a cause of these conditions (102–104). A Mendelian randomization study has examined the association between polymorphisms of the *CRP* gene and demonstrated that while serum CRP differences were highly predictive of blood pressure and hypertension, the CRP variants—which are related to sizeable serum CRP differences—were not associated with these same outcomes (105). It is likely that these divergent findings are explained by the extensive confounding between serum CRP and outcomes. Current evidence on this issue, though statistically underpowered, also suggests that CRP levels do not lead to elevated risk of insulin resistance (106) or CHD (107–109). Again, confounding and reverse causation—where existing coronary disease or insulin resistance may influence CRP levels—could account for this discrepancy. Similar findings have been reported for serum fibrinogen, variants in the beta fibrinogen gene and CHD (110). The CRP and fibrinogen examples demonstrate that Mendelian randomization can both increase evidence for a causal effect of an environmentally modifiable factor (as in the cases of alcohol and cholesterol levels discussed earlier) and also provide evidence against causal effects, which can help direct efforts away from targets of no preventative or therapeutic relevance.

Maternal Genotype as an Indicator of Intrauterine Environment

Maternal Folate Intake and Neural Tube Defects

Mendelian randomization studies can provide unique insights into the causal nature of intrauterine environment influences on later disease outcomes. In such studies, maternal genotype is taken to be a proxy for environmentally modifiable exposures mediated through the mother that influence the intrauterine environment. For example, it is now widely accepted that neural tube defects (NTDs) can in part be prevented by periconceptional maternal folate supplementation. RCTs of

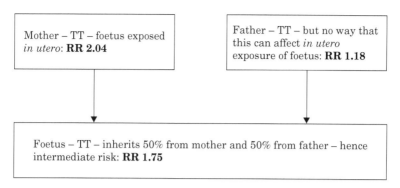

Figure 21.13 Inheritance of MTHFR polymorphism, and neural tube defects. Data derived from Botto and Yang (113).

folate supplementation have provided the key evidence in this regard (111,112). But could we have reached the same conclusion before the RCTs were carried out, if we had had access to evidence from genetic association studies? Using the *MTHFR* 677C→T polymorphism (a genetic variant that is associated with methyltetrahydrofolate reductase activity and circulating homocysteine levels; TT genotype being associated with higher homocysteine levels) as a marker of interuterine exposure in newborns with NTDs compared to controls, an increased risk in TT versus CC newborns has been found, with a relative risk of 1.75 (95% confidence interval (CI): 1.41–2.18) in a meta-analysis of all such studies (113). Using the same *MTHFR* variant in parents and examining the risk of NTD in their offspring, mothers who have the TT genotype have an increased risk of 2.04 (95% CI: 1.49–2.81) of having an offspring with a NTD compared to mothers who have the CC genotype. For TT fathers, the equivalent relative risk is 1.18 (95% CI: 0.65–2.12) (113). This pattern of associations suggests that it is the intrauterine environment—influenced by maternal TT genotype—rather than the genotype of offspring that is related to disease risk (Figure 21.13). As the *MTHFR* variant is being used as a marker for low maternal folate intake in pregnancy—which is associated with raised homocysteine—these findings support the hypothesis that maternal folate intake is the exposure of importance.

In this case, the findings from observational studies, genetic association studies, and an RCT are closely similar. Had the technology been available, the genetic association studies, with the divergent influence of maternal versus paternal genotype on NTD risk, would have provided strong evidence of the beneficial effect of folate supplementation, before the results of any RCT had been completed; although trials would still have been necessary to confirm the effect was causal for folate supplementation. Certainly, the genetic association studies would have provided better evidence than that given by conventional epidemiologic studies that had to cope with the problems of accurately assessing diet and also with the considerable confounding of maternal folate intake with a wide variety of lifestyle and socioeconomic factors that may also influence NTD risk. The association of genotype with NTD risk does not suggest that genetic screening is indicated; rather, it demonstrates that an environmental intervention may benefit the whole population, independent of the genotype of individuals receiving the intervention.

Studies utilizing maternal genotype as a proxy for environmentally modifiable influences on the intrauterine environment can be analyzed in a variety of ways. First, the mothers of offspring with a particular outcome can be compared to a control group of mothers who have offspring without the outcome, in a conventional case-control design, but with the mother as the exposed individual (or control) rather than the offspring with the particular health outcome (or the control offspring). Fathers could serve as a control group when autosomal genetic variants are being studied. If the exposure is mediated by the mother, maternal genotype, rather than offspring genotype, will be the appropriate exposure indicator. Clearly, maternal and offspring genotype are associated, but conditional on each other; it should be the maternal genotype that shows the association with the health outcome among the offspring. Indeed, in theory, it would be possible to simply compare genotype distributions of mothers and offspring, with a higher prevalence among mothers providing evidence that maternal genotype, through an intrauterine pathway, is of importance. However, the statistical power of such an approach is low, and an external control group, whether fathers or women who have offspring without the health outcome, is generally preferable.

Alcohol Intake and Offspring Development

The influence of alcohol intake by pregnant women on the health and development of their offspring is well recognized for very high levels of intake, in the form of fetal alcohol syndrome (115). However, the influence outside of this extreme situation is less easy to assess, particularly as higher levels of alcohol intake will be related to a wide array of potential sociocultural, behavioral, and environmental confounding factors. Furthermore, there may be systematic bias in how mothers report alcohol intake during pregnancy, which could distort associations with health outcomes. Therefore, outside of the case of very high alcohol intake by mothers, it is difficult to establish a causal link between maternal alcohol intake and offspring developmental characteristics. Some studies have approached this by investigating alcohol-metabolizing genotypes in mothers and offspring outcomes.

Although sample sizes have been low and the analysis strategies not optimum, they provide some evidence to support the influence of maternal genotype (116– 118). For example, in one study, mental development at age 7.5 was delayed among offspring of mothers possessing a genetic variant associated with less rapid alcohol metabolism. Among these mothers there would presumably be less rapid clearance of alcohol, and thus an increased influence of maternal alcohol on offspring during the intrauterine period (117). Offspring genotype was not independently related to these outcomes, indicating that the crucial exposure related to maternal alcohol levels. As in the *MTHFR* examples, these studies are of relevance because they provide evidence of the influence of maternal alcohol levels—unconfounded by socioeconomic position, smoking, and other variables—on offspring development, rather than because they highlight a particular maternal genotype that is of importance. In the absence of alcohol drinking, the maternal genotype would presumably have no influence on offspring outcomes. The association of maternal genotype and offspring outcome suggests that alcohol levels in mothers, and therefore their alcohol consumption, have an influence on offspring development.

Implications of Mendelian Randomization Study Findings

Establishing the causal influence of environmentally modifiable risk factors from Mendelian randomization designs informs policies for improving population health through population-level interventions targeting the modifiable risk factors. Such evidence does not imply that the appropriate strategy is genetic screening to identify those at high risk and the application of selective exposure reduction policies. For example, the implications of studies on maternal *MTHFR* genotype and offspring NTD risk is that population risk for NTDs can be reduced through increased folate intake peri-conceptionally and in early pregnancy. It does not suggest that women should be screened for *MTHFR* genotype and women with the TT variant treated with folate; women without the TT genotype but with low folate intake are still exposed to preventable risk of having babies with NTDs. Similarly establishing the association between genetic variants (such as familial defective ApoB) associated with elevated cholesterol level and CHD risk strengthens causal evidence that elevated cholesterol is a modifiable risk factor for CHD for the whole population. Thus, even though the population attributable risk for CHD of this variant is small, it usefully informs public health approaches to improving population health. It is this aspect of Mendelian randomization that illustrates its distinction from conventional risk identification and genetic screening applications of genetic epidemiology.

Mendelian Randomization and Randomized Controlled Trials

Randomized controlled trials are clearly the definitive means of obtaining evidence on the effects of modifying disease risk processes. There are similarities in the logical structure of RCTs and Mendelian randomization studies as illustrated in Figure 21.14, which draws attention to the unconfounded nature of exposures for which genetic variants serve as proxies (analogous to the unconfounded nature of a randomized intervention), the impossibility of reverse causation as an influence on exposure-outcome associations in both Mendelian randomization and randomized controlled trial settings, and the importance of intention to treat analyses—that is, analysis by group defined by genetic variant, irrespective of associations between the genetic variant and the exposure for which this is a proxy within any particular individual.

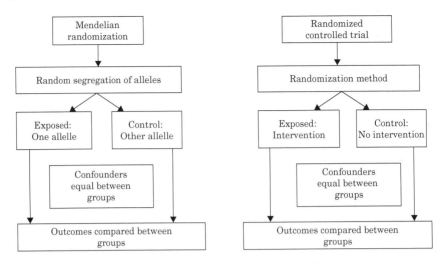

Figure 21.14 Mendelian randomization and randomized controlled trial designs compared.

The analogy with randomized controlled trials is also useful with respect to one objection that has been raised in conjunction with Mendelian randomization studies. This is that the environmentally modifiable exposure for which genetic variants serve as proxies (such as alcohol intake or circulating CRP levels) is influenced by many other factors in addition to the genetic variants (119). This is, of course, true. However, consider a randomized controlled trial (RCT) of blood pressure-lowering medication. Blood pressure is mainly influenced by factors other than taking blood pressure lowering medication—obesity, alcohol intake, salt consumption and other dietary factors, smoking, exercise, physical fitness, genetic factors, and early-life developmental influences are all of importance. However, the randomization that occurs in trials ensures that these factors are balanced between the groups that receive the blood pressure lowering medication and those that do not. Thus, the fact that many other factors are related to the modifiable exposure does not vitiate the power of RCTs; neither does it vitiate the strength of Mendelian randomization designs.

A related objection is that the genetic variants often explain only a trivial proportion of the variance in the environmentally modifiable risk factor for which the genetic variants are surrogate variables (120). Again, consider a RCT of blood pressure-lowering medication, where 50% of participants receive the medication and 50% received a placebo. If the antihypertensive therapy reduced blood pressure by a quarter of a standard deviation (i.e., 5 mmHg reduction in systolic blood pressure with blood pressure having a standard deviation of 20 mmHg), then within the whole study group, treatment assignment (i.e., antihypertensive use versus placebo) will explain 1.25% of the variance in blood pressure. In the example of *CRP* haplotypes used as instruments for CRP levels, these haplotypes explain 1.66% of the variance in CRP levels in the population (53). As can be seen, the quantitative

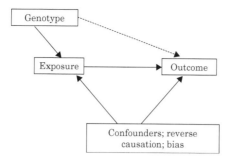

Figure 21.15 Mendelian randomization as an instrumental variables approach.

association of genetic variants as instruments can be similar to that of randomized treatments with respect to biological processes that such treatments modify. Both logic and quantification fail to support criticisms of the Mendelian randomization approach based on either the obvious fact that many factors influence most phenotypes of interest or that particular genetic variants only account for a small proportion of variance in the phenotype.

Mendelian Randomization and Instrumental Variable Approaches

As well as the analogy with RCTs, Mendelian randomization can also be likened to instrumental variable approaches that have been heavily utilized in econometrics and social science, although rather less so in epidemiology. In an instrumental variable approach, the instrument is a variable that is only related to the outcome through its association with the modifiable exposure of interest. The instrument is not related to confounding factors, nor is its assessment biased in a manner that would generate a spurious association with the outcome. Furthermore, the instrument will not be influenced by the development of the outcome (i.e., there will be no reverse causation). Figure 21.15 presents this basic schema, where the dotted line between genotype and the outcome provides an unconfounded and unbiased estimate of the causal association between the exposure for which the genotype is a proxy and the outcome. The development of instrumental variable methods within econometrics, in particular, has led to a sophisticated suite of statistical methods for estimating causal effects, and these have now been applied within Mendelian randomization studies (105,106,110). The parallels between Mendelian randomization and instrumental variable approaches are discussed in more detail elsewhere (53,122).

The instrumental variable method allows for the estimation of the causal effect size of the modifiable environmental exposure of interest and the outcome, together with estimates of the precision of the effect. Thus, in the example of alcohol intake (indexed by *ALDH2* genotype) and blood pressure discussed earlier, it is possible

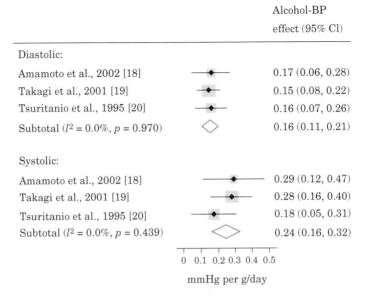

Figure 21.16 Association between alcohol intake and diastolic (top panel) and systolic (bottom panel) blood pressure estimated from instrumental variables analysis utilizing ALDH2 genotype as the instrument. Data from Chen et al. (81).

to utilize the joint associations of *ALDH2* genotype and alcohol intake and *ALDH2* genotype and blood pressure to estimate the causal influence of alcohol intake on blood pressure. Figure 21.16 reports such an analysis, showing that for a 1 g per day increase in alcohol intake, there are robust increases in diastolic and systolic blood pressure among men (81).

Mendelian Randomization and Gene by Environment Interaction

Mendelian randomization is one way in which genetic epidemiology can inform understanding about environmental determinants of disease. A more conventional approach has been to study interactions between environmental exposures and genotype (123,124). From epidemiologic and Mendelian randomization perspectives, several issues arise with gene–environment interactions.

The most reliable findings in genetic association studies relate to the main effects of polymorphisms on disease risk (66). The power to detect meaningful gene–environment interaction is low (125), with the result being that there are a large number of reports of spurious gene–environment interactions in the medical literature (2,126). Detection of the presence or absence of statistical interactions depends upon the scale used (e.g., linear or logarithmic with respect to the exposure-disease outcome) but the biological meaning of any observed deviation from either an additive or multiplicative model is generally uncertain (127). Mendelian randomization is most powerful when studying modifiable exposures that are difficult to

Table 21.1 Association of *NAT2* slow acetylation genotype with bladder cancer in never and ever smokers
and overall. Odds ratio (95% confidence intervals) Data
from Garcia-Closas et al. (128)

Overall	Never Smokers	Ever Smokers
1.4 (1.2–1.7)	0.9 (0.6–1.3)	1.6 (1.3–1.9)

measure and/or considerably confounded, such as dietary factors. Given measurement error—particularly if this is differential with respect to other factors influencing disease risk—interactions are both difficult to detect and often misleading
when, apparently, they are found (66).

The interpretation of interactions may be easier with exposures that differ qualitatively rather than quantitatively between individuals. Consider the issue of the
influence of smoking tobacco on bladder cancer risk. Observational studies suggest
an association, but clearly confounding and a variety of biases could generate such
an association. The potential carcinogens in tobacco smoke of relevance to bladder cancer risk include aromatic and heterocyclic amines, which are detoxified by
N-acetyl transferase 2 (*NAT2*). Genetic variation in *NAT2* leads to slower or faster
acetylation states. If the carcinogens in tobacco smoke do increase the risk of bladder cancer, then it would be expected that slow acetylators, who have a reduced
rate of detoxification of these carcinogens, would be at an increased risk of bladder
cancer if they were smokers, whereas if they were not exposed to these carcinogens
(and the major exposure route for those outside of particular industries is through
tobacco smoke) then an association of genotype with bladder cancer risk would not
be anticipated. Table 21.1 tabulates findings from the largest study to date reported
in a way that allows consideration of this simple hypothesis (128). As can be
seen, the influence of the *NAT2* slow acetylation genotype is only appreciable among
those also exposed to smoking. Since the genotype will be unrelated to confounders,
it is difficult to reason why this situation should arise unless smoking is a causal factor with respect to bladder cancer. Thus the presence of a sizable effect of genotype in
the exposed group but not in the unexposed group provides evidence as to the causal
nature of the environmentally modifiable risk factor, in this example, smoking. It must
be recognized, however, that gene–environment interactions interpreted within the
Mendelian randomization framework as evidence regarding the causal nature of environmentally modifiable exposures are not protected from confounding to the same
extent as main genetic effects. In the *NAT2*/smoking/bladder cancer example any factor related to smoking—such as social class—will tend to show a greater association
with bladder cancer within *NAT2* slow acetylators than within *NAT2* rapid acetylators.
Because there is not a one-to-one association of social class with smoking, this will
not produce the quantitative interaction of essentially no effect of the genotype in one
exposure stratum and an effect in the other, as in the *NAT2*/smoking interaction, but
rather a quantitative interaction of a greater effect of *NAT2* in the poorer social classes

(amongst whom smoking is more prevalent) and a smaller (but still evident) effect in the better-off social classes, amongst whom smoking tends to be less prevalent. Thus, situations in which both the biological basis of an expected interaction is well understood and in which a qualitative (effect vs no effect) interaction may be postulated are the ones that are most amenable to interpretations related to the general causal nature of the environmentally modifiable risk factor. Mendelian randomization interpretations of gene by environment interactions are discussed in detail elsewhere (125).

Problems and Limitations of Mendelian Randomization

We consider Mendelian randomization to be one of the brightest current prospects for improving causal understanding within population-based studies. There are, however, several potential limitations to the application of this methodology (49), which will now be discussed.

Failure to Establish Reliable Genotype-Intermediate Phenotype or Genotype-Disease Associations

If the associations between genotype and a potential intermediate phenotype, or between genotype and disease outcome, are not reliably estimated, then interpreting these associations in terms of their implications for potential environmental causes of disease will clearly be inappropriate. This is not an issue peculiar to Mendelian randomization, rather the nonreplicable nature of perhaps most apparent findings in genetic association studies is a serious limitation to the whole enterprise. This issue has been discussed elsewhere (2,129), and will not be dealt with further here. Instead, problems with the Mendelian randomization approach even when reliable genotype-phenotype associations can be determined will be addressed.

Confounding of Genotype—Environmentally Modifiable Risk Factor—Disease Associations

The power of Mendelian randomization lies in its ability to avoid the often substantial confounding seen in conventional observational epidemiology. However, confounding can be reintroduced into Mendelian randomization studies, and when interpreting the results, this possibility needs to be considered.

Linkage Disequilibrium

It is possible that the locus under study is in linkage disequilibrium—that is, is associated with another polymorphic locus, with the effect of the polymorphism under investigation being confounded by the influence of the other polymorphism. It may seem unlikely—given the relatively short distances over which linkage disequilibrium is seen in the human genome—that a polymorphism influencing, for instance,

CHD risk would be associated with another polymorphism influencing CHD risk (and thus producing confounding). There are, nevertheless, examples of different genes influencing the same metabolic pathway being in physical proximity. For example, different polymorphisms influencing alcohol metabolism appear to be in linkage disequilibrium (130).

Pleiotropy and the Multifunction of Genes

Mendelian randomization is most useful when it can be used to relate a single intermediate phenotype to a disease outcome. However, polymorphisms may (and probably often will) influence more that one intermediate phenotype, and this may mean they proxy for more than one environmentally modifiable risk factor. This can be the case through multiple effects mediated by their RNA expression or intermediate protein coding, through alternative splicing, where one polymorphic region contributes to alternative forms of more than one protein, or through other mechanisms. The most robust interpretations will be possible when the functional polymorphism appears to directly influence the level of the intermediate phenotype of interest (as in the CRP example), but such examples are probably going to be less common in Mendelian randomization than in cases where the polymorphism can influence several systems, with different potential interpretations of how the effect on outcome is generated.

How to Investigate Reintroduced Confounding within Mendelian Randomization

Linkage disequilibrium and pleiotropy can reintroduce confounding and thus vitiate the potential value of the Mendelian randomization approach. Genomic knowledge may help in estimating the degree to which these are likely to be problems in any particular Mendelian randomization study, through, for instance, explication of genetic variants that may be in linkage disequilibrium with the variant under study, or the function of a particular variant and its known pleiotropic effects. Furthermore, genetic variation can be related to measures of potential confounding factors in each study, and the magnitude of such confounding estimated. Empirical studies to date suggest that common genetic variants are largely unrelated to the behavioral and socioeconomic factors considered to be important confounders in conventional observational studies (70). However, relying on measurement of confounders does, of course, remove the central purpose of Mendelian randomization, which is to balance unmeasured as well as measured confounders (as randomization does in RCTs).

In some circumstances, the genetic variant will be related to the environmentally modifiable exposure of interest in some population subgroups but not in others. An example of this relates to the alcohol *ALDH2* genotype and blood pressure association affecting men but not women, discussed earlier (see Figure 21.8). If *ALDH2* genetic variation influenced blood pressure for reasons other than its influence on alcohol intake, for example, if it was in linkage disequilibrium with another genetic variant that influenced blood pressure through another pathway or if there was a pleiotropic effect of the genetic variant on blood pressure, the same genotype-blood pressure association should be seen among both men and women. If, however, the genetic variant only influences blood pressure through its effect on alcohol intake, an effect should only be seen in men, which is what is observed (see Figure 21.9). This further strengthens the evidence that the genotype-blood pressure association depends on the genotype influencing alcohol intake, and that the associations do indeed provide causal evidence of an influence of alcohol intake on blood pressure.

In some cases, it may be possible to identify two separate genetic variants, which are not in linkage disequilibrium with each other, but which both serve as proxies for the environmentally modifiable risk factor of interest. If both variants are related to the outcome of interest and point to the same underlying association, then it becomes much less plausible that reintroduced confounding explains the association, since it would have to be acting in the same way for these two unlinked variants. This can be likened to RCTs of different blood pressure lowering agents, which work through different mechanisms and have different potential side effects, but lower blood pressure to the same degree. If the different agents produce the same reductions in cardiovascular disease risk, then it is unlikely that this is through agent-specific effects of the drugs; rather, it points to blood pressure lowering as being key. Use of multiple variants in this way has been applied in the study of the association of body mass index with more mineral density (131).

Canalization and Developmental Stability

Perhaps a greater potential problem for Mendelian randomization than reintroduced confounding arises from the developmental compensation that may occur through a polymorphic genotype being expressed during fetal or early postnatal development, and thus influencing development in such a way as to buffer against the effect of the polymorphism. Such compensatory processes have been discussed since C.H. Waddington introduced the notion of canalization in the 1940s (132). Canalization refers to the buffering of the effects of either environmental or genetic forces attempting to perturb development, and Waddington's ideas have been well developed both empirically and theoretically (133–139). Such buffering can be achieved either through genetic redundancy (more than one gene having the same or similar function) or through alternative metabolic routes, where the complexity of metabolic networks allows recruitment of different pathways to reach the same phenotypic endpoint. In effect, a functional polymorphism expressed during fetal development or postnatal growth may influence the expression of a wide range of other genes, leading to changes that may compensate for the influence of the polymorphism. Put crudely, if a person has developed and grown from the intrauterine period onward within an environment in which one factor is perturbed (e.g., there is elevated CRP due to genotype) then they may be rendered resistant to the influence of lifelong elevated circulating CRP, through permanent changes in tissue structure and function that counterbalance its effects. In intervention trials—for example, hypothetical RCTs of CRP-lowering drugs—the intervention is generally randomized to participants during their middle age; similarly, in observational studies of this issue, CRP levels are ascertained during adulthood. In Mendelian randomization, on the other hand, randomization occurs before birth. This leads to important caveats when attempting to relate the findings of conventional observational epidemiologic studies to the findings of studies carried out within the Mendelian randomization paradigm.

The most dramatic demonstrations of developmental compensation come from knockout studies—where a functioning gene is essentially removed from an organism. The overall phenotypic effects of such knockouts have often been much lower than knowledge of the function of the genes would predict, even in the absence of other genes carrying out the same function as the knockout gene (140–143). For example, pharmacological inhibition demonstrates that myoglobulin is essential to maintain energy balance and contractile function in the myocardium of mice, yet disrupting the myoglobulin gene resulted in mice devoid of myoglobulin with no disruption of cardiac function (144).

In the field of animal genetic engineering studies—such as knockout preparations or transgenic animals manipulated so as to overexpress foreign DNA—the interpretive problem created by developmental compensation is well recognized (140–143). Conditional preparations—in which the level of transgene expression can be induced or suppressed through the application of external agents—are now being utilized to investigate the influence of such altered gene expression after the developmental stages during which compensation can occur (145). Thus, further evidence on the issue of genetic buffering should emerge to inform interpretations of both animal and human studies.

Most examples of developmental compensation relate to dramatic genetic or environmental insults; thus it is unclear whether the generally small phenotypic differences induced by common functional polymorphisms will be sufficient to induce compensatory responses. The fact that the large gene–environment interactions that have been observed often relate to novel exposures that have not been present during the evolution of a species (e.g., drug interactions) (125,146) may indicate that homogenization of response to exposures that are widely experienced—as would be the case with the products of functional polymorphisms or common mutations—has occurred; canalizing mechanisms could be particularly relevant in these cases. Further work on the basic mechanisms of developmental stability and how this relates to relatively small exposure differences during development will allow these considerations to be taken forward. Knowledge of the stage of development at which a genetic variant has functional effects will also allow the potential of developmental compensation to buffer the response to the variant to be assessed.

In some Mendelian randomization designs, developmental compensation is not an issue. For example, when maternal genotype is utilized as an indicator of the intrauterine environment, then the response of the fetus will not differ whether the effect is induced by maternal genotype or by environmental perturbation, and the effect on the fetus can be taken to indicate the effect of environmental influences during the intrauterine period. Also in cases where a variant influences an adulthood environmental exposure—for example, *ALDH2* variation and alcohol intake—developmental compensation to genotype will not be an issue. In many cases of gene–environment interaction interpreted with respect to causality of the environmental factor, the same applies. Solving the potential problem of canalization in some Mendelian randomization situations cannot currently be adequately assessed, but the lines of research described above are likely to help.

Complexity of Associations and Interpretations

The interpretation of findings from studies in which the Mendelian randomization approach has been adopted can often be complex. The association between *ALDH2* genotype and esophageal cancer, discussed earlier, provides one example. Genotype is related both to level of alcohol drinking and, given situations where some alcohol is consumed, also to levels of acetaldehyde at any given level of alcohol consumption. This leads to the situation where heterozygotes—who consume less alcohol than homozygous wild type individuals—have increased risk of esophageal cancer, because they experience higher acetaldehyde; despite less alcohol consumption and less acetaldehyde production, they are slower in clearing the acetaldehyde that is produced. As a second example, consider the association of extracellular superoxide dismutase (EC-SOD) and CHD. EC-SOD is an extracellular scavenger of superoxide anions, and thus genetic variants associated with higher circulating EC-SOD levels might be considered to mimic higher levels of antioxidants. However, findings are dramatically opposite to this—bearers of such variants have an increased risk of CHD (147). The explanation of this apparent paradox is that the higher circulating EC-SOD levels associated with the variant may arise from movement of EC-SOD from arterial walls; thus the *in situ* antioxidative properties of these arterial walls is lower in individuals with the variant associated with higher circulating EC-SOD. The complexity of these interpretations—together with their sometimes speculative nature—detracts from the transparency that otherwise makes the Mendelian randomization approach attractive.

Lack of Suitable Genetic Variants to Proxy for Exposure of Interest

An obvious limitation of Mendelian randomization is that it can only examine areas for which there are functional polymorphisms (or genetic markers linked to such functional polymorphisms) that are relevant to the modifiable exposure of interest. In the context of genetic association studies, it has been pointed out more generally that in many cases, even if a locus is involved in a disease-related metabolic process, there may be no suitable marker or functional polymorphism to allow study of this process (148). In an earlier paper on Mendelian randomization (49) we discussed the example of vitamin C, since observational epidemiology appeared to have got the wrong answer regarding associations between vitamin C levels and disease. We considered whether the association between vitamin C and CHD could have been studied utilizing the principles of Mendelian randomization. We stated that polymorphisms exist that are related to lower circulating vitamin C levels—for example, the haptoglobin polymorphism (149)—but in this case the effect on vitamin C is at some distance from the polymorphic protein and the other phenotypic differences could have an influence on CHD risk that would distort examination of the influence of vitamin C levels through relating genotype to disease. *SLC23A1*—a gene encoding for the vitamin C transporter SVCT1, which is involved in vitamin C transport by intestinal cells—would be an attractive candidate for Mendelian randomization studies. However, by 2003 (the date of our earlier paper) a search for variants had failed to find any common SNP that could be used in such a way (150). We therefore used this as an example of a situation where suitable polymorphisms for studying the modifiable risk factor of interest—in this case vitamin C—could not be located. However, since the earlier paper was written, functional variation in *SLC23A1* has been identified that is related to circulating vitamin C levels (Timpson et al., personal communication). We use this example not to suggest that the obstacle of locating relevant genetic variation for particular problems will always be overcome but to point out that rapidly developing knowledge of human genomics will identify more variants that can serve as instruments for Mendelian randomization studies.

Conclusions

Mendelian Randomization, What It Is and What It Isn't

Mendelian randomization is not predicated on the presumption that genetic variants are major determinants of health and disease within populations. There are many cogent critiques of genetic reductionism and the overselling of "discoveries" in genetics that reiterate obvious truths so clearly (albeit somewhat repetitively) that there is no need to repeat them here (e.g., 43,151–154). Mendelian randomization does not depend on there being "genes for" particular traits, and certainly not in the strict sense of a gene "for" a trait being one that is maintained by selection because of its causal association with that trait (155). The association of genotype and the environmentally modifiable factor that it proxies for will be like most genotype-phenotype associations, one that is contingent and cannot be reduced to individual level prediction, but within environmental limits will pertain at a group level (156). This is analogous to an RCT of antihypertensive agents, where at a collective level the group randomized to active medication will have lower mean blood pressure than the group randomized to placebo, but at an individual level many participants randomized to active treatment will have higher blood pressure than many individuals randomized to placebo. Indeed, in the phenocopy/genocopy example of pellagra and Hartnup disease discussed above, only a minority of the Hartnup gene carriers develop symptoms, but at a group level they have both a much greater tendency to such symptoms and a shift in amino acid levels that reflect this (157,158). These group level differences are what create the analogy between Mendelian randomization and RCTs, outlined in Figure 21.14.

Finally, the associations that Mendelian randomization depend upon do need to pertain to a definable group at a particular time, but do not need to be immutable. Thus, *ALDH2* variation will not be related to alcohol consumption in a society where alcohol is not consumed; the association will vary by gender, by cultural group, and may change over time (159,160). Within the setting of a study of a well-defined group, however, the genotype will be associated with group-level differences in alcohol consumption and group assignment will not be associated with confounding variables.

Mendelian Randomization and Genetic Epidemiology

Critiques of contemporary genetic epidemiology often focus on two features of findings from genetic association studies: that the population attributable risk of the genetic variants is low, and that in any case the influence of genetic factors is not reversible. Illustrating both of these criticisms, Terwilliger and Weiss suggest the following as reasons for considering that many of the current claims regarding genetic epidemiology are hype: (a) that alleles identified as increasing the risk of common diseases "tend to be involved in only a small subset of all cases of such diseases" and (b) that in any case "while the concept of attributable risk is an important one for evaluating the impact of removable environmental factors, for non-removable genetic risk factors, it is a moot point" (161). These evaluations of the role of genetic epidemiology are not relevant when considering the potential contributions of Mendelian randomization. This approach is not concerned with the population attributable risk of any particular genetic variant, but the degree to which associations between the genetic variant and disease outcomes can demonstrate the importance of environmentally modifiable factors as causes of disease, for which the population attributable risk is of relevance to public health prioritisation. Consider, for example, the case of familial hypercholesterolaemia or familial defective Apo B. The genetic mutations associated with these conditions will only account for a trivial percentage of cases of CHD within the population—that is, the population attributable risk will be low. For example, in a Danish population, the frequency of familial defective Apo B is 0.08% and, despite its sevenfold increased risk of CHD, will only generate a population attributable risk of 0.5% (162). However, by identifying blood cholesterol levels as a causal factor for CHD, the triangular association between genotype, blood cholesterol, and CHD risk identifies an environmentally modifiable factor with a very high population attributable risk—assuming that 50% of the population have raised blood cholesterol above 6.0 mmol/l and this is associated with a relative twofold risk, a population attributable risk of 33% is obtained. The same logic applies to the other examples discussed above—the attributable risk of the genotype is low, but the population attributable risk of the modifiable environmental factor identified as causal through the genotype–disease associations is large. The same reasoning applies when considering the suggestion that since genotype cannot be modified, genotype–disease associations are not of public health importance (161). The point of Mendelian randomization approaches is not to attempt to modify genotype, but to utilize genotype–disease associations to strengthen inferences regarding modifiable environmental risks for disease, and then reduce disease risk in the population through applying this knowledge.

Mendelian randomization differs from other contemporary approaches to genetic epidemiology in that its central concern is not with the magnitude of genetic variant influences on disease, but rather on what the genetic associations tell us about environmentally modifiable causes of disease. As David B. Abrams, former director of the Office of Behavioral and Social Sciences Research at the U.S. National Institutes of Health has said, "The more we learn about genes the more we see how important environment and lifestyle really are." Many years earlier, the pioneering geneticist Thomas Hunt Morgan articulated a similar sentiment in his Nobel Prize acceptance speech, when he contrasted his views with the then popular genetic approach to disease: eugenics. He thought that "through public hygiene and protective measures of various kinds we can more successfully cope with some of the evils that human flesh is heir to. Medical science will here take the lead— but I hope that genetics can at times offer a helping hand" (163). More than seven decades later, it might now be time for genetic research to strengthen the knowledge base of public health directly.

References

1. Phillips AN, Davey Smith G. Bias in relative odds estimation owing to imprecise measurement of correlated exposures. *Stats Med.* 1992;11:953–961.
2. Colhoun HM, McKeigue PM, Davey Smith G. Problems of reporting genetic associations with complex outcomes. *Lancet.* 2003;361:865–872.
3. NCI-NHGRI Working Group on Replication in Association Studies. Replicating genotype–phenotype associations. *Nature.* June 7, 2007;447:655–660.
4. Davey Smith G, Ebrahim S. Data dredging, bias, or confounding (editorial). *BMJ.* 2002;325:1437–1438.
5. Manson J, Stampfer MJ, Willett WC et al. A prospective study of antioxidant vitamins and incidence of coronary heart disease in women. *Circulation.* 1991;84(suppl II):II–546.
6. Rimm EB, Stampfer MJ, Ascherio A, et al. Vitamin E consumption and the risk of coronary heart disease in men. *N Engl J Med.* 1993;328:1450–1456.
7. Stampfer MJ, Hennekens CH, Manson JE, et al. Vitamin E consumption and the risk of coronary disease in women. *N Engl J Med.* 1993;328:1444–1449.
8. Osganian SK, Stampfer MJ, Rimm E, et al. Vitamin C and risk of coronary heart disease in women. *J Am Coll Cardiol.* 2003;42:246–252.
9. Stampfer MJ, Colditz GA. Estrogen replacement therapy and coronary heart disease: a quantitative assessment of the epidemiologic evidence. *Prev Med.* 1991;20:47–63 (reprinted *Int J Epidemiol.* 2004;33:445–453).
10. Omenn GS, Goodman GE, Thornquist MD, et al. Effects of a combination of beta carotene and vitamin A on lung cancer and cardiovascular disease. *N Engl J Med.* 1996;334:1150–1155.

11. Alpha-Tocopherol, Beta Carotene Cancer Prevention Study Group. The effect of vitamin E and beta carotene on the incidence of lung cancer and other cancers in male smokers. *N Engl J Med.* 1994;330:1029–1035.

12. Dietary supplementation with n-3 polyunsaturated fatty acids and vitamin E after myocardial infarction: results of the GISSI-Prevenzione Investigators (Gruppo Italiano per lo Studio della Sopravvivenza nell'Infarto miocardico). *Lancet.* 1999;354:447–455.

13. Heart Protection Study Collaborative Group. MRC/BHF Heart Protection Study of antioxidant vitamin supplementation in 20536 high-risk individuals: a randomised placebo-controlled trial. *Lancet.* 2002;360:23–33.

14. Beral V, Banks E, Reeves G. Evidence from randomized trials of the long-term effects of hormone replacement therapy. *Lancet.* 2002;360:942–944.

15. Manson JE, Hsia J, Johnson KC, et al. Estrogen plus progestin and the risk of coronary heart disease. *N Engl J Med.* 2003;349:523–534.

16. Steinberg D, Witztum JL. Is the oxidative modification hypothesis relevant to human atherosclerosis? Do the antioxidant trials conducted to date refute the hypothesis? *Circulation.* 2002;105:2107–2111.

17. Willett WC, Stampfer MJ. What vitamins should I be taking, doctor? *N Engl J Med.* 2001;345:1819–1824.

18. Stampfer MJ. Commentary: hormones, heart disease, and the definition of hormone "initiation." *Int J Epidemiol.* 2006;35:738–739.

19. Stampfer MJ, Rimm E, Willett W. Folate supplementation and cardiovascular disease. *Lancet.* 2006;367:1237–1238.

20. Davey Smith G, Ebrahim S. Epidemiology: is it time to call it a day? *Int J Epidemiol.* 2001;30:1–14.

21. Lawlor DA, Davey Smith G, Bruckdorfer KR, et al. Those confounded vitamins: what can we learn from the differences between observational versus randomised trial evidence? *Lancet.* 2004;363:1724–1727.

22. Vandenbroucke JP. Commentary: the HRT story: vindication of old epidemiological theory. *Int J Epidemiol.* 2004;33:456–457.

23. Davey Smith G, Ebrahim S. Folate supplementation and cardiovascular disease. *Lancet.* 2005;366:1679–1681.

24. Eidelman RS, Hollar D, Hebert PR, et al. Randomized trials of vitamin E in the treatment and prevention of cardiovascular disease. *Arch Intern Med.* 2004;164:1552–1556.

25. Radimer K, Bindewald B, Hughes J, et al. Dietary supplement use by US adults: data from the National Health and Nutrition Examination Survey, 1999–2000. *Am J Epidemiol.* 2004;160:339–349.

26. Millen AE, Dodd K, Subar A. Use of vitamin, mineral, nonvitamin, and nonmineral supplements in the United States: the 1987, 1992, and 2000 National Health Interview Survey results. *J Am Diet Assoc.* 2004;104:942–950.

27. Lawlor DA, Davey Smith G, Bruckdorfer KR, et al. Those confounded vitamins: what can we learn from the differences between observational versus randomised trial evidence? *Lancet.* 2004;363:1724–1727.

28. Lawlor DA, Ebrahim S, Kundu D, et al. Vitamin C is not associated with coronary heart disease risk once life course socioeconomic position is taken into account: prospective findings from the British Women's Heart and Health Study. *Heart.* 2005;91:1086–1087.

29. Berkson J. Limitations of the application of fourfold table analysis to hospital data. *Biometrics Bull.* 1946;2:47–53.

30. Thun MJ, Peto R, Lopez AD, et al. Alcohol consumption and mortality among middle-aged and elderly US adults. *N Engl J Med.* 1997;337:1705–1714.

31. Hart C, Davey Smith G, Hole D, et al. Alcohol consumption and mortality from all causes, coronary heart disease, and stroke: results from a prospective cohort study of Scottish men with 21 years of follow up. *Br Med J.* 1999;318:1725–1729.
32. Reynolds K, Lewis LB, Nolen JDL, et al. Alcohol consumption and risk of stroke: a meta-analysis. *JAMA.* 2003;289:579–588.
33. Spearman C. The proof and measurement of association between two things. *Am J Psychol.* 1904;15:72–101.
34. Davey Smith G, Phillips AN. Inflation in epidemiology: "the proof and measurement of association between two things" revisited. *Br Med J.* 1996;312:1659–1661.
35. Goldschmidt RB. *Physiological Genetics.* New York: McGraw Hill; 1938.
36. Baron DN, Dent CE, Harris H, et al. Hereditary pellagra-like skin rash with temporary cerebellar ataxia, constant renal amino-aciduria, and other bizarre biochemical features. *Lancet.* 1956;September 1:421–429.
37. Snyder LH. Fifty years of medical genetics. *Science.* 1959;129:7–13.
38. Guy JT. Oral manifestations of systematic disease. In: Cummings CW, Haughey B, Thomas JR, et al., eds. *Otolaryngology—Head and Neck Surgery.* Volume 2. Saint Louis, MO: Mosby-Year Book, Inc, 1993.
39. Kraut JA, Sachs G. Hartnup disorder: unravelling the mystery. *Trends Pharmacol Sci.* 2005;26:53–55.
40. Broer S, Cavanaugh JA, Rasko JEJ. Neutral amino acid transport in epithelial cells and its malfunction in Hartnup disorder. *Transporters.* 2004;33:233–236.
41. Gause GF. The relation of adaptability to adaption. *Q Rev Biol.* 1942;17:99–114.
42. Jablonka-Tavory E. Genocopies and the evolution of interdependence. *Evolutionary Theory.* 1982;6:167–170.
43. Rose S. The rise of neurogenetic determinism. *Nature.* 1995;373:380–382.
44. Lenz W. Phenocopies. *J Med Genet.* 1973;10:34–48.
45. Zuckerkandl E, Villet R. Concentration—affinity equivalence in gene regulation: convergence and envirnonmental effects. *Proc Natl Acad Sci USA.* 1988;85:4784–4788.
46. West-Eberhard MJ. *Developmental Plasticity and Evolution.* New York: Oxford University Press; 2003.
47. Leimar O, Hammerstein P, Van Dooren TJM. A new perspective on developmental plasticity and the principles of adaptive morph determination. *Am Nat.* 2006;167:367–376.
48. Cheverud JM. A comparison of genetic and phenotypic correlations. *Evolution.* 1988;42:958–968.
49. Davey Smith G, Ebrahim S. "Mendelian randomization": can genetic epidemiology contribute to understanding environmental determinants of disease? *Int J Epidemiology.* 2003;32:1–22.
50. Davey Smith G, Ebrahim S. Mendelian randomization: prospects, potentials, and limitations. *Int J Epidemiol.* 2004;33:30–42.
51. Davey Smith G, Ebrahim S. What can Mendelian randomization tell us about modifiable behavioural and environmental exposures. *BMJ.* 2005;330:1076–1079.
52. Davey Smith G. Cochrane Lecture: Randomised by (your) god: robust inference from an observational study design. *J Epidemiol Community Health.* 2006;60:382–388.
53. Davey Smith, G., Ebrahim, S. Mendelian randomization: genetic variants as instruments for strengthening causal inference in observational studies. In: Vaupel JW, Weinstein M, eds. *Bio-social Surveys: Current Insight and Future Promise.* National Research Council, Washington, DC: The National Academies Press; 2007;16:336–366.
54. Ebrahim S, Davey Smith G. Mendelian randomization: can genetic epidemiology help redress the failures of observational epidemiology? *Hum Genet.* 2008;123:15–33.
55. Davey Smith G, Timpson N, Ebrahim S. Strengthening causal inference in cardiovascular epidemiology through Mendelian randomization. *Ann Med.* 2008;12:1–18.

56. Palmer L, Cardon L. Shaking the tree: mapping complex disease genes with linkage disequilibrium. *Lancet.* 2005;366:1223–1234.
57. Bhatti P, Sigurdson AJ, Wang SS, et al. Genetic variation and willingness to participate in epidemiological research: data from three studies. *Cancer Epidemiol Biomarkers Prev.* 2005;14:2449–2453.
58. Fisher RA. Statistical methods in genetics. *Heredity.* 1952;6:1–2.
59. Birge SJ, Keutmann HT, Cuatrecasas P, Wheedon GD. Osteoporosis, intestinal lactase deficiency and low dietary calcium intake. *N Engl J Med.* 1976;276:445–448.
60. Newcomer AD, Hodgson SF, Douglas MD, Thomas PJ. Lactase deficiency: prevalence in osteoporosis. *Ann Intern Med.* 1978;89:218–220.
61. Lower GM, Nilsson T, Nelson CE Wolf H, Gamsky TE, Bryan GT. N-acetylransferase phenotype and risk in urinary bladder cancer: approaches in molecular epidemiology. *Environ Health Perspect.* 1979;29:71–79.
62. Honkanen R, Pulkkinen P, Järvinen R, et al. Does lactose intolerance predispose to low bone density? A population-based study of perimenopausal Finnish women. *Bone.* 1996;19:23–28.
63. Gray R, Wheatley K. How to avoid bias when comparing bone marrow transplantation with chemotherapy. *Bone Marrow Transplant.* 1991;7(Suppl 3):9–12.
64. Youngman LD, Keavney BD, Palmer A, et al. Plasma fibrinogen and fibrinogen genotypes in 4685 cases of myocardial infarction and in 6002 controls: test of causality by "Mendelian randomization." *Circulation.* 2000;102(Suppl II):31–32.
65. Fallon UB, Ben-Shlomo Y, Elwood P, Ubbink JB, Davey Smith G. Homocysteine and coronary heart disease—Author's reply. Heart, published online March 14, 2001 Available at: http://heart.bmjjournals.com/cgi/eletters/85/2/153.
66. Clayton D, McKeigue PM. Epidemiological methods for studying genes and environmental factors in complex diseases. *Lancet.* 2001;358:1356–1360.
67. Keavney B. Genetic epidemiological studies of coronary heart disease. *International Journal of Epidemiology.* 2002;31:730–736.
68. Davey Smith G. Capitalising on Mendelian randomization to assess the effects of treatments. *James Lind Library* (www.jameslindlibrary.org). 2006.
69. Wellcome Trust Case Control Consortium. Genome-wide association study of 14,000 cases of seven common diseases and 3,000 shared controls. *Nature.* 2007;447:661–678.
70. Davey Smith G, Lawlor D, Harbord R, Timpson N, Day I, Ebrahim S. Clustered environments and randomized genes: a fundamental distinction between conventional and genetic epidemiology. *PLoS Med.* 2008;4:1985–1992.
71. Marmot M. Reflections on alcohol and coronary heart disease. *Int J Epidemiol.* 2001;30:729–734.
72. Bovet P, Paccaud F. Alcohol, coronary heart disease and public health: which evidence-based policy? *Int J Epidemiol.* 2001;30:734–737.
73. Klatsky AL. Commentary: Could abstinence from alcohol be hazardous to your health? *Int J Epidemiol.* 2001;30:739–742.
74. Shaper AG. Editorial: alcohol, the heart, and health. *Am J Public Health.* 1993;83:799–801.
75. Rimm E. Commentary: alcohol and coronary heart disease—laying the foundation for future work. *Int J Epidemiol.* 2001;30:738–739.
76. Enomoto N, Takase S, Yasuhara M, Takada A. Acetaldehyde metabolism in different aldehyde dehydrogenase-2 genotypes. *Alcohol Clin Exp Res.* 1991;15:141–144.
77. Takagi S, Iwai N, Yamauchi R, et al. Aldehyde dehydrogenase 2 gene is a risk factor for myocardial infarction in Japanese men. *Hypertens Res.* 2002;25:677–681.
78. Chao Y-C, Liou S-R, Chung Y-Y, et al. Polymorphism of alcohol and aldehyde dehydrogenase genes and alcoholic cirrhosis in Chinese patients. *Hepatology.* 1994;19:360–366.

79. Haskell WL, Camargo C, Williams PT, et al. The effect of cessation and resumption of moderate alcohol intake on serum high-density-lipoprotein subfractions. *N Engl J Med.* 1984;310:805–810.

80. Burr ML, Fehily AM, Butland BK, Bolton CH, Eastham RD. Alcohol and high-density-lipoprotein cholesterol: a randomized controlled trial. *Br J Nutr.* 1986;56:81–86.

81. Chen L, Davey Smith G, Harbord R, Lewis S. Alcohol intake and blood pressure: a systematic review implementing Mendelian Randomization approach. *PLoS Med.* 2008;5:461.

82. Memik F. Alcohol and esophageal cancer, is there an exaggerated accusation? *Hepatogastroenterology.* 2003;54:1953–1955.

83. Lewis S, Davey Smith G. Alcohol, ALDH2 and esophageal cancer: a meta-analysis which illustrates the potentials and limitations of a Mendelian randomization approach. *Cancer Epidemiol Biomarkers Prev.* 2005;14:1967–1971.

84. Gutjahr E, Gmel G, Rehm J. Relation between average alcohol consumption and disease: an overview. *Eur Addict Res.* 2001;7:117–127.

85. LDL receptor mutation catalogue: http://www.ucl.ac.uk/fh. Accessed December 16, 2003.

86. Marks D, Thorogood M, Neil HAW, Humphries SE. A review on diagnosis, natural history and treatment of familial hypercholesterolaemia. *Atherosclerosis.* 2003;168:1–14.

87. Slack J. Risks of ischaemic heart disease in familial hyperlipoproteinaemic states. *Lancet.* 1969;2:1380–1382.

88. Scientific Steering Committee on behalf of the Simon Broome Register Group. Risk of fatal coronary heart disease in familial hyper-cholesterolaemia. *BMJ.* 1991;303:893–896

89. Steinberg D. Thematic review series: the Pathogensis of Athersclerosis. An interpretive history of the cholesterol controversy: part 1. *J Lipid Res.* 2004;45:1583–1593.

90. Steinberg D. Thematic review series: the Pathogensis of Athersclerosis. An interpretive history of the cholesterol controversy: part II: the early evidence linking hypercholes-trolemia to cornary disease in humans. *J Lipid Res.* 2005;46:179–190.

91. Færgeman O. *Coronary Artery Disease: Genes Drugs and the Agricultural Connection.* Netherlands: Elseveir; 2003.

92. Rose G. Incubation period of coronary heart disease. *BMJ.* 1982;284:1600–1601.

93. Cohen JC, Boerwinkle E, Mosely TH, Hobbs HH. Sequence variations in PSCK9, low LDL, and protection against coronary heart disease. *N Engl J Med.* 2006;354:1264–1272.

94. Linsel-Nitschke P, Götz A, Erdmann J, et al. Lifelong reduction of LDL-cholesterol related to a common variant in the LDL-receptor gene decreases the risk of coronary artery disease—a Mendelian Randomisation study. *Plos One.* 2008;3(8):e2986.

95. Kathiresan S, Melander O, Guiducci, Burtt NP, Roos C, Hirschhorn JN, Berglund G, Hedblad B, Groop L, Altshuler DM, Newton-Cheh C, Orho-Melander. Polymorphisms associated with cholesterol and risk of cardiovascular events. *NEJM.* 2008;358:1240–1249.

96. Danesh J, Wheller JB, Hirschfield GM, et al. C-reactive protein and other circulating markers of inflammation in the prediction of coronary heart disease. *N Engl J Med.* 2004;350:1387–1397.

97. Wu T, Dorn JP, Donahue RP, Sempos CT, Trevisan M. Associations of serum C-reactive protein with fasting insulin, glucose, and glycosylated hemoglobin: the Third National Health and Nutrition Examination Survey, 1988–1994. *Am J Epidemiol.* 2002;155:65–71.

98. Pradhan AD, Manson JE, Rifai N, Buring JE, Ridker PM. C-reactive protein, interleukin 6, and risk of developing type 2 diabetes mellitus. *JAMA.* 2001;286:327–334.

99. Han TS, Sattar N, Williams K, Gonzalez-Villalpando C, Lean ME, Haffner SM. Prospective study of C-reactive protein in relation to the development of diabetes and metabolic syndrome in the Mexico City Diabetes Study. *Diabetes Care.* 2002;25:2016–2021.

100. Sesso D, Buring JE, Rifai N, Blake GJ, Gaziano JM, Ridker PM. C-reactive protein and the risk of developing hypertension. *JAMA*. 2003;290:2945–2951.

101. Hirschfield GM, Pepys MB. C-reactive protein and cardiovascular disease: new insights from an old molecule. *Q J Med*. 2003;9:793–807.

102. Ridker PM, Cannon CP, Morrow D, et al. C-reactive protein levels and outcomes after statin therapy. *N Engl J Med*. 2005;352:20–28.

103. Sjöholm A, Nyström T. Endothelial inflammation in insulin resistance. *Lancet*. 2005;365:610–612.

104. Verma S, Szmitko PE, Ridker PM. C-reactive protein comes of age. *Nat Clin Pract*. 2005;2:29–36.

105. Davey Smith G, Lawlor DA, Harbord R, et al. Association of C-reactive protein with blood pressure and hypertension: life course confounding and mendelian randomization tests of causality. *Arterioscler Thromb Vasc Biol*. 2005;25(5):1051–1056.

106. Timpson NJ, Lawlor DA, Harbord RM, et al. C-reactive protein and its role in metabolic syndrome: Mendelian randomization study. *Lancet*. 2005;366:1954–1959.

107. Casas JP, Shah T, Cooper J, et al. Insight into the nature of the CRP–coronary event association using Mendelian randomization. *Int J Epidemiol*. 2006;35:922–931.

108. Lawlor DA, Harboard RM, Timpson NJ, et al. The association of C-reactive protein and CRP genotype with coronary heart disease: Findings from five studies with 4,610 cases amongst 18,637 participants. *PLoS One*. 2008;8:e3011.

109. Zacho J, Tybjærg-Hansen A, Skov Jensen, Grande P, Sillesen H, Nordestgaard BG. Genetically elevated C-reactive protein and ischemic vascular disease. *NEJM*. 2008;359:1897–1908.

110. Davey Smith G, Harbord R, Milton J, Ebrahim S, Sterne JAC. Does elevated plasma fibrinogen increase the risk of coronary heart disease: evidence from a meta-analysis of genetic association studies. *Arterioscler Thromb Vasc Biol*. 2005;25:2228–2233.

111. MRC Vitamin Study Research Group. Prevention of neural tube defects: Results of the Medical Research Council vitamin study. *Lancet*. 1991;338:131–137.

112. Czeizel AE, Dudás I. Prevention of the first occurrence of neural-tube defects by periconceptional vitamin supplementation. *N Engl J Med*. 1992;327:1832–1835.

113. Botto LD, Yang Q. 5, 10-Methylenetetrahydrofolate reductase gene variants and congenital anomalies: a HuGE Review. *Am J Epidemiol*. 2000;151:862–877.

114. Abel EL. Fetal alcohol syndrome: same old, same old. *Addiction*. 2009;104(8): 1274–1275.

115. Burd LJ. Interventions in FASD: we must do better. *Child Care Health Dev*. 2006;33:398–400.

116. Gemma S, Vichi S, Testai E. Metabolic and genetic factors contributing to alcohol induced effects and fetal alcohol syndrome. *Neurosci Biobehav Rev*. 2007;31:221–229.

117. Jacobson SW, Carr LG, Croxford J, Sokol RJ, Li TK, Jacobson JL. Protective effects of the alcohol dehydrogenase-ADH1B allele in children exposed to alcohol during pregnancy. *J Pediatr*. 2006;148:30–37.

118. Warren KR, Li TK. Genetic polymorphisms: impact on the risk of fetal alcohol spectrum disorders. *Birth Defects Res A Clin Mol Teratol*. 2005;73:195–203.

119. Jousilahti P, Salomaa V. Fibrinogen, social position, and Mendelian randomisation. *J Epidemiol Community Health*. 2004;58:883.

120. Glynn RK. Commentary: Genes as instruments for evaluation of markers and causes. *Int J Epidemiol*. 2006;35:932–934.

121. Lawlor DA, Harbord RM, Sterne JA, Timpson N, Davey Smith G. Mendelian randomization: using genes as instruments for making causal inferences in epidemiology. *Stat Med*. 2008;27(8):1133–1163.

122. Thomas DC, Conti DV. Commentary on the concept of "Mendelian Randomization." *Int J Epidemiol.* 2004;33:17–21.

123. Perera FP. Environment and cancer: who are susceptible? *Science.* 1997;278:1068–1073.

124. Mucci LA, Wedren S, Tamimi RM, Trichopoulos D, Adami HO. The role of gene-environment interaction in the aetiology of human cancer: examples from cancers of the large bowel, lung and breast. *J Intern Med.* 2001;249:477–493.

125. Davey Smith G. Mendelian randomization for strengthening casual interface in observational studies: application to gene by environment interaction. *Perspect Psychol Sci.* In press.

126. Ioannidis PA. Why most published research findings are false. *PLoS Med.* 2005;2(8):e124.

127. Thompson WD. Effect modification and the limits of biological inference from epidemiological data. *J Clin Epidemiol.* 1991;44:221–232.

128. Garcia-Closas M, Malats N, Silverman D, et al. NAT2 slow acetylation, GSTM1null genotype, and risk of bladder cancer: results from the Spanish Bladder Cancer Study and meta-analyses. *Lancet.* 2005;366:649–659.

129. Cardon LR, Bell JI. Association study designs for complex diseases. *Nat Rev Genet.* 2001;2:91–99.

130. Osier MV, Pakstis AJ, Soodyall H, et al. A global perspective on genetic variation at the ADH genes reveals unusual patterns of linkage disequilibrium and diversity. *Am J Hum Genet.* 2002;71:84–99.

131. Timpson NJ, Sayers A, Davey-Smith G, Tobias JH. How does body fat influence bone mass in childhood? A Mendelian randomization approach. *J Bone Miner Res.* 2009;24(3):522–533.

132. Waddington CH. Canalization of development and the inheritance of acquired characteristics. *Nature.* 1942;150:563–565.

133. Wilkins AS. Canalization: a molecular genetic perspective. *Bioessays.* 1997;19:257–262.

134. Rutherford SL. From genotype to phenotype: buffering mechanisms and the storage of genetic information. *Bioessays.* 2000;22:1095–1105.

135. Gibson G, Wagner G. Canalization in evolutionary genetics: a stabilizing theory? *Bioessays.* 2000;22:372–380.

136. Hartman JL, Garvik B, Hartwell L. Principles for the buffering of genetic variation. *Science.* 2001;291:1001–1004.

137. Debat V, David P. Mapping phenotypes: canalization, plasticity and developmental stability. *Trends Ecol Evol.* 2001;16:555–561.

138. Kitami T, Nadeau JH. Biochemical networking contributes more to genetic buffering in human and mouse metabolic pathways than does gene duplication. *Nat Genet.* 2002;32:191–194.

139. Hornstein E, Shomron N. Canalization of development by microRNAs. *Nat Genet.* 2006;38:S20–S24.

140. Morange M. *The Misunderstood Gene.* Cambridge: Harvard University Press; 2001.

141. Shastry BS. Gene disruption in mice: models of development and disease. *Mol Cell Biochem.* 1998;181:163–179.

142. Gerlai R. Gene targeting: technical confounds and potential solutions in behavioural and brain research. *Behav Brain Res.* 2001;125:13–21.

143. Williams RS, Wagner PD. Transgenic animals in integrative biology: approaches and interpretations of outcome. *J Appl Physiol.* 2000;88:1119–1126.

144. Garry DJ, Ordway GA, Lorenz JN, et al. Mice without myoglobulin. *Nature.* 1998;395:905–908.

145. Bolon B, Galbreath E. Use of genetically engineered mice in drug discovery and development: wielding Occam's razor to prune the product portfolio. *Int J Toxicol.* 2002;21:55–64.

146. Wright AF, Carothers AD, Campbell H. Gene-environment interactions—the BioBank UK study. *Pharmacogenomics J.* 2002;2:75–82.

147. Juul K, Tybjaerg-Hansen A, Marklund S, et al. Genetically reduced antioxidative protection and increased ischaemic heart disease risk: the Copenhagen city heart study. *Circulation.* 2004;109:59–65.

148. Weiss K, Terwilliger J. How many diseases does it take to map a gene with SNPs? *Nat Genet.* 2000;26:151–157.

149. Langlois MR, Delanghe JR, De Buyzere ML, Bernard DR, Ouyang J. Effect of haptoglobin on the metabolism of vitamin C. *Am J Clin Nutr.* 1997;66:606–610.

150. Erichsen HC, Eck P, Levine M, Chanock S. Characterization of the genomic structure of the human vitamin C transporter SVCT1 (*SLC23A2*). *J Nutr.* 2001;131:2623–2627.

151. Berkowitz A. Our genes, ourselves?. *Bioscience.* 1996;46:42–51.

152. Baird P. Genetic technologies and achieving health for populations. *Int J Health Serv.* 2000;30:407–424.

153. Holtzman NA. Putting the search for genes in perspective. *Int J Health Serv.* 2001;31:445.

154. Strohman RC. Ancient genomes, wise bodies, unhealthy people: the limits of a genetic paradigm in biology and medicine. *Perspect Biol Med.* 1993;37:112–145.

155. Kaplan JM. Pigliucci M. Genes "for" phenotypes: a modern history view. *Biol Philosophy.* 2001;16:189–213.

156. Wolf U. The genetic contribution to the phenotype. *Hum Genet.* 1995;95:127–148.

157. Scriver CR, Mahon B, Levy HL. The Hartnup phenotype: Mendelain transport disorder, multifactorial disease. *Am J Hum Genet.* 1987;40:401–412.

158. Scriver CR. Nutrient-gene interactions: the gene is not the disease and vice versa. *Am J Clin Nutr.* 1988;48:1505–1509.

159. Higuchi S, Matsuushita S, Imazeki H, Kinoshita T, Takagi S, Kono H. Aldehyde dehydrogenase genotypes in Japanese alcoholics. *Lancet.* 1994;343:741–742.

160. Hasin D, Aharonovich E, Liu X, et al. Alcohol and ADH2 in Israel: ashkenazis, sephardics, and recent Russian immigrants. *Am J Psychiatry.* August 2002;159(8):1432–1434.

161. Terwilliger JD, Weiss WM. Confounding, ascertainment bias, and the blind quest for a genetic "fountain of youth." *Ann Med.* 2003;35:532–544.

162. Tybjaerg-Hansen A, Steffensen R, Meinertz H, Schnohr P, Nordestgaard BG. Association of mutations in the apolipoprotein B gene with hypercholesterolemia and the risk of ischemic heart disease. *N Engl J Med.* 1998;338:1577–1584.

163. Morgan TH. The relation of genetics to physiology and medicine. *Sci Mon.* 1935;41:5–18.

22

Evaluation of predictive genetic tests for common diseases: bridging epidemiological, clinical, and public health measures

A. Cecile J. W. Janssens, Marta Gwinn,
and Muin J. Khoury

Introduction

Common diseases such as type 2 diabetes, osteoporosis, and cardiovascular disease are caused by a complex interplay of many genetic and nongenetic factors, each of which conveys a minor increase in the risk of disease. Although the genetic contributions to these multifactorial diseases are still poorly understood, enormous progress in the identification of susceptibility genes is expected from the large-scale genome-wide association studies (1,2) and biobank initiatives that have been launched worldwide (3). The vast amount of information issuing from these studies is fueling the search for useful applications of genetic testing to guide prevention and early detection of common diseases with substantial public health impact. One of the greatest expectations is that unraveling the genetic origins of common diseases will lead to individualized medicine, in which prevention and treatment strategies are personalized on the basis of the results of predictive genetic tests. Examples of multifactorial diseases showing promise for predictive genetic testing include type 2 diabetes and age-related macular degeneration (4,5).

Predictive genetic tests can be used to identify persons who have a disease at the time of testing (diagnosis) or who will develop the disease in the future (prediction). Genetic testing is useful when the value it adds to existing efforts to reduce morbidity or mortality (or to efficiency or effectiveness of health care programs) outweighs the additional costs. This evaluation includes not only measures of test performance, but also of health benefits, side effects, financial costs, and psychosocial, ethical, legal, and social implications (6). A brief assessment of the clinical validity and utility of a potential genetic test can help decide whether it merits further, in-depth evaluation.

In this chapter, we first explain how genetic contributions to monogenetic and complex diseases differ, and how these differences affect the predictive value of genetic tests. Then we review some measures for the clinical validity and utility of a single genetic test; we demonstrate that although they are based on the same epidemiological parameters, they provide different information about the usefulness of a genetic test.

Genetic Predisposition to Monogenic and Complex Diseases

Monogenic Diseases

Monogenic diseases such as Huntington disease, familial hypercholesterolemia, cystic fibrosis, and several hereditary forms of cancer are completely or predominantly caused by mutations in a single gene. Predictive testing for these mutations is very informative because disease risks differ substantially between carriers and noncarriers, as shown in Figure 22.1 for Huntington disease, hereditary breast cancer, and nonpolyposis colorectal cancer (7–9). These mutations are typically rare; thus, the risk of disease in carriers is substantially increased, whereas the risk of disease in noncarriers approximates the population average.

Because of the large difference in disease risk between carriers and noncarriers, genetic testing can be useful for targeting preventive or therapeutic interventions to the relatively small group of individuals at increased risk. Examples include intensive surveillance and prophylactic surgery for breast and ovarian cancer and prescription of statins for familial hypercholesterolemia. Genetic testing is also considered valuable in the absence of effective interventions to relieve uncertainty—even when test results are positive—and to prepare for the future.

Multifactorial Diseases

Because multifactorial diseases are caused by complex interactions of many genetic and nongenetic factors, the predictive value of testing for a single genetic variant is

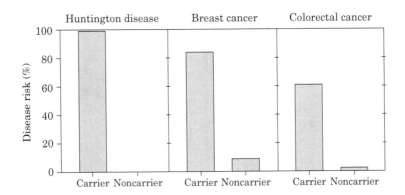

Figure 22.1 Disease risks of carriers and noncarriers in genetic testing for monogenic disorders (10). The genetic variants tested are CAG repeats in 4p16.3 for Huntington disease (7), BRCA1/BRCA2 mutations for breast cancer (8), and MLH1/hMSH2 mutations for colorectal cancer (9).

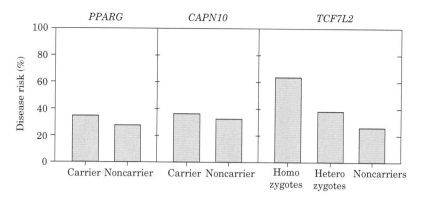

Figure 22.2 Disease risks of carriers and noncarriers in single genetic testing for multifactorial disorders (10). Data on the odds ratios of the genetic variants are obtained from the literature (PPARG (11), CAPN10 (12), TCF7L2 (13)). For the calculation of the disease risks from the published odds ratios, we assumed a lifetime risk of type 2 diabetes of 33% (14).

limited. The disease risk in carriers of the risk variant is only slightly higher than that in noncarriers. For example, several examples of genetic test results for predicting type 2 diabetes are shown in Figure 22.2. Because risk variants are generally common (>1%), carriers and noncarriers have disease risks that are only slightly higher or lower, respectively, than the population average. The differences in disease risk are small and noncarriers remain at risk.

Because multiple genetic and nongenetic factors each have only a minor role in the etiology of multifactorial diseases, researchers and test developers have turned their attention to genetic prediction of disease based on simultaneous testing for multiple genetic variants. This approach is called *genetic profiling*. A genetic profile describes the genotypes for all tested variants and predicts disease risk as a function of their combined effects. For example, when single genetic variants are equally associated with disease, predicted risk is simply proportional to the number of risk genotypes in the genetic profile, as illustrated in Figure 22.3. Figure 22.3a shows the expected distribution of the number of risk genotypes when 40 genes are tested simultaneously: all individuals have at least some risk genotypes but none have risk genotypes for all variants tested. Figure 22.3b shows the associated risk when each single risk genotype increases the risk of disease by 50% (odds ratio = 1.5): the greater the number of risk genotypes present, the higher the risk of disease. Genetic profiles associated with very high disease risks are rare. Most people have disease risks that are only slightly higher or lower than the average disease risk in the population.

In Figure 22.3c, we consider a more realistic scenario in which some genetic factors are stronger predictors of disease than others. The odds ratios of the individual genetic variants vary from 1.05 for genotypes that are more common to 2.0 for those that are less common. In this case, a person's disease risk depends on both the

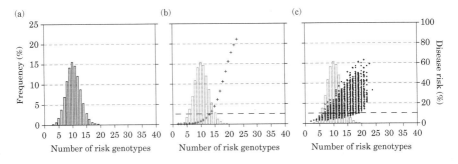

Figure 22.3 Disease risks associated with profiles in genetic testing for multifactorial disorders (10). Bars indicate the frequency distribution of the genetic profiles quantified by the number of risk genotypes in the profile. The frequencies are presented on the left axis. The scatter plots represent the disease risks associated with the genetic profiles when all individual variants have the same odds ratio (OR = 1.5; Figure 22.3b) and when the odds ratios vary (Figure 22.3c). The disease risks are presented on the right axis. Genetic profiles were constructed using a previously described method (15). We assumed that the disease risk in the population was 10% and that the frequencies of the risk genotypes varied between 1% and 60% (incremental from 1% to 19% by 1% and from 20% to 60% by 2%). In Figure 22.3c we assumed that the odds ratios varied from 1.05 to 2.0 (incremental from 1.05 to 1.19 by 0.01 and from 1.20 to 2.0 by 0.05).

number of risk genotypes carried and on each genotype-specific risk. Genotypes more strongly associated with disease contribute more to a person's disease risk than do those with weaker associations. The result is a scattering of disease risks rather than clearly distinguishable risk categories. Considering the role of environmental factors, as well as gene–environment interactions, would contribute to further variation in disease risks for individuals with the same genetic profile.

Evaluation of Single Genetic Tests

Clinical validity and clinical utility are key measures for evaluating genetic tests (6). Clinical validity defines the ability of a test to detect or predict disease; clinical utility focuses on health outcomes, both positive and negative, associated with testing. Several measures of clinical validity and clinical utility (Table 22.1) can be calculated from a basic 2×2 table summarizing the numbers of carriers and noncarriers of risk genotypes who will and will not develop the disease (Table 22.2). A 2×2 table simply assumes that the genetic marker has a risk genotype and a referent genotype (assuming a dominant or recessive effect), but three or more genotypes can be considered as well. The table is defined by basic epidemiological parameters: the population disease risk, the genotype frequencies, and the association between genotypes and the risk of disease (Table 22.1).

To illustrate the formulas of Table 22.1, we present examples of genetic testing for monogenic diseases in offspring of patients (Huntington disease) or of mutation carriers (hereditary breast and colorectal cancer) and for multifactorial diseases

Table 22.1 Overview of epidemiological, clinical, and public health measures in the evaluation of predictive genetic tests

Measure	Description	Formula
Epidemiological evaluation		
Genotype frequency	Frequency of genotype in total population	$P(g) = g/N$
Population risk	Disease risk in total population	$P(D) = D/N$
Penetrance	Disease risk conditional on genotype status	$P(D \mid g) = \dfrac{P(D \cap g)}{P(g)}$
Relative risk	Ratio of disease risks of carriers and noncarriers	$RR = P(D \mid G)/P(D \mid nG)$
Odds ratio	Ratio of odds of disease of carriers and noncarriers	$OR = \dfrac{P(D \mid G) * P(nD \mid nG)}{P(D \mid nG) * P(nD \mid G)}$
Risk difference	Difference between disease risks of carriers and noncarriers	$RD = P(D \mid G) - P(D \mid nG)$
Clinical validity		
Sensitivity	Proportion of carriers among affected	$Se = P(G|D)$
Specificity	Proportion of noncarriers among unaffected	$Sp = P(nG|nD)$
False positive rate	Proportion of carriers among unaffected	$FPR = 1-Sp = P(G|nD)$
False negative rate	Proportion of noncarriers among affected	$FNR = 1-Se = P(nG|D)$
Positive predictive value	Proportion of affected among carriers	$PPV = P(D|G)$
Negative predictive value	Proportion of unaffected among noncarriers	$NPV = P(nD|nG)$
Clinical or public health utility		
Likelihood ratio	Ratio of the genotype frequency in affected and the genotype frequency in unaffected	$LR_g = P(g|D)/P(g|nD)$
Population attributable fraction	Proportion of cases that is attributable to the genetic variant	$PAF = \dfrac{P(D) - P(D \mid nG)}{P(D)}$
Number needed to treat	Number needed to treat to prevent one case	$NNT = \dfrac{1}{RD}$
Number needed to screen	Number of cases needed to screen to prevent one case	$NNS = \dfrac{NNT}{P(G)}$

Persons with the risk genotype are called "carriers"; those without the risk genotype are "noncarriers." Persons who will develop the disease are called "affected"; those who will not are called "unaffected." The letter "g" represents the number of persons with a given genotype, which can be either the risk genotype (G) or the referent genotype (nG). N = the total number of persons in a population; D = the number of persons who will develop the disease; nD = the number of persons who will not develop the disease; P = probability. The symbol "|" stands for "conditional on": for example, $P(D|G)$ means "the probability of disease conditional on the risk genotype," or "the proportion of persons with the risk genotype who will develop disease." The symbol "∩" denotes "and." Although the examples refer to predictive testing for future disease, all measures can also be calculated for diagnostic tests that aim to identify persons with or without the disease.

Table 22.2 Basic table for the calculation of the clinical and public health measures of a single genetic test based on epidemiological data

	Will develop disease	Will not develop disease	Total
Carriers of risk genotype	True positive	False positive	G
Noncarriers	False negative	True negative	nG
Total	D	nD	N

Persons with the risk genotype are called "carriers"; those without the risk genotype are "noncarriers." The letter "g" represents the number of persons with a given genotype, which can be either the risk genotype (G) or the referent genotype (nG). N = the total number of individuals in a population; D = the number of individuals who develop the disease; nD = the number of individuals who will not develop the disease.

in the general population (type 2 diabetes) in Table 22.3. Note that examples refer to predictive testing for future disease, but all measures can also be calculated for diagnostic tests that aim to identify persons with or without the disease.

Epidemiological Parameters

The population disease risk is the probability that a member of a defined population will develop disease within a specified period of time (Table 22.1). Genotype frequencies are the population proportions of carriers and noncarriers of the risk genotype. Measures of association, such as the relative risk, risk difference, and odds ratio compare the risk or odds of disease in carriers and noncarriers of the risk genotype. Relative risk is the ratio of the disease risk in carriers divided by the disease risk in the noncarriers; risk difference is the absolute difference between the disease risk of carriers and noncarriers; and odds ratio is the ratio of the odds of disease in carriers divided by the odds of disease in noncarriers. Odds ratio is also the ratio of the odds of the risk genotype in individuals who will develop the disease and those who will not (referred to as affected and unaffected individuals in Table 22.1). In contrast to the relative risk and risk difference, the odds ratio is the same whether one looks from the genotype or from the disease perspective, that is, horizontally or vertically in Table 22.2 (16). Odds ratios may be used to approximate relative risks in rare diseases; however, odds ratios overestimate relative risks in common diseases.

In monogenic diseases such as Huntington disease, where disease develops in all carriers but in no noncarriers, the genotype frequency is equal to the disease risk in the population (17). In this situation, the disease risk is 100% for carriers and 0% for noncarriers (Figure 22.1; Table 22.3). In contrast, carriers of genetic variants associated with risk for complex diseases have risks that are only slightly higher than the risks in noncarriers (Figure 22.2).

Clinical Validity

Clinical validity measures the ability of genetic markers to detect or predict disease. Clinical validity comprises both the discriminative accuracy of the test and the

Table 22.3 Examples of the evaluation of predictive genetic tests for monogenic and multifactorial diseases

Disease		Huntington disease	Breast cancer	Colorectal cancer		Type 2 diabetes	
clinical scenario*		Offspring of patients	Offspring of patients	Offspring of mutation carriers		General population	
Gene		4p16.3	BRCA1/2	MLH1/MSH2	PPARG	CAPN10	TCF7L2
Marker		CAG repeats			P12A	SNP44	rs7903147
Genotype definition		Mutations	Mutations	Mutations	PP	TT	TT
	Referent				PA/AA	CC/CT	CC/CT
Epidemiological evaluation							
Genotype frequency	At-risk	50%	50%	50%	73% (18)	62% (18)	7% (13)
	Referent	50%	50%	50%	26%	38%	93%
Disease risk		50%	39%†	38%†	33% (14)	33% (14)	33% (14)
Penetrance	At-risk	100%	65% (19)	70% (9)	36%	36%	49%
	Referent	0%	13% (20)	6% (20)	24%	28%	32%
Odds ratio		∞	12.9	40.1	1.77 (18)	1.45 (18)	2.05 (13)
Relative risk		∞	5.13	12.6	1.49	1.29	1.54
Risk difference		100%	52%	64%	12%	8%	17%
Clinical validity and utility							
Sensitivity		100%	84%	93%	80%	68%	10%

(Continued)

Table 22.3 Continued

Disease		Huntington disease	Breast cancer	Colorectal cancer	Type 2 diabetes	
clinical scenario*		Offspring of patients	Offspring of mutation carriers		General population	
Specificity		100%	72%	76%	31%	41%	95%
False negative rate		0%	29%	24%	70%	59%	90%
False positive rate		0%	16%	7%	20%	32%	5%
Positive predictive value		100%	65%	70%	36%	36%	49%
Negative predictive value		100%	87%	94%	76%	72%	68%
Likelihood ratio	At-risk	∞	2.94	3.88	1.15	1.15	1.94
	Referent	0	0.23	0.1	0.65	0.79	0.95
Clinical or public health impact							
Population attributable fraction		100%	67%	85%	26%	15%	4%
Number needed to treat		1	2	2	8	12	6
Number needed to screen		2	4	3	11	20	84

Numbers are for illustration purposes only. Specific risk estimates may vary among populations. All calculations were performed according to the formulas from Table 22.2, by using the Risk Translator of the HuGE Navigator (www.hugenavigator.net).

*Clinical scenario specifies the target population for the genetic testing.

†Disease risks for offspring of mutation carriers, calculated as the average of the penetrances.

predictive value of the test results. The discriminative accuracy of a genetic marker is the extent to which the marker can discriminate between individuals who will develop the disease and those who will not. Key indicators of discriminative accuracy are sensitivity and specificity. Sensitivity is the proportion of carriers among persons who will develop the disease. Specificity is the proportion of noncarriers among persons who will not develop the disease. Sensitivity and specificity are measures of the genetic marker's ability to correctly classify persons according to their future disease status. Sensitivity, and specificity are also known as the true positive rate and the true negative rate. Conversely, the false positive rate is equal to one minus the specificity, and the false negative rate is equal to one minus the sensitivity.

The predictive value of a genetic marker is its ability to predict disease. Positive predictive value is the absolute risk of disease in carriers, and negative predictive value is the probability that noncarriers will *not* develop the disease. Positive predictive value is related to the genetic epidemiological concept of penetrance.

Clinical Utility

Clinical utility is defined in terms of the extent to which genetic testing improves disease prediction beyond conventional risk factors, improves population health outcomes, and improves health care services by increasing the efficiency of interventions. A comprehensive assessment of clinical utility further requires data on social, economic, and behavioral factors as well as knowledge of test performance and disease risks. Genetic testing is useful when it sufficiently changes the distribution of risks predicted before testing. When a genetic marker is associated with risk of disease, carriers of the risk genotype have a higher risk of disease and noncarriers a lower risk of disease compared to the average or pretest disease risk. The likelihood ratio is the magnitude of change from the pretest to the posttest disease risk. The likelihood ratio of a certain genotype differs from its odds ratio in that the odds ratio compares the odds of disease to a referent genotype, whereas the likelihood ratio compares to the pretest odds of disease. A likelihood ratio higher than 1.0 indicates that the genotype is associated with increased risk of disease, and a likelihood ratio lower than 1.0 with a decreased disease risk compared to the risk of disease before testing. When the likelihood ratio is approximately 1.0 (see Table 22.3 for the risk genotypes of *PPARG* and *CAPN10* and the referent genotype of *TCF7L2*), the penetrance approaches the pretest risk of disease. When the likelihood ratios of *all* genotypes approximate 1.0, their odds ratios approximate 1.0 and the test is uninformative.

Population-attributable fraction is an epidemiologic parameter that aims to assess the potential of a genetic test to improve population health outcomes. The population-attributable fraction is the proportion of cases that can be prevented when a particular risk factor is eliminated. Population-attributable fraction increases with higher frequency of the risk genotype and with stronger association of the risk genotype with disease risk. Common interpretations of the population-attributable fraction (Table 22.1) are based on assumptions that the risk factor can be eliminated and that there is no confounding by other risk factors. For risk factors that cannot be eliminated, such as genetic risk factors, population-attributable fraction is the proportion of cases that could be prevented by a preventive intervention that is 100% effective and is adopted by all carriers. Thus, population-attributable fraction can be interpreted as the maximum number of cases that could be prevented by eliminating the adverse effects of the genetic risk factor.

While population-attributable fraction indicates the proportion of cases that can be prevented, the efficiency of interventions to achieve this reduction is indicated by the number needed to treat and the number needed to screen. The number needed to treat is the number of at-risk persons who would need to adopt the preventive intervention to prevent one case. The number needed to screen is the number of persons who would have to be tested to find a sufficient number of persons needed to treat to prevent one case.

Evaluation of Genetic Profiling

Genetic profiles based on multiple variants can be evaluated for clinical validity and utility by the same measures used to evaluate single genetic tests; however, their calculation is sometimes more complex because testing at multiple loci yields a large number of different profiles (Figure 22.3). Regression modeling can be used to estimate some measures—such as the odds ratio, risk difference, predictive value, likelihood ratio, and population-attributable fraction—for specific profiles. Other measures, such as sensitivity and specificity, can only be calculated for genetic markers with two genotypes but have analogous measures for tests with continuous results. The area under the receiver operating characteristic curve (AUC) is a summary measure of discriminative accuracy for continuous tests that is related to the sensitivity and specificity.

Discussion

Several measures of clinical validity and clinical utility can be calculated when information is available for estimating genotype frequencies, disease risk in the population, and the association of genotypes with disease risk. We demonstrate that these different measures, though calculated from the same three epidemiological parameters, provide different and complementary information about the clinical validity and utility of a genetic test.

The measures of clinical validity and clinical utility that we have discussed are related; all of them can be calculated from the same 2×2 table, and hence each can be calculated from the others. For example, the likelihood ratio of the risk genotype is the odds of disease in genotype carriers divided by the odds of disease in the total population; it is also equivalent to the true positive rate divided by the false positive rate, or the sensitivity divided by (1-specificity). Likewise, the odds ratio is the likelihood ratio of the risk genotype divided by the likelihood ratio of the referent genotype. Although these indicators can be calculated from one another, they have different interpretations. For example, a genetic test with appreciable clinical validity may have a low population-attributable fraction when the frequency of the risk genotype is low. Furthermore, a test with a substantial population-attributable fraction may have poor clinical validity when the disease is very common and the odds ratio is low (e.g., as for *PPARG* in type 2 diabetes risk; see Table 22.3).

In this chapter, we present several key points relevant to the evaluation of genetic testing. Most important, we demonstrate that clinical validity and utility vary with differences in the same three epidemiological parameters, whether testing single or multiple genetic variants. Thus, a test that is useful for predicting disease in one population may not be useful in another population, for example, where the risk of disease is lower, the frequency of the risk genotype is lower, or the gene–disease association is weaker. Because disease risks, genotype frequencies, and risk ratios may vary among populations, the clinical validity and utility of a genetic test should be evaluated for each disease in every setting in which the test will be applied (6). For example, the frequency of *BRCA1/2* mutations and the risk of breast cancer in the general population are very different from the parameters for diseases included in Table 22.3; thus, their clinical validity and utility vary accordingly.

Sensitivity and specificity, as well as positive and negative predictive values, should be evaluated simultaneously in the context of one another. Table 22.3 demonstrates that a genetic marker with a frequent risk genotype by definition has good sensitivity. A test based on a genetic marker that is not associated with a disease will have sensitivity and 1-specificity equal to the frequency of the risk genotype. For example, the minimum sensitivity of the *PPARG P12A* polymorphism is 73%, irrespective of which disease is tested for and irrespective of whether the marker is associated with the disease. The same holds for the positive predictive value and 1-negative predictive value, which are at least equal to the population risk of disease. This means, for example, that the positive predictive value of any diabetes risk genotype is at least 33%, regardless of the strength of the association (see Table 22.3) (14).

By definition, a "risk genotype" is associated with a higher risk of disease compared with the referent genotypes; however, this does not mean that the posttest disease risk in carriers will be markedly higher than the average population disease risk (i.e., the probability of disease prior to testing). When the risk genotype is very common (>50%, such as the *PPARG* and *CAPN10* genotypes in Table 22.3), the absolute increase in risk among carriers is smaller than the decrease among non-carriers. Advocates for the potential clinical or public health impact of a genetic test often emphasize the proportion of the population that carries the risk genotype; however, a genetic test for a very common risk genotype might be more useful for identifying individuals at low risk of disease.

Deciding which measure of clinical validity or clinical utility is of primary interest is not an arbitrary decision, but instead is determined by the intended use of the test and the perspective of the user. For example, a test that is used for screening to select persons for further diagnostic testing should have high sensitivity and reasonably good specificity, so that it identifies most affected individuals without yielding an excessive number of false positives. Persons who undergo genetic testing want to know their own risks of disease based on genotype (indicated by the penetrance or predictive value) and the extent to which genetic test results change their estimated risk (indicated by the likelihood ratio). Policy makers or health care payers are likely more interested in the number of individuals that need to be screened or treated to achieve a certain reduction in disease risk and morbidity. Because different perspectives rely on different primary indicators, genetic testing can easily be useful from one perspective but not from another (21).

In summary, the clinical validity and clinical utility of a genetic test depend on the disease risk, the genotype frequency, and the association of a genetic marker with the risk of disease. Different performance measures can lead to different conclusions about the value of genetic testing; therefore, each of these measures should be reported and evaluated in the context of the others. The HuGE Navigator (www. hugenavigator.net; see Chapter 4) includes the HuGE Risk Translator, which can be used to calculate measures of clinical validity and clinical utility based on combinations of epidemiological parameters (measures of disease risk, genotype frequency, and association) supplied by the user. This concise but rigorous evaluation is a first step in determining whether a genetic test warrants further evaluation in terms of cost-effectiveness, policy implications, and ethical, legal, and social implications. This more comprehensive evaluation is required to justify introduction of the test in clinical care or public health practice.

Acknowledgments
The figures in this chapter have been published previously (10) and are reprinted with permission.

References

1. Herbert A, et al. A common genetic variant is associated with adult and childhood obesity. *Science.* 2006;312:279–283.
2. Klein RJ, et al. Complement factor H polymorphism in age-related macular degeneration. *Science.* 2005;308:385–389.
3. Davey Smith G, et al. Genetic epidemiology and public health: hope, hype, and future prospects. *Lancet.* 2005;366:1484–1498.
4. Weedon MN, et al. Combining information from common type 2 diabetes risk polymorphisms improves disease prediction. *PLoS Med.* 2006;3:e374.
5. Maller J, et al. Common variation in three genes, including a noncoding variant in CFH, strongly influences risk of age-related macular degeneration. *Nat Genet.* 2006;38:1055–1059.
6. Haddow JE, Palomaki GE. ACCE: a model process for evaluating data on emerging genetic tests. In: Khoury MJ, Little J, Burke W, eds. *Human Genome Epidemiology: A Scientific Foundation for Using Genetic Information to Improve Health and Prevent Disease.* New York: Oxford University Press; 2003:217–233.

7. Kremer B, et al. A worldwide study of the Huntington's disease mutation. The sensitivity and specificity of measuring CAG repeats. *N Engl J Med*. 1994;330:1401–1406.

8. Ford D, et al. Genetic heterogeneity and penetrance analysis of the BRCA1 and BRCA2 genes in breast cancer families. The Breast Cancer Linkage Consortium. *Am J Hum Genet*. 1998;62:676–689.

9. Vasen HF, et al. MSH2 mutation carriers are at higher risk of cancer than MLH1 mutation carriers: a study of hereditary nonpolyposis colorectal cancer families. *J Clin Oncol*. 2001;19:4074–4080.

10. Janssens ACJW, Khoury MJ. Predictive value of testing for multiple genetic variants in multifactorial diseases: implications for the discourse on ethical, legal and social issues. *Ital J Public Health*. 2006;3:35–41.

11. Zeggini E, et al. Examining the relationships between the Pro12Ala variant in PPARG and Type 2 diabetes-related traits in UK samples. *Diabet Med*. 2005;22:1696–1700.

12. McCarthy MI. Progress in defining the molecular basis of type 2 diabetes mellitus through susceptibility-gene identification. *Hum Mol Genet*. 2004;13 Spec No 1:R33–R41.

13. Grant SF, et al. Variant of transcription factor 7-like 2 (TCF7L2) gene confers risk of type 2 diabetes. *Nat Genet*. 2006;38:320–323.

14. Narayan KM, Boyle JP, Thompson TJ, Sorensen SW, Williamson DF. Lifetime risk for diabetes mellitus in the United States. *JAMA*. 2003;290:1884–1890.

15. Janssens ACJW, et al. Predictive testing for complex diseases using multiple genes: fact or fiction? *Genet Med*. 2006;8:395–400.

16. Bland JM, Altman DG. Statistics notes. The odds ratio. *BMJ*. 2000;320:1468.

17. Khoury MJ, Newill CA, Chase GA. Epidemiologic evaluation of screening for risk factors: application to genetic screening. *Am J Public Health*. 1985;75:1204–1208.

18. Lyssenko V, et al. Genetic prediction of future type 2 Diabetes. *PLOS Med*. 2005;2:e345.

19. Antoniou A, et al. Average risks of breast and ovarian cancer associated with BRCA1 or BRCA2 mutations detected in case Series unselected for family history: a combined analysis of 22 studies. *Am J Hum Genet*. 2003;72:1117–1130.

20. Ries LAG, Harkins D, Krapcho M, et al. *SEER Cancer Statistics Review, 1975–2003*. Bethesda, MD: National Cancer Institute; 2006.

21. Grosse SD, Khoury MJ. What is the clinical utility of genetic testing? *Genet Med*. 2006;8:448–450.

23

The Evaluation of Genomic Applications in Practice and Prevention (EGAPP) initiative: methods of the EGAPP Working Group

Steven M. Teutsch, Linda A. Bradley, Glenn E. Palomaki, James E. Haddow, Margaret Piper, Ned Calonge, W. David Dotson, Michael P. Douglas, and Alfred O. Berg

The Evaluation of Genomic Applications in Practice and Prevention (EGAPP) Initiative, established by the Office of Public Health Genomics at the Centers for Disease Control and Prevention, supports the development and implementation of a rigorous, evidence-based process for evaluating genetic tests and other genomic applications for clinical and public health practice in the United States. An independent, nonfederal EGAPP Working Group (EWG), a multidisciplinary expert panel selects topics, oversees the systematic review of evidence, and makes recommendations based on that evidence. This chapter describes the EGAPP processes and details the specific methods and approaches used by the EWG.

The completion of the Human Genome Project has generated enthusiasm for translating genome discoveries into testing applications that have potential to improve health care and usher in a new era of "personalized medicine" (1–4). For the past decade, however, questions have been raised about the appropriate evidentiary standards and regulatory oversight for this translation process (5–10). The U.S. Preventive Services Task Force (USPSTF) was the first established national process to apply an evidence-based approach to the development of practice guidelines for genetic tests, focusing on *BRCA1/2* testing (to assess risk for heritable breast cancer) and on *HFE* testing for hereditary hemochromatosis (11,12). The Centers for Disease Control and Prevention-funded ACCE Project piloted an evidence evaluation framework of 44 questions, which defines the scope of the review (i.e., disorder, genetic test, clinical scenario) and addresses the previously proposed (6,7) components of evaluation: *A*nalytic and *C*linical validity, *C*linical utility and associated *E*thical, legal, and social implications. The ACCE Project examined available evidence on five genetic testing applications, providing evidence summaries that could

Reprinted with permission from *Genet Med.* 2009;11(1):3–14.

be used by others to formulate recommendations (13–16). Systematic reviews on genetic tests have also been conducted by other groups (17–20).

Genetic tests tend to fit less well within "gold-standard" processes for systematic evidence review for several reasons (21–24). Many genetic disorders are uncommon or rare, making data collection difficult. Even greater challenges are presented by newly emerging genomic tests with potential for wider clinical use, such as genomic profiles that provide information on susceptibility for common complex disorders (e.g., diabetes, heart disease) or drug-related adverse events, and tests for disease prognosis (25,26). The actions or interventions that are warranted based on test results, and the outcomes of interest, are often not well defined. In addition, the underlying technologies are rapidly emerging, complex, and constantly evolving. Interpretation of test results is also complex, and may have implications for family members. Of most concern, the number and quality of studies are limited. Test applications are being proposed and marketed based on descriptive evidence and pathophysiologic reasoning, often lacking well-designed clinical trials or observational studies to establish validity and utility, but advocated by industry and patient interest groups.

The EGAPP Initiative

The EGAPP Working Group (EWG) is an independent panel established in April 2005, to develop a systematic process for evidence-based assessment that is specifically focused on genetic tests and other applications of genomic technology. Key objectives of the EWG are to develop a transparent, publicly accountable process, minimize conflicts of interest, optimize existing evidence review methods to address the challenges presented by complex and rapidly emerging genomic applications, and provide clear linkage between the scientific evidence and the subsequently developed EWG recommendation statements. The EWG is currently composed of 16 multidisciplinary experts in areas such as clinical practice, evidence-based medicine, genomics, public health, laboratory practice, epidemiology, economics, ethics, policy, and health technology assessment (27). This nonfederal panel is supported by the EGAPP initiative launched in late 2004 by the Office of Public Health Genomics at the Centers for Disease Control and Prevention (CDC). In addition to supporting the activities of the EWG, EGAPP is developing data collection, synthesis, and review capacity to support timely and efficient translation of genomic applications into practice, evaluating the products and impact of the EWG's pilot phase, and working with the EGAPP Stakeholders Group on topic prioritization, information dissemination, and product feedback (28). The EWG is not a federal advisory committee, but rather aims to provide information to clinicians and other key stakeholders on the integration of genomics into clinical practice. The EGAPP initiative has no oversight or regulatory authority.

Scope and Selection of Genetic Tests as Topics for Evidence Review

Much debate has centered on the definition of a "genetic test." Because of the evolving nature of the tests and technologies, the EWG has adopted the broad view articulated in a recent report of the Secretary's Advisory Committee on Genetics, Health, and Society (10):

> A genetic test involves the analysis of chromosomes, deoxyribonucleic acid (DNA), ribonucleic acid (RNA), genes, or gene products (e.g., enzymes and other proteins) to detect heritable or somatic variations related to disease or health. Whether a laboratory method is considered a genetic test also depends on the intended use, claim or purpose of a test.

Based on resource limitations, EGAPP focuses on tests having wider population application (e.g., higher disorder prevalence, higher frequency of test use), those with potential to impact clinical and public health practice (e.g., emerging prognostic and pharmacogenomic tests), and those for which there is significant demand for information. Tests currently eligible for EGAPP review include those used to guide intervention in symptomatic (e.g., diagnosis, prognosis, treatment) or asymptomatic individuals (e.g., disease screening), to identify individuals at risk for future disorders (e.g., risk assessment or susceptibility testing), or to predict treatment response or adverse events (e.g., pharmacogenomic tests) (Table 23.1). Though the methods developed for systematic review are applicable, EGAPP is not currently considering diagnostic tests for rare single gene disorders, newborn screening tests, or prenatal screening and carrier tests for reproductive decision making, as these tests are being addressed by other processes (10,29–39).

EGAPP-commissioned evidence reports and EWG recommendation statements are focused on patients seen in traditional primary or specialty care clinical settings, but may address other contexts, such as direct web-based offering of tests to consumers without clinician involvement (e.g., direct-to-consumer or DTC genetic testing). EWG recommendations may vary for different applications of the same test or for different clinical scenarios, and may address testing algorithms that include preliminary tests (e.g., family history or other laboratory tests that identify high risk populations).

Candidate topics (i.e., applications of genetic tests in specific clinical scenarios to be considered for evidence review) are identified through horizon scanning in the published and unpublished literature (e.g., databases, web postings), or nominated by EWG members, outside experts and consultants, federal agencies, healthcare providers and payers, or other stakeholders (40). Like the USPSTF (23), the EWG does not have an explicit process for ranking topics. EGAPP staff prepares background summaries on each potential topic, which are reviewed and given preliminary priorities by an EWG Topics Subcommittee, based on specific criteria and aimed at achieving a diverse portfolio of topics that also challenge the evidence

Table 23.1 Categories of genetic test applications and some characteristics of how clinical validity and utility are assessed

Application of test	Clinical validity	Clinical utility
Diagnosis (symptomatic patient)	Association of marker with disorder	Improved clinical outcomes[*]—health outcomes based on diagnosis and subsequent intervention or treatment
		Availability of information useful for personal or clinical decision making
		End of diagnostic odyssey
Disease screening (asymptomatic patient)	Association of marker with disorder	Improved health outcome based on early intervention for screen positive individuals to identify a disorder for which there is intervention or treatment, or provision of information useful for personal or clinical decision making
Risk assessment/ susceptibility	Association of marker with future disorder (consider possible effect of penetrance)	Improved health outcomes based on prevention or early detection strategies
Prognosis of diagnosed disease	Association of marker with natural history benchmarks of the disorder	Improved health outcomes, or outcomes of value to patients, based on changes in patient management
Predicting treatment response or adverse events (pharmacogenomics)	Association of marker with a phenotype/metabolic state that relates to drug efficacy or adverse drug reactions	Improved health outcomes or adherence based on drug selection or dosage

[*]Clinical outcomes are the net health benefit (benefits and harms) for the patients and/or population in which the test is used.

review methods (Table 23.2). Final selections are determined by vote of the full EWG. EGAPP is currently developing a more systematic and transparent process for prioritizing topics that is better informed by stakeholders.

Review of the Evidence

Evidence Review Strategies

When topics are selected for review by the EWG, CDC commissions systematic reviews of the available evidence. These reviews may include meta-analyses and economic evaluations. New topics are added on a phased schedule as funding and staff capacity allow. All EWG members, review team members, and consultants disclose potential conflicts of interest for each topic considered. Following the identification of the scope and the outcomes of interest for a systematic review, key questions and an analytic framework are developed by the EWG, and later refined by the review team in consultation with a technical expert panel (TEP). The EWG assigns members to serve on the TEP, along with other experts selected by those conducting the review; these members constitute the EWG "topic team" for that review. Based on

Table 23.2 Criteria for preliminary ranking of topics

Criteria related to health burden	What is the potential public health impact based on the prevalence/incidence of the disorder, the prevalence of gene variants, or the number of individuals likely to be tested?
	What is the severity of the disease?
	How strong is the reported relationship between a test result and a disease/drug response?
	Is there an effective intervention for those with a positive test or their family members?
	Who will use the information in clinical practice (e.g., health care providers, payers) and how relevant might this review be to their decision making?
Criteria related to practice issues	What is the availability of the test in clinical practice?
	Is an inappropriate test use possible or likely?
	What is the potential impact of an evidence review or recommendations on clinical practice? On consumers?
Other considerations	How does the test add to the portfolio of EGAPP evidence-based reviews? As a pilot project, EGAPP aims to develop a portfolio of evidence reviews that adequately tests the process and methodologies.
	Will it be possible to make a recommendation, given the body of data available? EGAPP is attempting to balance selection of somewhat established tests versus emerging tests for which insufficient evidence or unpublished data are more likely.
	Are there other practical considerations? For example, avoiding duplication of evidence reviews already underway by other groups.
	How does this test contribute to diversity in reviews? In what category is this test? As a pilot project, EGAPP aims to consider different categories of tests (e.g., pharmacogenomics or cancer), mutation types (e.g., inherited or somatic) or test types (e.g., predictive or diagnostic).

the multidisciplinary nature of the panel, selection of EWG topic teams aims to include expertise in evidence-based medicine and scientific content.

For five of eight testing applications selected by the EWG to date, CDC-funded systematic evidence reviews have been conducted in partnership with the Agency for Healthcare Research and Quality (AHRQ) Evidence-based Practice Centers (EPCs) (41). Based on expertise in conducting comprehensive, well-documented literature searches and evaluation, AHRQ EPCs represent an important resource for performing comprehensive reviews on applications of genomic technology. However, comprehensive reviews are time and resource intensive, and the numbers of relevant tests are rapidly increasing. Some tests have multiple applications and require review of more than one clinical scenario (7,10).

Consequently, the EWG is also investigating alternative strategies to produce shorter, less expensive, but no less rigorous, systematic reviews of the evidence needed to make decisions about immediate usefulness and highlight important gaps in knowledge. A key objective is to develop methods to support "targeted" or "rapid" reviews that are both timely and methodologically sound (13,17–20,42). Candidate topics for such reviews include situations when the published literature base is very limited, when it is possible to focus on a single evaluation component (e.g., clinical validity) that is most critical for decision making, and when information is urgently needed on a test with immediate potential for great benefit or harm. Three such targeted reviews are being coordinated by CDC-based EGAPP staff in collaboration with technical contractors, and with early participation of expert core consultants who can identify data sources and provide expert guidance on the interpretation of results (43). Regardless of the source, a primary objective for all evidence reviews is that the final product is a comprehensive evaluation and interpretation of the available evidence, rather than summary descriptions of relevant studies.

Structuring the Evidence Review

"Evidence" is defined as peer-reviewed publications of original data or systematic review or meta-analysis of such studies; editorials and expert opinion pieces are not included (23,44). However, EWG methods allow for inclusion of peer-reviewed unpublished literature (e.g., information from Food and Drug Administration [FDA] Advisory Committee meetings), and for consideration on a case-by-case basis of other sources, such as review articles addressing relevant technical or contextual issues, or unpublished data. Topics are carefully defined based on the *medical disorder*, the *specific test* (*or tests*) to be used, and the specific *clinical scenario* in which it will be used.

The medical "disorder" (a term chosen as more encompassing than "disease") should optimally be defined in terms of its clinical characteristics, rather than by the laboratory test being used to detect it. Terms such as condition or risk factor generally designate intermediate or surrogate outcomes or findings, which may be of interest in some cases; for example, identifying individuals at risk for atrial fibrillation as an intermediate outcome for preventing the clinical outcome of cardiogenic stroke. In pharmacogenomic testing, the disorder, or outcome of interest, may be a reduction in adverse drug events (e.g., avoiding severe neutropenia among cancer patients to be treated with irinotecan via *UGT1A1* genotyping and dose reduction in those at high risk), optimizing treatment (e.g., adjusting initial warfarin dose using *CYP2C9* and *VKORC1* genotyping to more quickly achieve optimal anticoagulation in order to avoid adverse events), or more effectively targeting drug interventions to those patients most likely to benefit (e.g., herceptin for *HER2* overexpressing breast cancers).

Characterizing the genetic test(s) is the second important step. For example, the American College of Medical Genetics defined the genetic testing panel for cystic fibrosis in the context of carrier testing as the 23 most common *CFTR* mutations (i.e., present at a population frequency of 0.1% or more) associated with classic, early onset cystic fibrosis in a U.S. pan-ethnic study population. This allowed the subsequent review of analytic and clinical validity to focus on a relatively small subset of the 1,000 or more known mutations (45). Rarely, a nongenetic test may be evaluated, particularly if it is an existing alternative to mutation testing. An example would be biochemical testing for iron overload (e.g., serum transferrin saturation, serum ferritin) compared with *HFE* genotyping for identification of hereditary hemochromatosis.

A clear definition of the clinical scenario is of major importance, as the performance characteristics of a given test may vary depending on the intended use of the test, including the clinical setting (e.g., primary care, specialty settings), how the test will be applied (e.g., diagnosis or screening), and who will be tested (e.g., general population or selected high risk individuals). Preliminary tests should also be considered as part of the clinical scenario. For example, when testing for Lynch syndrome among newly diagnosed colorectal cancer cases, it may be too expensive to sequence two or more mismatch repair genes (e.g., *MLH1*, *MSH2*) in all patients. For this reason, preliminary tests, such as family history, microsatellite instability, or immunohistochemical testing, may be evaluated as strategies for selecting a smaller group of higher risk individuals to offer gene sequencing.

Methods

Methods of the EWG for reviewing the evidence share many elements of existing processes, such as the USPSTF (23), the AHRQ Evidence-based Practice Center Program (46), the Centre for Evidence Based Medicine (47), and others (44,48–53). These include the use of analytic frameworks with key questions to frame the evidence review; clear definitions of clinical and other outcomes of interest; explicit search strategies; use of hierarchies to characterize data sources and study designs; assessment of quality of individual studies and overall certainty of evidence; linkage of evidence to recommendations; and minimizing conflicts of interest throughout the process. Typically, however, the current evidence on genomic applications is limited to evaluating gene–disease associations, and is unlikely to include randomized controlled trials that evaluate test-based interventions and patient outcomes. Consequently, the EWG must rigorously assess the quality of observational studies, which may not be designed to address the questions posed.

In this new field, direct evidence to answer an overarching question about the effectiveness and value of testing is rarely available. Therefore, it is necessary to construct a chain of evidence, beginning with the technical performance of the test (analytic validity) and the strength of the association between a genotype and disorder of interest. The strength of this association determines the test's ability to diagnose a disorder, assess susceptibility or risk, or provide information on prognosis or variation in drug response (clinical validity). The final link is the evidence that test results can change patient management decisions and improve net health outcomes (clinical utility).

To address some unique aspects of genetic test evaluation, the EWG has adopted several aspects of the ACCE model process, including formal assessment of analytic validity; use of unpublished literature for some evaluation components when published data are lacking or of low quality; consideration of ethical, legal, and social implications as integral to all components of evaluation; and use of questions from the ACCE analytic framework to organize collection of information (13). Important concepts that underlie the EGAPP process and add value include (i) providing a venue for multidisciplinary independent assessment of collected evidence; (ii) conducting reviews that maintain a focus on medical outcomes that matter to patients, but also consider a range of specific family and societal outcomes when appropriate (54); (iii) developing and optimizing methods for assessing individual study quality, adequacy of evidence for each component of the analytic framework, and certainty of the overall body of evidence; (iv) focusing on summarization and synthesis of the evidence and identification of gaps in knowledge; and (v) ultimately, providing a foundation for evidentiary standards that can guide policy decisions. Although evidentiary standards will necessarily vary depending on test application (e.g., for diagnosis or to guide therapy) and the clinical situation, the methods and approaches described in this chapter are generally applicable; further refinement is anticipated as experience is gained.

The Analytic Framework and Key Questions

After the selection and structuring of the topic to be reviewed, the EWG Methods Subcommittee drafts an analytic framework for the defined topic that explicitly illustrates the clinical scenario, the intermediate and health outcomes of interest, and the key questions to be addressed. Table 23.1 provides generic examples of clinical scenarios. However, analytic frameworks for genetic tests differ based on clinical scenario, and must be customized for each topic. Figure 23.1 shows the example of an analytic framework used to develop the first EWG recommendation, *Testing for Cytochrome P450 Polymorphisms in Adults with Nonpsychotic Depression Prior to Treatment with Selective Serotonin Reuptake Inhibitors (SSRIs)*; numbers in the figure refer to the key questions listed in the legend (55,56).

The first key question is an overarching question to determine whether there is direct evidence that using the test leads to clinically meaningful improvement in outcomes or is useful in medical or personal decision making. In this case, EGAPP uses the USPSTF definition of direct evidence, "a single body of evidence establishes the connection" between the use of the genetic test (and possibly subsequent tests or interventions) and health outcomes (23). Thus, the overarching question addresses clinical utility, and specific measures of the outcomes of interest. For genetic tests, such direct evidence on outcomes is most commonly not available or of low quality, so a "chain of evidence" is constructed using a series of key questions. EGAPP follows the convention that the chain of evidence is indirect if, rather than answering the overarching question, two or more bodies of evidence (linkages in the analytic framework) are used to connect the use of the test with health outcomes (23,57).

After the overarching question, the remaining key questions address the components of evaluation as links in a possible chain of evidence: *analytic validity* (technical test performance), *clinical validity* (the strength of association that determines the test's ability to accurately and reliably identify or predict the disorder of interest),

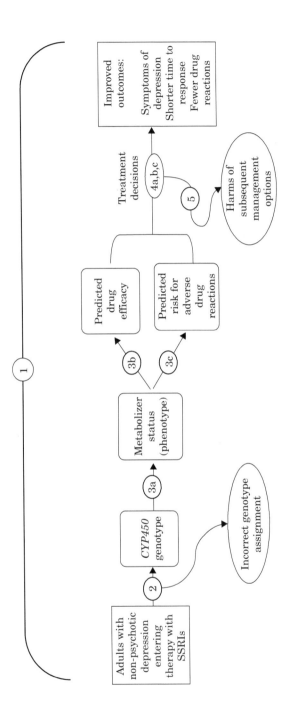

Figure 23.1 Analytic framework and key questions for evaluating one application of a genetic test in a specific clinical scenario: Testing for Cytochrome P450 Polymorphisms in Adults with Nonpsychotic Depression Treated With Selective Serotonin Reuptake Inhibitors (SSRIs); modified from Reference 56. The numbers correspond to the following key questions:

1. Overarching question: Does testing for cytochrome P450 (CYP450) polymorphisms in adults entering selective serotonin reuptake inhibitor (SSRI) treatment for nonpsychotic depression lead to improvement in outcomes, or are testing results useful in medical, personal, or public health decision making?
2. What is the analytic validity of tests that identify key CYP450 polymorphisms?
3. Clinical validity: (a). How well do particular CYP450 genotypes predict metabolism of particular SSRIs? (b). How well does CYP450 testing predict drug efficacy? (c). Do factors such as race/ethnicity, diet, or other medications, affect these associations?
4. Clinical utility: (a). Does CYP450 testing influence depression management decisions by patients and providers in ways that could improve or worsen outcomes? (b). Does the identification of the CYP450 genotypes in adults entering SSRI treatment for nonpsychotic depression lead to improved clinical outcomes compared to not testing? (c). Are the testing results useful in medical, personal, or public health decision making?
5. What are the harms associated with testing for CYP450 polymorphisms and subsequent management options?

and *clinical utility* (balance of benefits and harms when the test is used to influence patient management). Determining whether a chain of indirect evidence can be applied to answer the overarching question requires consideration of the quality of individual studies, the adequacy of evidence for each link in the evidence chain, and the certainty of benefit based on the quantity (i.e., number and size) and quality (i.e., internal validity) of studies, the consistency and generalizability of results, and understanding of other factors or contextual issues that might influence the conclusions (23,57). The USPSTF has recently updated its methods and clarified its terminology (57). Because this approach is both thoughtful and directly applicable to the work of EGAPP, the EWG has adopted the terminology; an additional benefit will be to provide consistency for shared audiences.

Evidence Collection and Assessment

The review team considers the analytic framework, key questions, and any specific methodological approaches proposed by the EWG. As previously noted, the report will focus on clinical factors (e.g., natural history of disease, therapeutic alternatives) and outcomes (e.g., morbidity, mortality, quality of life), but the EWG may request that other familial, ethical, societal, or intermediate outcomes also be considered for a specific topic (54). The EWG may also request information on other relevant factors (e.g., impact on management decisions by patients and providers) and contextual issues (e.g., cost effectiveness, current use, or feasibility of use).

Methods for individual evidence reviews will differ in small ways based on the reviewers (AHRQ EPC or other review team), the strategy for review (e.g., comprehensive, targeted/rapid), and the topic. These differences will be transparent because all evidence reviews describe methods and follow the same general steps: framing the specific questions for review; gathering technical experts and reviewers; identifying data sources, searching for evidence using explicit strategies and study inclusion/exclusion criteria; specifying criteria for assessing quality of studies; abstracting data into evidence tables; synthesizing findings; and identifying gaps and making suggestions for future research.

All draft evidence reports are distributed to the TEP and other selected experts for technical review. After consideration of reviewer comments, EPCs provide a final report that is approved and released by AHRQ and posted on the AHRQ web site; the EPC may subsequently publish a summary of the evidence. Non-EPC review teams submit final reports to CDC and the EWG, along with the comments from the technical reviewers and how they were addressed; the EWG approves the final report. Final evidence reports (or links to AHRQ reports) are posted on the http://www.egappreviews.org Web site. When possible, a manuscript summarizing the evidence report is prepared to submit for publication along with the clinical practice recommendations developed by the EWG (56).

Grading Quality of Individual Studies

Table 23.3 provides the hierarchies of data sources for analytic validity, and of study designs for clinical validity and utility, designated for all as Level 1 (highest) to Level 4. Table 23.4 provides a checklist of questions for assessing the quality of individual studies for each evaluation component based on the published literature (5,13,23,48,58,59). Different reviewers may provide a quality rating for individual studies that is based on specified criteria, or derived using a more quantitative algorithm. The EWG ranks individual studies as *Good*, *Fair*, or *Marginal* based on critical appraisal using the criteria in Tables 23.3 and 23.4. The designation *Marginal* (rather than *Poor*) acknowledges that some studies may not have been "poor" in overall design or conduct, but may not have been designed to address the specific key question in the evidence review.

Table 23.3 Hierarchies of data sources and study designs for the components of evaluation

Level*	Analytic validity	Clinical validity	Clinical utility
1	Collaborative study using a large panel of well-characterized samples	Well-designed longitudinal cohort studies	Meta-analysis of randomized controlled trials (RCT)
	Summary data from well-designed external proficiency testing schemes or interlaboratory comparison programs	Validated clinical decision rule[†]	
2	Other data from proficiency testing schemes	Well-designed case-control studies	A single randomized controlled trial
	Well-designed peer-reviewed studies (e.g., method comparisons, validation studies)		
	Expert panel reviewed FDA summaries		
3	Less well-designed peer-reviewed studies	Lower quality case-control and cross-sectional studies Unvalidated clinical decision rule[†]	Controlled trial without randomization Cohort or case-control study
4	Unpublished and/or nonpeer-reviewed research, clinical laboratory, or manufacturer data	Case series	Case series
	Studies on performance of the same basic methodology, but used to test for a different target	Unpublished and/or nonpeer-reviewed research, clinical laboratory or manufacturer data	Unpublished and/or nonpeer-reviewed studies
		Consensus guidelines	Clinical laboratory or manufacturer data
		Expert opinion	Consensus guidelines
			Expert opinion

*Highest level is 1.
[†]A clinical decision rule is an algorithm leading to result categorization. It can also be defined as a clinical tool that quantifies the contributions made by different variables (e.g., test result, family history) in order to determine classification/interpretation of a test result (e.g., for diagnosis, prognosis, therapeutic response) in situations requiring complex decision making (55).

Table 23.4 Criteria for assessing quality of individual studies (internal validity) (55)

Analytic validity	Clinical validity	Clinical utility
Adequate descriptions of the index test (test under evaluation)	*Clear description of the disorder/phenotype and outcomes of interest*	*Clear description of the outcomes of interest*
Source and inclusion of positive and negative control materials	Status verified for all cases Appropriate verification of controls	What was the relative importance of outcomes measured; which were prespecified primary outcomes and which were secondary?
Reproducibility of test results	*Verification does not rely on index test result*	*Clear presentation of the study design*
Quality control/assurance measures	Prevalence estimates are provided	Was there clear definition of the specific outcomes or decision options to be studied (clinical and other endpoints)?
Adequate descriptions of the test under evaluation	*Adequate description of study design and test/methodology*	Was interpretation of outcomes/endpoints blinded?
Specific methods/platforms evaluated	*Adequate description of the study population*	*Were negative results verified?*
Number of positive samples and negative controls tested	Inclusion/exclusion criteria	*Was data collection prospective or retrospective?*
Adequate descriptions of the basis for the "right answer"	Sample size, demographics	If an experimental study design was used, were subjects randomized? Were intervention and evaluation of outcomes blinded?
Comparison to a "gold standard" referent test	Study population defined and representative of the clinical population to be tested	Did the study include comparison with current practice/empirical treatment (value added)?
Consensus (e.g., external proficiency testing)	Allele/genotype frequencies or analyte distributions known in general and subpopulations	*Intervention*
Characterized control materials (e.g., NIST, sequenced)	*Independent blind comparison with appropriate, credible reference standard(s)*	What interventions were used?
Avoidance of biases	Independent of the test	What were the criteria for the use of the interventions?
Blinded testing and interpretation	Used regardless of test results	*Analysis of data*
Specimens represent routinely analyzed clinical specimens in all aspects (e.g., collection, transport, processing)	Description of handling of indeterminate results and outliers	Is the information provided sufficient to rate the quality of the studies?
Reporting of test failures and uninterpretable or indeterminate results	Blinded testing and interpretation of results	Are the data relevant to each outcome identified?
Analysis of data	*Analysis of data*	Is the analysis or modeling explicit and understandable?
Point estimates of analytic sensitivity and specificity with 95% confidence intervals	Possible biases are identified and potential impact discussed	Are analytic methods prespecified, adequately described, and appropriate for the study design?
Sample size/power calculations addressed	Point estimates of clinical sensitivity and specificity with 95% confidence intervals	Were losses to follow-up and resulting potential for bias accounted for?
	Estimates of positive and negative predictive values	Is there assessment of other sources of bias and confounding?
		Are there point estimates of impact with 95% CI?
		Is the analysis adequate for the proposed use?

NIST = National Institute of Standards and Quality.

469

Components of Evaluation

Analytic Validity. EGAPP defines the analytic validity of a genetic test as its ability to accurately and reliably measure the genotype (or analyte) of interest in the clinical laboratory, and in specimens representative of the population of interest (13). Analytic validity includes analytic sensitivity (detection rate), analytic specificity (1-false positive rate), reliability (e.g., repeatability of test results), and assay robustness (e.g., resistance to small changes in preanalytic or analytic variables) (13). As illustrated by the "ACCE wheel" figure (http://www.cdc.gov/genomics/gtesting/ACCE.htm), these elements of analytic validity are themselves integral elements in the assessment of clinical validity (13,42). Many evidence-based processes assume that evaluating clinical validity will address any analytic problems, and do not formally consider analytic validity (23). The EWG has elected to pursue formal evaluation of analytic validity because genetic and genomic technologies are complex and rapidly evolving, and validation data are limited. New tests may not have been validated in multiple sites, for all populations of interest, or under routine clinical laboratory conditions over time. More importantly, review of analytic validity can also determine whether clinical validity can be improved by addressing test performance.

Tests kits or reagents that have been cleared or approved by the FDA may provide information on analytic validity that is publicly available for review (e.g., FDA submission summaries) (60). However, most currently available genetic tests are offered as laboratory developed tests not currently reviewed by the FDA, and information from other sources must be sought and evaluated. Different genetic tests may use a similar methodology, and information on the analytic validity of a common technology, as applied to genes not related to the review, may be informative. However, general information about the technology cannot be used as a substitute for specific information about the test under review. Based on experience to date, access to specific expertise in clinical laboratory genetics and test development is important for effective review of analytic validity.

Table 23.3 (column 1) provides a quality ranking of data sources that are used to obtain unbiased and reliable information about analytic validity. The best information (quality Level 1) comes from collaborative studies using a single large, carefully selected panel of well-characterized samples (both cases and controls) that are blindly tested and reported, with the results independently analyzed. At this time, such studies are largely hypothetical, but an example that comes close is the Genetic Testing Quality Control Materials Program at CDC (61). As part of this program, samples precharacterized for specific genetic variants can be accessed from Coriell Cell Repositories (Camden, NJ) by other laboratories to perform in-house validation studies (62). Data from proficiency testing schemes (Levels 1 or 2) can provide some information about all three phases of analytic validity (i.e., analytic, pre- and postanalytic), as well as interlaboratory and intermethod variability. ACCE questions 8 through 17 are helpful in ensuring that all aspects of analytic validity have been addressed (42).

Table 23.4 (column 1) lists additional criteria for assessing the quality of individual studies on analytic validity. Assessment of the overall quality of evidence for analytic validity includes consideration of the quality of studies, the quantity of data (e.g., number and size of studies, genes/alleles tested), and the consistency and generalizability of the evidence (also see Table 23.5, column 1). The consistency of findings can be assessed formally (e.g., by testing for homogeneity), or by less formal methods (e.g., providing a central estimate and range of values) when sufficient data are lacking. One or more internally valid studies do not necessarily provide sufficient information to conclude that analytic validity has been established for the test. Supporting the use of a test in routine clinical practice requires data on analytic validity that are generalizable to use in diverse "real world" settings.

Clinical Validity. EGAPP defines the clinical validity of a genetic test as its ability to accurately and reliably predict the clinically defined disorder or phenotype of interest. Clinical validity encompasses clinical sensitivity and specificity (integrating analytic validity), and predictive values of positive and negative tests that take into account the disorder prevalence (the proportion of individuals in the selected setting who have, or will develop, the phenotype/clinical disorder of interest). Clinical validity may also be affected by reduced penetrance (i.e., the proportion of individuals with a disease-related genotype or mutation who develop disease), variable expressivity (i.e., variable severity of disease among individuals with the same genotype), and other genetic (e.g., variability in allele/genotype frequencies or gene–disease association in racial/ethnic subpopulations) or environmental factors. ACCE questions 18 through 25 are helpful in organizing information on clinical validity (42).

Table 23.3 (column 2) provides a hierarchy of study designs for assessing quality of individual studies (13,23,44,46–48,50,53,63). Published checklists for reporting studies on clinical validity are reasonably consistent, and Table 23.4 (column 2) provides additional criteria adopted for grading the quality of studies (e.g., execution, minimizing bias) (5,13,23,44,46–51,53,58,59,63). As with analytic validity, the important characteristics defining overall quality of evidence on clinical validity include the number and quality of studies, the representativeness of the study population(s) compared with the population(s) to be tested, and the consistency and generalizability of the findings (Table 23.5). The quantity of data includes the number of studies, and the number of total subjects in the studies. The overall consistency of clinical validity estimates can be determined by formal methods such as meta-analysis. Minimally, estimates of clinical sensitivity and specificity should include confidence intervals (63). In pilot studies, initial estimates of clinical validity may be derived from small data sets focused on individuals known to have, versus not have, a disorder, or from case/control studies that may not represent the wide range or frequency of results that will be found in the general population. Although important to establish proof of concept, such studies are insufficient evidence for

Table 23.5 Grading the quality of evidence for the individual components of the chain of evidence (key questions) (57)

Adequacy of information to answer key questions	Analytic validity	Clinical validity	Clinical utility
Convincing	*Studies that provide confident estimates of analytic sensitivity and specificity using intended sample types from representative populations*	*Well-designed and conducted studies in representative population(s) that measure the strength of association between a genotype or biomarker and a specific and well-defined disease or phenotype*	*Well-designed and conducted studies in representative population(s) that assess specified health outcomes*
	Two or more Level 1 or 2 studies that are generalizable, have a sufficient number and distribution of challenges, and report consistent results	Systematic review/meta-analysis of Level 1 studies with homogeneity	Systematic review/meta-analysis of randomized controlled trials showing consistency in results
			At least one large randomized controlled trial (Level 2)
	One Level 1 or 2 study that is generalizable and has an appropriate number and distribution of challenges	Validated Clinical Decision Rule High quality Level 1 cohort study	
Adequate	Two or more Level 1 or 2 studies that	Systematic review of lower quality studies	Systematic review with heterogeneity
	Lack the appropriate number and/or distribution of challenges	Review of Level 1 or 2 studies with heterogeneity	One or more controlled trials without randomization (Level 3)
	Are consistent, but not generalizable	Case-control study with good reference standards	Systematic review of Level 3 cohort studies with consistent results
	Modeling showing that lower quality (Level 3, 4) studies may be acceptable for a specific well-defined clinical scenario	Unvalidated Clinical Decision Rule (Level 2)	
Inadequate	Combinations of higher quality studies that show important unexplained inconsistencies	Single case-control study Nonconsecutive cases Lacks consistently applied reference standards	Systematic review of Level 3 quality studies or studies with heterogeneity
	One or more lower quality studies (Level 3 or 4)	Single Level 2 or 3 cohort/case-control study	Single Level 3 cohort or case-control study Level 4 data
	Expert opinion	Reference standard defined by the test or not used systematically Study not blinded Level 4 data	

clinical application; additional data are needed from the entire range of the intended clinical population to reliably quantify clinical validity before introduction.

Clinical Utility. EGAPP defines the clinical utility of a genetic test as the evidence of improved measurable clinical outcomes, and its usefulness and added value to patient management decision making compared with current management without genetic testing. If a test has utility, it means that the results (positive or negative) provide information that is of value to the person, or sometimes to the individual's family or community, in making decisions about effective treatment or preventive strategies. Clinical utility encompasses effectiveness (evidence of utility in real clinical settings), and the net benefit (the balance of benefits and harms). Frequently, it also involves assessment of efficacy (evidence of utility in controlled settings like a clinical trial).

Tables 23.3 and 23.4 (column 3) provide the hierarchy of study designs for clinical utility, and other criteria for grading the internal validity of studies (e.g., execution, minimizing bias) adopted from other published approaches (13,23,46–48,57). Paralleling the assessment of analytic and clinical validity, the three important quality characteristics for clinical utility are quality of individual studies and the overall body of evidence, the quantity of relevant data, and the consistency and generalizability of the findings (Table 23.5). Another criterion to be considered is whether implementation of testing in different settings, such as clinician ordered versus direct-to-consumer, could lead to variability in health outcomes.

Grading the Quality of Evidence for the Individual Components in the Chain of Evidence (Key Questions)

Table 23.5 provides criteria for assessing the quality of the body of evidence for the individual components of evaluation, analytic validity (column 2), clinical validity (column 3), and clinical utility (column 4) (23,44,47,48,64). The adequacy of the information to answer the key questions related to each evaluation component is classified as *Convincing, Adequate,* or *Inadequate.* This information is critical to assess the "strength of linkages" in the chain of evidence (57). The intent of this approach is to minimize the risk of being wrong in the conclusions derived from the evidence. When the quality of evidence is *Convincing,* the observed estimate or effect is likely to be real, rather than explained by flawed study methodology; when *Adequate,* the observed results may be influenced by such flaws. When the quality of evidence is *Inadequate,* the observed results are more likely to be the result of flaws in study methodology rather than an accurate assessment; availability of only *Marginal* quality studies always results in *Inadequate* quality.

Based on the evidence available, the overall level of certainty of net health benefit is categorized as *High, Moderate,* or *Low* (57). *High* certainty is associated with consistent and generalizable results from well-designed and conducted studies, making it unlikely that estimates and conclusions will change based on future studies. When the level of certainty is *Moderate*, some data are available, but limitations in data quantity, quality, consistency, or generalizability reduce confidence in the results, and, as more information becomes available, the estimate or effect may change enough to alter the conclusion. *Low* certainty is associated with insufficient or poor quality data, results that are not consistent or generalizable, or lack of information on important outcomes of interest; as a result, conclusions are likely to change based on future studies.

Translating Evidence into Recommendations. Based on the evidence report, the EWG's assessment of the magnitude of net benefit and the certainty of evidence, and consideration of other clinical and contextual issues, the EWG formulates clinical practice recommendations (Table 23.6). Although the information will have value to other stakeholders, the primary intended audience for the content and format of the recommendation statement is clinicians. The information is intended to provide transparent, authoritative advice, inform targeted research agendas, and underscore the increasing need for translational research that supports the appropriate transition of genomic discoveries to tests, and then to specific clinical applications that will improve health or add other value in clinical practice.

Key factors considered in the development of a recommendation are the relative importance of the outcomes selected for review, the benefits (e.g., improved clinical outcome, reduction of risk) that result from the use of the test and subsequent

Table 23.6 Recommendations based on certainty of evidence, magnitude of net benefit, and contextual issues

Level of certainty	Recommendation
High or moderate	**Recommend for...**
	. . . if the magnitude of net benefit is Substantial, Moderate, or Small*, unless additional considerations warrant caution.
	Consider the importance of each relevant contextual factor and its magnitude or finding.
	Recommend against...
	. . . if the magnitude of net benefit is zero or there are net harms.
	Consider the importance of each relevant contextual factor and its magnitude or finding.
Low	**Insufficient evidence...**
	. . . if the evidence for clinical utility or clinical validity is insufficient in quantity or quality to support conclusions or make a recommendation.
	Consider the importance of each contextual factor and its magnitude or finding.
	Determine whether the recommendation should be Insufficient (neutral), Insufficient (encouraging), or Insufficient (discouraging).
	Provide information on key information gaps to drive a research agenda.

*Categories for the "magnitude of effect" or "magnitude of net benefit" used are *substantial, moderate, small,* and *zero* (57).

actions or interventions (or if not available, maximum potential benefits), the harms (e.g., adverse clinical outcome, increase in risk or burden) that result from the use of the test and subsequent actions/interventions (or if not available, largest potential harms), and the efficacy and effectiveness of the test and follow-up compared with currently used interventions (or doing nothing). Simple decision models or outcomes tables may be used to assess the magnitudes of benefits and harms, and estimate the net effect. Consistent with the terminology used by the USPSTF, the magnitude of net benefit (benefit minus harm) may be classified as *Substantial, Moderate, Small,* or *Zero* (57).

Considering Contextual Factors

Contextual issues include clinical factors (e.g., severity of disorder, therapeutic alternatives), availability of diagnostic alternatives, current availability and use of the test, economics (e.g., cost, cost effectiveness, and opportunity costs), and other ethical and psychosocial considerations (e.g., insurability, family factors, acceptability, equity/fairness). Cost-effectiveness analysis is especially important when a recommendation for testing is made. Contextual issues that are not included in preparing EGAPP recommendation statements are values or preferences, budget constraints, and precedent. Societal perspectives on whether use of the test in the proposed clinical scenario is ethical are explored before commissioning an evidence review.

The ACCE analytic framework considers as part of clinical utility the assessment of a number of additional elements related to the integration of testing into routine practice (e.g., adequate facilities/resources to support testing and appropriate follow-up, plan for monitoring the test in practice, availability of validated educational materials for providers and consumers) (13). The EWG considers that most of these elements constitute information that should not be included in the consideration of clinical utility, but may be considered as contextual factors in developing recommendation statements and in translating recommendations into clinical practice.

Recommendation Language

Standard EGAPP language for recommendation statements uses the terms: *Recommend For, Recommend Against,* or *Insufficient Evidence* (Table 23.6). Because the types of emerging genomic tests addressed by EGAPP are more likely to have findings of *Insufficient Evidence*, three additional qualifiers may be added. Based on the existing evidence and consideration of contextual issues and modeling, *Insufficient Evidence* could be considered "Neutral" (not possible to predict with current evidence), "Discouraging" (discouraged until specific gaps in knowledge are filled *or* not likely to meet evidentiary standards even with further study), and "Encouraging" (likely to meet evidentiary standards with further studies or reasonable to use in limited situations based on existing evidence while additional evidence is gathered).

As a hypothetical example of how the various components of the review are brought together to reach a conclusion, consider the model of a pharmacogenetic test proposed for screening individuals who are entering treatment with a specific drug. The intended use is to identify individuals who are at risk for a serious adverse reaction to the drug. The analytic validity and clinical validity of the test are established and are adequately high. However, the specific adverse outcomes of interest are often clinically diagnosed and treated as part of routine management, and clinical studies have not been conducted to show the incremental benefit of the test in improving patient outcomes. Because there is no evidence to support improvement in health outcome or other benefit of using the test (e.g., more effective, more acceptable to patients, or less costly), the EWG would consider the recommendation to be *Insufficient Evidence* (Neutral). In a second scenario, a genetic test is proposed for testing patients with a specific disorder to provide information on prognosis and treatment. Clinical trials have provided good evidence for benefit to a subset of patients based on the test results, but more studies are needed to determine the validity and utility of testing more generally. The EWG is likely to consider the recommendation to be *Insufficient Evidence* (Encouraging).

Products and Review

Draft evidence reports are distributed by the EPC or other contractor for expert peer review. Objectives for peer review of draft evidence reports are to ensure accuracy, completeness, clarity, and organization of the document; assess modeling, if present, for parameters, assumptions, and clinical relevance; and to identify scientific or contextual issues that need to be addressed or clarified in the final evidence report. In general, the selection of reviewers is based on expertise, with consideration given to potential conflicts of interest.

When a final evidence report is received by the EWG, a writing team begins development of the recommendation statement. Technical comments are solicited from test developers on the evidence report's accuracy and completeness, and are considered by the writing team. The recommendation statement is intended to summarize current knowledge on the validity and utility of an intended use of a genetic test (what we know and do not know), consider contextual issues related to implementation, provide guidance on appropriate use, list key gaps in knowledge, and suggest a research agenda. Following acceptance by the full EWG, the draft EGAPP recommendation statement is distributed for comment to peer reviewers selected from organizations expected to be impacted by the recommendation, the EGAPP Stakeholders Group, and other key target audiences (e.g., healthcare payers, consumer organizations). The objectives of this peer review process are to ensure the accuracy and completeness of the evidence summarized in the recommendation statement and the transparency of the linkage to the evidence report, improve the clarity and organization of information, solicit feedback from different perspectives, identify contextual issues that have not been addressed, and avoid unintended consequences. Final drafts of recommendation statements are approved by the EWG and submitted for publication in *Genetics in Medicine*. Once published, the journal provides open access to these documents, and the link is also posted on the www.egappreviews.org. web site Announcements of recommendation statements are distributed by email to a large number of stakeholders and the media. The newly established EGAPP Stakeholders Group will advise on and facilitate dissemination of evidence reports and recommendation statements.

Summary

This document describes methods developed by the EWG for establishing a systematic, evidence-based assessment process that is specifically focused on genetic tests and other applications of genomic technology. The methods aim for transparency, public accountability, and minimization of conflicts of interest, and provide a framework to guide all aspects of genetic test assessment, beginning with topic selection and concluding with recommendations and dissemination. Key objectives are to optimize existing evidence review methods to address the challenges presented by complex and rapidly emerging genomic applications, and to establish a clear linkage between the scientific evidence, the conclusions/recommendations, and the information that is subsequently disseminated.

In combining elements from other internationally recognized assessment schemes in its methods, the EWG seeks to maintain continuity in approach and nomenclature, avoid confusion in communication, and capture existing expertise and experience. The panel's methods differ from others in some respects, however, by calling for formal assessment of analytic validity (in addition to clinical validity and clinical utility) in its evidence reviews, and including (on a selective basis) nontraditional sources of information such as gray literature, unpublished data, and review articles that address relevant technical or contextual issues. The methods and process of the EWG remain a work in progress and will continue to evolve as knowledge is gained from each evidence review and recommendation statement.

Future challenges include modifying current methods to achieve more rapid, less expensive, and targeted evidence reviews for test applications with limited literature, without sacrificing the quality of the answers needed to inform practice decisions and research agendas. A more systematic horizon scanning process is being developed to identify high priority topics more effectively, in partnership with the EGAPP Stakeholders Group and other stakeholders. Additional partnerships will need to be created to develop evidentiary standards and build additional evidence review capacity, nationally. Finally, the identification of specific gaps in knowledge in the evidence offers the opportunity to raise awareness among researchers, funding entities, and review panels, and thereby focus future translation research agendas.

Acknowledgments

Members of the EGAPP Working Group are Alfred O. Berg, MD, MPH, Chair; Katrina Armstrong, MD, MSCE; Jeffrey Botkin, MD, MPH; Ned Calonge, MD, MPH; James E. Haddow, MD; Maxine Hayes, MD, MPH; Celia Kaye, MD, PhD; Kathryn A. Phillips, PhD; Margaret Piper, PhD, MPH; Sue Richards, PhD; Joan A. Scott, MS, CGC; Ora Strickland, PhD; Steven Teutsch, MD, MPH.

References

1. Burke W, Psaty BM. Personalized medicine in the era of genomics. *JAMA.* 2007; 298:1682–1684.
2. Gupta P, Lee KH. Genomics and proteomics in process development: opportunities and challenges. *Trends Biotechnol.* 2007;25:324–330.
3. Topol EJ, Murray SS, Frazer KA. The genomics gold rush. *JAMA.* 2007;298:218–221.
4. Feero WG, Guttmacher AE, Collins FS. The genome gets personal—almost. *JAMA.* 2008;299:1351–1352.
5. Burke W, Atkins D, Gwinn M, et al. Genetic test evaluation: information needs of clinicians, policy makers, and the public. *Am J Epidemiol.* 2002;156:311–318.
6. Holtzman NA, Watson MS. Promoting safe and effective genetic testing in the United States. Final Report of the National Institute of Health -Department of Energy (DOE) Task Force on Genetic Testing. Available at http://www.genome.gov/10001733. Accessed December 12, 2007.
7. Secretary's Advisory Committee on Genetics, Health and Society. Enhancing oversight of genetic tests: recommendations of the SACGT. Available at http://www4.od.nih.gov/oba/sacgt/reports/oversight_report.pdf. Accessed December 12, 2007.
8. Huang A. Genetics & Public Policy Center, Issue Briefs. Who regulates genetic tests? Available at http://www.dnapolicy.org/policy.issue.php?action=detail&issuebrief_id=10. Accessed December 12, 2007.
9. Secretary's Advisory Committee on Genetics, Health and Society. Coverage and reimbursement of genetic tests and services. Available at http://www4.od.nih.gov/oba/SACGHS/reports/CR_report.pdf. Accessed December 12, 2007.
10. U.S. System of Oversight of Genetic Testing. A response to the charge of the secretary of health and human services. Report of the Secretary's Advisory Committee on Genetics, Health, and Society. April, 2008. Department of Health and Human Services. Available at http://oba.od.nih.gov/oba/SACGHS/reports/SACGHS_oversight_report.pdf. Accessed June 13, 2009.
11. USPSTF. Genetic risk assessment and BRCA mutation testing for breast and ovarian cancer susceptibility: recommendation statement. *Ann Intern Med.* 2005;143:355–361.
12. Whitlock EP, Garlitz BA, Harris EL, Beil TL, Smith PR. Screening for hereditary hemochromatosis: a systematic review for the U.S. Preventive Services Task Force. *Ann Intern Med.* 2006;145:209–223.
13. Haddow J, Palomaki G. ACCE: a model process for evaluating data on emerging genetic tests. In: Khoury M, Little J, Burke W, editors. *Human Genome Epidemiology: A Scientific Foundation for Using Genetic Information to Improve Health and Prevent Disease.* New York: Oxford University Press; 2003:217–233.
14. Palomaki GE, Haddow J, Bradley L, Fitzsimmons SC. Updated assessment of cystic fibrosis mutation frequencies in non-Hispanic Caucasians. *Genet Med.* 2002;4: 90–94.

15. Palomaki G, Bradley L, Richards C, Haddow J. Analytic validity of cystic fibrosis testing: a preliminary estimate. *Genet Med.* 2003;5:15–20.

16. Palomaki G, Haddow J, Bradley L, Richards CS, Stenzel TT, Grody WW. Estimated analytic validity of HFE C282Y mutation testing in population screening: the potential value of confirmatory testing. *Genet Med.* 2003;5: 440–443.

17. Gudgeon J, McClain M, Palomaki G, Williams M. Rapid ACCE: experience with a rapid and structured approach for evaluating gene-based testing. *Genet Med.* 2007;9:473–478.

18. McClain M, Palomaki G, Piper M, Haddow J. A rapid ACCE review of *CYP2C9* and *VKORC1* allele testing to inform warfarin dosing in adults at elevated risk for thrombotic events to avoid serious bleeding. *Genet Med.* 2008;10:89–98.

19. Piper MA. Blue Cross and Blue Shield Special Report. Genotyping for cytochrome P450 polymorphisms to determine drug-metabolizer status. Available at www.bcbs.com/tec/Vol19/19_09.pdf. Accessed July 6, 2006.

20. Piper MA. Blue Cross Blue Shield TEC Assessment. Gene expression profiling of breast cancer to select women for adjuvant chemotherapy. Available at http://www.bcbs.com/blueresources/tec/vols/22/22_13.pdf. Accessed August 18, 2008.

21. Briss P, Zaza S, Pappaioanou M, et al. Developing an evidence-based Guide to Community Preventive Services—methods. The Task Force on Community Preventive Services. *Am J Prev Med.* 2000;18:35–43.

22. Briss P, Brownson R, Fielding J, Zaza S. Developing and using the Guide to Community Preventive Services: lessons learned about evidence-based public health. *Annu Rev Public Health.* 2008;25:281–302.

23. Harris R, Helfand M, Woolf S, et al. Current methods of the US Preventive Services Task Force: a review of the process. *Am J Prev Med.* 2001;20:21–35.

24. Zaza S, Wright-De A, Briss P, et al. Data collection instrument and procedure for systematic reviews in the Guide to Community Preventive Services. Task Force on Community Preventive Services. *Am J Prev Med.* 2000;18: 44–74.

25. Hunter D, Khoury M, Drazen J. Letting the genome out of the bottle—will we get our wish? *N Engl J Med.* 2008;358:105–107.

26. Kamerow D. Waiting for the genetic revolution. *BMJ.* 2008;336:22.

27. EGAPPreviews.org Homepage. Available at http://www.egappreviews.org/. Accessed March 20, 2008.

28. National Office of Public Health Genomics, CDC Web site. Available at http://www.cdc.gov/genomics. Accessed March 20, 2008.

29. Maddalena A, Bale S, Das S, et al. Technical standards and guidelines: molecular genetic testing for ultra-rare disorders. *Genet Med.* 2005;7:571–583.

30. Faucett WA, Hart S, Pagon RA, Neall LF, Spinella G. A model program to increase translation of rare disease genetic tests: collaboration, education, and test translation program. *Genet Med.* 2008;10:343–348.

31. Gross SJ, Pletcher BA, Monaghan KG. Carrier screening in individuals of Ashkenazi Jewish descent. *Genet Med.* 2008;10:54–56.

32. Driscoll DA, Gross SJ. First trimester diagnosis and screening for fetal aneuploidy. *Genet Med.* 2008;10:73–75.

33. Grody WW, Cutting GR, Klinger KW, et al. Laboratory standards and guidelines for population-based cystic fibrosis carrier screening. *Genet Med.* 2001;3:149–154.

34. Richards CS, Bradley LA, Amos J, et al. Standards and guidelines for CFTR mutation testing. *Genet Med.* 2002;4:379–391.

35. Evidence-based evaluation and decision process for the Advisory Committee on Heritable Disorders and Genetic Diseases in Newborn and Children: a workgroup meeting summary. October 23, 2006. Advisory Committee on Heritable Disorders and Genetic

Diseases in Newborns and Children. Available at ftp://ftp.hrsa.gov/mchb/genetics/reports/MeetingSummary23Oct2006.pdf. Accessed June 13, 2009.

36. Advisory Committee on Heritable Disorders and Genetic Diseases in Newborns and Children. U.S. Department of Health and Human Services, Health Resources and Services Administration. Available at http://www.hrsa.gov/heritabledisorderscommittee/. Accessed June 13, 2009.

37. National Newborn Screening and Genetics Resource Center. Available at http://genes-r-us.uthscsa.edu/. Accessed June 10, 2008.

38. American College of Obstetricians and Gynecologists News Release. ACOG's screening guidelines on chromosomal abnormalities: what they mean to patients and physicians. Available at http://www.acog.org/from_home/publications/press_releases/nr05-07-07-1.cfm. Accessed June 13, 2009.

39. Genetic advances and the rarest of rare diseases: genetics in medicine focuses on genetics and rare diseases. Available at http://www.acmg.net/AM/Template.cfm?Section=Home3&Template=/CM/HTMLDisplay.cfm&ContentID=3049. Accessed June 11, 2008.

40. National Office of Public Health Genomics—EGAPP Stakeholders Group. Available at http://www.cdc.gov/genomics/gtesting/egapp_esg.htm. Accessed January 15, 2008.

41. Agency for Healthcare Research and Quality Evidence-based Practice Centers. Available at http://www.ahrq.gov/clinic/epc/. Accessed January 15, 2008.

42. National Office of Public Health Genomics, CDC. ACCE model system for collecting, analyzing and disseminating information on genetic tests. Available at http://www.cdc.gov/genomics/gtesting/ACCE.htm. Accessed December 12, 2007.

43. EGAPP Reviews.org Topics. Available at http://www.egappreviews.org/workingrp/topics.htm. Accessed October 9, 2007.

44. Ebell M, Siwek J, Weiss B, et al. Strength of recommendation taxonomy (SORT): a patient-centered approach to grading evidence in the medical literature. *J Am Board Fam Pract.* 2004;17:59–67.

45. ACCE. Population-based prenatal screening for cystic fibrosis via carrier testing—introduction. Available at http://www.cdc.gov/genomics/gtesting/ACCE/FBR/CF/CFIntro.htm. Accessed January 16, 2008.

46. AHRQ. Systems to rate the strength of scientific evidence. Evidence Report/Technology Assessment. Available at http://www.ncbi.nlm.nih.gov/books/bv.fcgi?rid=hstat1.chapter.70996. Accessed December 12, 2007.

47. Centre for Evidence Based Medicine. Levels of evidence and grades of recommendation. Available at http://www.cebm.net/levels_of_evidence.asp. Accessed December 12, 2007.

48. Atkins D, Best D, Briss PA, et al. Grading quality of evidence and strength of recommendations. *BMJ.* 2004;328:1490.

49. Bossuyt P, Reitsma J, Bruns D, et al. Towards complete and accurate reporting of studies of diagnostic accuracy: the STARD initiative. *Ann Intern Med.* 2003;138:40–44.

50. Deeks JJ. Systematic reviews in health care: systematic reviews of evaluations of diagnostic and screening tests. *BMJ.* 2001;323:157–162.

51. Tatsioni A, Zarin D, Aronson N, et al. Challenges in systematic reviews of diagnostic technologies. *Ann Intern Med.* 2005;142:1048–1055.

52. US Food and Drug Administration. Draft guidance for industry, clinical laboratories, and FDA staff. In vitro diagnostic multivariate index assays. Available at http://www.fda.gov/cdrh/oivd/guidance/1610.pdf. Accessed January 15, 2008.

53. Whiting P, Rutjes A, Reitsma J, Bossuyt PM, Kleijnen J. The development of QUADAS: a tool for the quality assessment of studies of diagnostic accuracy included in systematic reviews. *BMC Med Res Methodol.* 2003;3:25.

54. Botkin JR, Teutsch SM, Kaye CI, et al. Examples of types of health-related outcomes. Table 5–2 in: U.S. System of Oversight of Genetic Testing: a response to the Charge of the Secretary of Health and Human Services. Report of the Secretary's Advisory Committee on Genetics, Health, and Society, 2008:122–123. Available at http://www4.od.nih.gov/oba/SACGHS/reports/SACGHS_oversight_report.pdf. Accessed June 12, 2008.

55. Evaluation of Genomic Applications in Practice and Prevention (EGAPP) Working Group. Recommendations from the EGAPP Working Group: testing for cytochrome P450 (*CYP450*) polymorphisms in adults with nonpsychotic depression treated with selective serotonin reuptake inhibitors. *Genet Med.* 2007;9:819–825.

56. Matchar DB, Thakur ME, Grossman I, et al. Testing for cytochrome P450 polymorphisms in adults with non-psychotic depression treated with selective serotonin reuptake inhibitors (SSRIs). Evidence Report/Technology Assessment No. 146. (Prepared by the Duke Evidence-based Practice Center under Contract No. 290–02-0025.) AHRQ Publication No. 07-E002. Rockville, MD: Agency for Healthcare Research and Quality. Available at http://www.ahrq.gov/downloads/pub/evidence/pdf/cyp450/cyp450.pdf. Accessed January 23, 2007.

57. Sawaya GF, Guirguis-Blake J, LeFevre M, et al. Update on methods of the U.S. Preventive Services Task Force: estimating certainty and magnitude of net benefit. *Ann Intern Med.* 2007;147:871–875.

58. Lijmer JG, Mol BW, Heisterkamp S, et al. Empirical evidence of design-related bias in studies of diagnostic tests. *JAMA.* 1999;282:1061–1066.

59. Little J, Bradley L, Bray M, et al. Reporting, appraising, and integrating data on genotype prevalence and gene–disease associations. *Am J Epidemiol.* 2002;156:300–310.

60. U.S. Food and Drug Administration. 510(k) Substantial equivalence determination decision summary for Roche AmpliChip *CYP450* microarray for identifying CYP2D6 genotype (510(k) Number k042259). Available at http://www.fda.gov/cdrh/reviews/k042259.pdf. Accessed April 19, 2006.

61. Genetic Testing Reference Materials Coordination Program (GeT-RM)—Home. Available at http://wwwn.cdc.gov/dls/genetics/rmmaterials/default.aspx. Accessed January 17, 2008.

62. Cell lines typed for CYP2C9 and VKORC1 alleles. Available at http://www.cdc.gov/dls/genetics/rmmaterials/pdf/CYP2C9_VKORC1.pdf. Accessed January 17, 2008.

63. American College of Medical Genetics. C8—test validation. Standards and guidelines for clinical genetics laboratories: general policies. Available at http://www.acmg.net/Pages/ACMG_Activities/stds-2002/c.htm. Accessed December 12, 2007.

64. Clinical evidence: the international source of the best available evidence for effective healthcare. Available at http://clinicalevidence.bmj.com/ceweb/about/index.jsp. Accessed January 16, 2008.

24

Rapid, evidence-based reviews of genetic tests

James M. Gudgeon, Glenn E. Palomaki,
and Marc S. Williams

Introduction

Genetic and genomic tests are rapidly emerging from the efforts of the Human
Genome Project. As of August 2009, GeneTests (www.genetests.org) listed 599 laboratories testing for 1,772 diseases, of which 1,498 are offered clinically. Between
1997 and 2007, the number of clinically offered tests has increased at an annual rate
of about 25%. Even this is an underestimate, since registration is voluntary and tests
for somatic mutations are not included. Many more tests are in the development
pipeline, and as they enter the medical marketplace, clinicians, policy makers, and
health care payers must make decisions about provision or coverage in a timely and
affordable manner.

Evidence Reviews

In the United States, evaluation of such testing falls generally into two categories:
comprehensive and *ad hoc*. Comprehensive evaluations are resource intensive,
highly structured, transparent, and usually take many months to years to complete.
At present, many of the comprehensive evidence reviews are commissioned or performed by government entities. *Ad hoc* reviews include those performed by a number
of health insurers, medical delivery systems, professional organizations, technology
assessments entities (for-profit and not-for-profit), and other entities that are required
or compelled to examine the evidence about the effectiveness of genetic tests. In the
authors' experience, *ad hoc* reviews are more variable with respect to their structure, transparency, objectiveness, timeliness, and thoroughness.

Two notable organizations in the United States that perform comprehensive tech-
nology reviews include the US Preventive Services Task Force (USPSTF) and the
Medicare Evidence Development and Coverage Advisory Committee (MEDCAC).
The USPSTF focuses on evaluating screening tests for public health (1). The
MEDCAC was established to provide independent guidance and expert advice to the
Center for Medicare and Medicaid Services (2). Neither has an evaluative process
specific for genetic/genomic tests. The US National Institutes of Health-Department
of Energy (NIH-DOE) Task Force on Genetic Testing (TFGT) and the Health and

Human Services Secretary's Advisory Committee on Genetic Testing (SACGT) proposed the adoption of the ACCE criteria, which subsequently led to the ACCE and EGAPP models (see separate discussion, below).

In the United Kingdom, the National Institute for Clinical Excellence (NICE) is the principal entity responsible for directing the review of new medical technologies, and supports both a "global standard [comprehensive] process" as well as the current development of their Single Technology Appraisal process for more rapid review of "life-saving drugs." Neither is specific for genetic/genomic tests (or even diagnostics). The Cochrane Collaboration (with Cochrane Centers throughout the world) has developed a general model for evaluating medical interventions. This comprehensive model is designed to evaluate clinical utility via the assessment of results from randomized trials. Recently, the Cochrane Collaboration has begun efforts to develop methods to guide systematic reviews of diagnostic test performance (3). In the past several years, the United Kingdom's Department of Health, via its Genetic Testing Network (UKGTN), has developed a standardized methodology for the rapid review of genetic tests for single-gene disorders (4). No doubt, organizations in many other developed countries have review processes, both comprehensive and *ad hoc*, to address the evaluation of medical technologies.

Private Sector Evidence Reviews

Various private organizations (e.g., ECRI Institute, Hayes Inc.) also conduct and sell technology assessment reports. Their efforts to review genetic tests have expanded commensurate with demand. Hayes has developed a model and now provides a service for purchase, specifically for evaluating genetic tests based on ACCE and EGAPP model concepts. Their reviews emphasize clinical utility. Some large payers (e.g., Aetna, Blue Cross/Blue Shield, Cigna) have the resources to support and maintain dedicated personnel to perform comprehensive technology assessments, and may have proprietary methods for evaluating genetic tests. The Blue Cross and Blue Shield Association Technology Evaluation Center currently has a strong focus on genomics. Aetna, Cigna, and others have also reviewed many genetic/genomic tests, many of which are publicly available via the Internet. Smaller payers apply a variety of methods, within their resource and time constraints.

The ACCE Model

Beginning with the 1997 NIH-DOE Task Force on Genetic Testing report, *Promoting Safe and Effective Genetic Testing* (5), followed by the SACGT report, *Enhancing the Oversight of Genetic Tests* (6) in 2000, evidence regarding genetic tests was divided into four broad areas: analytic validity (does the test accurately measure the target), clinical validity (do test results correlate with the disorder of interest), clinical utility (what are the harms and medical benefits), and ethical, legal, and social implications (what safeguards have been implemented and are they effective). Subsequently, the Office of Public Health Genomics at the Centers for Disease

Control and Prevention (CDC) requested proposals aimed at addressing some of the deficits in evaluating genetic tests that had been identified by these and other reports. This resulted in the CDC-funded ACCE project (an acronym of Analytic validity, Clinical validity, Clinical utility, and Ethical, legal and social implications). The ACCE project culminated in an evaluation framework comprising 44 questions that address the four components of evaluation for a specified disorder, test, and clinical scenario that was tested in a wide range of settings, using various methodologies, to produce evidence-based reviews of five genetic tests (7). All of the completed sections were placed into the public domain for review and comment. The ACCE model has since become the backbone of most formal efforts to evaluate genetic tests, including those performed in Europe (8,9).

The EGAPP Process

In 2005 the Evaluation of Genomic Applications in Practice and Prevention (EGAPP) program was established to extend and refine the ACCE model by formalizing assessment of the strength of evidence and by adding an independent, multidisciplinary EGAPP Working Group (EWG), whose primary function is to make evidence-based recommendations. Key objectives of the EWG are to develop a transparent, publicly accountable process, minimize conflicts of interest, optimize existing evidence review methods to address the challenges presented by complex and rapidly emerging genomic applications, and provide clear linkage between the scientific evidence and the subsequently developed EWG recommendation statements (10). While the ACCE framework is a useful construct when considering the completeness of any technology assessment for EGAPP, EGAPP is a process that incorporates additional steps to develop, ultimately, formal recommendation statements. The EGAPP initiative is currently the premier model in the United States for evaluation of genetic tests; however, its current format generally requires extensive resources and time to complete.

Thus, there are multiple review formats being used by a variety of different stakeholders but, as yet, no universally accepted standard. In our experience, nearly all genetic/genomic test-specific evaluation approaches are based on at least some elements of the ACCE model. This chapter aims at encapsulating the most important elements for the performance of rapid reviews of genetic and genomic tests, and suggests one possible recipe for performing a rapid review. We have recently published a methods paper on a rapid ACCE model for evaluating genetic tests, based on our early experiences using a modification of the ACCE approach to evaluate two genetic tests (11). More recently, Burke and Zimmern, in a report funded by the United Kingdom's Department of Health for the UK Genetic Testing Network (UKGTN), and based on extensive experience with rapid reviews of genetic tests, published (online) an Expanded Framework for Genetic Test Evaluation (based on the ACCE model) that addresses additional elements and issues (12). However, those reviews are aimed at rare genetic disorders that pose their own unique problem set.

Rapid Evidence Reviews

Proposed Uses and Stakeholders of Rapid Reviews

Rapid reviews of genetic tests are necessary when circumstances require relatively quick decisions about test use or reimbursement. In the United States, this is primarily among payers, and secondarily among health care delivery systems (especially integrated ones). Implicit in the need for a relatively quick decision is a limitation in resources for evaluation. In addition, rapid reviews can be applied when resources are limited, the literature is limited, or when the review can be focused on specific portions of the question (e.g., clinical utility).

In the United Kingdom, there is a well-coordinated and relatively mature process for reviewing genetic tests for single-gene (Mendelian) disorders. All emerging genetic tests for Mendelian disorders that might be used by the NHS are submitted as "gene dossiers" for review. Such submissions are generally made by providers within molecular diagnostics laboratories. These reviews are now performed rapidly using a consistent framework, with favorable decisions implemented, albeit imperfectly, into routine NHS care delivery.

Decisions about reimbursement and clinical use may require only a subset of questions for review, defined by decision makers' needs, whereby the scope of the questions addressed and/or the published literature is limited (i.e., "targeted"). Providers and clinicians often focus only on the clinical utility, with the belief that if a test has demonstrated utility, then its analytic validity and clinical validity are likely to be acceptable as well. More comprehensive reviews are performed by public policy makers, guideline developers, and those wanting to describe completely the current state of a given test, including identifying gaps in knowledge.

It is important to differentiate between a "targeted" review, which is compatible with being done rapidly, and a comprehensive review, that will take considerably more resources. The Roche AmpliChip™ for *CYP2D6* and *CYP2C19* analysis can be used as an example. The United States Food and Drug Administration (FDA) evaluated this test under its regulatory authority for medical devices, specifically the In Vitro Diagnostic Multivariate Index Analysis (IVDMIA) draft guidelines. FDA reviews tend to focus principally on safety considerations; therefore, the data demonstrating analytic validity and clinical validity are the main focus. There is limited information required for clinical utility beyond the plausibility that the test could improve health. The recent FDA clearance of the Roche AmpliChip demonstrated analytic validity by comparing the chip results with sequencing results. Limited information was provided about clinical validity, relying mostly on relating the metabolic phenotype (defined by probe drugs) to the *CYP* genotype. This is an example of a targeted review. More recently, a comprehensive review commissioned by the EGAPP Working Group found little or no association of *CYP2D6* genotypes and SSRI levels in patients with depression (13). Not only was there no evidence of clinical utility in the literature, but there was poor correlation of blood levels of the SSRI drugs with the polymorphisms under study (i.e., clinical validity).

Box 24.1

Completed rapid ACCE reviews:
   • *BMPR2* testing for idiopathic pulmonary hypertension (14)
   • *CYP2C9* and *VKORC1* variant testing to aid initial dosing of warfarin (15)

In contrast to the FDA, a payer is interested in how the result of this test would impact care of their members (i.e., clinical utility). If an evidence review found no evidence addressing this question, it would likely conclude that the test is experimental/investigational, and therefore not provide insurance coverage. To take it a step further, a medical delivery system would likely consider the test as part of a clinical process, whereby the resources and activities required to provide and fund the test, with interpretation, to its patients would also be considered in decision making.

While professional societies and support groups would prefer to have a comprehensive review in order to develop guidelines, many emerging tests have an incomplete base of evidence. Box 24.1 contains two recent examples of rapid ACCE reviews, one requested by a disease-specific support group, the other by a professional society.

If timely, evidence-based reviews are performed and made publicly available, then other stakeholders will likely emerge, including clinicians and delivery systems, policy makers at various levels, and the public. This has been seen in the EGAPP program with the establishment of the EGAPP Stakeholder's Group (ESG) (16). However, if these reviews are only available through the private sector, their accessibility will be limited.

How Might Requests for Reviews Come About?
The majority of industrialized countries have a form of universal health care delivery and payment. With this comes centralized medical decision making, where emerging modalities of diagnosis and treatment are prioritized and reviewed systematically. The fragmented nature of health care decision making in the United States leads to different stakeholder perspectives as well as different reasons for reviews.

In the case of public health indications such as newborn screening, professional society guideline development, and national coverage decisions (e.g., Medicare), comprehensive evidence review processes are preferred, though such reviews may, at times, be targeted.

In the private health care sector, most technology assessment activity regarding new genetic tests is by payers, secondarily by health care delivery systems (especially integrated ones), and medical specialty societies. The stimulus to perform a technology review in these settings is often an impending or a recent FDA approval, provider or multiple patient requests for a new test, or a new marketing effort to providers or direct to consumers. There is little literature that systematically evaluates how health care entities perform technology assessment for any purpose, much less specific to genetic testing (17). This was examined in detail in a presentation at the Institute of Medicine in 2007, and the interested reader is referred here for a full discussion (18).

How Rapid Is "Rapid Review"?

The timeframe for a rapid review of a genetic test is established by those making a recommendation for its use, provision, or coverage. This is dictated by the availability of the test, its impact within the jurisdiction of the decision-making entity, the resources available for the evaluation, and the complexity or magnitude of the evaluation. We suggest that a rapid review be defined as one that can be completed in a matter of several weeks or months from the time of topic identification, applying adequate resources to ensure that the evidence collected is suitable for decision making. Overall, less than 200 hours of research time would normally be required. Substantially less time (e.g., 20–40 hours) and resources may be needed to complete a rapid review for the purpose of an insurance coverage decision (given that the focus is mostly around evidence of clinical utility), compared with a more comprehensive evidence review commissioned by a medical specialty society for the purposes of guideline development.

Performing a Rapid ACCE Review

Expertise Required

The expertise required for a rapid, evidence-based review of genetic tests is essentially the same as that for any medical intervention, with the caveat being that the analyst be well versed in evaluating screening and diagnostic testing, commensurate with the complexity of the analytic challenges and decision needs of the stakeholders. Given several unique aspects of genetic tests, including results that are frequently probabilistic rather than deterministic, impact on other family members, as well as the relatively high rate of uninformative or equivocal test results, the reviewers will need familiarity specific to these issues. It may be highly desirable to have a clinical and/or molecular geneticist on the review team. Content experts play a key role by providing clinical context, clarifying competing testing modalities, and explaining specialized language and/or nomenclature. Complete interpretation of results may require expertise from related fields such as medical education, social science, ethics, and the law.

Understanding the Test and Clinical Setting

Prior to beginning any systematic review, the specific clinical disorder, test, and setting for which the test is intended must be articulated carefully and thoughtfully, including the exact nature of the proposed test and the alternatives to the test (19).

Box 24.2

Expertise required for a rapid ACCE review:
   Clinical laboratory science
   Epidemiology/biostatistics
   Clinical medicine
   Genetics

And Preferred:
   Economics
   Education and the law
   Social science/ethics

Implicit in this process is the recognition that there is a chain of events linking the use of the test and its results to decisions that ultimately lead to the primary outcomes of interest (e.g., changes in health care that result in improvements in quality of life, morbidity, or mortality). Often the test results are intermediate or surrogate outcomes which may, or may not, lead to improvement in primary medical outcomes. For example, it is clear that *CYP2C9* genotypes are related to warfarin dose at stable INR. However, current evidence is lacking that adjusting initial dosing based on genotype would result in improved outcomes (15). Policy makers must determine whether knowledge of secondary outcomes is sufficient to drive decisions or whether knowledge of primary health outcomes is required. In either case, broader issues may also be important to address, not the least of which could be ethical, legal, and social issues (ELSI) as well as operational issues. These choices will shape the entire evaluation process.

The Review Process

Once the topic is clearly specified, the review should begin with a systematic search of published literature. If stakeholders are based in the United States and decisions are "local," then a search of PubMed may suffice. However, due to the extensive literature published elsewhere in the world not indexed in PubMed; it may be important to also search other databases including the Euro-centric EMBASE literature base, Science Citation Index, and BIOSIS.

When the literature base is small and/or incomplete, as will frequently be the case with emerging genetic/genomic tests, it may be useful to search for and include analysis of data that has not been through a peer review process. The sources of this type of data are sometimes referred to as "gray literature." Such data may be available from academic laboratories that are doing the leading-edge work in this area, from manufacturers or support groups, or as part of publicly available FDA submissions. The SACGT Oversight report previously referenced has called for

---

Box 24.3

Rapid ACCE review checklist:
- Assemble knowledgeable stakeholders/content experts
- Define the disorder, setting, and test
- Review the literature using a structured approach
- Interpret the results (knowledge synthesis)
- Summarize the identified gaps in knowledge
- Make decisions/recommendations using transparent methods
- Communicate results

---

increased transparency and availability of these data to the public. This may provide information needed to answer important analytic questions via application of standard statistical methods. Regardless of the source, analysts must be cautious when using gray data due to the possibility of multiple biases (not unlike published and peer-reviewed literature). There may also be financial or intellectual investment in the test as well as inadequate information about methods used to obtain the data. Another alternative to gray data is the use of expert opinion. The use of multiple content experts from different institutions, with outside reviewers when possible, may reduce the risk of bias and improve the credibility of the review. However, if experts are the only source of information, a gap in knowledge should be acknowledged.

The Basic Formula

For clinicians and payers, here is one possible step-by-step approach to a rapid ACCE review of an emerging genetic/genomic test:

1. Assemble a knowledgeable group of stakeholders and content experts along with the team performing the review and those developing recommendations or making coverage decisions.
2. Begin the discussion by clarifying the details of the review. This is often a discovery process, as the evaluation team clarifies the issues and evidence. Central to this (iterative) process is determination of the outcome(s) that drive(s) the decision-making process. It is important to understand fully the role of the testing in the chain of events leading to the primary outcomes in order to assess the value of the testing.
3. Define and agree on key terms and definitions related to the review and decisions.
4. Carefully define the disorder of interest, the setting (or clinical scenario), and the specific test that will be used. The analyst might ask the clinician and

    laboratory expert for key references, and whether they have access to relevant unpublished data pertinent to the emerging, key questions.

5. The analyst then performs a thorough review of literature, perhaps in consultation with clinical and/or laboratory experts, with a clear focus on gathering data to address the key questions upon which the decision will be based.

6. The analyst links the data extracted from the literature with key questions and evaluates study strengths and level of confidence (when decision-makers expect this). If the literature base is small, a quantitative analysis of available data may be relatively simple (20,21).

7. The analyst begins building the evidence review, based on a format that meets the needs of the stakeholders. Internal, and ideally external, review is then solicited as a way of ensuring that the data review and interpretation are complete and correct.

8. Steps 5–7 can be repeated as needed to support completion of answers to key questions. Outside experts can provide value to the final report, upon which a decision to provide or cover is made.

9. Communicate to stakeholders the conclusions of the review, with a summary of gaps in evidence in a consistent and useful format. One such format has been proposed by Ramsey et al. (22), who also suggested making and communicating information about pricing/reimbursement of tests.

This simple sequence of steps is not substantially different from how one would evaluate a non-genetic application, whether simple (e.g., serum cholesterol) or complex/expensive (e.g., imaging test). Some of the issues that do distinguish genetic/genomic tests from non-genetic tests include the discovery of genomic elements heretofore undiscovered and thus not understood, a far higher magnitude of complexity in test interpretation, familial issues that may, at times, supersede those of the patient, and complex ethical, legal, and social implications.

The timeframe for the review is often defined by decision-makers' needs. Principal among these needs are the time, often a few weeks to a few months, to make a decision, and the limited experience of staff to conduct the review. Regardless of the timeframe and resources, a consistent, structured and, preferably transparent, methodology is desired. The ACCE questions and structure may be helpful in guiding reviewers' initial efforts.

We suggest that perhaps a partial distinction of "rapid" versus "comprehensive" is that time (relatively short) and resources (limited) are the defining issues of a rapid review, while completeness distinguishes a comprehensive review, the consequence of which is often a considerable commitment to time and resources.

Analytic Challenges

There will be many challenges as genetic/genomic tests become even more complex, and are applied in predicting the risk of complex conditions such as heart disease or diabetes. Principal among these is the lack of adequate amounts of relevant data leading to gaps in evidence. This is a common problem impacting the evaluation of virtually all new technologies and is not unique to the evaluation of genetic tests. Second is what might be called the "gold standard" problem. Many new genetic/ genomic tests measure things that have never been measured before, or to a degree of detail not previously possible. Thus, a true reference standard may not exist.

As an example, molecular cytogenetic techniques, such as array-Comparative Genomic Hybridization (a-CGH), when applied to the evaluation of a patient with developmental delay, has much higher "resolution" than the current standard diagnostic test (microscopic analysis of banded chromosomes—a karyotype). Thus, a-CGH will detect copy number changes that are undetectable by the "gold standard" methodology it may supplant. These new findings are not always able to be unambiguously assigned to any phenotype of interest. This reflects the "open-ended" nature of some of the new methods, where the test "looks for" any abnormality, not all of which are known in advance, and for which the clinical significance is indeterminate. This contrasts with "closed" assays, which look only for specified abnormalities (12).

Additionally, the qualitative or informational nature of some patient (i.e., final) outcomes, as well as ELSI issues resulting from and associated with genetic tests, provide substantial challenges in quantifying benefits. Payne et al. have made a substantial contribution in this regard by determining, of all outcomes related to genetic services reported in the literature, which are most important to providers, patients, and families (23).

There are several situations that pose difficult challenges for those charged with assessing the value of a test in a specific clinical application. These include tests with a high level of analytic and/or conceptual complexity (e.g., multiplex testing platforms, testing for complex disorders); tests where evidence and experience are changing extremely rapidly; rare disorders where there will always be limited analytic and clinical data; and predictive testing where the phenotype of interest may not appear for many years. Given the rapid progress in testing methods, it is likely these challenges will only increase as analytics are introduced that include molecular "signatures" (e.g., expression and protein arrays), combining with a variety of clinical factors and biomarkers (multivariate analysis), and ultimately systems biomedicine (24,25) to better stratify diagnosis, prognosis, and treatment selection. It is also likely that the results of these analyses will not be directly related to the primary outcomes of clinical interest, but rather to secondary outcomes that can be linked to the primary outcomes by a chain of evidence that must also be assessed for its strength and integrity. For example, in pharmacogenomic testing for warfarin, the outcomes most frequently studied are prediction of the dose at sample INR, time to stable dosing, and time in INR target range. These are intermediate outcomes for which evidence exists that links them to the primary outcomes of interest: adverse drug events such as bleeding and clotting (see Chapter 31 in this volume for a full discussion of this issue). These challenges, and others, may prevent analysts from estimating the classic measures of test performance such as sensitivity and specificity. Rather, analysts may have to settle for measures such as diagnostic yield, false positive rate (26), or other metrics of performance, including some as yet undeveloped. New ways to model the clinical and cost effectiveness of these new tests may be needed (22).

Completeness of Evidence—When Do We Know Enough?

There is no standard answer to this question. However, Eddy (1997) captured the essence of this question when he suggested that available evidence must be sufficient to enable appropriately trained, motivated, and impartial people to draw conclusions about the magnitudes of the effects of the treatment, compared with no treatment, on all the health outcomes they consider important. If not, the technology (test) can reasonably be considered "investigational" (27). Aronson (2008) addressed this issue specifically when she stated that establishing clinical utility generally relies heavily on indirect evidence, using a causal chain of logic, inference, and linkage of various bodies of literature, from the diagnostic performance of the test to the effect on patient management and, ultimately, to the effect on health outcomes (28).

The functional answer to the question is that it depends upon the decision-makers and the context within which they make decisions, which can be quite complex and involve more issues than just "do we know enough."

For rare genetic tests, the Collaboration, Education and Test Translation (CETT) program, sponsored by the National Institutes of Health (NIH) Office of Rare Diseases (ORD), has addressed this issue by establishing a standard process of distilling current evidence, assessing utility based on that evidence, and reviewing the testing procedure to make sure it is consistent with the best evidence (29). They take this one step further by partnering with researchers in the field and requiring submission of clinical and test data to a publicly available database for at least five years. While this seems to work well for rare tests, this process is neither appropriate nor scalable for higher volume or complex testing models, given the potentially large impact on patient outcomes and cost. However, the concept of post-market data collection to increase the knowledge base is highly desirable. As such, many (including the SACGT Oversight Report), are advocating the development of such systems.

As Ramsey et al. (22) and others suggest, and Aronson implies (above), decision-analytic methods often are necessary to piece together available data to estimate the effectiveness and cost effectiveness of genetic tests. Such methods help clarify the important questions, illustrate and quantify relationships between relevant variables, and identify gaps in evidence, thereby encouraging transparent and rational decision making. Burke and Zimmern also suggest, in their discussion of optimality of services, that when budgets are constrained, costly new genomic testing services or those with limited benefits should undergo formal cost-effectiveness studies (12). Similarly so for low-cost but high-volume tests such as *CYP2C9* and *VKORC1* for warfarin dosing.

In the United States, however, the Centers for Medicare and Medicaid Services (CMS) federal agency is explicitly prohibited from basing coverage decisions for Medicare and Medicaid on cost effectiveness. Likewise, state regulations universally prohibit health insurers from using cost effectiveness as a coverage criterion but do not prohibit the use of economic analyses (e.g., cost consequences) that demonstrate cost comparisons when the effectiveness of interventions is considered equivalent (28). These limitations seem to be vulnerable to change. The crux of the issue is that any measure considered must reflect the realities of the (local) decision-making environment and that an economic measure, if chosen for evaluation, can be legally applied and provide some potential to influence thinking and decision-making that ultimately leads to more efficient yet equitable provision of health care services (30).

Summary

Table 24.1 lists and compares selected characteristics of rapid versus comprehensive reviews. Many of these decisions and challenges facing stakeholders who

Table 24.1 Comparison of selected characteristics of rapid versus comprehensive evidence-based reviews

	TYPE OF EVIDENCE-BASED REVIEW	
Characteristic	*Rapid*	*Comprehensive*
Elapsed time	Several weeks/months	One year or more
Cost (dollars)	Thousands	One hundred thousand or more
Cost (hours of time)	<200	Possibly 1,000 or more
Structure	Variable; may be targeted to specific questions	Structured analytic framework or complete set of 44 ACCE questions
Methodology	May vary in rigor depending on the reviewing group	Often well described and conscientiously followed
Topics addressed	Emerging, or highly focused on established topics	Wide-ranging, from established to emerging
ACCE components addressed	One or more, but often not all four	All four components customarily reviewed
Gaps in knowledge	May or may not be addressed	Usually a relatively complete list of gaps
Target audience	Often narrowly focused to those funding the review	Aimed at a wider general audience
Literature review	Structured, but may be limited in scope	Broader scope of sources with more formal review of included/excluded studies
Size of literature base	Usually 100 or fewer references considered	Hundreds or even thousands of references considered
Use of gray literature	Often useful, as data for emerging tests are limited	May be difficult because of the highly structured methodology
Use of modeling	Limited, although simple modeling may be applied to address targeted questions (e.g., "affordability")	Possible modeling of benefits versus harms as well as economics

must choose between these two review types may be substantially reduced, if not eliminated, if a technology assessment service specific to genetic testing becomes available. This assumes that a review process uses an accepted and transparent methodology, is credible, timely, accessible, addresses the clinically relevant questions, and is affordable. The EGAPP Stakeholders' Group is advising the EGAPP Working Group on these issues. Results from this interaction may have broad applicability to the field.

Additionally, stakeholders must bear in mind that a genetic test, if implemented, becomes part of a process that includes many parts. Thus, the technical merits of the test or assay itself are only part of the delivery of care. Ability of providers to access test results in a timely and useful format, interpret them accurately, to guide appropriate modifications to care, including patient compliance, can all impact the optimal performance of a test. Modeling and decision analysis may be useful to "put it all together," especially when there are gaps in information, as will generally be the case both for emerging as well as established genetic tests.

References

1. U.S. Preventive Services Task Force. Available at http://www.ahrq.gov/clinic/uspstfix. htm. Accessed December 29, 2008.
2. Center for Medicare & Medicaid Services (CMS). Available at http://www.cms.hhs.gov/ FACA/02_MEDCAC.asp. Accessed December 29, 2008.
3. Leeflang MMG, Deeks JJ, Gatsonis C, Bossuyt PMM; on behalf of the Cochrane Diagnostic Test Accuracy Working Group. Systematic reviews of diagnostic test accuracy. *Ann Intern Med*. December 2008;149(12):889–897.
4. UK Department of Health Genetic Testing Network (UKGTN). Available at http://www. ukgtn.nhs.uk/gtn/Home. Accessed December 29, 2008.
5. National Institutes of Health-Department of Energy (NIH-DOE) Task Force on Promoting Safe and Effective Genetic Testing in the United States. Available at http:// www.genome.gov/10001733. Accessed December 29, 2008.
6. Department of Health and Human Services (DHHS), Secretary's Advisory Committee on Genetic Testing, Enhancing the Oversight of Genetic Tests. Available at http://oba. od.nih.gov/oba/sacgt/reports/oversight_report.pdf. Accessed December 29, 2008.
7. Haddow J, Palomaki G. ACCE: a model process for evaluating data on emerging genetic tests. In: Khoury M, Little J, Burke W, editors. *Human Genome Epidemiology: A Scientific Foundation for Using Genetic Information to Improve Health and Prevent Disease*. New York: Oxford University Press; 2003:217–233.
8. Sanderson S, Zimmern R, Kroese M, et al. How can the evaluation of genetic tests be enhanced? Lessons learned from the ACCE framework and evaluating genetic tests in the United Kingdom. *Genet Med*. September 2005;7(7):495–500.
9. Márquez-Calderón S, Pérez de la Blanca EB. *Framework for the Assessment of Genetic Testing in the Andalusian Public Health System*. Sevilla: Agencia de Evaluación de Tecnologías Sanitarias de Andalucía; 2006.
10. Teutsch SM, Bradley LA, Palomaki GE, et al. The Evaluation of Genomic Applications in Practice and Prevention (EGAPP) initiative: methods of the EGAPP Working Group. *Genet Med*. January 2009;11(1):3–14.

11. Gudgeon JM, McClain MR, Palomaki GE, Williams MS. Rapid ACCE: experience with a rapid and structured approach for evaluating gene-based testing. *Genet Med.* July 2007;9(7):473–478.
12. Burke W, Ron Zimmern. Moving Beyond ACCE: An Expanded Framework for Genetic Test Evaluation. A paper for the United Kingdom Genetic Testing Network, September 2007. Available at http://www.phgfoundation.org/pages/work7.htm. Accessed December 29, 2008.
13. Recommendations from the EGAPP Working Group: testing for cytochrome P450 polymorphisms in adults with nonpsychotic depression treated with selective serotonin reuptake inhibitors. EGAPP Recommendation Statement. *Genet Med.* December 2007;9(12):819–825. Evaluation of Genomic Applications in Practice and Prevention (EGAPP) Working Group. Available at http://www.geneticsinmedicine.org/pt/re/gim/abstract.00125817-200712000-00004.htm;jsessionid=HpBJ2fZ2GMqnpWXJh7DnzpQLYJ3DKq3kyGQCmknt9GT0ZncTPJRL!1219373867!181195629!8091!-1. Accessed December 29, 2008.
14. McClain MR, Palomaki GE, Haddow JE. An Abbreviated ACCE Review of BMPR2 Mutation Testing Among Individuals Diagnosed with Familial or Idiopathic Pulmonary Arterial Hypertension. Institute for Preventive Medicine, Gray, Maine. Available at http://www.ipmms.org/PUBS/ACCE%20review.pdf. Accessed December 29, 2008.
15. McClain MR, Palomaki GE, Piper M, Haddow JE. Commissioned by American College of Medical Genetics (ACMG). A rapid ACCE review of CYP2C9 and VKORC1 allele testing to inform warfarin dosing in adults at elevated risk for thrombotic events to avoid serious bleeding. Updated August 20, 2007. See Chapter 31, A rapid ACCE review of *CYP2C9* and *VKORC1* allele testing to inform warfarin dosing in adults at elevated risk for thrombotic events to avoid serious bleeding in this volume.
16. EGAPP stakeholder's group. Available at http://www.cdc.gov/genomics/gtesting/egapp_esg.htm. Accessed December 29, 2008.
17. Williams MS. Insurance coverage for pharmacogenomic testing. *Per Med.* 2007;4:479–487.
18. Teutsch S. Issues in Adjusting the Evidence to Decision Needs. Presentation during the Institute of Medicine Workshop: Judging the Evidence: Standards for Determining Clinical Effectiveness, February 5, 2007. Available at http://www.iom.edu/Object.File/Master/40/367/Steve%20Teutsch.pdf. Accessed December 29, 2008.
19. Burke W, Zimmern RL, Kroese M. Defining purpose: a key step in genetic test evaluation. *Genet Med.* October 2007;9(10):675–681.
20. Gatsonis C, Paliwal P. Meta-analysis of diagnostic and screening test accuracy evaluations: methodologic primer. *AJR Am J Roentgenol.* August 2006;187(2):271–281.
21. Zamora J, Abraira V, Muriel A, Khan K, Coomarasamy A. Meta-DiSc: a software for meta-analysis of test accuracy data. *BMC Med Res Methodol.* July 12, 2006;6:31.
22. Ramsey SD, Veenstra DL, Garrison LP, Jr, et al. Toward evidence-based assessment for coverage and reimbursement of laboratory-based diagnostic and genetic tests. *Am J Manag Care.* April 2006;12(4):197–202.
23. Payne K, Nicholls SG, McAllister M, et al. Outcome measures for clinical genetics services: a comparison of genetics healthcare professionals and patients' views. *Health Policy.* November 2007;84(1):112–122.
24. Loscalzo J, Kohane I, Barabasi AL. Human disease classification in the postgenomic era: a complex systems approach to human pathobiology. *Mol Syst Biol.* 2007;3:124.
25. From Wikipedia, the free encyclopedia: "Systems biology." Available at http://en.wikipedia.org/wiki/Systems_biology. Accessed December 29, 2008.
26. Subramonia-Iyer S, Sanderson S, Sagoo G, et al. Array-based comparative genomic hybridization for investigating chromosomal abnormalities in patients with learning

disability: systematic review meta-analysis of diagnostic and false-positive yields. *Genet Med.* February 2007;9(2):74–79.

27. Eddy DM. Investigational treatments. How strict should we be? *JAMA.* July 16, 1997;278(3):179–185.

28. Aronson N. Assessing technology for use in health and medicine. In: Hernandez LM (Reporter), *Institute of Medicine of the National Academies. Diffusion and Use of Genomic Innovations in Health and Medicine.* Washington DC: The National Academies Press; 2008:29–33.

29. The Collaboration, Education and Test Translation (CETT) Program. Available at http://www.cettprogram.org/default.aspx. Accessed December 18, 2007.

30. Grosse SD, Wordsworth S, Payne K. Economic methods for valuing the outcomes of genetic testing: beyond cost-effectiveness analysis. *Genet Med.* September 2008;10(9):648–654.

25

Role of social and behavioral research in assessing
the utility of genetic information

Saskia C. Sanderson, Christopher H. Wade,
and Colleen M. McBride

The completion of the sequence of the human genome has led to the discovery of a
growing number of genetic variants associated with common, complex diseases and
traits. This improved understanding of the role that genetic variants play in common
health conditions is anticipated to benefit public health through several routes. First,
such research will shed light on mechanisms of disease and accelerate the development of new therapeutic interventions. Second, it will increase diagnostic precision and enable individualized therapies (e.g., pharmacogenomics). Third, and the
focus for this chapter, is that new genomic information will allow for personalized
risk prediction in ways that might motivate healthy individuals to engage in risk-
reducing behavioral changes. For the purposes of this chapter, we are considering
behavior change to include cancer screening, quitting smoking, improving diet, and
increasing physical activity.

Common, complex diseases such as heart disease, cancer, and diabetes, as well as
the precursors to these diseases such as obesity, hypertension, and hypercholesterolemia, represent a global health epidemic (1). This epidemic is attributed largely to
population trends in poor diet (e.g., calorie-dense, nutrient-deficient foods) and physical inactivity (e.g., physical environments that discourage walking). Additionally,
despite significant reductions in cigarette smoking in Western countries in the past
few decades, many people still struggle unsuccessfully to quit, and a significant proportion of adolescents and young adults worldwide continue to start smoking. There
are numerous evidence-based interventions to help individuals modify these health-
harming behaviors. However, successfully producing long-term behavior changes
and motivating individuals to avail themselves of behavior change interventions
continues to be extremely challenging (2).

Throughout this chapter, we use the term "genetic information" to refer to general information about single gene variants or personalized information based on a
genetic test result for a single gene variant. By contrast, we use the term "genomic
information" to refer to general or personalized information that considers multiple
genetic variants, gene–gene interactions or gene–environment interactions. We use

"social and behavioral research" to refer to the broad field of research concerned with applying theoretical models (e.g., Theory of Planned Behavior, Self-Regulation Theory, Protection Motivation Theory) to explain health behaviors and suggest behavior change strategies. Application of these models enables hypothesis-driven analyses of posited associations among social and psychological factors that can influence behavioral outcomes (3,4). Social and behavioral research employs a range of measures and study designs that are suitable to varying degrees to address different research questions at different stages in the research process (5,6).

Social and behavioral research has given a good deal of focus to the development and evaluation of disease risk communication approaches with the aim to motivate risk-reducing behavior changes. Social and behavioral theory suggests that the advantage of genomic information over other types of feedback (e.g., other biomarkers or behavioral risk assessments) is its highly personalized nature and its potential for greater motivational potency. Proponents of genomic information suggest that such feedback could be provided to healthy, asymptomatic individuals or populations and contribute substantially to primary prevention of common chronic diseases (7).

On the other hand, there is considerable skepticism being voiced about the potential of genomic information to motivate behavior change. Skeptics argue, for example, that the biology underlying these gene–disease risk estimates will be unclear or complex and that the low levels of risk conferred by common genetic risk variants (often ranging from 10% to 30% increased risk) for most common health conditions will result in confusion or, worse yet, create unnecessary concerns or provide false reassurances (8). However, relatively little social and behavioral research has been conducted to inform the debate about the potential utility of genomic information for motivating behavior change.

The ongoing debate raises important questions and testable hypotheses about the mechanisms through which genomic information might be more motivational than existing risk feedback approaches. For example, can genomic risk information improve upon state-of-the-art risk communications by personalizing risk in different or better ways than other risk indicators (e.g., blood pressure, cholesterol level, or family history) to motivate adoption of healthy behaviors? And can personalized genomic information inspire risk reduction above that achieved with current intervention approaches, given that the disease risk conferred by individual, common gene variants is modest? Indeed, rigorous social and behavioral research is needed to address these and other questions in order to evaluate whether and how genomic information can be translated into public health benefit through improved communication strategies and behavior change interventions.

In this chapter, we describe and critique the state of the science with respect to understanding how genetic information has been, and how genomic information might in the future be used to improve health by encouraging health behaviors that decrease chronic disease risk. To this end, we review studies in which the impact of providing genetic information has been evaluated as a means to influence behavioral outcomes. We then identify gaps in the research and recommend new conceptual and methodological directions to accelerate this field of research. Lastly, we recommend roles that social and behavioral science can play in the next generation of research to consider the translation potential of genomic information for public health benefit. We have organized the chapter to address three broad questions: Does the available evidence indicate that genetic information motivates behavior change? What research gaps can social and behavioral science fill with respect to gauging the utility of genomic information to change behavior? What future roles should social and behavioral research play in the evaluation of the utility of genomic information to improve public health?

In selecting the content for this chapter we have made the following decisions and assumptions. First, we excluded studies that explore treatment matching based on *post hoc* comparisons of the relative efficacy of pharmacological treatments by genotype (see for example References 9 and 10). These studies have not provided genetic information to individuals to influence their behaviors. Additionally, we assume it to be unlikely that genetic or genomic information will stand alone as a risk communication and behavior change strategy. Instead, we anticipate that such information will be combined with other risk factors such as gender, family history, and behavior and that these amalgamated risk assessments will be provided in the context of multicomponent complex interventions—that is, those that are "made up of various interconnecting parts" (11). Examples of complex interventions include programs to prevent heart disease and health promotion interventions directed at individuals to support dietary change (11). To limit the scope of the chapter, we have not included discussion of the opportunities and challenges of family history-based risk assessments but direct the reader to other thorough reviews on this subject (12–17). Lastly, with the rapid pace of genome-wide association studies (GWAS), we assume that clinically valid genetic or genomic "markers" of disease risk will be forthcoming and that individually these markers will have relatively modest associations with disease risk.

Does the Available Evidence Indicate that Genetic Information Motivates Behavior Change?

The best answer to this first question that can be distilled from the literature is that there is not yet enough evidence to determine whether genomic information can motivate behavior change. To date, most of the work in this area has focused on whether feedback of mutation carrier status for hereditary breast, ovarian, and colon cancers influences behaviors such as cancer screening. A less developed but emerging area of research is exploring how lifestyle behaviors such as smoking, unhealthy diet, and physical inactivity are affected by personalized genetic information relating to common health conditions that have more complex etiologies, such as heart disease and lung cancer. This latter area of research has focused primarily on genetic information as a tool to motivate smoking cessation, but is starting to move toward examining other behavior changes, such as making improvements in dietary habits. We will briefly describe the evidence regarding whether personal genomic information influences each of these behaviors (cancer screening, smoking cessation, diet, and exercise).

Cancer Screening

Several comprehensive reviews have been published summarizing the evidence regarding the impact of genetic information on behavioral outcomes such as cancer screening (9,18–20). As reviewed in these articles, early studies of the impact of genetic information on cancer screening focused primarily on the impact of providing individuals with personal test results indicating the presence or absence of *BRCA1* and *BRCA2* gene mutations. While rare, these mutations are strongly associated with increased risk (35–85% increased lifetime risk) of hereditary breast and ovarian cancer (HBOC).

The most recent review (20) included 32 studies on HBOC, hereditary nonpolyposis colorectal cancer (HNPCC), or both HBOC and HNPCC. Most of these studies were conducted in tertiary care cancer centers with populations at high family history-based risk of, or already diagnosed with, cancer. The findings from these studies generally indicate that, after receiving genetic test results, individuals informed that they are carriers of a *BRCA1/2* mutation are significantly more likely than noncarriers to have a mammogram (21,22) and to undergo appropriate ovarian cancer screening (23) in the recommended time interval. Similarly, individuals informed that they carry an HNPCC-related gene mutation are more likely than noncarriers to have a colonoscopy in the recommended time interval (24–27). In most cases, the between-group differences are accounted for by maintenance of already high rates of screening among mutation carriers, and appropriately decreased rates of screening among noncarriers (27).

These studies have generally provided participants with intensive genetic counseling sessions (an hour or more in duration) conducted by certified genetic counselors both before and after delivery of personal test results. The sample sizes for these studies have been quite small, and descriptive study designs have predominated and rarely include randomization of participants to different genetic information delivery formats.

Smoking Cessation

To date, 13 studies have explored the impact of genetic information on motivation to quit smoking or smoking cessation. Figure 25.1 illustrates that the studies spanned over a decade in their execution (1997–2008), a time of rapid developments in genetics research and of considerable change in public awareness of genetic testing. As Figure 25.1 shows, four of these studies were randomized controlled trials (RCTs) where the effects of actual genetic test result feedback on cessation outcomes were compared with a nontested control condition (28–31). All four studies tested individuals for a single genetic variant believed to be associated with increased

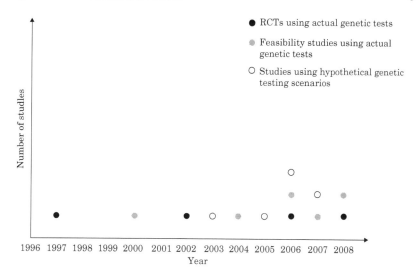

Figure 25.1 Studies examining the impact of genetic information on smoking cessation and related outcomes.

susceptibility to lung cancer and used this as the basis for their personal risk feedback, although three different genetic variants were used (*CYP2D6, GSTM1,* and *L-myc*). In addition, the studies varied greatly in their approach.

The four RCT studies differed in the intensity of interpersonal support provided to participants, which has been associated positively with successful smoking cessation. For example, Lerman and colleagues (28) provided smokers with a 60-minute comprehensive face-to-face quit smoking consultation. Two-thirds of participants were then randomized to receive an additional 10-minute motivational discussion based on either results of breath samples analyzed for carbon monoxide, or personal genetic test results based on *CYP2D6* genotyping. Those identified as "extensive metabolizers" based on *CYP2D6* testing were told that they were more susceptible to lung cancer than poor metabolizers.

McBride and colleagues (29) randomly assigned participants to either a standard-of-care self-help smoking cessation intervention alone or in combination with *GSTM1* genetic testing and telephone counseling. Smokers who underwent genetic testing for the *GSTM1* gene received an in-person explanation from a health educator about the *GSTM1* gene prior to testing and a personalized *GSTM1* genetic test result booklet along with four follow-up counseling calls from a health educator. Use of the *GSTM1* gene for feedback enabled comparisons between those who received higher than average genetic risk feedback (about one-third of the participants in this study) and those who received "not at higher" risk feedback.

Ito and colleagues (30) randomly assigned participants (a third of whom already had cancer) to either a control condition in which no smoking cessation intervention was delivered, or a genetic information condition in which participants received a blood test, a face-to-face 10-minute explanation about the effects of the *L-myc* poly-morphism on cancer risk due to smoking and an *L-myc* genetic test result by mail. Participants who had the LL genotype received a "non-risky" test result and partici-pants who had the LS/SS genotypes received a "risky" test result. The participants received no other assistance with smoking cessation.

Most recently, Sanderson and colleagues (31) provided all participating smokers with a brief 20-minute in-person smoking cessation intervention. Two-thirds of the participants were subsequently randomized to an in-person explanation of lung can-cer risk associated with the *GSTM1* genotype using a 17-page illustrated guide to *GSTM1*, smoking, and lung cancer, were offered genetic testing for *GSTM1* using a cheek-cell DNA swab, and received a copy of the *GSTM1* information booklet to take home. These participants received their *GSTM1* test results in person two weeks later, and received another copy of the *GSTM1* booklet that had their per-sonal test result marked in it. The Ito and Sanderson study designs (30, 31) had the advantage over previous trials of enabling pair-wise comparisons of cessation rates and associated cognitive and affective outcomes between a nontested control condi-tion, a "risky/higher-risk" genetic test result condition, and a "non-risky/lower-risk" genetic test result condition.

Cessation rates for these randomized trials were measured at different time points with inconsistent outcomes. Lerman and colleagues (28) found no effect of personal genetic test result feedback on smoking cessation rates at a 2-month or a 1-year fol-low-up. McBride and colleagues (29) reported a significantly greater cessation rate in the genetic testing group compared to the nontested comparison group at 6-month follow-up, but the independent contribution of genetic risk feedback could not be dis-entangled from the known positive effects of telephone counseling. Within the genetic testing group, cessation rates did not differ between those who received "high" ver-sus "not high" risk results. Ito and colleagues (30) found a significant difference in cessation rates at one of the follow-ups within the subgroup of participants who had not had cancer: 8% of the no-intervention control group and 9% of the group receiv-ing the "non-risky genotype" feedback who had quit smoking, compared to 21% of the group receiving the "risky genotype" feedback had quit smoking, at the 9-month follow-up. Sanderson and colleagues (31) found significantly higher cessation rates in the "higher-risk" group than control group at 1-week follow-up, but no difference at a 2-month follow-up (although note that this study was considerably smaller than the others and so was underpowered to detect a difference at this later follow-up).

An observational study (32) recruited smokers to participate in genetic testing for alpha-1 antitrypsin deficiency (AATD), a condition exacerbated by smoking that can lead to early-onset emphysema and hepatic impairment. This intervention was conducted almost entirely by mail with no face-to-face contact. Smokers who took the genetic test and were subsequently informed that their test results indicated they were severely AAT deficient were no more likely to have quit smoking at 3-month follow-up than those informed that their test results indicated they had normal AAT levels.

All of the above studies evaluated genetic risk information based on a single common gene variant. This risk communication approach grossly oversimplifies what is a complex etiology involving multiple genes and multiple facets of smoking topography. Hamajima and colleagues (33,34) therefore made initial steps toward using more complex genomic information, by providing smokers with information and feedback about cancer susceptibility based on three common variants in genes that code for enzymes involved in the detoxification of carcinogens: *GSTM1, GSTT1,* and *NQO1*. Participants who received personal information that they had more high-risk gene variants were more likely to quit smoking than those who received personal information that they had fewer high-risk variants (4% of those with 0 or 1 genotypes with no enzyme activity quit smoking, compared to 17% of those with 2 or 3 genotypes with no enzyme activity).

In a recent observational study (35), relatives of patients with late-stage lung cancer were offered a web-based decision aid and *GSTM1* genetic testing. Results indicated that smokers receiving "higher-risk" genetic test results were no more likely than those receiving "lower-risk" genetic test results to take up offered free smoking cessation services (35). However, participants in the study were highly motivated to quit smoking prior to seeking genetic testing.

It is difficult to draw conclusions from these studies due to the multiple methodological differences between the studies. Moreover, these studies offer little insight into the immediate emotional and cognitive responses participants may have had to genetic feedback. For several of the studies, it is not clear how individuals responded to the feedback, only that such feedback did not prompt changes in their success at quitting smoking (29, 32). More in-depth information about immediate responses to genetic feedback could be informative in guiding the development of alternative approaches to be tested in future RCTs. The studies suggest future directions for research and provide the groundwork for RCTs that, for example, compare different types of genetic information content and delivery. Such preliminary research often is essential to establish the probable active ingredients of complex interventions (11).

The "experimental analog" method that uses hypothetical genetic testing scenarios rather than real genetic testing, may have a number of advantages for early phase formative research. Currently, the use of real genetic testing is costly, and time-consuming (return of feedback can take 3 months or more). Experimental analog methods allow researchers to: anticipate reactions to genetic tests that are not yet a clinical reality, have greater experimental control than is possible in a clinical situation to reduce differences between experimental conditions, and allow researchers to assign equal numbers of participants to each genetic test result condition (36). In experimental analog studies generally, participants are asked to imagine themselves in a situation and to respond as if they had experienced the events described (37).

Four studies have used experimental analog methodology to evaluate the potential effect of genetic information on psychological antecedents of smoking cessation such as perceived personal control or ability to quit smoking and/or motivation to quit smoking (36–39). Wright and colleagues (38) asked smokers to imagine they had received a high-risk genetic test result for nicotine addiction. They found that smokers who received the high-risk test results were more likely to choose a pharmacological intervention over their own willpower than those in a control condition, a finding the authors suggested might be indicative of lower perceived personal control also referred to as "genetic fatalism." Moreover, in a second study (36), smokers who received similar genetic test results for heart disease risk were no more motivated to quit smoking than those who did not receive personal genetic test results. In the third experimental analog study (37), smokers receiving Crohn's disease risk assessments were no more motivated to quit smoking when the risk assessment included genetic information than when it was based on family history and smoking status alone. In contrast, Sanderson and Michie (39) found that smokers who imagined receiving a high-risk genetic test result for heart disease risk reported greater intention to quit smoking than those whose personal results indicated a low-risk genetic test result or a high-risk result based on an oxidative stress test. Additionally, Sanderson and Wardle (40) included questions in a mailed survey to explore whether genetic information about different diseases might be more or less motivational to smokers. When imagining receiving a high-risk test result, smokers who considered a hypothetical scenario about personal cancer genetic information did not differ in motivation to quit smoking from those who considered a scenario about personal heart disease genetic information (40).

While it is difficult to draw any firm conclusions about the impact of genetic information on smoking cessation and related outcomes, the research to date has suggested a range of methodological approaches and research questions that can be applied and explored in future research.

Diet and Exercise

Only five studies have examined the impact of genetic testing on lifestyle behaviors other than smoking, such as eating a healthy diet and exercising (41–45). As with the research on smoking cessation, the studies exploring the effects of genetic information on motivation to improve diet and to be physically active have varied in behavioral outcomes, disease or trait phenotypes tested, timing of follow-ups, and control conditions.

Two studies have explored genetic information with respect to its potential to motivate or demotivate weight loss. Harvey-Berino and colleagues (41) evaluated genetic risk information based on a variant in the beta-3-adrenergic receptor (beta-3-AR) gene, which was believed to negatively influence weight loss and energy expenditure. In this small pilot study conducted with 30 obese women who were participating in a weight loss program, women who were told they had the adverse variant showed no differences over time in reported confidence in their ability to lose weight compared to those who were told they did not have the adverse variant. Frosch and colleagues (44) used an experimental analog design in which participants were randomly assigned to review one of four hypothetical vignettes in a 2×2 experimental design (genetic versus hormone test, and increased versus average risk of obesity). There was no effect of test type on the primary outcome, intention to eat a healthy diet.

Hicken and Tucker (42) evaluated the effect of genetic risk feedback about a fictitious disease called Asch syndrome on intentions to adopt risk-reducing behaviors, including reducing dietary fat, and consuming soy products. Participants were informed that they had a positive family history for Asch syndrome, and were then randomly assigned to one of three experimental conditions: increased risk (30–40%) based on "positive family history" alone; increased risk (30–40%) based on "positive family history" plus a "positive genetic test result"; or average risk (10–12%) conferred by a "positive family history" plus a "negative genetic test result." Participants who were told that their increased risk was based on a genetic test were no more likely to report intending to engage in any of the recommended behaviors than those who were informed that their increased risk was based on family history alone.

Marteau and colleagues (43) evaluated whether genetic information negatively influenced adherence to cholesterol-lowering medication, diet, physical activity, and smoking cessation. Participants with familial hypercholesterolemia (a hereditary form of heart disease) and their relatives were randomized to one of two groups: routine clinical diagnosis or routine clinical diagnosis plus genetic testing. Results indicated no support for the supposition that genetic confirmation of the condition was associated with lowered personal control, nor were there any differences on any of the behavioral outcomes.

Roberts and colleagues (45,46) randomly assigned first-degree relatives of Alzheimer patients to receive either individualized numerical risk assessment based on family history and gender alone (control group) or an individualized numerical risk assessment based on family history, gender, and *APOE* genotype (intervention group). Control participants were given lifetime risk estimates of 18% through 29%, and intervention participants received estimates of 13% through 57%. Although participants were informed that there were no proven preventive measures for Alzheimer disease, those receiving the higher-risk ε4-positive result were significantly more likely than both ε4-negative participants (52% versus 24%) and control participants (52% versus 30%) to self-report at least one of three health behavior changes (diet, exercise, or medications and/or vitamins). Use of medications or vitamins, and adding vitamin E specifically, were the most commonly reported behavior changes amongst ε4-positive participants.

The differences between these studies limit the conclusions that can be drawn. However, as in the case of smoking cessation, genetic feedback, even for conditions such as Alzheimer disease, does not appear to demoralize individuals. However, these results also suggest that such feedback may not consistently be a motivator for behavior change.

Gaps in the Research

With only a few years having passed since the completion of the Human Genome Project, it is not surprising that there are significant gaps in public health applications of genomics and related social and behavioral research. In this section, we outline four particularly noteworthy and interrelated gaps. Attending to these gaps now could advance the social and behavioral research field significantly, and in turn improve the chances that genomic discoveries will result in public health benefit.

Few Studies Have Examined the Psychological Impact of Genomic Information About Common, Complex Diseases and Traits

Social and behavioral translational research in the genetics field has to date been heavily influenced by early discoveries of gene variants that independently confer very high lifetime risks of familial cancer syndromes. This has had several effects on the emerging research agenda to evaluate the potential of genomic information related to common complex diseases and traits. First, the majority of studies directed to common complex diseases have continued in the tradition of evaluating genetic information based on single genetic variants, rather than multiple genetic variants or genomic information. This clearly belies the genetic, behavioral, and environmental complexity of these conditions. Additionally, this means that risk messages have been based on odds ratios of 1.2–1.5, with little understanding of how these lower probabilities, as compared to Mendelian-inherited conditions, might influence the motivational potency of these messages.

Second, the Mendelian inheritance paradigm has influenced selection of psychological (cognitive, affective, and behavioral) outcomes that have been assessed. Research to understand the impact of genomic information on social and behavioral outcomes has fallen largely under the aegis of the Ethical, Legal, and Social Implications (ELSI) research, which has to date focused more on the potential harms than benefits of developments in genetics. Thus, rather than focusing on affective and behavioral outcomes suggested by behavior change theories, the research has emphasized the potential negative implications, for instance, measures of traumatic distress such as the impact of events scale. While concerns about genomics must be taken seriously, even highly predictive genetic tests (e.g., *BRCA1/2* and *APOE*) have not been shown to lead to any sustained adverse emotional outcomes such as depression and worry (45,47,48). Despite this, there remains a general perception that the potential for personal genomic information to lead to adverse outcomes is high. Consequently, research that explores possible benefits of personal genomic information, such as the potential to lead to much-needed improvements in lifestyle behaviors, has lagged behind that focusing on potential harms.

Third, concerns about the possibly exceptional nature of genomic information also have influenced selection of target populations. For example, much of the research has targeted adult patient populations already known to have or be at very high risk of disease. Asymptomatic general-public populations have rarely been the focus of this research. However, the preventive potential of genomic risk information suggests that such healthy individuals may be the most appropriate targets of this research. This also raises the thorny issue of the appropriate age to introduce the possibility of genetic testing. Expert panels have recommended against genetic testing of minors to assess susceptibility for adult-onset conditions (49) although some have argued that it is unethical to deny the option of testing when it may be beneficial (50). Given that early adoption of preventive behaviors might have the greatest benefit to health for minors (51), the question of at which age it is appropriate to start genetic testing requires greater exploration.

Methodological Rigor Has Been Limited

The research to date has had notable methodological weaknesses. Here we focus on three that raise questions about the veracity of the research findings: (i) small, highly self-selected samples; (ii) over-reliance on self-reported outcomes; and (iii) inadequately or inappropriately timed follow-up assessments.

Populations studied. Study samples have over-represented females, whites, highly educated individuals with health insurance, and those who have access to medical care. Moreover, the majority of studies have had sample sizes of less than 100, with most underpowered to evaluate behavioral outcomes. Study recruitment has been conducted in settings serving predominantly high-risk populations. Few studies have recruited from the general population or primary care settings where health promotion and disease prevention efforts typically take place. Base rates of screening behaviors and other health behaviors of high-risk populations such as those with familial cancer syndromes are not likely to be comparable to those found among general populations. Moreover, general population groups are likely to have lower genetic literacy (52) and lower awareness of the availability of genetic testing than high-risk populations. The general lack of population-based recruitment approaches that would enable comparison of characteristics of those who do and do not seek genetic testing makes it difficult to evaluate the external validity of study findings. Additionally, attrition rates are rarely described, raising additional questions about external validity. These limitations make it hard to draw inferences from the current research about the motivational potential of genomic information.

Over reliance on self-reported outcomes. Almost all of the studies to date have relied on self-reported behavioral outcomes, such as individuals telling survey interviewers after participating in an intervention whether they have or have not changed the target behavior. Few of the smoking cessation studies used gold standard biochemical validation of abstinence such as cotinine assays. Studies relying on hypothetical vignettes about genetic information necessarily have relied on self-reports of motivation and intention to change behavior. The hypothetical nature of these studies and the social desirability of reporting motivation to behave in a healthier manner might explain in part the higher rates of favorable effects of genetic information on motivation and intentions in these studies, which have less often been found in studies using actual genetic testing.

Timing of follow-up assessments. The studies to date have varied greatly in the time points at which follow-up data have been collected. Additionally, many of the studies have timed follow-up assessments at 3-, 6-, and 12-month follow-ups, the standard follow-up points for behavior change interventions. While this timing makes good conceptual sense for assessing standard behavioral outcomes (e.g., smoking cessation, improvements in physical activity), it is less well suited to tap into more immediate cognitive and motivational changes that might accompany consideration of genetic testing and interpretation of test results, and precede behavioral changes. A case in point is that the few randomized controlled trials to date included standard follow-up points for assessing behavioral outcomes. These trials not only found no benefit of genetic information for behavioral outcomes but also provided few clues for developing the next generation of genetic information for testing. Immediate and early cognitive and emotional responses to genetic information in the hours, days, and weeks following genetic testing are needed to gain insight into how they influence behavioral outcomes further downstream. The frequency of assessment also must be considered carefully so as not to encourage response bias that could result from too frequent or too closely timed assessments.

Research is Too Narrowly Focused on Perceived Risk and Fatalism

Perceived disease risk has been considered almost exclusively as the mediating cognitive mechanism through which genomic information might influence behavior. However, although people who feel threatened are somewhat more likely to take action and change their behavior than people who do not feel threatened, simply raising an individual's perception of personal risk is not always sufficient in and of itself to directly motivate behavior change (53). Other important cognitions and emotions associated with behavior include: "perceived response-efficacy" or confidence that the recommended behavior can reduce the threat (53,54), "perceived self-efficacy" or confidence in ability to change the behavior (55,56), beliefs about the causes and consequences of the threat (57), and self-esteem (58).

To date, when these other cognitions have been addressed, research questions have usually been posed in a negative frame, asking whether genetic information might induce feelings of fatalism, lack of personal control, or reduced self-efficacy. However, self-esteem (positive self-image or feelings of self-worth) could be increased by providing individuals with information indicating that their tendency to "eat in the absence of hunger" (59) is influenced by dopamine gene variants, not simply a "lack of willpower." Whether genomic information can be used to enhance positive feelings of self-worth, improve positive self-image and reduce stigma, guilt, and self-blame has yet to be explored. Clearly, the cognitive and emotional pathways through which genomic information might influence behavioral outcomes are far more complex than the impact on perceived disease risk alone.

The Social and Behavioral Research Agenda Has Not Been Guided by Consensus Priorities or Strategic Planning

There is currently no systematic planning effort underway to understand whether and how genomic information might best be applied to address public health priorities related to multifactorial, complex conditions (e.g., heart disease, type 2 diabetes, asthma, and obesity) that are influenced by multiple genetic, behavioral, and environmental factors (60). As a result, the "tail has wagged the dog," with most genomic information research focusing on the latest genetic variant to accrue sufficient evidence base for an association with a disease outcome. Study outcomes have focused on disease risk, the genetic risk variants used to indicate risk have differed between studies even when studying the same disease, and study designs and outcome measures have varied widely. Additionally, the literature is largely dominated by descriptive studies of genetic test uptake, and the cognitive and emotional responses to genetic test results measured have usually been negative, such as depression, anxiety, worry, and fatalism.

Roles for Social and Behavioral Research

Based on the gaps outlined above, we recommend four roles for future social and behavioral research to increase understanding of the utility of genomic information to improve public health through behavior change means.

ROLE 1: *Building a bridge between basic science, medicine, and public health*

Dr. Elias Zerhouni, former Director of the NIH, suggests that we are in a time of "revolutionary and rapid changes in science" (http://nihrecord.od.nih.gov/news-letters/03_16_2004/story01.htm) and that currently researchers are not organized optimally for tackling the complexity and scale of biological problems. He suggests that "multidisciplinary research teams of the future" are needed to address contemporary health problems. Public health genomics is one such new field concerned with the responsible and effective translation of genome-based knowledge and technologies for the benefit of population health (61). Researchers from all backgrounds will increasingly need to be prepared and able to talk across disciplinary boundaries, and to arrive at mutual understandings of methodologies and conceptual models that can be used to translate basic science most effectively into public health benefit. More programs in public health genomics such as the flagship interdepartmental undergraduate and graduate training programs at the University of Michigan (see http://www.sph.umich.edu/genetics/) and the University of Washington (see http://depts.washington.edu/phgen) are needed to train scientists in translation and the conduct of high-quality research into the potential utility of genomic information.

Additionally, it will be essential that the genetic literacy of medical students and the frontline primary care providers of the future be improved far beyond what it is today. It may also be useful for there to be a paradigm shift within the genetic counseling training programs to incorporate preventive health education and behavior change counseling.

ROLE 2: Expanding research emphasis to include both distal disease phenotypes and more proximal intermediate phenotypes

Evaluation of the utility of genetic information has almost completely focused on information based on genetic variations associated with distal disease phenotypes such as heart disease and cancer. However, genetic variants are now starting to be associated with more proximal intermediate phenotypes such as obesity (62), satiety (63), airway reactivity (64), and physiological response to exercise (65). Each of these traits or biological processes plays a role in not one but many diseases. Social and behavioral research approaches are needed to evaluate the utility of providing individuals with personal genomic information about these emerging intermediate phenotypes. This research will require a focus not only on the potential cognitive, affective, and behavioral outcomes of providing individuals with this information, but also how to communicate the information effectively and appropriately for the general population as well as different subgroups. Whether personal genomic information about variants associated with intermediate phenotypes, such as appetite or responses to physical activity, is more, less, or equally motivating compared to personal genomic information about heart disease or cancer risk is an important question that also remains to be answered.

ROLE 3: Priority setting and planning horizon-scanning research agendas that consider future technologies

The rapid progression and decreasing cost of genetic technologies and GWAS have had a profound effect on the pace at which the genetic risk factors for diseases and traits are being identified (66). Computational advances will enable increasingly comprehensive and accurate "genomic risk portraits" of individuals based on proteomic, transcriptomic, lifestyles, and environmental factors. The resultant risk algorithms and personal risk messages will be much more complex than those based on traditional risk factors or single genetic variants in isolation.

Social and behavioral research provides useful theoretical frameworks for advancing hypothesis-driven research to understand how these increasing levels of personalization might best be communicated to target audiences, how such information might influence behavioral outcomes, and how this information might improve upon current public health interventions. A few of the research questions that need to be addressed include: Can genomic information be integrated with existing widely available risk prediction and communication tools (e.g., www.yourdiseaserisk. harvard.edu) to increase their efficacy for motivating behavior change? Can individuals make sense of these complex risk profiles? How should messages be framed when information appears to contradict itself, for example, when an individual has both risk-reducing and risk-conferring gene variants for the same disease or trait? Given the wide range of research questions that will be generated by these new and emerging technologies, priority setting based on what has been learned previously about the dissemination of technological innovations related to public health will be essential.

New planning mechanisms need to be developed to begin these conversations. The CDC's Office of Public Health Genomics has played a critical role to date in increasing attention to these important issues. The American Public Health Association (APHA) and the Society of Behavioral Medicine (SBM) are examples of additional leading organizations that also could play a central role in developing forums for setting priorities for social and behavioral research on the utility of genomic information. Integrating genomics into the scientific programs and publications of these influential organizations will be useful in directing research to understand the potential translation of genomic information into public health benefit.

ROLE 4: *Implementing appropriately phased programs of applied research*

The increasing recognition of the complex biopsychosocial nature of health means that interventions designed to improve health will likely increase in complexity as well. Social and behavioral research into changing behavior suggests that complex, multicomponent, sustained interventions are most successful in promoting enduring behavior change. However, arriving at the optimal combinations of intervention components that are efficacious, cost-effective and not overly burdensome for individuals will continue to require a good deal of research. Campbell and colleagues (11,67) speak to this eloquently in calling for a more systematic, phased approach to research to understand and shape improvements in complex health promotion interventions. As Campbell and others show, there are several phases to the research process that can be conducted linearly or simultaneously. Figure 25.2 illustrates that this type of phased framework is useful in guiding structured research programs to assess how best to integrate new genomic discoveries into existing public health interventions.

As shown in Figure 25.2, the first step, the Preclinical or Theory Phase (11, 67), is to explore relevant models and theories to suggest mechanisms by which genomic information might have beneficial impact on motivation, emotions, cognitions, and ultimately behavior change. For example, Marteau and Weinman (68) adapted Leventhal's common sense model of the self-regulation of health and illness to suggest hypotheses about whether and how individual beliefs about disease causation may influence psychological responses to genomic information (68).

In the Phase I "Modeling" step, interviews and surveys, as well as focus groups, experimental analog (hypothetical scenarios) studies, case studies, and observational studies are conducted to define the components of the intervention and to provide evidence that the underlying mechanisms through which genomic information exerts its effects, as well as how it interacts with other components of the intervention, can be predicted. It is important to highlight that this Phase I research is viewed not as being conducted in isolation, but rather, where appropriate, as part of comprehensive research programs in which the results are directly used to inform the design of subsequent studies using actual genetic tests.

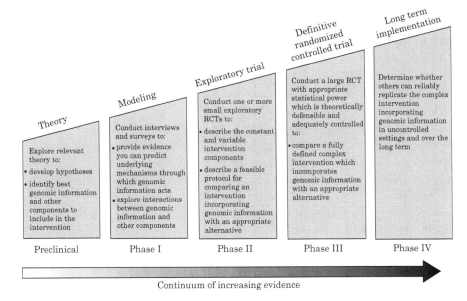

Figure 25.2 Adaptation of the MRC framework (11) to illustrate the sequential phases of developing complex interventions that incorporate genomic information to improve health.

In Phase II, the information gathered in Phase I is used to develop the optimum intervention and study design, and one or more small exploratory RCTs are conducted to describe a feasible protocol for comparing an intervention incorporating genomic information using real genetic testing with an appropriate alternative. When is it appropriate to move from hypothetical scenario methods to studies that use actual genetic testing and feedback of real personal genomic information? The planning strategies laid out (see Role 3 above) should be helpful in addressing this critical question. Additionally, Phase II trials can be useful as an intermediate step between Phase I hypothetical studies and large fully powered Phase III trials. Phase II trials are useful in the development and evaluation of different delivery formats, appropriate genomic feedback information materials, and determining appropriate comparison conditions. A Phase II methodological approach also enables increased methodological rigor allowing greater internal validity to consider and refine best practices for delivering interventions and considering the individual contributions of components of these interventions.

In Phase III, a theoretically defensible and adequately controlled RCT with appropriate statistical power is conducted comparing a fully defined complex intervention that incorporates a genomic information component with an appropriate alternative. Large Phase III trials might be considered once enough Phase I and II data demonstrate the safety and optimal interventions on which to base a large-scale trial.

Finally, the purpose of Phase IV is to examine the implementation of the intervention into practice, paying particular attention to the rate of uptake, the stability of the intervention, any broadening of subject groups, and the possible existence of adverse effects (11, 67). As suggested more generally by Campbell and colleagues, implementing appropriately phased programs of applied research in this way will give researchers and funding bodies reasonable confidence that appropriately designed and relevant studies are being proposed, which examine the potential utility of genomic information as part of complex interventions to improve health (11).

Concluding Comment: What *Is* the Role of Social and Behavioral Research in Assessing Utility of Genetic Information?

In this chapter, we have provided an overview of the social and behavioral research that has been conducted to date assessing the potential utility of genetic information, pointed out some of the gaps in this research, and made some recommendations about how to move the field forward. We suggest that social and behavioral science has multiple roles to play in assessing the utility of genetic information, including research agenda setting, collaborating, training, and matching appropriate methodologies and conceptual models to important questions. All these activities are essential and needed now if we are to begin to amass the empirical evidence needed to inform whether and how genomics can be translated and incorporated into multicomponent behavior change interventions to produce benefit for the health of all.

Note: No statement in this article should be construed as an official position of the National Human Genome Research Institute, NIH, or the Department of Health and Human Services.

References

1. Strong K, Mathers C, Epping-Jordan J, Beaglehole R. Preventing chronic disease: a priority for global health. *Int J Epidemiol.* 2006;35:492–494.
2. Smith TW, Orleans CT, Jenkins CD. Prevention and health promotion: decades of progress, new challenges, and an emerging agenda. *Health Psychol.* 2004;23:126–131.
3. Conner M, Norman P. *Predicting Health Behaviour: Research and Practice with Social Cognition Models*, 1 ed. Buckingham: Open University Press; 1999.
4. Glanz K, Rimer BK, Lewis FM. *Health Behavior and Health Education: Theory, Research and Practice*, 3 ed. San Francisco: John Wiley & Sons; 2002.
5. Streiner DL, Norman GR. *Health Measurement Scales: A Practical Guide to Their Development and Use*, 2 ed. New York: Oxford University Press; 1995.
6. Stone AA, Turkkan JS, Bachrach CA, Jobe JB, Kurtzman HS, Cain VS. *The Science of Self-Report: Implications for Research and Practice*, 1 ed. Mahwah: Lawrence Erlbaum Associates; 2000.
7. McCabe LL, McCabe ER. Genetic screening: carriers and affected individuals. *Annu Rev Genomics Hum Genet.* 2004;5:57–69.
8. Carlsten C, Burke W. Potential for genetics to promote public health: genetics research on smoking suggests caution about expectations. *JAMA.* 2006;296:2480–2482.
9. Lerman C, Croyle RT, Tercyak KP, Hamann H. Genetic testing: psychological aspects and implications. *J Consult Clin Psychol.* 2002;70:784–797.

10. Berrettini WH, Lerman CE. Pharmacotherapy and pharmacogenetics of nicotine dependence. *Am J Psychiatry.* 2005;162:1441–1451.

11. Campbell M, Fitzpatrick R, Haines A, et al. Framework for design and evaluation of complex interventions to improve health. *BMJ.* 2000;321:694–696.

12. Burke W, Fesinmeyer M, Reed K, Hampson L, Carlsten C. Family history as a predictor of asthma risk. *Am J Prev Med.* 2003;24:160–169.

13. Bowen DJ, Ludman E, Press N, Vu T, Burke W. Achieving utility with family history: colorectal cancer risk. *Am J Prev Med.* 2003;24:177–182.

14. Guttmacher AE, Collins FS, Carmona RH. The family history—more important than ever. *N Engl J Med.* 2004;351:2333–2336.

15. Matakidou A, Eisen T, Houlston RS. Systematic review of the relationship between family history and lung cancer risk. *Br J Cancer.* 2005;93:825–833.

16. Butterworth AS, Higgins JP, Pharoah P. Relative and absolute risk of colorectal cancer for individuals with a family history: a meta-analysis. *Eur J Cancer.* 2006;42:216–227.

17. Valdez R, Greenlund KJ, Khoury MJ, Yoon PW. Is family history a useful tool for detecting children at risk for diabetes and cardiovascular diseases? A public health perspective. *Pediatrics.* 2007;120(Suppl 2):S78–S86.

18. Marteau TM, Lerman C. Genetic risk and behavioural change. *BMJ.* 2001; 322:1056–1059.

19. Lerman C, Shields AE. Genetic testing for cancer susceptibility: the promise and the pitfalls. *Nat Rev Cancer.* 2004;4:235–241.

20. Beery TA, Williams JK. Risk reduction and health promotion behaviors following genetic testing for adult-onset disorders. *Genet Test.* 2007;11:111–123.

21. Watson M, Foster C, Eeles R, et al. Psychosocial impact of breast/ovarian (BRCA1/2) cancer-predictive genetic testing in a UK multi-centre clinical cohort. *Br J Cancer.* 2004;91:1787–1794.

22. Kinney AY, Simonsen SE, Baty BJ, et al. Risk reduction behaviors and provider communication following genetic counseling and BRCA1 mutation testing in an African American kindred. *J Genet Couns.* 2006;15:293–305.

23. Lynch HT, Snyder C, Lynch JF, et al. Patient responses to the disclosure of BRCA mutation tests in hereditary breast-ovarian cancer families. *Cancer Genet Cytogenet.* 2006;165:91–97.

24. Halbert CH, Lynch H, Lynch J, et al. Colon cancer screening practices following genetic testing for hereditary nonpolyposis colon cancer (HNPCC) mutations. *Arch Intern Med.* 2004;164:1881–1887.

25. Hadley DW, Jenkins JF, Dimond E, de CM, Kirsch I, Palmer CG. Colon cancer screening practices after genetic counseling and testing for hereditary nonpolyposis colorectal cancer. *J Clin Oncol.* 2004;22:39–44.

26. Claes E, Denayer L, Evers-Kiebooms G, et al. Predictive testing for hereditary nonpolyposis colorectal cancer: subjective perception regarding colorectal and endometrial cancer, distress, and health-related behavior at one year post-test. *Genet Test.* 2005;9:54–65.

27. Collins V, Meiser B, Gaff C, St John DJ, Halliday J. Screening and preventive behaviors one year after predictive genetic testing for hereditary nonpolyposis colorectal carcinoma. *Cancer.* 2005;104:273–281.

28. Lerman C, Gold K, Audrain J, et al. Incorporating biomarkers of exposure and genetic susceptibility into smoking cessation treatment: effects on smoking-related cognitions, emotions, and behavior change. *Health Psychol.* 1997;16:87–99.

29. McBride CM, Bepler G, Lipkus IM, et al. Incorporating genetic susceptibility feedback into a smoking cessation program for African-American smokers with low income. *Cancer Epidemiol Biomarkers Prev.* 2002;11:521–528.

30. Ito H, Matsuo K, Wakai K, et al. An intervention study of smoking cessation with feedback on genetic cancer susceptibility in Japan. *Prev Med.* 2006;42:102–108.
31. Sanderson SC, Humphries SE, Hubbart C, Hughes E, Jarvis MJ, Wardle J. Psychological and behavioural impact of genetic testing smokers for lung cancer risk: a phase II exploratory trial. *J Health Psychol.* 2008;13:481–494.
32. Carpenter MJ, Strange C, Jones Y, et al. Does genetic testing result in behavioral health change? Changes in smoking behavior following testing for alpha-1 antitrypsin deficiency. *Ann Behav Med.* 2007;33:22–28.
33. Hamajima N, Atsuta Y, Goto Y, Ito H. A pilot study on genotype announcement to induce smoking cessation by Japanese smokers. *Asian Pac J Cancer Prev.* 2004;5:409–413.
34. Hamajima N, Suzuki K, Ito Y, Kondo T. Genotype announcement to Japanese smokers who attended a health checkup examination. *J Epidemiol.* 2006;16:45–47.
35. Sanderson SC, O'Neill SC, White DB, et al. Responses to online *GSTM1* genetic test results amongst smokers related to patients with lung cancer: a pilot study. . *Cancer Epidemiol Biomarkers Prev.* 2009;18:1953–1961.
36. Wright AJ, French DP, Weinman J, Marteau TM. Can genetic risk information enhance motivation for smoking cessation? An analogue study. *Health Psychol.* 2006;25:740–752.
37. Wright AJ, Takeichi C, Whitwell SC, Hankins M, Marteau TM. The impact of genetic testing for Crohn's disease, risk magnitude and graphical format on motivation to stop smoking: an experimental analogue study. *Clin Genet.* 2008;73:306–314.
38. Wright AJ, Weinman J, Marteau TM. The impact of learning of a genetic predisposition to nicotine dependence: an analogue study. *Tob Control.* 2003;12:237–230.
39. Sanderson SC, Michie S. Genetic testing for heart disease susceptibility: potential impact on motivation to quit smoking. *Clin Genet.* 2007;71:501–510.
40. Sanderson SC, Wardle J. Will genetic testing for complex diseases increase motivation to quit smoking? Anticipated reactions in a survey of smokers. *Health Educ Behav.* 2005;32:640–653.
41. Harvey-Berino J, Gold EC, West DS, et al. Does genetic testing for obesity influence confidence in the ability to lose weight? A pilot investigation. *J Am Diet Assoc.* 2001;101:1351–1353.
42. Hicken BL, Tucker D. Impact of genetic risk feedback: perceived risk and motivation for health protective behaviours. *Psychol Health Med.* 2002;7:25–36.
43. Marteau T, Senior V, Humphries SE, et al. Psychological impact of genetic testing for familial hypercholesterolemia within a previously aware population: a randomized controlled trial. *Am J Med Genet A.* 2004;128A:285–293.
44. Frosch DL, Mello P, Lerman C. Behavioral consequences of testing for obesity risk. *Cancer Epidemiol Biomarkers Prev.* 2005;14:1485–1489.
45. Roberts JS, Cupples LA, Relkin NR, Whitehouse PJ, Green RC. Genetic risk assessment for adult children of people with Alzheimer's disease: the Risk Evaluation and Education for Alzheimer's Disease (REVEAL) study. *J Geriatr Psychiatry Neurol.* 2005;18:250–255.
46. Chao S, Roberts JS, Marteau TM, Silliman R, Cupples LA, Green RC. Health behavior changes after genetic risk assessment for Alzheimer disease: the REVEAL Study. *Alzheimer Dis Assoc Disord.* 2008;22:94–97.
47. Meiser B, Dunn S. Psychological effect of genetic testing for Huntington's disease: an update of the literature. *West J Med.* 2001;174:336–340.
48. Meiser B. Psychological impact of genetic testing for cancer susceptibility: an update of the literature. *Psychooncology.* 2005;14:1060–1074.
49. Borry P, Stultiens L, Nys H, Cassiman JJ, Dierickx K. Presymptomatic and predictive genetic testing in minors: a systematic review of guidelines and position papers. *Clin Genet.* 2006;70:374–381.

50. Rhodes R. Why test children for adult-onset genetic diseases? *Mt Sinai J Med.* 2006; 73:609–616.

51. Segal ME, Sankar P, Reed DR. Research issues in genetic testing of adolescents for obesity. *Nutr Rev.* 2004;62:307–320.

52. Kutner M, Greenberg E, Jin Y, Paulsen C. *The Health Literacy of America's Adults: Results from the 2003 National Assessment of Adult Literacy* (NCES 2006–483). US Department of Education, Washington DC: National Center for Education Statistics; 2006.

53. Rogers RW. Cognitive and physiological processes in fear appeals and attitude change: a revised theory of protection motivation. In: Cacioppo JT, Petty RE, editors. *Social Psychophysiology: A Sourcebook.* New York: Guilford Press; 1983:153–176.

54. Witte K, Allen M. A meta-analysis of fear appeals: implications for effective public health campaigns. *Health Educ Behav.* 2000;27:591–615.

55. Bandura A. Self-efficacy: toward a unifying theory of behavioral change. *Psychol Rev.* 1977;84:191–215.

56. Ajzen I. The theory of planned behavior. *Organ Behav Hum Decis Process.* 1991; 50:179–211.

57. Leventhal H, Brissette I, Leventhal EA. The common-sense model of self-regulation of health and illness. In: Katouzian HD, Cameron LD, Leventhal H, editors. *The Self-Regulation of Health and Illness Behaviour.* Routledge; 2003:42–65.

58. Muhlenkamp AF, Sayles JA. Self-esteem, social support, and positive health practices. *Nurs Res.* 1986;35:334–338.

59. Faith MS, Berkowitz RI, Stallings VA, Kerns J, Storey M, Stunkard AJ. Eating in the absence of hunger: a genetic marker for childhood obesity in prepubertal boys? *Obesity (Silver Spring).* 2006;14:131–138.

60. McBride CM, Brody LC. Point: genetic risk feedback for common disease time to test the waters. *Cancer Epidemiol Biomarkers Prev.* 2007;16:1724–1726.

61. Burke W, Khoury MJ, Stewart A, Zimmern RL. The path from genome-based research to population health: development of an international public health genomics network. *Genet Med.* 2006;8:451–458.

62. Frayling TM, Timpson NJ, Weedon MN, et al. A common variant in the FTO gene is associated with body mass index and predisposes to childhood and adult obesity. *Science.* 2007;316:889–894.

63. Rosado EL, Bressan J, Martins MF, Cecon PR, Martinez JA. Polymorphism in the PPARgamma2 and beta2-adrenergic genes and diet lipid effects on body composition, energy expenditure and eating behavior of obese women. *Appetite.* 2007;49:635–643.

64. Chae SC, Li CS, Kim KM, et al. Identification of polymorphisms in human interleukin-27 and their association with asthma in a Korean population. *J Hum Genet.* 2007;52:355–361.

65. Ingelsson E, Larson MG, Vasan RS, et al. Heritability, linkage, and genetic associations of exercise treadmill test responses. *Circulation.* 2007;115:2917–2924.

66. Revill P. Genomics of common diseases. *Drug News Perspect.* 2007;20:475–479.

67. Campbell NC, Murray E, Darbyshire J, et al. Designing and evaluating complex interventions to improve health care. *BMJ.* 2007;334:455–459.

68. Marteau TM, Weinman J. Self-regulation and the behavioural response to DNA risk information: a theoretical analysis and framework for future research. *Soc Sci Med.* 2006;62:1360–1368.

26

Assessing the evidence for clinical utility in newborn screening

Scott D. Grosse

The first newborn screening programs to use dried blood spots collected on filter paper cards and sent to biochemical screening laboratories to screen for phenylketonuria (PKU) began in the United States in 1962 (1). Most screening programs before the early 2000s screened for only a handful of disorders, chiefly PKU and congenital hypothyroidism (CH). In the United States, most screening panels at the time also included galactosemia and hemoglobinopathies (2), but these were rarely included in other countries (3). In recent years, programs in many countries have used tandem mass spectrometry (MS/MS) to screen for a number of rare metabolic disorders (2,4).

This chapter outlines key methodological issues in collecting and analyzing data on outcomes in individuals with genetic disorders that are candidates for inclusion in screening panels and reviews the relevant literature for two disorders that have relatively abundant evidence. One disorder is medium-chain acyl-CoA dehydrogenase deficiency (MCADD), which is a fatty acid oxidation disorder that is the most common of the new disorders detected by mass-throughput MS/MS technology (5). MCADD has been the "poster child" for expanded newborn screening. The other disorder is cystic fibrosis (CF), which is also increasingly being added to screening panels (6).

Sources of Evidence on Clinical Utility of Newborn Screening

The clinical utility of a screening test is commonly defined as the balance of benefits and harms in terms of health and psychosocial outcomes (7). Psychosocial issues include potential harms of false-positive or carrier screening results on anxiety, misunderstanding, and parent-child bonding (8,9). Leaving these issues aside, the effect of newborn screening on health status for a given disorder can be assessed by comparing outcomes observed among cohorts of individuals born with a given disorder, some of whom received newborn screening and some of whom did not. Potential sources of data are randomized trials and observational cohort studies, with most available data coming from observational data. For the latter, challenges lie in ensuring that both cases and outcomes are reliably ascertained, particularly in unscreened cohorts. These challenges, a number of which are reviewed in this section, are not unique to genetic disorders.

Randomized controlled trials (RCTs), which are the most reliable source of evidence for evaluating effectiveness (10), have been conducted for only one newborn screening test, cystic fibrosis, and those trials involved small numbers of cases (11,12). An RCT of screening for less common metabolic disorders would require millions of infants to be enrolled, which is not practical even if ethically tolerable (13). Also, the close monitoring of patients in RCT can lessen the external validity or generalizability of results to individuals receiving care in the community (14).

Observational data are challenging to analyze because there are multiple potential sources of bias that need to be considered. In particular, unscreened cohorts of individuals identified with a genetic disorder are not necessarily equivalent to screened cohorts because of underascertainment. Underascertainment can have two opposite effects. First, disorders that often go undiagnosed because certain individuals are either asymptomatic or have only mild signs and symptoms can result in relatively severely affected individuals being overrepresented among those who are clinically detected relative to the population of those with the disorder. If this is the case, the frequency of poor outcomes among those clinically detected with the disorder could be overstated. On the other hand, if affected individuals who have not been clinically diagnosed experience sudden death, perhaps during an infectious episode, the death might be attributed to an infectious agent or to unknown cause, thereby leading to an underestimation of the risk of death due to the disorder. One way to adjust for the first type of bias is to examine the differences in the distributions of genetic variants associated with differences in phenotypes between screened and unscreened cohorts. This presumes that genotype–phenotype associations are already established.

A potential source of unbiased estimates of outcomes in unscreened cohorts is the retrospective analysis of stored dried blood spot specimens collected by newborn screening programs that did not screen for the disorder of interest at the time the specimens were collected (15). Such specimens need to be linked to databases containing either information on outcomes or information permitting families to be contacted to obtain those data. This type of method is particularly valuable for investigating the frequency of sudden death in the absence of diagnosis for those disorders for which the analytes are sufficiently stable for retrospective testing to be reliably done. Also, screening randomly selected specimens for rare disorders, for example, prevalence of 1 in 20,000 births would require testing of a very large number of specimens in order to detect more than a handful of cases. Furthermore, certain disorders are difficult to reliably identify with simple tests, and confirmation by genotyping can be very expensive if feasible. If the primary endpoint for a disorder is mortality, a less expensive alternative is to link stored blood spot specimens with infant and child death records and test only those specimens for the disorder, along with a matched sample of control specimens. Ideally, specimens should be retrieved for all children who died in infancy or early childhood, since deaths caused by a disorder might be incorrectly attributed to infectious or other causes.

An excellent example of a retrospective screening study is one that analyzed 100,239 stored dried blood spot specimens collected in Sweden prior to the initiation of screening for CH and followed up with families to confirm diagnoses and assess outcomes (16). Alm et al. linked 32 specimens positive for CH by thyroid stimulating hormone (TSH) screening to children's records, and 31 of these children could be tracked at 5 years of age. Medical records revealed that 15 of the children had been clinically diagnosed with CH, and an additional 7 children were found by the investigators to have undiagnosed hypothyroidism. The Griffiths Mental Development Scales were administered to 26 of the 31 children. Two of 14 (14%) children who had been clinically detected with CH had a developmental quotient (DQ), equivalent to IQ, of < 70, indicative of developmental delay and probable intellectual disability. No child with untreated CH was found to have low overall cognitive test scores, although statistically significant reductions on specific test scales were observed even among that group.

Many studies report improved outcomes in screened cohorts using historical cohorts as comparison groups, but it is often difficult to distinguish the effects of screening from that of improved treatments. The "natural history" of a disorder is the course of disease in the absence of treatment. Disease outcomes often improve over time as a result of changes in clinical awareness and diagnostic and therapeutic practices. Consequently, estimates based on historical cohorts born prior to the introduction of screening and effective treatment are likely to overstate the benefits of early identification (17,18). For example, U.S. adults for whom PKU was not detected at birth by newborn screening but who were put on a low phenylalanine diet beginning in the first several years of life mostly did not experience severe disability as adults, although they did experience some degree of disability (17,19). Comparisons from different geographic areas are likewise subject to bias if the availability of screening is correlated with the clinical awareness and management of a disorder (18).

Another common challenge to the identification of the effectiveness of screening is a lack of long-term follow-up for both screened and unscreened cohorts. Few long-term follow-up studies of screened cohorts have been reported, with the exceptions of PKU, CH, and CF. Cognitive testing is unreliable in infants and toddlers, and hence studies with follow-up of 1 or 2 years after birth (20) are difficult to interpret. The best-studied fatty acid oxidation disorder included in expanded screening panels, MCADD, has only had cognitive outcomes tracked up to 4 years of age (21).

Evidence on the Clinical Utility of Screening: Case Studies

Cystic Fibrosis

Cystic fibrosis is an autosomal recessive disorder affecting chiefly the lungs and the gastrointestinal tract that is caused by mutations in the *CFTR* gene (OMIM 602421).

A single common mutation, ΔF508, accounts for two-thirds of all CF alleles world-wide (22). Approximately 15–20% of newborns with CF develop meconium ileus (MI), an intestinal obstruction present at birth that generally requires surgery to correct. The most common presenting symptoms among infants with CF but without MI are respiratory (recurrent cough, wheezing) and gastrointestinal, including loose stools and failure to thrive (23). Because symptoms are nonspecific, it is common for a diagnosis of CF not to be reached until after an infant is 12 months of age, and after multiple work-ups (24). Growth failure is secondary to maldigestion caused by insufficiency of pancreatic enzymes among most children with CF. As children age, growth retardation, chronic cough, lung infections, and decreased lung function become increasingly common. Spirometry is the method used to measure lung function, with the standard metric being forced expiratory volume in 1 second, or FEV_1 as a percentage of predicted values based on height and age. However, FEV_1 cannot be reliably measured in children less than 6 years of age, and it is not a sensitive measure of early-stage lung disease in children, reducing its utility as an outcome measure for evaluating CF newborn screening (25). Mortality in CF generally is associated with chronic obstructive pulmonary disease, with respiratory failure being the primary cause of death in more than 90% of people with CF (26).

A relative abundance of data exists to evaluate the clinical utility of newborn screening for CF, including two randomized trials in Wisconsin and England, four cohort studies with data on both screened and unscreened cohorts, and several analyses of two national patient registries in the United States and the United Kingdom (6,27). Summaries of findings from the two trials and two cohort studies follow, along with registry analyses. Because the focus is on data sources and methods of analysis to control for bias, results are presented study by study rather than by outcome. Findings relating to nutritional status and growth (12), which have consistently favored screened cohorts (6,27), are not discussed.

Randomized trials. The Wisconsin CF Neonatal Screening Project randomly assigned neonates born in Wisconsin during 1985–1994 to either a screened or control group (12). CF screening was performed for all children, but positive results were reported only to families in the screened group. Positive results were released to families in the control group if parents requested the results or when the child reached 4 years of age. Subjects with a diagnosis of CF were recruited into a protocol with follow-up every 6 weeks during the first year of life and every 3 months through 17 years of age. All children received care at one of two centers. Despite randomization, significantly more subjects with no ΔF508 allele (p <0.001) were in the control group (12). The Wisconsin study found significantly better growth status among those in the screened group (12), but no significant difference in either lung function (spirometry) or chest radiography, which is a more sensitive measure of lung disease (25). Endpoints not originally targeted but assessed in response to suggestions from experts (28) were health-related quality of life (no difference; 29) and cognitive ability (a significant difference among the subset of children with a vitamin E deficiency during infancy; 30). The Wisconsin study was not powered to evaluate mortality as an endpoint (28). Perhaps because of the close follow-up provided in the RCT, no deaths prior to 10 years of age were observed in either group among those without MI, unlike in the general pediatric population with CF (31).

In the United Kingdom, all neonates born in Wales and the West Midlands during 1985–1989 were randomly allocated to undergo or not undergo CF screening on an alternate-week basis (11). Because no screening was performed for those in the control group, an unknown number of undiagnosed cases of CF were not ascertained and no unbiased comparison of clinical outcomes could be undertaken; no differences in lung function were observed (11). Investigators subsequently reviewed registry and death certificate data to identify CF-related deaths among children in the unscreened group (32). No early deaths were reported among 78 children without MI in the screened group compared with four CF-related deaths before 5 years of age among 71 children without MI in the unscreened cohort (5.6 per 100) ($p < .05$). Two of the four deaths occurred among children who had received a clinical diagnosis of CF by 7 weeks of age based on the development of symptoms, and it was not clear whether the deaths would have been averted by screening (32).

Cohort studies. A historical cohort study in Australia compared 57 children with CF without MI who were born in New South Wales during the 3 years before July 1981, before screening was available, and 60 born during July 1981 to July 1984, when screening was available (33). All analyses were conducted on an intent-to-treat basis, with children included in the screened cohort if they were born while screening was offered, including three children not detected through screening. All subjects were followed at a single clinic. Significant differences in favor of the screened cohort were observed in hospitalizations during the first 2 years of life, in height at ages 1 and 5 years, in lung function at ages 5, 10, and 15 years, in chest radiographs at age 15 years, and in survival at age 10 years (33–35). The investigators acknowledged changes in treatment introduced during 1981–1983 could potentially have biased outcomes in favor of the screened cohort (34). However, no differences in outcomes were reported among children with CF and MI. Also, most of the differences in the Australian study have been confirmed by subsequent studies, with the exception of the lung function findings (6).

A concurrent geographical cohort study from northern France compared children with CF born during 1989–1998 in Brittany, which screened newborns for CF, with a comparison group of newborns in a neighboring region, Loire-Atlantique, which did not implement screening for CF and was said to have had comparable CF care (36). Standardized follow-up and therapeutic management was provided for patients in both regions who received a diagnosis of CF. Differential ascertainment did not appear to be a major problem, because the same birth prevalence of CF was observed in both areas. False-negative screening results ($n = 5$) were excluded by the investigators from the screened cohort, which is a potential source of bias and a weakness of the study design. Significant differences in favor of the screened cohort were reported for hospitalizations, height at ages 1, 3, and 5 years, chest radiographs and clinical scores, and mortality, although no differences were observed in lung function among the limited subset of individuals with spirometry measures (36). The investigators reported three CF-related deaths among 36 children without MI born in Loire-Atlantique (8.3 per 100), and no deaths among 77 children without MI born in Brittany ($p < .05$).

Patient registries. Three analyses (two published and one unpublished) of U.S. data from the Cystic Fibrosis Foundation National Patient Registry (CFFPR) reported evidence of improved lung function, although the first one in particular had biased case ascertainment. Wang et al. analyzed children at least 6 years of age in 1996 who were born during 1987–1990 and were diagnosed with CF by 36 months of age or the end of 1990, whichever came sooner (37). They classified CF cases without MI into four categories: early asymptomatic diagnosis (EAD), early symptomatic diagnosis (ESD), later asymptomatic diagnosis (LAD), and later symptomatic diagnosis (LSD), each on the basis of two dichotomous variables: age of diagnosis before or after 6 weeks of age and the presence of clinical signs and symptoms at the time of diagnosis. Asymptomatic diagnosis was defined as diagnosis by family history, genotype, prenatal diagnosis, or neonatal screening in the absence of clinical signs or symptoms recorded at the time of diagnosis. Children in the EAD group had significantly higher FEV_1 scores. However, this finding was due to truncation of the late diagnosis groups. An unpublished analysis of data from the 2002 CFFPR by Grosse, Devine, and Rosenfeld found that the difference in mean lung function was attenuated when the 1990 diagnosis cutoff was removed and was eliminated when the arbitrary 36 month diagnostic cutoff was removed. In any case, the EAD group primarily consisted of infants diagnosed based on family history, and the majority of children detected based on newborn screening either had symptoms at diagnosis or were diagnosed after 6 weeks of age.

An analysis of data from the 2002 CFFPR by Accurso et al. compared lung function in relation to four types of diagnosis: newborn screening, symptomatic, MI, and prenatal diagnosis (24). The analysis excluded individuals diagnosed on the basis of a family history of CF, which was the leading source of asymptomatic diagnoses during the period. Children who had both newborn screening and symptoms checked were assigned to the newborn screening group (Marci Sontag, personal communication, February 13, 2008). Individuals at 6–10 and 11–20 years of age classified as diagnosed through newborn screening had significantly higher FEV_1 scores than those in the symptomatic diagnosis group (24). Mean FEV_1 for those with prenatal diagnoses did not differ from those with symptomatic or MI diagnoses, even though prenatal and newborn screening both enabled early detection and preventive care. The high FEV_1 scores in the newborn screening group might have been due to unmeasured confounding or selection bias.

In an unpublished analysis of 2002 CFFPR data, Grosse, Devine, and Rosenfeld used the presence of newborn screening for CF in a state at the time of birth as a predictor variable in regression analysis on FEV_1 scores among children 6–10 years of age. Children born in states with CF newborn screening programs had significantly better lung function, controlling for other predictors of lung function. Only a small number of states at the time screened for CF and it was not possible to determine whether states with better management of CF were more likely to have adopted screening, early treatment made possible by screening causally improved lung function, or both.

Three analyses of CFFPR data examined the association of newborn screening with survival. First, Lai et al. used the 2000 registry data to compare children or adults with a newborn or prenatal screening diagnosis recorded and those diagnosed with MI or with symptoms other than MI (23). They reported significantly longer survival among those in the screening group compared with those in both the MI and symptom groups. However, most of the difference in survival was estimated to have occurred after 20 years of age. This is unlikely, since neither newborn nor prenatal screening was available before the 1980s (6). The CFFPR contains records in which a newborn screening diagnosis was listed for children born in states without screening programs at the time or which occurred after 1 year of age. The same investigators subsequently published an analysis that restricted the analysis to individuals diagnosed after 1986 and to deaths occurring before 14 years of age (38). That analysis reported that the association with mortality remained but was of borderline statistical significance ($p < .10$).

Finally, Grosse et al. compared the cumulative risk of death to 10 years of age among children with CF who were born during 1987–1991 in states with or without CF statewide newborn screening programs (31). The former group consisted of Colorado, Wisconsin, and Wyoming; children born in three states with voluntary private screening programs with incomplete coverage (Connecticut, Montana, and Pennsylvania) were excluded from the analysis. The analysis found an absolute difference in risk of 1.7 per 100 (0.65 versus 2.35 per 100), with a rate ratio of 3.6 ($p= .13$). Although not statistically significant, the difference in risk was only slightly smaller than that reported in the individual-level analysis (38). The small number of children born in states with screening programs made the results difficult to interpret. It is possible that better quality of care provided in states with screening programs could have accounted for the lower mortality rates observed. On the other hand, there is a greater likelihood that children with CF born in states without screening could have died due to complications of the disorder, such as electrolyte imbalance under heat stress, without a diagnosis having been established or recorded. Only a retrospective screening study conducted using stored specimens from a cohort not screened for CF at birth could quantify such deaths.

The 2002 UK Cystic Fibrosis Database (UKCFD) has been analyzed in several publications to compare outcomes for children 1–9 years of age without MI who were identified either through newborn screening or manifestation of symptoms and who were diagnosed beginning in 1994 (39–41). The investigators reported that children in the newborn screening group did not differ in terms of FEV_1 scores but differed significantly in chest radiography at 6 years of age. They focused on the finding that children in the screened group were less likely to have received intensive or longterm therapies, which was regarded as indicative of less lung disease and a lower need for aggressive treatment (39). The percentage of children homozygous for the ΔF508 mutation was similar for each group (about 50%), and results of analyses stratified by genotype to test for potential confounding were comparable with those of the overall analysis. The one exception was that pancreatic enzyme replacement therapy was significantly more common in the clinically detected group overall but not among ΔF508 homozygotes (39). At the time children were born, screening for CF was universal in Wales and Northern Ireland, limited in England, and not available in Scotland. An analysis restricted to observations from seven English CF centers that treated appreciable numbers of children in both groups generated findings comparable with those in the overall sample (39).

Finally, the UKCFD was used to assess potential harm from unnecessary treatment. It was found that those with CF diagnosed through newborn screening have not been prematurely introduced to aggressive therapies, including pancreatic enzyme replacement therapy prior to the emergence of pancreatic insufficiency (40,41). This question has not been studied in the United States. A concern expressed in the United States is that many individuals are identified with borderline or atypical CF and have an unknown prognosis with unknown benefit (or harm) of treatment (42).

The potential harms of screening for CF include a risk that infants with newly diagnosed CF might be exposed to other CF patients with established *Pseudomonas aeruginosa* lung infections and become infected themselves (6). This almost certainly happened in one of the two centers in the Wisconsin trial, causing infants diagnosed with CF who were treated in that center and born during the first part of the trial to develop serious, chronic lung infections at an earlier age (27). However, CF centers have since instituted safeguards against exposure of CF patients to other patients to minimize this risk, and there is no evidence that this harm has subsequently been repeated (24).

Medium-Chain Acyl-CoA Dehydrogenase Deficiency

Medium-chain acyl-coA dehydrogenase deficiency (MCADD) is an autosomal recessive mitochondrial fatty acid oxidation disorder that is caused by mutations on the *ACADM* or *MCAD* gene (OMIM 607008). Deficiency in the MCAD protein reduces the formation of ketone bodies in the liver that provide an alternative energy source during periods of prolonged fasting or increased energy demands. Consequently, clinical presentation is usually related to hypoglycemia brought about by fasting and increased metabolic stress and can result in encephalopathy or sudden death. Although most patients present during infancy or early childhood, acute crises can occur throughout life. Most studies reported high mortality (16–26%) and variable levels of neurological sequelae among survivors of an acute metabolic crisis (43,44). Clinical case series have reported permanent sequelae in up to one-fourth to one-third of survivors in symptomatic MCADD (45,46).

The highest quality outcomes data for MCADD that are currently available come from one retrospective screening study conducted in England (47) and from studies of outcomes among screened and unscreened cohorts born in different states in Australia and followed to 4 years of age using a standardized protocol (21,48). Ascertainment bias in unscreened cohorts is a major problem. Population-based surveillance data from Australia and Western Europe indicated that in the absence of screening 35–60% of cases of MCADD were detected based on clinical signs or family history (21,49–51). MCADD was more rarely diagnosed in the United States prior to screening (52). Furthermore, children detected clinically have been reported to be more likely to be homozygotes for the relatively severe common mutation than are those detected through screening programs (5,49). Consequently, extrapolation of the frequency of sequelae among individuals with MCADD diagnosed in unscreened cohorts to all individuals with MCADD detected by screening will almost inevitably overstate the potential benefits of screening (53).

At least 25% of children with MCADD appear to remain asymptomatic and a similar percentage of affected children are likely to display relatively limited clinical signs and symptoms (44,47). Conversely, in the absence of screening an important percentage of children with MCADD experience fatal decompensation episodes that are likely to go undiagnosed, approximately 5–6% according to a retrospective analysis of stored blood spot specimens for unexplained child deaths in Virginia (54). Consequently, a count of child deaths attributed to MCADD in an unscreened population could understate the actual number of deaths caused by the disorder. In addition, sudden deaths among adults with MCADD can occur.

One retrospective MCADD screening study assessed outcomes for a random sample of stored specimens. Pourfarzam et al. analyzed 100,600 stored dried blood spot specimens collected from infants born in the northern United Kingdom during 1991–1993 and found that 14 screened positive for MCADD (47). They followed up with an examination of medical records and family surveys for all 14 children, including 12 children who were still alive at 7–9 years of age. They identified eight children as having MCADD, including three who had been clinically diagnosed prior to the study. One of the latter three had died at 17 months of age and was diagnosed post mortem. Three of the seven survivors with MCADD had experienced episodes of encephalopathy, two had had milder symptoms, and two had no symptoms recorded, although one of the latter had learning difficulties that might have been unrelated to the metabolic disorder. None of the survivors had a developmental disability that could be linked to a metabolic decompensation crisis. The number of observations was too restricted to provide precise estimates of the frequency of death or sequelae.

The frequency with which children with biochemical MCADD develop serious, life-threatening symptoms can also be assessed by using information on the older siblings of probands detected as newborns through screening. For example, Waisbren et al., through testing family members of 20 infants detected through screening, identified seven older surviving siblings with MCADD, of whom four had shown symptoms (hypoglycemia and extreme lethargy) of MCADD (the other three remained asymptomatic) (20). That study did not consider older siblings who might have died of MCADD. In another study, Pollitt and Leonard reported that four of six older siblings confirmed to have MCADD had experienced symptoms, and that an additional four siblings died with symptoms compatible with MCADD, although it could not be confirmed that they had MCADD (44).

The most informative study to date on MCADD outcomes utilized contemporaneous population-based screened and unscreened cohorts with MCADD born in Australia during 1994–2002 (21). A unique feature of the study was the reportedly complete ascertainment of all diagnosed cases of MCADD in Australia including those states that did not screen for the disorder at the time. Wilcken et al. analyzed the frequency of death and developmental delay among children followed to 4 years of age. They reported deaths among 6 (17%) of 35 children with the disorder diagnosed through clinical presentation or after diagnosis of a sibling, compared with 1 (4%) of 24 in those diagnosed through screening, as noted in an accompanying commentary (53). The latter death occurred in the first 3 days of life, before laboratory screening was done (55).

The death rate among the approximately 50% of the Australian MCADD unscreened cohort who were not diagnosed with the disorder based on clinical manifestations was probably lower than among those who did come to clinical attention. Wilcken et al. proposed that the death rate was perhaps only half as high in that group, which implies an overall unscreened cohort death rate of 12% (21). The 12% estimate can be compared with a death rate of 25% that is often cited on the basis of clinical case series but was the same as that reported in a retrospective study of stored blood spot specimens (47). Surprisingly, a subsequent publication from the same group that compared health care utilization for the screened and unscreened cohorts did not make an adjustment for ascertainment bias among the unscreened cohort (48).

A recent study of 137 Dutch individuals identified with MCADD from the late 1970s to 2003 based on clinical symptoms or family history, including individuals diagnosed post mortem, found a 20% death rate (56). However, mortality was lower, 15%, when restricted to the 110 probands, and no deaths were observed among 18 individuals detected in the newborn period through testing prompted by family history. The investigators made no adjustment for asymptomatic individuals with MCADD who were not included in their observations.

Although the risk of mortality is reduced through newborn screening for MCADD, it is not eliminated (21,55). First, infants with MCADD can die during the first 3 days after birth, before screening results can be reported (55,57). Second, reports from the United States and Germany discussed children diagnosed with MCADD who died despite receiving treatment (58,59). An analysis on the first 46 children diagnosed with MCADD through screening of 713,552 infants in four New England states identified two deaths (4%) at 11 and 33 months of age that were attributed to MCADD (59). The California newborn screening program reported two deaths in screened infants with MCADD that occurred in the first week after birth (Fred

Lorey, personal communication, February 21, 2008). A retrospective screening study would be required to reliably ascertain the risk of death in an unscreened cohort.

Another endpoint in MCADD is disability among survivors of metabolic decompensation crises. However, clinical case reports are likely to be affected by ascertainment bias due to more severely affected children being more likely to be referred to specialized centers. Another problem is a lack of standardization in developmental assessments. In particular, there is a tendency for case series to cite poorly defined neurological sequelae and to fail to report the number of children affected rather than the number of symptoms. Sequelae resulting in intellectual disability typically occurred in 5–6% of all children with MCADD, with milder sequelae affecting perhaps a similar number of additional children (5). Those estimates take into account the probability that one-quarter to one-half of children with MCADD do not experience a metabolic crisis during childhood that would put them at risk of neurological disability.

Two recent publications reported on neurological sequelae among unscreened individuals with MCADD. The Australian study found no developmental delay in either screened or unscreened children at least 4 years of age who were administered cognitive assessments (21,48). The finding that unscreened children did not have serious problems was more favorable than had been previously reported for unscreened children with MCADD, not only in Australia but in other countries as well (5,53). This finding reflected improved clinical awareness of MCADD in Australia in recent years (21).

Van der Hilst et al. reported that five (4%) of 116 Dutch patients with MCADD born during 1985–2003 had been institutionalized, three of whom required permanent institutional care (60). This is slightly lower than the 6% frequency of severe disability reported by the same investigators for a sample of 155 patients that presumably included 39 born prior to 1985 (56). The latter sample included 18 subjects identified neonatally through family history, one (5%) of whom had a mild neurological impairment. No information was presented as to the ages of individuals who were classified as having severe disability, the criteria that were used, or cognitive assessments.

One potential harm from screening for MCADD is unnecessary treatment for children who would have remained asymptomatic or without sequelae. The Australian study cited previously reported that children in the screened cohort were less likely to have been hospitalized than were those in the unscreened cohort, 42% versus 71%, respectively (48). However, compared with the frequency of MCADD in states with screening, probably only 60% of children in the unscreened cohort were diagnosed. If those who did not come to clinical attention were not hospitalized, the rates of hospitalization among the screened and unscreened cohorts would have been approximately equal. Consequently, these data do not provide evidence of reduced rates of hospitalization with screening. At least these data do suggest that screening does not cause excess hospitalizations in screened children.

Lessons Learned

Evaluating the cumulative evidence of clinical utility from multiple epidemiologic studies is even more challenging than interpreting the results of a single study. Ioannidis et al. have proposed three types of criteria: amount of evidence in terms of total numbers of observations, consistency in findings among studies, and study quality in terms of protection from bias (61). In addition, it seems reasonable to take into account effect size. Other things constant, a larger effect size in terms of proportional improvement in outcomes is associated with greater clinical utility.

The cumulative evidence of clinical utility from newborn screening is uneven. Among the two disorders reviewed here, the greatest amount and quality of evidence exists for CF, with two randomized trials of screening, several cohort studies, and analysis of two national patient registries. However, consistency of findings in CF studies of screening is variable. The most consistent evidence among study findings is for growth and the weakest evidence is for lung function. Most studies, including one randomized trial, have found significant differences in mortality, but the highest quality trial did not.

For MCADD, one small retrospective screening study and two pilot screening studies with long-term follow-up are available. In addition to the Australian study, a large-scale MCADD screening study in the United Kingdom has collected outcomes data that will be reported at a later date. There has been a lack of consistency of findings in terms of both mortality and disability. Although studies have consistently reported deaths among at least 10% of children with MCADD in the absence of screening, this percentage is variable and subject to ascertainment bias in both directions. Also, there are persistent reports of deaths from MCADD even with screening, occurring among as many as 4% of children born with MCADD (55,59), but the numbers involved are very small. Finally, to the extent that cognitive impairment in MCADD can be prevented without screening, as suggested by the Australian study, the number of cases of disability prevented by screening is context specific.

The MCADD case study illustrates the challenge of evaluating rare disorders; most other disorders being added to newborn screening panels are even less common. Because of the rarity of MCADD, about 1 in 15,000 births, comprehensive follow-up data on millions of children screened for MCADD are needed in order to generate reliable data on outcomes of screening (53). The Australian data suggest that perhaps 70% of child deaths from MCADD are prevented by newborn screening (21). Although this is less than 100%, it is still important evidence of the clinical utility of screening for MCADD. In the absence of pooling of long-term follow-up data from multiple screening programs utilizing a standard protocol (50), all assessments of clinical utility of screening must remain tentative.

A long lead time is needed before a fully evidence-based decision about the clinical utility of screening can be reached. The first statewide screening programs for CF began in 1981 in Australia and 1982 in the United States. The first statewide screening programs for MCADD began in 1997 in the United States and in 1998 in Australia. Two U.K. health technology assessments published in 1997 concluded that screening for MCADD met all or almost all recognized criteria for screening programs (62,63). A subsequent U.K. report (64) confirmed and expanded on the first assessment (62). However, it was only in 2007 that the National Health Service decided to adopt universal screening for MCADD in England, after preliminary results from a pilot screening study confirmed findings from other countries. In the United States, Massachusetts adopted universal screening for MCADD in 1998 (65,66), based in large part on one of the U.K. reviews (62). Numerous other states followed subsequently (67).

Given what is known now, the early adopters of screening for CF and MCADD appear to have been justified in their decisions. There is a societal cost of delaying the initiation of screening tests that can save lives and prevent disability, which needs to be balanced against the cost of deciding to screen for disorders that might eventually be shown to not provide clear benefit. Large-scale pilot screening programs with rigorous evaluation protocols are essential to contribute to the evidence base. In addition, policy makers should be prepared to discontinue screening tests for which evidence of utility is ultimately lacking.

Acknowledgments

I thank Ingeborg Blancquaert, Anne Comeau, Philip Farrell, Alex Kemper, Martin Kharrazi, Fred Lorey, Lisa Prosser, Marci Sontag, Esther Sumartojo, John Thompson, and Bridget Wilcken for their helpful comments.

References

1. MacCready R. Phenylketonuria screening program. *N Engl J Med.* 1963;269:52–56.
2. Therrell BL, Adams J. Newborn screening in North America. *J Inherit Metab Dis.* 2007;30:447–465.
3. Loeber JG. Neonatal screening in Europe; the situation in 2004. *J Inherit Metab Dis.* 2007;30:430–438.
4. Bodamer OA, Hoffmann GF, Lindner M. Expanded newborn screening in Europe 2007. *J Inherit Metab Dis.* 2007;30:439–444.
5. Grosse SD, Khoury MJ, Greene C, Crider KS, Pollitt RJ. The epidemiology of medium chain acyl-coA dehydrogenase deficiency (MCADD): an update. *Genet Med.* 2006;8:205–212.
6. Grosse SD, Boyle CA, Botkin JR, et al. Newborn screening for cystic fibrosis: evaluation of benefits and risks and recommendations for state newborn screening programs. *MMWR Recomm Rep.* 2004;53(RR–13):1–36.
7. Grosse SD, Khoury MJ. What is the clinical utility of genetic testing? *Genet Med.* 2006;8:448–450.
8. Hewlett J, Waisbren SE. A review of the psychosocial effects of false-positive results on parents and current communication practices in newborn screening. *J Inherit Metab Dis.* 2006;29:677–682.
9. Green JM, Hewison J, Bekker HL, Bryant LD, Cuckle HS. Psychosocial aspects of genetic screening of pregnant women and newborns: a systematic review. *Health Technol Assess.* 2004;8(33):1–109.

10. Dezateux C. Newborn screening for medium chain acyl-CoA dehydrogenase deficiency: evaluating the effects on outcome. *Eur J Pediatr.* 2003;162:S25–S28.

11. Chatfield S, Owen G, Ryley HC, et al. Neonatal screening for cystic fibrosis in Wales and the West Midlands: clinical assessment after five years of screening. *Arch Dis Child.* 1991;66:29–33.

12. Farrell PM, Kosorok MR, Rock MJ, et al. Early diagnosis of cystic fibrosis through neonatal screening prevents severe malnutrition and improves long-term growth. *Pediatrics.* 2001;107:1–13.

13. Wilcken B. Ethical issues in newborn screening and the impact of new technologies. *Eur J Pediatr.* 2003;162:S62–S66.

14. Weiss NS, Koepsell TD, Psaty BM. Generalizability of the results of randomized trials. *Arch Intern Med.* 2008;168:133–135.

15. Nørgaard-Pedersen B, Simonsen H. Biological specimen banks in neonatal screening. *Acta Paediatr Suppl.* 1999;88(432):106–109.

16. Alm J, Hagenfeldt L, Larsson A, Lundberg K. Incidence of congenital hypothyroidism: retrospective study of neonatal laboratory screening versus clinical symptoms as indicators leading to diagnosis. *BMJ.* 1984;289:1171–1175.

17. Grosse SD. Late-treated phenylketonuria and partial reversibility of intellectual disability. *Child Develop.* In press.

18. Castellani C. Evidence for newborn screening for cystic fibrosis. *Paediatr Respir Rev.* 2003;4:278–284.

19. Koch R, Moseley K, Ning J, Romstad A, Guldberg P, Guttler F. Long-term beneficial effects of the phenylalanine-restricted diet in late-diagnosed individuals with phenylketonuria. *Mol Genet Metab.* 1999;67:148–155.

20. Waisbren SE, Albers S, Amato S, et al. Effect of expanded newborn screening for biochemical genetic disorders on child outcomes and parental stress. *JAMA.* 2003;290:2564–2572.

21. Wilcken B, Haas M, Joy P, et al. Outcome of neonatal screening for medium-chain acyl-CoA dehydrogenase deficiency in Australia: a cohort study. *Lancet.* 2007;369:37–42.

22. Bobadilla JL, Macek M, Jr, Fine JP, Farrell PM. Cystic fibrosis: a worldwide analysis of CFTR mutations—correlation with incidence data and application to screening. *Hum Mutat.* 2002;19:575–606.

23. Lai HJ, Cheng Y, Cho H, Kosorok MR, Farrell PM. Association between initial disease presentation, lung disease outcomes, and survival in patients with cystic fibrosis. *Am J Epidemiol.* 2004;159:537–546.

24. Accurso FJ, Sontag MK, Wagener JS. Complications associated with symptomatic diagnosis in infants with cystic fibrosis. *J Pediatr.* 2005;147:S37–S41.

25. Farrell PM, Li Z, Kosorok MR, et al. Longitudinal evaluation of bronchopulmonary disease in children with cystic fibrosis. *Pediatr Pulmonol.* 2003;36:230–240.

26. Welsh MJ, Ramsey BW, Accurso F, Cutting GR. Cystic fibrosis. In: Scriver CR, et al., editors. *The Metabolic and Molecular Basis of Inherited Disease*, 8th ed. New York: McGraw-Hill; 2001:5121–5188.

27. McKay KO. Cystic fibrosis: benefits and clinical outcome. *J Inherit Metab Dis.* 2007;30:544–555.

28. Centers for Disease Control and Prevention. Newborn screening for cystic fibrosis: a paradigm for public health genetics policy development: proceedings of a 1997 workshop. *MMWR.* 1997;46(No. RR–16):1–24.

29. Koscik RL, Douglas JA, Zaremba K, et al. Quality of life of children with cystic fibrosis. *J Pediatr.* 2005;147:S64–S68.

30. Koscik RL, Farrell PM, Kosorok MR, et al. Cognitive function of children with cystic fibrosis: deleterious effect of early malnutrition. *Pediatrics.* 2004;113:1549–1558.

31. Grosse SD, Rosenfeld M, Devine OJ, Lai HJ, Farrell PM. Potential impact of newborn screening for cystic fibrosis on child survival: a systematic review and analysis. *J Pediatr.* 2006;149:362–366.

32. Doull IJ, Ryley HC, Weller P, Goodchild MC. Cystic fibrosis-related deaths in infancy and the effect of newborn screening. *Pediatr Pulmonol.* 2001;31:363–366.

33. Wilcken B, Chalmers G. Reduced morbidity in patients with cystic fibrosis detected by neonatal screening. *Lancet.* 1985;2:1319–1321.

34. Waters DL, Wilcken B, Irwing L, et al. Clinical outcomes of newborn screening for cystic fibrosis. *Arch Dis Child Fetal Neonatal Ed.* 1999;80:F1–F7.

35. McKay KO, Waters DL, Gaskin KJ. The influence of newborn screening for cystic fibrosis on pulmonary outcomes in new South Wales. *J Pediatr.* 2005;147:S47–S50.

36. Siret D, Bretaudeau G, Branger B, et al. Comparing the clinical evolution of cystic fibrosis screened neonatally to that of cystic fibrosis diagnosed from clinical symptoms: a 10-year retrospective study in a French region (Brittany). *Pediatr Pulmonol.* 2003;35:342–349.

37. Wang SS, O'Leary LA, Fitzsimmons SC, Khoury MJ. The impact of early cystic fibrosis diagnosis on pulmonary function in children. *J Pediatr.* 2002;141:804–810.

38. Lai HJ, Cheng Y, Farrell PM. The survival advantage of patients with cystic fibrosis diagnosed through neonatal screening: evidence from the United States Cystic Fibrosis Foundation registry data. *J Pediatr.* 2005;147:S57–S63.

39. Sims EJ, McCormick J, Mehta G, Mehta A. Newborn screening for cystic fibrosis is associated with reduced treatment intensity. *J Pediatr.* 2005;147:306–311.

40. Sims EJ, McCormick J, Mehta G, Mehta A. Neonatal screening for cystic fibrosis is beneficial even in the context of modern treatment. *J Pediatr.* 2005;147:S42–S46.

41. Sims EJ, Clark A, McCormick J, et al. Cystic fibrosis diagnosed after 2 months of age leads to worse outcomes and requires more therapy. *Pediatrics.* 2007;119:19–28.

42. Parad RB, Comeau AM. Diagnostic dilemmas resulting from the immunoreactive trypsinogen/DNA cystic fibrosis newborn screening algorithm. *J Pediatr.* 2005;147:S78–S82.

43. Wilcken B, Hammond J, Silink M. Morbidity and mortality in medium-chain acyl coenzyme A dehydrogenase deficiency. *Arch Dis Child.* 1994;70:410–412.

44. Pollitt RJ, Leonard JV. Prospective surveillance study of medium-chain acyl-CoA dehydrogenase deficiency in the UK. *Arch Dis Child.* 1998;79:116–119.

45. Iafolla AK, Thompson RJ, Jr, Roe CR. Medium-chain acyl-coenzyme A dehydrogenase deficiency: clinical course in 120 affected children. *J Pediatr.* 1994;124:409–415.

46. Venditti LN, Venditti CP, Berry GT, et al. Newborn screening by tandem mass spectrometry for medium-chain Acyl-CoA dehydrogenase deficiency: a cost-effectiveness analysis. *Pediatrics.* 2003;112:1005–1015.

47. Pourfarzam M, Morris A, Appleton M, et al. Neonatal screening for medium-chain acyl-CoA dehydrogenase deficiency. *Lancet.* 2001;358:1063–1064.

48. Haas M, Chaplin M, Joy P, Wiley V, Black C, Wilcken B. Healthcare use and costs of medium-chain acyl-CoA dehydrogenase deficiency in Australia: screening versus no screening. *J Pediatr.* 2007;151:121–126.

49. Carpenter K, Wiley V, Sim KG, et al. Evaluation of newborn screening for medium chain acyl-CoA dehydrogenase deficiency in 275 000 babies. *Arch Dis Child Fetal Neonatal Ed.* 2001;85:F105–F109.

50. Liebl B, Nennstiel-Ratzel U, Roscher A, von Kries R. Data required for the evaluation of newborn screening programmes. *Eur J Pediatr.* 2003;162:S57–S61.

51. Hoffmann GF, von Kries R, Klose D, et al. Frequencies of inherited organic acidurias and disorders of mitochondrial fatty acid transport and oxidation in Germany. *Eur J Pediatr.* 2004;163:76–80.

52. Schoen EJ, Baker JC, Colby CJ, To TT. Cost-benefit analysis of universal tandem mass spectrometry for newborn screening. *Pediatrics.* 2002;110:781–786.

53. Grosse SD, Dezateux C. Newborn screening for inherited metabolic disease. *Lancet.* 2007;369:5–6.

54. Dott M, Chace D, Fierro M, et al. Metabolic disorders detectable by tandem mass spectrometry and unexpected early childhood mortality: a population-based study. *Am J Med Genet A.* 2006;140:837–842.

55. Wilcken B. Medium-chain acyl-coenzyme A dehydrogenase deficiency in a neonate. *N Engl J Med.* 2008;358:647.

56. Derks TG, Reijngoud DJ, Waterham HR, et al. The natural history of medium-chain acyl CoA dehydrogenase deficiency in the Netherlands: clinical presentation and outcome. *J Pediatr.* 2006;148:665–670.

57. Cyriac J, Venkatesh V, Gupta C. A fatal neonatal presentation of medium-chain acyl coenzyme A dehydrogenase deficiency. *J Int Med Res.* 2008;36:609–610.

58. Nennstiel-Ratzel U, Arenz S, Maier EM, et al. Reduced incidence of severe metabolic crisis or death in children with medium chain acyl-CoA dehydrogenase deficiency homozygous for c. 985A = G identified by neonatal screening. *Mol Genet Metab.* 2005;85:157–159.

59. Hsu HW, Zytkovicz TH, Comeau AM, et al. Spectrum of medium chain acyl-coA dehydrogenase (MCAD) deficiency detected by newborn screening. *Pediatrics.* 2008;121:e1108–e1114.

60. van der Hilst CS, Derks TG, Reijngoud DJ, Smit GP, TenVergert EM. Cost-effectiveness of neonatal screening for medium chain acyl-CoA dehydrogenase deficiency: the homogeneous population of The Netherlands. *J Pediatr.* 2007;151:115–120.

61. Ioannidis JP, Boffetta P, Little J, et al. Assessment of cumulative evidence on genetic associations: interim guidelines. *Int J Epidemiol.* 2008;37:120–132.

62. Pollitt RJ, Green A, McCabe CJ, et al. Newborn screening for inborn errors of metabolism: a systematic review. *Health Technol Assess.* 1997;1(7):1–202.

63. Seymour CA, Thomason MJ, Chalmers RA, et al. Newborn screening for inborn errors of metabolism: a systematic review. *Health Technol Assess.* 1997;1(11):1–95.

64. Pandor A, Eastham J, Beverley C, et al. Clinical effectiveness and cost-effectiveness of neonatal screening for inborn errors of metabolism using tandem mass spectrometry: a systematic review. *Health Technol Assess.* 2004;8(12):1–121.

65. Atkinson K, Zuckerman B, Sharfstein JM, et al. A public health response to emerging technology: expansion of the Massachusetts newborn screening program. *Public Health Rep.* 2001;116:122–131.

66. Grosse S, Gwinn M. Assisting states in assessing newborn screening options. *Public Health Rep.* 2001;116:169–172.

67. Therrell BL, Adams J. Newborn screening in North America. *J Inherit Metab Dis.* 2007;30:447–465.

27

The role of epidemiology in assessing the potential clinical impact of pharmacogenomics

David L. Veenstra

Introduction

A promising area of genomics is the use of information about genetic variation to guide drug therapy, a field known as pharmacogenomics. Pharmacogenomic applications can be broadly categorized into (a) those related to variation in drug metabolism and disposition genes, which affect the levels of active drug or metabolites in the body and thus both effectiveness and side effects, and (b) those related to variation in genes for drug targets, which primarily influence the effectiveness of a drug (1,2). These categories can be applied to both inherited and acquired variation. There has been significant excitement about the potential of this field over the past decade, but pharmacogenomics actually has an extensive 50-year history. Arno Motulsky proposed in 1957 that the inheritance of acquired traits could explain individual differences in drug efficacy and adverse drug reactions (ADRs) (3,4). The majority of early research focused on common polymorphisms in the drug metabolizing enzymes, which were identified using a candidate gene approach in patients with an unusual drug response (1). More recently, with technological advances in DNA analysis, rarer variants and those affecting drug effectiveness have been evaluated (2). In this chapter, the role of epidemiology in assessing pharmacogenomic associations is discussed, as well as approaches utilizing epidemiologic data to quantify the potential benefits and harms of pharmacogenomic tests in clinical use.

Epidemiology and Pharmacogenomics

A multitude of potential pharmacogenomic applications have been investigated over the past decade, including the relationship between genetic variation and drug treatment outcomes in asthma, hyperlipidemia, hypertension, and oncology (1,2). However, as with disease genetics, various widely cited association studies have not been reproduced and validated. For example, one study indicated a significant relationship between an alpha-adducin gene variant and diuretic antihypertensive response (5), but several recent, larger studies failed to identify such an association (6–9). The association between the *CETP* polymorphisms and statin therapy outcomes has been widely studied, but a recent meta-analysis failed to validate the association (10). Pharmacogenomic associations that have not been consistently replicated include: *ACE* gene polymorphisms and antihypertensives (11), beta-receptor polymorphisms and both asthma (12,13) and heart failure medications (14), and serotonin transporters and antidepressants (15–17). The importance of sound epidemiologic approaches to assessing genetic associations has been verified by this experience, including appropriately powered studies, assessment of potential selection bias and confounding, adjustment for multiple comparisons, careful assessment of phenotypes, and caution regarding publication bias (18–20). Multicenter, multinational consortiums will serve as a critical mechanism for providing the necessary sample sizes to identify and validate pharmacogenomic associations, for example, the International Warfarin Pharmacogenetics Consortium (IWPC).

Validated Examples—Current "State of the Science"

Drug Metabolism Genes

Despite these challenges, several important pharmacogenomic associations have been established (Table 27.1). Validated examples of genetic variants related to drug metabolism include: (a) *TPMT* variants and toxicity to the anticancer drug 6-mercaptopurine in children with acute lymphoblastic leukemia (21,22), (b) *CYP2C9* variants and dose requirements of the blood thinner drug warfarin in patients with clotting disorders (23,24), and (c) *UGT1A1* variants and toxicity to the anticolon cancer drug irinotecan (25).

These associations have been reproduced in various studies and are generally accepted in the scientific and clinical community as valid. In addition, the U.S. Food and Drug Administration (FDA) has added information about pharmacogenomic effects to the labeling of these drugs although testing has not been required to date (26,27). Another interesting example is the association between the *CYP2D6* drug metabolism gene and response to tamoxifen therapy in breast cancer. Patients with low-activity *CYP2D6* variants actually receive less benefit because tamoxifen requires modification by *CYP2D6* in the body to active forms (28–30). *CYP2D6* poor metabolizer genotypes have also been associated with decreased efficacy of codeine, which similarly requires activation in the body by *CYP2D6* (31). Conversely, ultra-rapid *CYP2D6* metabolizer status in mothers of breastfeeding infants has been associated with cases of infant mortality (32). The antiplatelet drug clopidogrel is yet another drug that requires activation by drug metabolizing enzymes—in this case, *CYP2C19*. A recent study found that patients with a lower activity variant (30% of the population) had lower levels of active metabolites, and a 50% higher risk of the composite primary efficacy outcome of the risk of death from cardiovascular causes, myocardial infarction, or stroke (33).

Table 27.1   Selected examples of pharmacogenomic associations

Category	Gene	Drug	Association/Outcome
Inherited genetic variation			
Drug metabolism	CYP2C9	Warfarin	dose requirement, drug response, and severe bleeding events
	CYP2C19	Clopidogrel	major cardiovascular outcomes
	CYP2D6	Codeine	variation in effect (pain control and respiratory depression)
	CYP2D6	Tamoxifen	disease recurrence in early stage breast cancer (some contradictory study findings)
Hypersensitivity reactions	HLA	Abacavir	hypersensitivity reaction
	HLA	Carbamazepine	Stevens-Johnson syndrome
Drug targets	VKORC1	Warfarin	dose requirement and initial drug response
Acquired genetic variation			
	HER2-neu	Trastuzumab	treatment response in early stage and metastatic breast cancer
	various (OncotypeDx)	Chemotherapy	risk score predicts breast cancer recurrence and chemotherapy response
	various (MammaPrint)	Chemotherapy	risk score predicts breast cancer recurrence
	KRAS	Cetuximab, panitumumab	treatment response in colon cancer

See text for references.

Hypersensitivity Reactions

The relationship between an HLA variant and hypersensitivity reactions to the anti-HIV drug abacavir has been well established in various studies and populations, and is likely clinically useful (34,35). The antiseizure drug carbamazepine has a rare risk of an extremely serious hypersensitivity reaction—Stevens-Johnson syndrome and toxic epidermal necrolysis. The association has been established in Chinese but not Caucasian populations—potentially due to the higher prevalence of the relevant variant in many Asian populations (36).

Drug Targets

There are relatively few well-validated examples of variation in a drug target influencing drug outcomes. The effect of *VKORC1* variants on warfarin dose requirements is probably the most well known. Variation in the promoter region (explained by a single SNP) explains approximately 25% of dosing variability, and influences anticoagulation levels in the initial days of therapy (37,38). In another emerging example, heart failure patients with a specific beta-1 adrenergic receptor genotype had a significant response to bucindolol; the FDA is evaluating these findings (39).

Acquired Genetic Variation

Evaluation of tumor cell lines is often used for guiding chemotherapy in oncology. A now classic example of using genetic information to do so is assessment of variation in the growth factor receptor gene *HER2/neu*, which is overexpressed in approximately 25% of metastatic breast tumors. Patients with tumors that overexpress *HER2/neu* are eligible for treatment with the targeted monoclonal antibody drug trastuzumab (Herceptin) (40). More recent examples include two gene expression profiles designed to help identify women with early-stage breast cancer who are at higher risk of disease recurrence and thus better candidates for adjuvant chemotherapy. Both the MammaPrint and OncotypeDx tests have been validated using retrospective analyses—in particular, both tests have been associated with recurrence risk, while the latter has also been associated with chemotherapy response (41–44). Recent studies suggest that colorectal cancer patients with *KRAS* mutations are not responsive to the EGFR-antibody drugs cetuximab and panitumumab, based on retrospective analyses of several clinical trials (45,46). Lastly, responses to the small molecule EGFR tyrosine kinase inhibitors erlotinib and gefitinib in nonsmall cell lung cancer have been correlated with gene mutations, protein expression, and gene copy number, although samples were available from only 30–40% of patients in the key Phase III trials, and further data and evaluation are needed (47).

The Translational Challenge: Evidence of Clinical Utility

Despite the promising examples discussed above, pharmacogenomics is currently rarely used in clinical practice (48). For example, a pharmacogenomic test is routinely used with only one drug (trastuzumab) of the top 200 drugs by sales, and none of the top 200 drugs by prescription volume (49,50). Although valid associations have been identified and tests are available, routine pharmacogenomic testing with 6-mercaptopurine, warfarin, and irinotecan therapy is conducted in a relatively limited number of settings—primarily academic research centers.

A major challenge for clinicians and policy makers is the general lack of direct evidence—that is, data from a randomized controlled trial (RCT)—indicating that testing improves patient outcomes compared to usual care. In the first prospective RCT designed to evaluate the outcomes of pharmacogenomic testing, investigators compared *HLA* testing to guide abacavir drug selection versus usual care in the treatment of HIV infection (51). Screening eliminated immunologically confirmed hypersensitivity reaction (0% in the prospective screening group versus 2.7% in the control group, $p < 0.001$). Other pharmacogenomic-based RCTs are currently being conducted with warfarin therapy (52,53) and the breast cancer gene expression profiles (54). However, results from these studies will not be available for several years, and for some pharmacogenomic tests, such studies may never be conducted because of (a) the lack of financial incentives for private industry to invest in such trials, (b) the challenges in identifying valid associations, (c) limited availability of a test kit or test results within a clinical decision-making timeframe, and lastly (d) genetic variation may not account for the majority of variation in drug-related therapeutic outcomes (48,55). Developing treatment and reimbursement guidelines for genetic tests thus promises to be challenging. Although prognostic and predictive information derived from genetic testing is not necessarily unique compared to phenotypic assays, there are important differences: (a) first, and most obvious, is the volume of data—genome-wide scans provide data on hundreds of thousands of variants; (b) there are relatively low regulatory barriers to the provision of test results and marketing claims—genetic tests have been marketed within days of the report of a novel genetic association; and (c) costs are dramatically decreasing, with genome-wide evaluations now available at costs similar to tests for a few SNPs. Thus, combined with the general lack of direct evidence of clinical utility, policy makers and clinicians are faced with significant uncertainty about a large number of potential applications of genetic information.

Approaches to Evaluating Pharmacogenomics with Indirect Evidence

It is helpful to consider the context and evidence framework used to evaluate drugs when considering evidence criteria for pharmacogenomic tests. As outlined in the FDA document *Guidance for Industry: Providing clinical evidence of effectiveness for human drugs and biological products*, two well-conducted, independent RCTs are generally required to provide sufficient direct evidence of efficacy (56). However, the *Guidance for Industry* also states "it may be possible to conclude that a new dose, regimen, or dosage form is effective on the basis of pharmacokinetic data without an additional clinical efficacy trial." These guidelines imply that the level of evidence for a pharmacogenomic test could depend on the specifics of the case. For example, when the intervention based on a test result is a dosage change, "indirect" evidence such as the association between variants and clinically relevant outcomes, mechanistic plausibility, and pharmacokinetic-pharmacodynamic modeling could be considered (57). The challenge is to integrate this approach with well-established methods for evidence-based assessment of health care technologies.

The U.S. Centers for Disease Control and Prevention (CDC) has sponsored an assessment process for pre- and post-market evaluation of the effectiveness for DNA-based genetic tests through the *Evaluation of Genomic Applications in Practice and Prevention (EGAPP)* initiative and the independent EGAPP Working Group (58). EGAPP has sponsored evidence reviews of several pharmacogenomic tests, including gene expression profiling in breast cancer, and *CYP2D6* genotyping in the treatment of depression (17,44). These assessments, in conjunction with Human Genome Epidemiology (HuGE) reviews, serve a critical role in establishing the validity of claimed associations and their clinical relevance (59). Another primary goal of the EGAPP process, as the name suggests, is to identify evidence gaps. Given a general lack of direct evidence of clinical utility, a conclusion of "insufficient evidence to recommend for or against use" will be reached frequently. Indeed, in the case of *CYP2D6* genotyping to guide the use of antidepressants, EGAPP found insufficient evidence—even of a valid association between *CYP2D6* variants and antidepressant response or dose requirements (60).

Despite a lack of comparative effectiveness data on clinical utility (or even valid associations), however, it is possible to estimate a range of potential benefits—and harms—of pharmacogenomic tests using clinical and epidemiologic data in both a qualitative approach and a quantitative decision modeling framework. These approaches can provide bounds for the potential clinical utility of a pharmacogenomic test, as well as highlight critical data gaps that should be the focus of future research efforts.

Qualitative Framework for Assessing Pharmacogenomic Tests

A qualitative framework based on decision modeling and risk–benefit analysis has been developed for situations in which an expedient, preliminary estimate of clinical utility is needed (61). The genetic, clinical, and epidemiologic considerations comprising this framework are discussed below, using some of the examples presented in Table 27.1 to illustrate its application.

Comparison to the Next-Best Alternative
An important tenet of decision modeling in health care is that the outcomes of an intervention be assessed compared to the next best alternative—in what is called an "incremental analysis" (62). The comparator strategy for a pharmacogenomic test is the ability to monitor patients for toxic effects or drug response and individualize their therapy accordingly—without the use of pharmacogenomic testing. Two examples highlight this issue. Variation in the *CYP2C9* and *VKORC1* genes clearly impact warfarin dosing requirements, but given that anticoagulation status is (or should be) already closely monitored and individualized in warfarin patients, the incremental benefits of pharmacogenomics knowledge are less clear (38,63). In contrast, *CYP2D6* variants may be predictive for lack of response to tamoxifen, and in this case, women and their physicians do not have any way to assess whether treatment is effective—other than monitoring for breast cancer recurrence (28,30). Furthermore, aromatase inhibitors provide a viable treatment alternative to tamoxifen.

Validity and Clinical Relevance of Genetic Associations
As discussed above, it is clearly important to follow recent recommendations for validating genetic associations, particularly with the advent of genome-wide association studies and the risk of false-positive findings (64,65). In addition, the nature of the clinical outcome for which a valid association has been identified should be carefully considered. For example, *VKORC1* variants explain approximately 25% of

warfarin dose requirement variability, compared to approximately 10% for *CYP2C9* variants (37). Yet *CYP2C9* variants have been associated with a 2–4 times higher risk of major bleeding in several independent studies, while *VKORC1* variants do not appear to confer as significant a risk (23,66,67). These findings could be explained by the influence of *CYP2C9* variants on warfarin elimination half-life or an as yet unknown independent association of *CYP2C9* variants with bleeding risk, but most importantly, they illustrate the challenge of relying on intermediate outcomes (such as dose requirements, or anticoagulation level) to model (or implicitly infer) the influence of genetic variants on clinical events, life expectancy, and quality of life.

Prevalence of Genomic Variation

The frequency of the variant of interest in the target patient populations can have important effects on (a) the positive and negative predictive value of a test and (b) the efficiency (cost-effectiveness) of testing. Variants that have a low prevalence (e.g., <1%) will have poorer positive predictive value, and require that significantly more tests be conducted per variant identified in a population.

The relationship between genomic variation and geographic origin may present some significant challenges for health care delivery. For instance, will a patient's race or ethnicity implicitly be incorporated into treatment guidelines or drug reimbursement policies (e.g., drug formularies) that account for such pharmacogenomic effects? These issues may be exacerbated by the lack of data in traditionally underserved populations. In a recent systematic review, Jaja and colleagues did not identify a single study that evaluated the prevalence of *CYP* variants in an American Indian population (68). In contrast, it appears variation in *VKORC1* explains a significant portion of observed differences in warfarin dosing requirements across races, which may lead to more accurate dosing for patients of all races (37).

Availability, Risks, and Benefits of an Intervention Based on Test Results

Genomic variation associated with drug response has the advantage of providing relatively clear potential interventions: (a) change drug dosing, (b) change drugs, or (c) change monitoring. Estimating the effectiveness of these interventions compared to alternative approaches may be challenging, as discussed above, but the potential impacts are likely clearer than for interventions based on genetic tests for disease risk (such as lifestyle modification). A particular issue that will have a tremendous impact on the outcomes of testing is the actions of patients and providers in response to test results. For example, if a woman is categorized as having a low risk of breast cancer recurrence using a gene expression profile, yet chooses to undergo adjuvant chemotherapy, potential cost and quality of life benefits would be lost.

Outcomes Severity

The severity of the outcome that is the target for improvement will impact the absolute benefit derived from the test information. The morbidity (including patient quality of life), mortality, and likelihood of the clinical event are all important. For example, with warfarin therapy, the type of bleed that might be prevented—minor, major, fatal—is critically important, as are the probabilities of each of these events.

In summary, each of these factors should be carefully considered in the evaluation of a pharmacogenomic test—primarily to identify tests that are not likely to be beneficial, those that may be, and tests that have a relatively strong set of indirect data supporting their use. This approach has the advantage of being relatively expedient, but there are several important limitations. First, how is the balance of risks versus benefits weighted to determine if there is an overall net benefit? For example, how does the avoidance of chemotherapy compare to the risk of cancer recurrence? Second, particularly for genetic tests, there is a significant degree of uncertainty in many of the data elements—how can this be assessed? Lastly, it is important to ensure that all relevant comparators and clinical events have been included and communicated clearly to decision makers—doing so without a formal framework is challenging.

Quantitative Risk–Benefit Assessment

Recently, there has been heightened interest in the use of approaches to quantitatively assess risk–benefit tradeoffs. These efforts have been driven in part by drug safety concerns. A recent Institute of Medicine (IOM) study initiated by the FDA and the Department of Health and Human Services (DHHS), *The Future of Drug Safety: Promoting and Protecting the Health of the Public*, advised that the FDA's Center for Drug Evaluation and Research (CDER) "develop and continually improve a systematic approach to risk–benefit analysis" (69). One of the approaches being considered by the FDA is a decision-analytic, health-outcomes based approach (70).

Decision Modeling

Decision-analytic modeling provides an explicit framework for incorporating data from various sources in a quantitative and transparent fashion. Weinstein and Fineberg describe the decision-analytic approach as: (i) identify and bound the decision problem, (ii) structure the decision problem over time by developing a decision tree, (iii) characterize the information needed to inform the structure, and (iv) choose a preferred course of action (71,72). For example, decision-analytic techniques could be applied to gene expression profiling in breast cancer, where the test result is used to identify women at lower risk of cancer recurrence and thus decrease their likelihood of receiving adjuvant chemotherapy (54). Decision modeling could be used to incorporate

a) the association between test result and disease recurrence risk,
b) the association between test result and response to chemotherapy,
c) the baseline risk of disease recurrence, and
d) baseline treatment effect.

These data potentially would be derived from four or more separate studies, and be used to generate an estimate of the outcomes for women who utilize gene expression profiling versus those that do not.

There are two important, and related, limitations to decision-analytic modeling: lack of transparency and subjectivity. The approach requires judgment about which data to incorporate and estimates about the effect of the intervention on long-term outcomes such as disease progression and life expectancy. Because multiple data sources are incorporated in potentially complex models, there is often concern about the validity of the analysis and the potential for bias in the results. These are valid concerns, and can only be addressed through clear presentation of data inputs, model structure, assumptions, and analysis, in conjunction with rigorous peer review.

Evaluation of Uncertainty

A valuable component of decision modeling is the ability to explicitly evaluate uncertainty—particularly related to uncertainty in the data inputs, referred to as parameter uncertainty (72,73). Analysts can calculate not only expected or mean values for the probability and magnitude of benefits and risks, but also the variance surrounding these estimates. Parameter uncertainty for individual inputs can be derived from 95% confidence intervals of specific studies or meta-analyses, the range of point estimates reported in the literature, or expert opinion. Decision makers can evaluate and revise these estimates, thus making any implicit assumptions explicit. Analytically, the uncertainty in the various parameters in the analysis (including probabilities, life expectancy, and quality of life) is evaluated using a variety of approaches. In one-way sensitivity analyses, a single parameter is varied over a specified range and the impact on results evaluated. This is typically done for all inputs to identify the key parameters. The overall uncertainty in a decision analysis can be evaluated using probabilistic sensitivity analysis, in which distributions are assigned to the model inputs, and Monte Carlo simulation used to repeatedly draw sets of model inputs from these distributions (74). The distribution of results can provide decision makers with a more comprehensive assessment of the range and likelihood of various outcomes.

A Summary Measure of Net Benefit (Clinical Utility)

A decision model can be used to quantify the likelihood of various clinical events given different courses of action—including patient morbidity and mortality—but a framework to assess the relative value of morbidity and length of life is needed to derive a summary measure of clinical benefit. The fields of outcomes research and health economics utilize the quality-adjusted life year (QALY) to address this need (70). Patients' quality of life is accounted for by weighting life expectancy in a certain state of health by people's preferences for that state of health. These preferences are derived using several quantitative approaches, and fundamentally involve asking respondents to trade quality of life for life expectancy (or risk of death) (62). Preferences range from 0 = death to 1 = perfect health. For example, a life expectancy of 2.0 years with a quality of life preference rating of 0.8 would give 1.6 QALYs.

Net risk-benefit can be expressed either as a ratio or a difference, with the latter being more clinically intuitive. The incremental net health benefit (INHB) for one technology versus another is thus:

$$INHB = (B_2 - B_1) - (R_2 - R_1)$$

where B_2 and R_2 are the effectiveness and risk of the new intervention being evaluated and B_1 and R_1 are the effectiveness and risk of the standard therapy, and both effectiveness and risk are measured in QALYs. A positive INHB would be considered favorable—that is, the clinical benefits of the intervention outweigh the clinical risks in terms of their impact on QALYs, and the test would be deemed to have "clinical utility."

The advantages of using QALYs to measure both risks and benefits are that different clinical events are weighted according to their impact on life expectancy and quality of life, and a summary measure can be calculated. The challenges in applying and interpreting QALY-based risk–benefit analysis include heterogeneity in people's preferences for specific risks and benefits, modeling complexity, and including qualitative social factors that may arise, particularly with genomics, such as impact on family members and the value of "information for information's sake" (75,76). Given these challenges, it is useful to present projected clinical events (e.g., heart attacks or GI bleeds) rather than relying only on QALYs, and allow decision makers to implicitly weigh these outcomes in comparison to the projected QALY impacts.

Risk-Benefit Analysis and Decision Making

Once decision makers have available quantitative estimates of the potential net benefit, the amount of uncertainty in this estimate, and identification of the most important data gaps, they will be better positioned to ascertain not only the likely clinical utility of the test, but assess the evidence requirements that should be established for that specific test. For example, indirect evidence may be sufficient for a test with a high likelihood of benefit and low risk, whereas a test with uncertain benefit and potential downsides might require direct evidence (e.g., RCT-level) of clinical utility before it could be recommended for use.

Example: Pharmacogenomics of Aminoglycoside-Induced Hearing Loss

Background and Rationale

A genetic test to identify patients with a mitochondrial mutation (*A1555G*) that may predispose patients to aminoglycoside-induced hearing loss has recently been developed and marketed (77). Although the *A1555G* variant is rare, it appears to confer a high risk of severe hearing loss in patients exposed to aminoglycosides. The question arises: in what population might this test be most useful? Aminoglycosides are a cornerstone of first-line therapy in cystic fibrosis (CF) patients with acute *Pseudomonas aeruginosa* respiratory infections, yet aminoglycoside-induced hearing loss (ranging from mild to severe) may occur in 1–15% of CF patients (78,79). The benefit of a proven, first-line agent for a serious and potentially life-threatening infection must be weighed against the risk of developing drug-induced hearing loss. To gain a better understanding of the potential outcomes associated with *A1555G* mitochondrial testing to guide aminoglycoside use in this patient population, we previously developed and evaluated a decision analytic model of this approach (80).

Approach

The structure of the decision model is shown in Figure 27.1. The two strategies evaluated are standard of care (no testing) versus *A1555G* testing. In patients receiving the genetic test, those with the mutation were assumed to be treated with IV ciprofloxacin and ceftazidime while those testing negative were assumed to be treated with tobramycin and ceftazidime. Patients in the standard care group received tobramycin and ceftazidime.

Data were derived from the literature, data from the U.S. Cystic Fibrosis Foundation National Patient Registry, and expert clinical opinion as needed. It was assumed in the base case that there was no difference in mortality between patients receiving quinolones + β-lactam versus those receiving aminoglycoside + β-lactam. This assumption was based on evidence from one randomized clinical trial suggesting equivalent efficacy of quinolones to aminoglycosides at eradicating gram-negative bacterial infections (81). However, because there is evidence of higher rates of quinolone resistant *Pseudomonas* infections compared to tobramycin-resistant infections in CF patients (82), we used a scenario analysis to assess the potential negative impacts of this drug switch by estimating a 10% relative increase in lifetime mortality with ciprofloxacin versus tobramycin to obtain a higher absolute risk of death of 2.8% attributable to lifetime use of a second-line therapy.

The systematic review of association studies revealed few data, with much of the available data of relatively poor quality. Most studies were small (<50 people) and conducted on either large high-risk pedigrees of maternally inherited hearing loss or conducted on individuals who already had severe to profound hearing loss. For variant positive individuals, the probability of mild hearing loss as a result of aminoglycoside exposure was estimated at 66% (83). The estimated prevalence in the U.S. population was approximately 1 in 1,000 (84), although two studies investigating the prevalence of the variant in populations worldwide have reported widely varying estimates, from 5 to 500 per 1,000 (85,86). The sensitivity and specificity of the *A1555G* test were estimated to be 99.9% and 87.0% based on communications with the test provider.

Results

In the base-case evaluation of the decision model, *A1555G* testing decreased the lifetime absolute risk of severe aminoglycoside-induced hearing loss by 0.12%. Because of the low prevalence of the mutation, over 800 patients would have to be tested to prevent one case of severe hearing loss, and in combination with a test

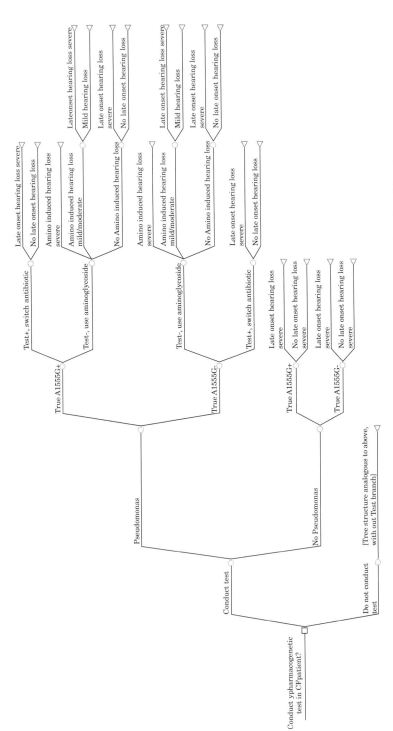

Figure 27.1 Decision model of pharmacogenomic testing to avoid aminoglycoside-induced hearing loss.

specificity of 87%, over 95% of patients that tested positive would be false-positives. The magnitude of the benefit in terms of quality of life was relatively small, with an expected increase of 0.0043 QALYs (1.6 days).

Given the uncertainty in the data informing the model, there was significant variability in the results. For instance, if avoidance of aminoglycosides in patients testing positive leads to an absolute increase in the lifetime risk of death from *Pseudomonas* infection of 0.8% or greater (e.g., as a result of increased drug resistance), *A1555G* testing could lead to a *decrease* in QALYs—that is, the risks would outweigh the benefits (Table 27.2). Several other model inputs influenced the results, most notably the probability of exposure to an aminoglycoside, test specificity, the quality of life impact of hearing loss, and mutation prevalence. Figure 27.2 shows the impact of both the risk of switching drug therapy, and test specificity, on the overall benefit (difference in QALYs) of the testing versus not testing strategies.

Implications

The results of the decision analysis indicate that there are significant data gaps and uncertainty in the outcomes with *A1555G* testing, and that it could lead to worse patient outcomes overall due to the avoidance of first-line therapy in the great majority of patients who are false positives. These findings have important policy implications. For example, a recent editorial in *BMJ* stated:

> We recommend that the true prevalence of the mutation...be ascertained to determine the cost effectiveness of screening everyone prescribed aminoglycoside antibiotics. In the meantime, patients who are likely to receive multiple courses of aminoglycosides...should be screened. (87)

In contrast, the decision analysis suggests additional data should be collected *before* eliminating a first-line agent used to treat often life-threatening infections.

Table 27.2 Evaluation of uncertainty for decision model of pharmacogenomic testing to avoid aminoglycoside-induced hearing loss

Model Input	INPUT VALUE		RESULT (QALYs)	
	Low	High	Range	
Absolute increase in mortality risk from avoiding first-line therapy	0.000	0.028	−0.012	0.004
Probability of exposure to aminoglycoside	0.300	0.800	0.003	0.007
Test specificity	0.830	0.930	0.002	0.006
Quality of life impact of mild hearing loss	0.850	0.950	0.003	0.006
Mutation prevalence	0.000	0.005	0.004	0.006
Quality of life of severe hearing loss (cochlear implant)	0.750	0.850	0.004	0.005

QALY, quality-adjusted life year

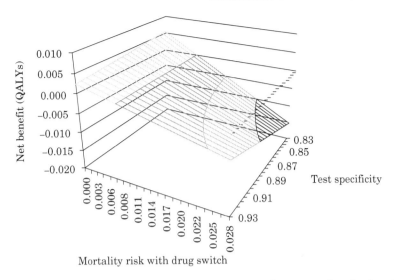

Figure 27.2   Influence of risk of drug switch and test specificity on net benefit of testing.

This example highlights the ability of decision-analytic techniques to synthesize disparate data, assess uncertainty resulting from a paucity of data, and provide quantitative estimates of risk–benefit tradeoff through the use of a QALY health outcomes framework.

Summary

Pharmacogenomics is a promising yet complex application of human genomics to health care. Although identification of valid genetic associations and establishment of the clinical utility of pharmacogenomic applications has unfolded at a measured pace, promising clinical applications are beginning to emerge. A paucity of data will be an ongoing challenge, and an opportunity exists to utilize clinical and epidemiologic data within quantitative modeling frameworks to evaluate the likely health benefits and risks of pharmacogenomic tests and the uncertainty surrounding these estimates, and identify critical data gaps. These analyses can provide guidance for patients, providers, and policy makers in a genomic era of many possibilities yet little evidence.

References

1. Weinshilboum R. Inheritance and drug response. *N Engl J Med.* 2003;348(6):529–537.
2. Evans WE, McLeod HL. Pharmacogenomics—drug disposition, drug targets, and side effects. *N Engl J Med.* 2003;348(6):538–549.
3. Motulsky AG. Drug reactions enzymes, and biochemical genetics. *J Am Med Assoc.* 1957;165(7):835–837.

4. Gurwitz D, Motulsky AG. "Drug reactions, enzymes, and biochemical genetics": 50 years later. *Pharmacogenomics.* 2007;8(11):1479–1484.
5. Manunta P, Bianchi G. Pharmacogenomics and pharmacogenetics of hypertension: update and perspectives—the adducin paradigm. *J Am Soc Nephrol.* 2006; 17(4_suppl_2):S30–S35.
6. Davis B. Absence of an interaction between the alpha-adducin polymorphism and anti hypertensive treatment on cardiovascular risk in high-risk hypertensives: the GenHAT study. *J Hypertens.* 2005;23:S272–S272.
7. Gerhard T, GongY, Beitelshees AL, et al., Association between CV outcomes, diuretic use and the alpha-adducin gene; results from the INternational VErapamil SR-Trandolapril STudy (INVEST). *Circulation.* 2005;112(Suppl.II):608.
8. Davis BR, Arnett DK, Boerwinkle E, Ford CE, Leiendecker-Foster C, Miller MB, et al. Antihypertensive therapy, the alpha-adducin polymorphism, and cardiovascular disease in high-risk hypertensive persons: the Genetics of Hypertension-Associated Treatment Study. *Pharmacogenomics J.* 2007;7(2):112–122.
9. Schelleman H, Klungel OH, Witteman JC, Hofman A, van Duijn CM, de Boer A, et al. The influence of the alpha-adducin G460W polymorphism and angiotensinogen M235T polymorphism on antihypertensive medication and blood pressure. *Eur J Hum Genet.* 2006;14(7):860–866.
10. Boekholdt SM, Sacks FM, Jukema JW, Shepherd J, Freeman DJ, McMahon AD, et al. Cholesteryl ester transfer protein TaqIB variant, high-density lipoprotein cholesterol levels, cardiovascular risk, and efficacy of pravastatin treatment: individual patient meta-analysis of 13 677 subjects. *Circulation.* 2005;111(3):278–287.
11. Mellen PB, Herrington DM Pharmacogenomics of blood pressure response to antihypertensive treatment. *J Hypertens.* 2005;23(7):1311–1325.
12. Tantisira KG, Weiss ST The pharmacogenetics of asthma: an update. *Curr Opin Mol Ther.* 2005;7(3):209–217.
13. Ferdinands JM, et al. ADRB2 Arg16Gly polymorphism, lung function, and mortality: results from the Atherosclerosis Risk in Communities study. *PLoS ONE.* 2007;2(3):e289.
14. Feldman DS, et al. Mechanisms of disease: beta-adrenergic receptors--alterations in signal transduction and pharmacogenomics in heart failure. *Nat Clin Pract Cardiovasc Med.* 2005;2(9):475–483.
15. Binder EB, Holsboer F. Pharmacogenomics and antidepressant drugs. *Ann Med.* 2006;38(2):82–94.
16. Matchar DB, et al. Testing for cytochrome P450 polymorphisms in adults with nonpsychotic depression treated with selective serotonin reuptake inhibitors (SSRIs). *Evid Rep Technol Assess (Full Rep).* 2007(146):1–77.
17. Evaluation of Genomic Applications in Practice and Prevention (EGAPP) Working Group. Recommendations from the EGAPP Working Group: testing for cytochrome P450 polymorphisms in adults with nonpsychotic depression treated with selective serotonin reuptake inhibitors. *Genet Med.* 2007;9(12):819–825.
18. Ioannidis JP, et al. A network of investigator networks in human genome epidemiology. *Am J Epidemiol.* 2005;162(4):302–304.
19. Ioannidis JP, et al. A road map for efficient and reliable human genome epidemiology. *Nat Genet.* 2006;38(1):3–5.
20. Khoury MJ, et al. Reporting of systematic reviews: the challenge of genetic association studies. *PLoS Med.* 2007;4(6):e211.
21. Relling MV, et al. Mercaptopurine therapy intolerance and heterozygosity at the thiopurine S-methyltransferase gene locus. *J Natl Cancer Inst.* 1999;91(23):2001–2008.
22. Rocha JC, et al. Pharmacogenetics of outcome in children with acute lymphoblastic leukemia. *Blood.* 2005;105(12):4752–4758.

23. Higashi MK, et al. Association between CYP2C9 genetic variants and anticoagulation-related outcomes during warfarin therapy. *JAMA*. 2002;287(13):1690–1698.

24. Gage B, Eby C, Johnson JA, Deych E, Rieder MJ, Ridker PM, et al. Use of pharmacogenetic and clinical factors to predict the therapeutic dose of warfarin. *Clin Pharmacol Ther*. September 2008;84(3):326–331.

25. Evaluation of Genomic Applications in Practice and Prevention (EGAPP) Working Group. Recommendations from the EGAPP Working Group: can UGT1A1 genotyping reduce morbidity and mortality in patients with metastatic colorectal cancer treated with irinotecan? *Genet Med*. 2009;11(1):15–20.

26. Haga SB, Thummel KE, Burke W. Adding pharmacogenetics information to drug labels: lessons learned. *Pharmacogenet Genomics*. 2006;16(12):847–854.

27. Frueh FW, et al. Pharmacogenomic biomarker information in drug labels approved by the United States food and drug administration: prevalence of related drug use. *Pharmacotherapy*. 2008;28(8):992–998.

28. Goetz MP, et al. Pharmacogenetics of tamoxifen biotransformation is associated with clinical outcomes of efficacy and hot flashes. *J Clin Oncol*. 2005;23(36):9312–9318.

29. Goetz MP, Kamal A, Ames MM. Tamoxifen pharmacogenomics: the role of CYP2D6 as a predictor of drug response. *Clin Pharmacol Ther*. 2008;83(1):160–166.

30. Schroth W, et al. Breast cancer treatment outcome with adjuvant tamoxifen relative to patient CYP2D6 and CYP2C19 genotypes. *J Clin Oncol*. 2007;25(33):5187–5193.

31. Lotsch J, et al. Genetic predictors of the clinical response to opioid analgesics: clinical utility and future perspectives. *Clin Pharmacokinet*. 2004;43(14):983–1013.

32. Madadi P, et al. Pharmacogenetics of neonatal opioid toxicity following maternal use of codeine during breastfeeding: a case-control study. *Clin Pharmacol Ther*. 2009;85(1):31–35.

33. Mega JL, et al. Cytochrome p-450 polymorphisms and response to clopidogrel. *N Engl J Med*. 2009;360(4):354–362.

34. Martin AM, et al. Predisposition to abacavir hypersensitivity conferred by HLA-B*5701 and a haplotypic Hsp70-Hom variant. *Proc Natl Acad Sci USA*. 2004;101(12):4180–4185.

35. Hughes AR, et al. Pharmacogenetics of hypersensitivity to abacavir: from PGx hypothesis to confirmation to clinical utility. *Pharmacogenomics J*. 2008;8(6):365–374.

36. Ferrell PB, Jr, McLeod HL. Carbamazepine, HLA-B*1502 and risk of Stevens-Johnson syndrome and toxic epidermal necrolysis: US FDA recommendations. *Pharmacogenomics*. 2008;9(10):1543–1546.

37. Rieder MJ, et al. Effect of VKORC1 haplotypes on transcriptional regulation and warfarin dose. *N Engl J Med*. 2005;352(22):2285–2293.

38. Schwarz UI, et al. Genetic determinants of response to warfarin during initial anticoagulation. *N Engl J Med*. 2008;358(10):999–1008.

39. Liggett SB, et al. A polymorphism within a conserved beta(1)-adrenergic receptor motif alters cardiac function and beta-blocker response in human heart failure. *Proc Natl Acad Sci USA*. 2006;103(30):11288–11293.

40. Genentech I. *Herceptin® (Trastuzumab) [full prescribing information]*. South San Francisco, CA: Genentech, Inc; 2005.

41. Paik S, et al. A multigene assay to predict recurrence of tamoxifen-treated, node-negative breast cancer. *N Engl J Med*. 2004;351(27):2817–2826.

42. van de Vijver MJ, et al. A gene-expression signature as a predictor of survival in breast cancer. *N Engl J Med*. 2002;347(25):1999–2009.

43. van 't Veer LJ, et al. Gene expression profiling predicts clinical outcome of breast cancer. *Nature*. 2002;415(6871):530.

44. Evaluation of Genomic Applications in Practice and Prevention (EGAPP) Working Group. Recommendations from the EGAPP Working Group: can tumor gene expression profiling improve outcomes in patients with breast cancer? *Genet Med*. 2009;11(1):66–73.

45. Amado RG, et al. Wild-type KRAS is required for panitumumab efficacy in patients with metastatic colorectal cancer. *J Clin Oncol.* 2008;26(10):1626–1634.

46. Jimeno A, Messersmith WA, Hirsch FR, Franklin WA, Eckhardt SG. KRAS mutations and sensitivity to epidermal growth factor receptor inhibitors in colorectal cancer: practical application of patient selection. *J Clin Oncol.* 2009;27(7):1130–1136.

47. Tsao MS, et al. Erlotinib in lung cancer—molecular and clinical predictors of outcome. *N Engl J Med.* 2005;353(2):133–144.

48. Garrison LP, et al. *Backgrounder on Pharmacogenomics for the Pharmaceutical and Biotechnology Industries: Basic Science, Future Scenarios, Policy Directions.* University of Washington, Pharmaceutical Outcomes Research and Policy Program; 2007.

49. *Top 200 brand-name drugs by retail dollars in 2005*, in *Drug Topics.* 2006.

50. *Top 200 brand-name drugs by units in 2004*, in *Drug Topics.* 2005.

51. Mallal S, et al. HLA-B*5701 screening for hypersensitivity to abacavir. *N Engl J Med.* 2008;358(6):568–579.

52. Hillman MA, et al. A prospective, randomized pilot trial of model-based warfarin dose initiation using CYP2C9 genotype and clinical data. *Clin Med Res.* 2005;3(3):137–145.

53. Voora D, et al. Prospective dosing of warfarin based on cytochrome P-450 2C9 genotype. *Thromb Haemost.* 2005;93(4):700–705.

54. Sparano JA, Paik S. Development of the 21-gene assay and its application in clinical practice and clinical trials. *J Clin Oncol.* 2008;26(5):721–728.

55. Garrison LP, Austin MJ. The economics of personalized medicine: a model of incentives for value creation and capture. *Drug Inf J.* 2007;41(4):501–509.

56. *Guidance for Industry: Providing Clinical Evidence of Effectiveness for Human Drugs and Biological Products.* FDA, Editor. 1998. Available at: http://www.fda.gov/downloads/Drugs/GuidanceComplianceRegulatoryInformation/Guidances/ucm078749.pdf

57. Hamberg AK, et al. A PK-PD model for predicting the impact of age, CYP2C9, and VKORC1 genotype on individualization of warfarin therapy. *Clin Pharmacol Ther.* 2007;81(4):529–538.

58. CDC. *Evaluation of Genomic Applications in Practice and Prevention (EGAPP): Implementation and Evaluation of a Model Approach.* Atlanta; 2006. http://www.cdc.gov/genomics/gtesting/egapp/about.htm

59. Khoury MJ, et al. On the synthesis and interpretation of consistent but weak gene-disease associations in the era of genome-wide association studies. *Int J Epidemiol.* 2007;36(2):439–445.

60. EGAPP. Recommendations from the EGAPP Working Group: testing for cytochrome P450 polymorphisms in adults with nonpsychotic depression treated with selective serotonin reuptake inhibitors. *Genet Med.* 2007;9(12):819–825.

61. Flowers CR, Veenstra D. The role of cost-effectiveness analysis in the era of pharmacogenomics. *Pharmacoeconomics.* 2004;22(8):481–493.

62. Gold MR, et al., eds. *Cost-Effectiveness in Health and Medicine.* New York: Oxford University Press; 1996.

63. Eckman MH, et al. Cost-effectiveness of using pharmacogenetic information in warfarin dosing for patients with nonvalvular atrial fibrillation. *Ann Intern Med.* 2009;150(2):73–83.

64. Ioannidis JP, et al. Assessment of cumulative evidence on genetic associations: interim guidelines. *Int J Epidemiol.* 2008;37(1):120–132.

65. Little J, Higgins JP, Ioannidis JP, Moher D, Gagnon F, von Elm E, et al. Strengthening the reporting of genetic association studies (STREGA): an extension of the STROBE statement. *Eur J Epidemiol.* 2009;24(1):37–55.

66. Limdi NA, McGwin G, Goldstein JA, Beasley TM, Arnett DK, Adler BK, et al. Influence of CYP2C9 and VKORC1 1173C/T genotype on the risk of hemorrhagic complications

in African-American and European-American patients on warfarin. *Clin Pharmacol Ther.* February 2008;83(2):312–321.

67. Meckley LM, et al. An analysis of the relative effects of VKORC1 and CYP2C9 variants on anticoagulation related outcomes in warfarin-treated patients. *Thromb Haemost.* 2008;100(2):229–239.

68. Jaja C, et al. Cytochrome p450 enzyme polymorphism frequency in indigenous and native american populations: a systematic review. *Community Genet.* 2008;11(3):141–149.

69. (IOM), I.o.M. *The Future of Drug Safety: Promoting and Protecting the Health of the Public.* Washington, DC: Institute of Medicine of the National Academies; 2006.

70. Garrison LP, Jr, Towse A, Bresnahan BW. Assessing a structured, quantitative health outcomes approach to drug risk-benefit analysis. *Health Aff (Millwood).* 2007;26(3):684–695.

71. Weinstein M, Fineberg H. *Clinical Decision Analysis.* Philadelphia: Saunders; 1980.

72. Briggs A, Claxton K, and Sculpher M. Decision modelling for health economic evaluation. In: Gray A, Briggs A, eds. *Health Economic Evaluation.* New York: Oxford University Press; 2007.

73. Briggs AH. Handling uncertainty in cost-effectiveness models. *Pharmacoeconomics.* 2000;17(5):479–500.

74. Briggs A. Probabilistic analysis of cost-effectiveness models: statistical representation of parameter uncertainty. *Value Health.* 2005;8(1):1–2.

75. Grosse SD, Wordsworth S, Payne K. Economic methods for valuing the outcomes of genetic testing: beyond cost-effectiveness analysis. *Genet Med.* 2008;10(9):648–654.

76. Payne K, et al. Outcome measurement in clinical genetics services: a systematic review of validated measures. *Value Health.* 2008;11(3):497–508.

77. Athena Diagnostics. *OtoDx aminoglycoside hypersensitivity test.* http://www.athenadiagnostics.com/content/diagnostic-ed/hearing-loss/otodx Accessed June 18, 2009.

78. Gibson RL, Burns JL, Ramsey BW. Pathophysiology and management of pulmonary infections in cystic fibrosis. *Am J Respir Crit Care Med.* 2003;168(8):918–951.

79. Mulheran M, et al. Occurrence and risk of cochleotoxicity in cystic fibrosis patients receiving repeated high-dose aminoglycoside therapy. *Antimicrob.Agents Chemother.* 2001;45(9):2502–2509.

80. Veenstra DL, et al. Pharmacogenomic testing to prevent aminoglycoside-induced hearing loss in cystic fibrosis patients: potential impact on clinical, patient, and economic outcomes. *Genet Med.* 2007;9(10):695–704.

81. Church D, et al. Sequential ciprofloxacin therapy in pediatric cystic fibrosis: comparative study vs. ceftazidime/tobramycin in the treatment of acute pulmonary exacerbations. *Pediatr Infect Dis J.* 1997;16(1):97–105.

82. Shawar R, et al. Activities of Tobramycin and six other antibiotics against Pseudomonas aeruginosa isolates from patients with Cystic Fibrosis. *Antimicrob Agents Chemother.* 1999;43(12):2877–2880.

83. Usami S-i, et al. Prevalence of mitochondrial gene mutations among hearing impaired patients. *J Med Genet.* 2000;37:38–40.

84. Tang HY, et al. Genetic susceptibility to aminoglycoside ototoxicity: how many are at risk? *Genet Med.* 2002;4(5):336–345.

85. Fischel-Ghodsian N. Mitochondrial deafness. *Ear Hear.* 2003;24(303):313.

86. Lehtonen M, et al. Frequency of mitochondrial DNA point mutations among patients with familial sensorineural hearing impairment. *Eur J Pediatr.* 2000;8:315–319.

87. Bitner-Glindzicz M, Rahman S. Ototoxicity caused by aminoglycosides. *BMJ.* 2007;335(7624):784–785.

28

The human epigenome and cancer

Mukesh Verma

Introduction

Epigenetics, the study of mechanisms that involve mitotically heritable changes in DNA other than changes in nucleotide sequence, represents a new frontier in research, especially in cancer. Most of our cells contain the same DNA, yet gene expression varies dramatically among different tissues. Epigenetic mechanisms establish and maintain this tissue-specific gene expression. Information in the genome exists in at least two forms, genetic and epigenetic. The genetic information provides the blueprint for the manufacture of all the proteins necessary to create a living organism, whereas the epigenetic information provides additional instructions on how, where, and when the genetic information will be used.

The DNA methylation and histone modification patterns associated with the development and progression of cancer have potential clinical use. The functional importance of epigenetic changes lies in their ability to regulate gene expression. Three major steps in epigenetic regulation are promoter methylation, histone acetylation/deacetylation, and chromatin conformation changes. Recently, the role of small noncoding RNAs has been included as an epigenetic mechanism (1). DNA methylation is one of the most common epigenetic events taking place in the human genome. Of the various types of epigenetic regulations, DNA methylation is a complex process where DNA methyltransferases (DNMTs) catalyze the addition of a methyl group to the 5-carbon position of the cytosine. DNA methylation of cytosine occurs when a guanine base follows cytosine, so the dinucleotide (CpG) gets methylated. Clusters of CpGs are called "CpG islands," which are predominantly located in the promoter region. Three DNMTs (DNMT1, DNMT3a, and DNMT3b) have been identified and recent studies have revealed that a functional cooperation between DNMT1 and DNMT3b is needed to maintain methylation status in cancer cells (2).

A variety of chemicals (such as nickel, arsenic, cadmium), certain base analogs, radiation, smoke, stress, hormones (such as estradiol), and reactive oxygen species can alter the phenotypes of mammalian cells, via epigenetic mechanisms, without changing the underlying DNA sequence (3). These agents can alter the methylation and/or acetylation state of the DNA. Contrary to mutations, epigenetic changes can be reversed by chemicals and thus provide opportunities for development of intervention and treatment strategies. Epigenetic markers could be used in cancer detection, diagnosis, prognosis, and epidemiology. Research opportunities at the National Cancer Institute (NCI), one of the 27 Institutes and Centers at the National Institutes of Health (NIH) and efforts to complete human epigenome are discussed.

Epigenetic Mechanisms

Our understanding of the role of epigenetic abnormalities in disease processes is still in its infancy. Epigenetic controls can become dysregulated in cancer cells. Such dysregulation can affect a variety of gene types, including tumor suppressor genes, oncogenes, and cancer-associated viral genes, all of which are subject to regulation by epigenetic mechanisms (4–6). Genomic methylation patterns are frequently altered in tumor cells, with global hypomethylation accompanying region-specific hypermethylation events. When hypermethylation occurs within the promoter of a tumor suppressor gene, silencing of expression of the associated gene can occur, providing the cell with a growth advantage in a manner akin to deletions or mutations. Examples of such genes are *APC, RAR, DAPK, E-cadherin, GSTP1, LKB1, MGMT,* and *TIMP3.* Conversely, hypomethylation of oncogenes leads to upregulation of genes associated with cell proliferation in cancer tissues. Examples of oncogenes activated by hypomethylation are *Raf, c-fos, c-myc, c-Ha-ras,* and *c-k-ras.* Importantly, the change in methylation patterns is considered an early event in cancer development. Selected genes regulated by epigenetic mechanism in cancer are shown in Table 28.1. The components of epigentic mechanism and gene expression are shown in Figure 28.1.

Epigenetic mechanisms have been studied in many seemingly disparate areas of scientific investigations from organ development to gene regulation. The importance of pursuing such investigations has come to the forefront, following the completion of the Human Genome Project. The challenge now is to understand the regulation of gene function, an activity that is dependent to a large extent on epigenetic control. One area of scientific investigation into epigenetic controls involves histone deacetylation. Histone deacetylation leads to chromatin condensation, with concomitant transcriptional repression. Conversely, the covalent addition of acetyl groups to the lysines in the tails of histones appears to result in decondensed chromatin that is associated with upregulation of gene expression. Histone acetylation and deacetylation function in a dynamic equilibrium in a manner that is regulated by histone acetyltransferases (HATs) and histone deacetylases (HDACs) (7). The quantitative balance between HATs and HDACs, and thus the dynamics of histone acetylation can be altered by exogenous agents. Those epigenetic agents that alter net acetylation so as to favor chromatin decondensation and gene expression are only effective in the context of previously "competent" chromatin, that is, partially transcriptionally active chromatin.

Table 28.1 Epigenetic modifications in different cancers

Cancer Type	Genes	Epigenetic Change and Comments	Reference
Bladder cancer	*CDKN2A*, p16^{INK4A}, *RASSF1A*, *PRSS3*	Hypermethylation (detected in tissue as well as in exfoliated cells from urine)	Marsit et al., 2006 (129)
Brain cancer	*MGMT, TIMP-3*	Hypermethylation in glioblastoma, could be used for diagnosis and prognosis	(60,130,131)
Breast cancer	*APC, BRCA1, CDH1, CXCL12, Cyclin D2, HIC-1, PROX1, RARbeta, RASSF1a, RUNX3, TMS1*	Hypermethylation	(90,132–139)
B-cell acute lymphoblastic leukemia (BALL)	Interleukin-12 receptor beta2 (IL-12Rbeta2)	Hypermethylation for tumor escape to B ALL	(140)
Cervical cancer	*SPARC, TFPI2, RRAD, SFRP1, MT1G, NMES1*	Hypermethylated in invasive cancer	(49)
Colon cancer	*APC, CDKN2A,CRBP1, DAPK, MGMT, MLH1, TIMP-3*	Hypermethylation	(28,40,51–54,58,141)
Endometrial cancer	*MLH1, TITF1, SESN3*	Hypermethylation	(142,143)
Esophageal cancer	*APC, CDKN2A, CALCA, MGMT, TIMP3p, p14ARF*	Hypermethylation	(58,144)
Gastric cancer	*ATM, p16INK4a(CDKN2A), hMLH1, MGMT, DAPK, CDH1(ECAD)*	Hypermethylation, *H. pylori* infection in 80% cases	(80,145)
Head and neck cancer	*DAPK, MGMT*, p16^{INK4A}	Hypermethylation	(146)
Kidney (renal) cancer	*RASSF1, RSSA3, TIMP-3*, p16^{INK4A}	Hypermethylation	(33–35)
Liver cancer	*T-cadherin*, p16^{INK4A}	Hypermethylation of *p16* and *T-cadherin*; functional assay of *T-cadherin* shows reduction in *T-cadherin* level which is correlated with the progression of liver cancer	(56,146,147)
Lung cancer	*RASSF1, RARbeta, DAPK*, p16^{INK4A}, *p15, MGMT*	Hypermethylation	(51,52,146,148)
Nasopharyngeal carcinoma	*RASSF1A, p16/INK4A, p14/ARF*	Hypermethylation	(149)

(*Continued*)

Table 28.1 Continued

Cancer Type	Genes	Epigenetic Change and Comments	Reference
Non-Hodgkin Lymphoma (NHL)	DLC-1, PCDHGB7, CYP27B1, EFNA5, CCND1 and RARbeta2	Hypermethylation	(150)
Ovarian cancer	FANCF, IGFBP-3, GSTP1, ER-alpha, hMLH1	Member of Fanconi gene family involved in DNA repair, genes involved in detoxification, and tumor suppressor genes	(41,151,152)
Pancreatic cancer	p14, p16^{INK4A}	Hypermethylation	(32,45–47)
Prostate cancer	GSTP1	Hypermethylation	(146)
Skin cancer	CDH1, p73, SOCS (suppressors of cytokine signaling)	Hypermethylation	(153–156)
Thyroid cancer	RASSF1	Hypermethylation	(157)
Wilms' tumors	glioma pathogenesis-related 1/ related to testis-specific, vespid, and pathogenesis proteins 1 (GLIPR1/RTVP-1)	Hypomethylation	(30)

Note: In most cases, tissue samples were analyzed for epigenetic changes, and in a few cases biofluids containing either circular DNA or exfoliated cells were used.

Investigations into the manner in which DNA methylation influences gene expression have revealed proteins that bind specifically to the methylated DNA. Binding of such proteins to methylated DNA leads to the suppression of gene expression. Only a few methylated DNA binding proteins have been identified thus far. One of these, MeCP2, binds to methylated DNA, leading to inhibition of gene expression.

Another context in which methylation of DNA exerts important control over gene expression involves viral genes. For example, methylation of the promoter region of the Epstein-Barr Virus (EBV) genome maintains latency of the virus thereby preventing the expression of viral antigens. The absence of viral antigens enables EBV to escape immune surveillance. Evasion of the host immune system may well explain the observed association of EBV infection with certain lymphomas and nasopharyngeal carcinomas.

The organization of DNA into chromatin presents the cell with the opportunity to use powerful regulatory mechanisms broadly defined as epigenetics (8). Research designed to characterize the molecular basis of disease tends to be gene-centric and may therefore miss important sources of variation of expression. Increasing evidence demonstrates that epigenetic mechanisms are linked to gene activation, gene silencing, and chromosomal instability (9–12). Thus, a

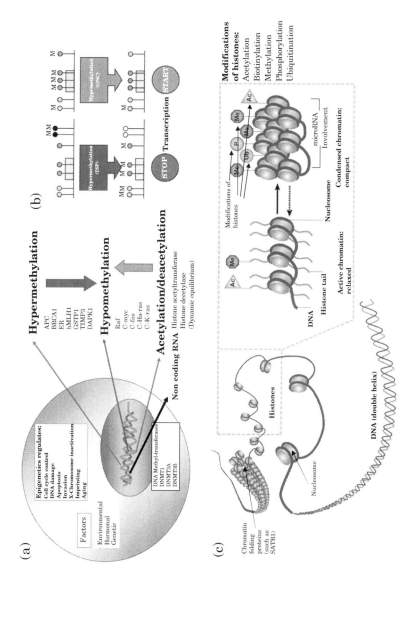

Figure 28.1 Schematic representation of the epigenetic mechanism. (a). Major players in epigenetic regulation are DNA methylation, histone modification, chromatin compaction and noncoding small RNAs. (b). Hypermethylation of tumor suppressor genes and hypomethylation of oncogenes. (c). Histone modification and chromatin compactation.

purely DNA sequence-based approach (naked DNA snapshot) may be insufficient
to explain pathogenesis of diseases that have a heritable component, but are modulated by other nongenetic or extragenetic mechanisms. For example, genomic
imprinting silences one parental allele in the zygotes of gametes via DNA methylation and histone modification (8). Imprinting in the germline via gene methylation
is heritable, and can result in transgenerational effects. Only about 1% of genes
are imprinted by this mechanism (13–21). Among the human diseases associated
with dysfunctional epigenetic regulation and/or deregulation of imprinted genes
are Beckwidth-Wiedeman syndrome, Prader-Willi/Angelman syndrome, placental
overgrowth, neurological and behavioral disorders, neuroblastoma, breast cancer, acute myeloblastic leukemia, Wilms' tumor, and rhabdomyosarcoma (15–21).
Evidence suggests that deregulation of imprinting also may impact immunological disorders such as type 1 diabetes, rheumatoid arthritis, lupus, inflammatory
bowel disease, and selective IgA deficiency.

Epigenetics and Its Potential Applications in Epidemiology

The study of the associations between epigenetic variation and risk of disease has
been called epigenetic epidemiology (22). Although methylation markers have been
studied in different populations at high risk of developing cancer, histone and other
epigenetic markers have not been evaluated for the same purpose. There is an urgent
need to identify epigenetic biomarkers for epidemiologic purposes. A biomarker is
a phenotypic parameter (generally a protein or other molecule, a structure or a process) that is measured and evaluated as an indicator of normal or pathogenic biological processes, or pharmacologic responses to a therapeutic intervention. In cancer
epidemiology, it is sometimes not possible to obtain DNA from study participants.
Fortunately, emerging evidence suggests that aberrantly methylated DNA can be
measured noninvasively. In addition, if epigenetic biomarkers can be found and validated for use not only as surrogates for epigenetic characteristics but also as indicators of the effects of epigenetic characteristics, their study will facilitate further
research into the role of epigenetic factors in cancer etiology.

It is critical that sensitive, quantitative, high-throughput techniques should be
used to identify epigenetic changes in the large number of samples required for population-based research and for the identification and validation of biomarkers. Such
technologies now exist and are important for the comparison of cancer risk between
groups of people with different epigenetic patterns. Current technologies to detect
epigenetic changes are quantitative, robust, inexpensive, sensitive, and applicable for
the analysis of a large number of samples (23). Methylation markers can be detected
in tissues, exfoliated cells (buccal cells), serum, and other body fluids (urine, pancreatic fluid, and nipple aspirate) (24–27). Since the assays are based on polymerase
chain reaction (PCR), only a small amount of cells (or DNA) are needed for testing. Primers are designed to either cover sites of potential methylation or to cover

nonmethylation sites. The PCR product is then analyzed by sequencing (multiplex PCR), restriction analysis (RLGS, Restriction Landmark Genomic Scanning), or differential methylation hybridization. The advantage of PCR-based quantitative high-throughput assays for methylation is that a panel of tests could be used to generate methylation profiles. Similarly, technologies to detect the acetylation status of histones have also been developed.

Evidence from epidemiologic studies of colon cancer suggests that epigenetic factors may play a critical role in the development of colon cancer (28). However, colon cancer is the only cancer for which the role of epigenetics is evaluated in detail. A large number of cancer genes reportedly carry a high level of methylation in a normally unmethylated promoter. Examples from the scientific literature include *RASSF1, RARbeta, DAPK, p16, p15, MGMT*, and *GSTP1* in lung cancer; *CDKN2A, CALCA, MGMT*, and *TIMP3p* in esophageal cancer; *14^{ARF}* in ulcerative colitis; *MGMT* in glioblastoma, *GSTP1* in prostate cancer; and *HIC-1* and *p53* in breast cancer (Table 28.1). It is not yet established whether methylation is the initiating event or the secondary event in gene silencing. Irrespective of the role of methylation in the initiation of tumor development, methylation plays a key role in an epigenetically mediated loss-of-gene function for tumorigenesis, similar to the role of mutations in coding regions (29). For instance, hypomethylation of the glioma pathogenesis-related 1 (related to testis-specific, vespid, and pathogenesis proteins 1 [GLIPR1/RTVP-1]) gene compared to normal tissues has been reported in more than 80% of Wilms' tumors with a complex etiology (30). RNA expression data supports gene activation data confirming epigenetic regulation in this tumor type.

Epigenetics has seen a recent surge of interest among cancer researchers as alterations in DNA methylation has emerged as one of the most consistent molecular changes in various neoplasms (31). Population-based studies involving environmental and occupational exposure, infectious agents, personal susceptibility factors, and acquired genetic factors may identify high-risk populations likely to develop cancer; additionally, such studies are very informative and significant in designing future community-based health initiatives. Epigenetic biomarkers could be used to identify high-risk populations that may benefit from interventions. Furthermore, since familial cancer comprises only 10–15% of all cancers, epigenetic approaches may help understand the remaining 85–90% of cancers.

Gene silencing and the formation of methylation patterns in the genome can teach us about mechanisms that operate in cancer progression as well as the study of the etiology of other diseases. In those cancers where the incidence rate and survival rate are similar, such as pancreatic cancer, methylation patterns of *p16* and *p14* in pancreatic fluid have been crucial in distinguishing normal subjects from those with pancreatitis and pancreatic cancer. In a study conducted by Klump et al. (32), pancreatic fluid was used to detect pancreatic cancer. In addition, methylation profiles may help identify a group of genes that can be used as markers of preneoplastic lesions. Epigenetic processes have been implicated in mechanisms of cancer progression (e.g., cell cycle control, DNA damage, apoptosis, and invasion) in bladder cancer. In bladder cancer, arsenic and smoking exposure have been shown to contribute to cancer development based on the methylation profile of $p16^{INK4A}$, *RASSF1A*, and *RSS3* genes in a case-control study (33–35). Bladder cancer occurs about three times more in males than in females. Exfoliated cells in urine have been successfully used in methylation analysis to detect bladder cancer. Among the three most commonly studied genes in bladder cancer, *RASSF1A* has been linked with invasive cancer. After lung cancer, tobacco exposure has been identified as a prominent etiological factor for bladder cancer. While lung cancer incidence depends on dose of smoking, such a relationship has not been observed in bladder cancer.

An important distinction between genetic and epigenetic changes in cancer is that the latter might be more easily reversed using therapeutic interventions. There is a critical need to understand epigenetic alterations in precancerous lesions that lead to cancer development. This knowledge could then be applied to risk assessment and early detection efforts, and provide molecular targets for chemopreventive interventions.

Epigenetic changes appear to serve as an alternative to mutations in selected genes, and such changes have emerged as particularly common in human leukemias. Strategies should be developed for epidemiologic studies to identify causal associations between early exposures, long-term changes in epigenetic regulation, and cancer. This may help to develop early interventions and ultimately improve health.

One example in the field of cancer epigenetics and epidemiology is described below. To understand the relationship between genetic variation, global methylation patterns, and regional hypermethylation of tumor suppressor genes, a case-control study was conducted in acute lymphoblastic leukemia (ALL), non-Hodgkin's lymphoma (NHL), and Multiple Myeloma (MM). The selected genes for studies were methylenetetrahydrofolate reductase (*MTHFR*) (a key methyl-group metabolism gene), and the *de novo* DNA methyl transferase gene *DNM3b* (2,36,37). In these genes, polymorphisms were observed in diseased samples. Results from this ongoing study will help us identify the association between genetic polymorphisms and gene-specific or global methylation changes. If abnormal methylation of a group of promoters is found to be associated with a specific polymorphism, it may serve as an early marker to identify individuals at high risk of developing the disease.

Clinical Implications

Methylation and histone deacetylation markers have implication in cancer detection, diagnosis, response to therapy, and disease stratification (11,38–40). At the early onset of disease, the number of epigenetic events exceed the number of genetic events (41–43). A number of methylation markers have been evaluated for early detection of cancer and have shown promising results (1). Some of these markers may also serve as risk assessment tools for disease. For example, *GSTP1* hypermethylation has been reported in about 90% of prostate cancer patients but not in benign hyperplastic prostate tissue (44). Thus *GSTP1* methylation could be used to distinguish between prostate cancer and benign tissue.

Table 28.2 Samples suitable for epigenetic studies

Sample	Comments	Reference
Bronchoalveolar lavage	Lung cancer detection	(146,163)
Buccal cells	Oral and lung cancer detection	(164,165)
Ductal lavage fluid	*Cyclin D2, RARbeta, Twist* hypermethylation in breast cancer	(146)
Cervical swab	Cervical cancer detection	(166,167)
Duodenal fluid	Pancreatic cancer detection	(24,27)
Ejaculate	*GSTP1* methylation in prostate cancer	(146)
Exfoliated cells	Bladder, cervical. and gastric cancer detection by methylation analysis	(168–170)
Nipple aspirate	*RASSF1A, DAPK* methylation in breast cancer	(146)
Pleural lavage	Lung cancer detection	(26,146)
Saliva	*MGMT* hypermethylation in head and neck cancer	(146,171)
Sputum	Sputum was collected from a population of smokers and nonsmokers and analyzed for double-strand breaks and DNA repair capacity to evaluate correlation with methylation index in a set of seven genes	(66,146,172,173)
Stool	*SFRP2* hypermethylation in colorectal cancer	(25,146,174)
Urine	*GSTP1* methylation in prostate cancer; *APC, RASSF1A, p14* methylation in bladder cancer	(146,175,176)

Note: Tissue and blood cells have been used to detect epigenetic markers in several studies (5,177,178).

For cancer detection in solid tissue, biofluids, exfoliated cells (detached tumor cells in circulation), and imaging techniques are used (Table 28.2). It is difficult to detect cancer in many solid tumors until it has metastasized. Visual detection and direct palpation are possible when the affected site is accessible. However, in some cases, such as pancreatic cancer, this is not possible due to the anatomical location of the organ. In such cases, biomarkers (methylation of *p14* and *p16*) detected in the biofluid (pancreatic fluid for detecting pancreatic cancer) would be very useful (32,45–47). Prostate cancer has been detected by analyzing urine from patients (based on hypermethylation of *GSTP1*) (48). A few examples of epigenetics and its clinical implications are described below.

In invasive cervical cancer (ICC), genome-wide methylation analysis was performed in samples from controls and cases. More than 200 genes were hypermethylated in cervical cancer samples (49). A set of six genes (*SPARC, TFPI2, RRAD, SFRP1, MT1G,* and *NMES1*) was proposed as screening markers, as these genes were shown to become hypermethylated in follow-up studies. These methylation markers are useful for cancer detection as well as disease stratification. Cell lines made from ICC were responsive to epigenetic inhibitors, which further confirmed epigenetic regulation of gene expression. In another study, exfoliated cells isolated from urine of cervical cancer patients were used for methylation profiling. Samples were taken from normal, carcinoma *in situ* (CS), and cervical intraepithelial neoplasia grade 1

(CIN-1), grade 2 (CIN-2), and grade 3 (CIN-3) (50). Results indicated a differential methylation pattern in samples from different grades.

Shame et al. completed a low-resolution genome-wide methylation profile of several human samples and demonstrated promoter hypermethylation of major cancers: breast, colon, lung, and prostate (51,52). One hundred thirty two genes were identified, which were hypermethylated in these cancers. The authors theorize that there is a common promoter methylation signature for major cancers although gene expression may vary for different genes in different tumor types.

The identification and characterization of genetic and epigenetic changes that drive cancer development and progression is of high interest in order to better understand carcinogenesis (28). Some investigators have studied genetic and epigenetic alterations in the same samples. In one such study Laird et al. evaluated microsatellite instability (MSI), *BRAFF* mutations, and the methylation profile of selected genes in colon cancer (40,53,54). Their results indicated a high risk of colon cancer in samples with high MSI that also had hypermethylation of genes. Thus, genomic instability correlates with epigenetic regulation (28). Whether some small noncoding RNAs also contribute to this instability remains to be seen.

In one preliminary study, Belinsky's group followed a methylation pattern of *p162A*, *CDH13*, and *RASSF1a* in the recurrence of nonsmall cell lung cancer (NSCLC) (55). Patients who underwent curative resection were followed for cancer recurrence within 40 months. An association was observed between the methylation profile and recurrence of the disease.

Recently, *T-cadherin* levels and promoter methylation were followed during progression of hepatocellular carcinoma (56). Results were compared with results from a normal liver. Decreased levels of *T-cadherin* and hypermethylation of the gene correlated with cancer progression. Cell lines made from diseased tissue were responsive to 5-aza-2-deoxycytidine treatment in restoring *T-cadherin* activity. This could be an excellent screening marker to identify populations with high risk of liver cancer.

More than 90% of prostate cancer cases have *GSP1* methylation and more than 90% of esophageal adenocarcinoma cases have *APC* methylation (39,44,57,58). Laird's group has demonstrated that targeted luminal sources of DNA are better than serum or plasma for methylation analysis in esophageal cancer samples (11). Methylation marker analysis, along with information about genomic makeup and lifestyle, are important for disease stratification and treatment. For example, a thymidylate synthase homozygous patient with colorectal cancer shows better response to treatment with 5-fluouracil than normal subjects (59). A number of cancer methylation markers have also been reported for prognosis of glioblastoma (60).

Environmental Factors and Epigenetics

Environmental exposure/agents include any environmental agent, to which there is significant human exposure, including but not limited to metals, pesticides/

Table 28.3 Potential environmental agents and their possible effects on human health

Name	Possible Effect	Reference
Aromatic amines	Bladder cancer	(179)
Air pollutants, such as carbon monoxide (CO), sulfur dioxide (SO(2)), nitrogen oxides (NOx), volatile organic compounds (VOCs), ozone (O(3)), heavy metals, and respirable particulate matter (PM2.5 and PM10), arsenic	Upper respiratory irritation to chronic respiratory and heart disease, lung cancer, acute respiratory infections in children and chronic bronchitis in adults, aggravating preexisting heart and lung disease, or asthmatic attacks	(3,180)
Asbestos	Gastric and lung cancer	(181,182)
Environmental estrogens	Breast cancer	(183)
Nickel	Multiple cancers	(184)
Pesticides, air pollutants, industrial chemicals, and heavy metals	Cancer, diabetes and obesity, infertility, respiratory diseases, allergies, and neurodegenerative disorders such as Parkinson and Alzheimer diseases	(185)
Polychlorinated biphenyls (PCBs)	Exposure to PCBs suppresses the immune system, thereby increasing the risk of acquiring several human diseases	(186)
Bisphenol A (BPA)	Exposure to fetus *in utero* may contribute to disease development (proposed mechanism is hypomethylation)	(187)
Smoke and fumes	Urothelial cancer	(188)
Trichloroethylene	Renal cancer	(189)

Note: Activity of these environmental agents is regulated epigenetically.

herbicides, organics, plasticizers, endocrine-disrupting chemicals, and air pollutants. Human gene expression is influenced by environmental components, which may be either toxic, carcinogenic, or both (61). Some exogenous mutagens or carcinogens are from pollution of air, water, and soil (Table 28.3). The sources range from motor vehicle emissions, pesticides, industrial effluents, radiation (radon, diagnostic X-rays), occupational exposure (petrochemicals), diet (substances in food preservatives), and various consumer products (tobacco, smoke, cosmetics). Among exposure to known carcinogens, the most widely studied to date are asbestos and tobacco. The malignant mesothelia (MM) epidemic was reported in workers exposed to asbestos (62,63). Increased genomic instability, disturbed apoptosis, poor DNA repair, increased genotoxicity (characterized by formation of aneuploid cells, abnormal anaphases, chromosomal aberrations, DNA single strand break), increased intracellular oxidation, and epigenetic changes were observed (61). According to current understanding, the interaction of asbestos with cells generates free radicals and deactivation of pathways for detoxification of environmental carcinogens. Epigenetic mechanisms are involved in altered gene expression influenced by environmental factors (64,65).

Tobacco and tobacco products are other carcinogens that affect human health. The cytochrome P450 family of enzymes are needed for the metabolism of such substances. Cytochrome P450 enzymes catalyze the oxidation of a large number of endogenous and exogenous chemicals. Endogenous chemicals include hormones and fatty acids, whereas exogenous chemicals include polycyclic aromatic hydrocarbons (PAH), aromatic amines, and mycotoxins. It could be argued that most cancers could be preventable because the factors that determine them are largely exogenous (66).

Environmental factors also include infectious agents (67–73). Infectious agents alter gene expression at the genetic, epigenetic, and proteomic levels. Epigenetic regulation has been reported in cancer-associated infectious agents (74,75). For example, infection of host cells by EBV and human papilloma virus (HPV) results in altered methylation patterns of a number of genes associated with cancer initiation and progression (70,76). Involvement of histone modifications in viral latency has also been proposed (71). In gastric cancer, *Helicobacter pylori* (*H.pylori*) infection plays a crucial role and cancer development is regulated genetically as well as epigenetically (72,77–79). In one study, hypermethylation of six genes was observed in tissues from patients with gastric lymphoma and 80% of the cancer tissues from patients in the study were positive for *H. pylori* (80). However, the levels of methylation did not correlate with percent infection in this study. In the case of Burkitt's lymphoma, the reversal of *E-cadherin* could be observed by Zebularine treatment but latency could not be converted to lytic phase (76). It is emphasized here that recurrent EBV infection is associated with increased incidence of Burkitt's lymphoma.

A specific example of environmental exposures/agents that alter imprinting comes from an examination of the effects of maternal nutrition on offspring phenotypes. Dietary methyl supplementation of pregnant dams with extra folic acid, vitamin B12, choline, and betaine has been shown to alter the phenotype of offspring via increased CpG methylation at specific genetic loci (81). Another example of environmental disruption of imprinting comes from the study of *in utero* exposure of pregnant rats to either methoxychlor or vinclozolin resulting in a phenotype of reduced sperm count and motility in the adult that is transmitted via the male germline through at least four generations (82–85). This remarkable effect occurs via epigenetic imprinting of unknown genes that affect the next generation(s) without loss of penetrance. The transgenerational nature of this effect is specific to a window of exposure that coincides with the time of imprinting of the germline.

The second mechanism, gene silencing or activation in somatic cells, influences gene expression in a temporal and tissue-specific manner. Alterations in normal gene silencing or activation result in inappropriate gene activation or deactivation, leading to tissue dysfunction and disease. Indeed, there are significant data showing that inappropriate activation of oncogenes or inactivation of tumor suppressor genes may underlie many malignancies, including some ovarian and breast cancers (86–91). There is also mounting evidence that environmentally induced perturbations in these epigenetic processes are involved in the development of a number of diseases, for example, autoimmune disorders, reproductive disorders, and neurobehavioral and cognitive dysfunctions. *In utero* or neonatal exposures to environmental agents are particularly vulnerable periods for alterations in epigenetic programming due to tissue development and result in a permanently altered gene expression in a tissue-specific manner related to increased disease susceptibility (92). For example, neonatal exposure to diethylstilbestrol (DES) results in altered methylation of specific genes that result in their continued expression in the uterus. This occurrence has been related to increased uterine cancers in a rodent model (93).

There are also human data that reinforce the importance of epigenetics. The Barker hypothesis is based on the correlation of undernutrition during development that results in lower birth weight and increased susceptibility to diseases later in life, including diabetes and cardiovascular diseases (94). It has been proposed that these effects are due to altered programming during development. In addition, human breast tumors have altered methylation of many genes that are related to tumor growth and promotion (86–91). Finally, recent data indicate that twins at a young age have similar gene methylation patterns across the genome. With age and exposure to different environments, including nutrition, the methylation pattern of their genomes diverges (7,95,96). This evidence suggests a need to examine human samples for epigenetic changes following exposure to environmental agents and the subsequent role this plays in human disease progression. It also indicates that epigenetic modulation of gene expression can occur at any time throughout life (65,97).

While the mechanisms responsible for adding and removing the epigenetic marks are not clearly defined at this point, it is clear that this phenomenon is critically important in normal developmental biology and disease development/progression, and that epigenetic markers can be modified by environmental exposures and lead to increased susceptibility to disease and dysfunction.

To better understand epigenetic mechanism and its role in disease and dysfunction due in part to environmental exposure, further investigations are needed to examine any and all aspects of epigenetic regulation. A greater understanding of epigenetics is needed in the following areas: imprinting, DNA methylation at promoter and other sites, chromatin modifications, gene silencing induced by small noncoding RNAs, and other novel epigenetic mechanisms (10,98–102). Additionally, state-of-the-art technologies should be employed to analyze the epigenetic changes in single genes, signaling pathways, or the entire genome in response to various exposures (61).

Epigenetics in Cancer Management

Epigenetic changes (sometimes called epimutations), such as the hypermethylation, histone deacetylation, and epigenetic silencing of tumor suppressor genes, have revealed a new area for cancer treatment using inhibitors of methylation and deacetylation (103). The precise anticancer mechanism of action of these inhibitors is not yet well defined and the rapid advancement of these classes of compounds in clinical trials, at least in part, reflects the urgency for new mechanism-based

Table 28.4 Epigenetic inhibitors used in different cancers

Inhibitor	Comments	Reference
5-Azacytidine	DNMT1 inhibitor	(111)
Butyric acid	Deacetylation inhibitor in gastric cancer	(158)
Decitabine	DNMT inhibitor	(111)
Depsipeptide	• HDAC inhibitor • Tested in leukemia/lymphoma	(118,119)
Suberoylanilide Hydroxamic Acid (SAHA)	• HDAC inhibitor • Promising results in cutaneous T-cell lymphoma (CTCL) phase II trial • Also has been used in breast cancer • SAHA reacts with and blocks the catalytic site of HDAC	(104,107,116,120)
Trichostatin A (TSA)	HDAC inhibitor	(121)
Valproic acid (VPA)	• HDAC inhibitor • Induces differentiation • Tested in leukemia • Potential to revert chemotherapy resistance in breast cancer patients (proof of principle study)	(109,121,125,126)
Zebularine (1-(®-D-ribofuranosyl)-1,2-dihydropyrimidin-2-one)	DNMT1 inhibitor Compared to 5-azacytidine (5-Aza-CR) and 5-aza-2′-deoxycytidine (5-Aza-CdR), Zebularine is less toxic and can be given orally to patients	(127,159,160)

Notes:
• Dietary HDAC inhibitors have weak ligands compared to pharmacologic agents.
• Several other inhibitors, such as PXD101 (phase I), LBH589 (phase I), Pyroxamide (phase I), MS-275 (phase I, II), Cl-994 (phase I, II, III) are showing promising results as epigenetics inhibitors (161).
• A combination of HDAC inhibitors and methylation inhibitors has been successful in a few cases (161,162).

therapeutics for cancers that are not adequately treated by conventional therapies (10,104,105). These inhibitors can induce differentiation, cell cycle, growth arrest, and in certain cases apoptosis in cancer cells (105). A few examples are discussed in the following section and in Table 28.4. Studies using DNA methyltransferase inhibitors such as procaine, hydralazine, and RG108 have had promising outcomes against cancer.

Recently, melatonin, one of the most versatile molecules in nature, has been shown to have a potential role in the inhibition of DNA methyltransferase (106). Whether gene promoter hypermethylation is the cause or consequence for the tumor suppressor gene silencing is still a matter of controversy; nevertheless, these views are not mutually exclusive. That DNA methylation is causal has been shown by the ability of diverse pharmacologic compounds and molecular techniques to reactivate gene expression upon inhibition of DNA methylation in cancer cells.

Histone deacetylase inhibitors (HDACIs) represent one of the most promising epigenetic treatments for cancer (107). HDACIs have emerged as promising targets for cancer therapy because they reactivate the transcription of multiple genes that are silenced in human tumors and they show pleiotropic antitumor effects selectively in cancer cells. HDACIs are well tolerated and several show promising antitumor activity. While gene transcription has been considered to be the major target of HDACIs, inhibition of acetylation of nonhistone proteins is now emerging as a novel basis for their antitumor effects (108). Table 28.4 presents selected epigenetic inhibitors. Suberoylanilide Hydroxamic Acid (SAHA) has shown anticancer activity and the Food and Drug Administration (FDA) has approved a new drug application for vorinostat to treat cutaneous T-cell lymphoma (104,107). In a proof-of-principle study of breast cancer, reversion of chemotherapy resistant by valproic acid, a HDAC inhibitor, has been reported (109). *RhoB* has been identified as a gene widely involved in lung carcinogenesis, which regulates diverse cellular processes including cytoskeletal organization, gene transcription, cell cycle progression, and cytokinesis. A decrease in *RhoB* expression has been observed in lung cancer. When cells were treated with HDAC inhibitors, reexpression of *RhoB* was observed (110). Thus it may be proposed that *RhoB* regulation of expression occurs mainly by histone deacetylation rather than by promoter hypermethylation and that this process can be modulated by specific 5' sequences within the promoter.

Optimum reexpression of most genes silenced through epigenetics requires sequential application of DNA methyl transferase inhibitors followed by HDAC inhibitors. Gore et al. (111) have demonstrated that treatment with aza-CR followed by sodium butyrate treatment results in activation of the *p16* gene in myeloid neoplasms. In addition to the potential use of these inhibitors as standalone therapeutics for cancer, there is excitement about the possibility of combining these classes of drugs with other conventional chemotherapeutics and biologics (112–115). Examples where HDAC inhibitors have additive or synergistic effects include the following: anthracyclins, tumor necrosis factor-related apoptosis inducing ligand, and all-trans retinoic acid (116–121). In clinical settings, few compounds (SAHA, valproic acid, and depsipeptides) show promising results, whereas others (benzamide derivative in pancreatic cancer) need improvement, especially in efficacy (122–126). Zebullarine is a stable compound that can be administered orally and shows higher efficiency than all other existing inhibitors (127).

Areas of Research Opportunities

Some of the research opportunities within epigenetic gene regulation and disease development are described below:

- Determination of epigenetic targets in the genome sensitive to modification by environmental exposures;
    - Examination of the changes in epigenetic markers over time and correlation of these changes with environmental exposures;
    - Identification of genes whose imprinting is modified by environmental exposures on paternal or maternal genomes;
    - Determination of genes modulated by environmental exposures that are targets for activation/inactivation by DNA methylation and/or chromatin remodeling;

- Determination of predictive biomarkers of altered epigenetic regulation due to exposures to environmental chemicals;
- Examination of the role of epigenetic modification of gene expression due to environmental exposures in the etiology or progression of disease of cardiovascular, pulmonary, immune/autoimmune, reproductive, nervous systems and different cancers, obesity, and any other disease for which there is a known or suspected exposure component;
  - Examination of the impact of nutrition on imprinting and epigenetically regulated gene expression;
  - Examination of the associations between epigenetic modulation as a result of environmental exposures, such as low-dose radiation, and the anticancer properties of dietary constituents;
  - Examination of the role of epigenetic changes in the regulation of transcription by environmental agents that mimic hormone or antagonists;
  - Examination of alterations in the normal imprinting of genes due to environmental exposures, including diet and bioactive food components, and the subsequent effect on disease dysfunction;
  - Examination of the role of epigenetics in the transgenerational effects of exposure to environmental agents;
  - Examination of the role of epigenetics in *in utero* or neonatal exposure to environmental agents and the subsequent increase in disease susceptibility later in life;
  - Examination and comparison of the windows of susceptibility to epigenetic changes, including neonatal, puberty, and adult;
  - Utilization of cell lines from diseased tissues to examine epigenetic markers that distinguish control from environmental exposures in animals or humans;
- Utilization of existing tools or development of new tools to elucidate the role of epigenetic modifications of DNA or chromatin in the etiology of environmentally induced disease;
  - Address development of bioinformatics resources and tools that aid in the analysis of epigenetic pathways;
  - Design therapeutic agents to modify environmentally induced epigenetic markers;
- Determination of the mechanisms of environmentally induced alterations in epigenetic markers via examination of the epigenetic pathways of DNA methylation and chromatin remodeling;
  - Study transcriptional gene silencing (TSG) induced by short interfering RNAs (siRNA) via DNA methylation;
  - Examination of the effects of environmental agents, including dietary factors, on the DNA methyltransferases (DNMTs), histone acetyltransferases (HATs), histone deacetylases (HDACs), and other critical enzymes;

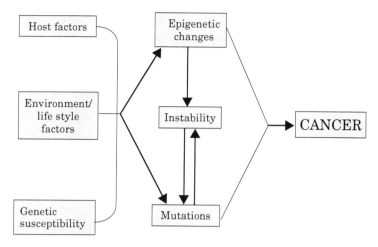

Figure 28.2 Environment influences genetics and epigenetics.

- Determination of the role of physical, chemical, and infectious agents and behavioral factors on the types and levels of epigenetic changes in human populations;
- Determination of the role of epigenetic changes in the risk of cancer in human populations;
- Identification of genetic, environmental, and host susceptibility factors that modify the risk of cancer associated with epigenetic changes;
- Improve sensitivity and specificity of epigenetic markers in cohort and case-control studies to identify high-risk populations;
- Evaluate epigenetic factors and disparities in cancer incidence in various populations.

Cancer markers can be categorized into markers of risk assessment, early detection, progression, and prognosis. On the other hand, markers can be categorized into genetic, epigenetic, imaging, and metabolomic markers. A schematic representing environmental factors contributing to disease development is shown in Figure 28.2.

Conclusions and Perspectives: The Road Ahead

The field of cancer epigenetics is evolving rapidly on several fronts, including cancer epidemiology. Now that the Human Genome Project is completed, the Human Epigenome project is underway. It is expected to generate genome-wide methylation and histone maps (http://nihroadmap.nih.gov/epigenomics/index.asp) (29). A comparison of such maps between healthy and diseased tissue will be made to identify specific genomic regions that are involved in development, tissue-specific expression, environmental susceptibility, and pathogenesis. Future epigenetic maps will help researchers and clinicians develop interventions and therapeutic strategies.

Due to the development of high-throughput methods of detecting epigenetic modifications, it is now possible to identify high-risk populations, as discussed above, for colon cancer. Epigenetic markers could be used in clinics for classification of a few cancer types. These markers also are useful for assessment of risk of developing cancer.

An area of epigenetics that is less developed is that of histone modifiers. For several histone modifiers, we do not know the mechanisms of action. Technological advancements in microarray technologies and proteomics may shed some light on this area. Genome-wide mapping approaches of histones provide new opportunities to decipher histone code. Integration of datasets and improved technologies will also provide future opportunities for research. The major challenge in the area of cancer diagnosis and epigenetic markers is validation of markers that have been studied by one or few groups. As always, this will be a very big project in which the collaborative efforts of biochemists, proteomic and genomic experts, clinicians, epidemiologists, and molecular biologists will be needed.

Additional research is needed in the area of developing new compounds or improving existing compounds that can inhibit methylation and histone deacetylation. It is important to remember that we cannot reverse mutations but we can reverse epigenetic changes and impact health. Inhibitors described in this article are not gene-specific. Use of inhibitors has the risk of inducing demethylation of normally methylated sequences, retrotransposons, resulting in retrotransposition. Furthermore, nonspecific methylation has the risk of inducing silencing of tumor suppressor genes. Efforts are underway to make epigenetic inhibitors gene-specific (116,128). The potential synergism between radiotherapy, chemotherapy, and biologicals in cancer treatment is also a topic for future research.

DNA methylation could be useful for disease diagnosis in certain cancers, or for screening in body fluids. DNA hypermethylated gene promoter sequences are extremely promising cancer markers. Their potential use for risk assessment, early diagnosis, or prognosis depends on the timing of gene expression changes during tumor progression. Technologies to follow up these markers with tumor progression studies are now well developed. A sensitive screening approach for cancer could markedly reduce the high mortality rate for this disease.

To investigate the effects of environmental agents and their effect on disease development via epigenetic gene regulation, it is recommended that researchers evaluate changes in methylation and histone profiles over time in the same set of individuals. Yet studies documenting epigenetic marker profiles over the lifespan, the vulnerability of these markers due to environmental insults, and the subsequent effects on cancer development, have been limited to date due to the absence of properly stored biospecimens.

Finally, current modalities of assessing patients at high risk of cancer are limited and the identification of novel and robust biomarkers is an important next step in the clinical management of cancer.

Acknowledgments

I appreciate Debbie Winn, Brit Reid, and Christine Kaefer of the Epidemiology and Genetics Research Program of the Division of Cancer Control and Population Sciences, NCI for critical evaluation of this manuscript.

References

1. Esteller M. Epigenetics in cancer. *N Engl J Med.* 2008;358:1148–1159.
2. Rhee I, Bachman KE, Park BH, et al. DNMT1 and DNMT3b cooperate to silence genes in human cancer cells. *Nature.* 2002;416:552–556.
3. Chen WT, Hung WC, Kang WY, Huang YC, Chai CY. Urothelial carcinomas arising in arsenic-contaminated areas are associated with hypermethylation of the gene promoter of the death-associated protein kinase. *Histopathology.* 2007;51:785–792.
4. Verma M, Manne U. Genetic and epigenetic biomarkers in cancer diagnosis and identifying high risk populations. *Crit Rev Oncol Hematol.* 2006;60:9–18.
5. Verma M, Maruvada P, Srivastava S. Epigenetics and cancer. *Crit Rev Clin Lab Sci.* 2004;41:585–607.
6. Verma M, Srivastava S. Epigenetics in cancer: implications for early detection and prevention. *Lancet Oncol.* 2002;3:755–763.
7. Esteller M. Cancer epigenomics: DNA methylomes and histone-modification maps. *Nat Rev Genet.* 2007;8:286–298.
8. Feinberg AP, Tycko B. The history of cancer epigenetics. *Nat Rev Cancer.* 2004;4:143–153.
9. Eads CA, Lord RV, Wickramasinghe K, et al. Epigenetic patterns in the progression of esophageal adenocarcinoma. *Cancer Res.* 2001;61:3410–3418.
10. Jones PA, Baylin SB. The epigenomics of cancer. *Cell.* 2007;128:683–692.
11. Laird PW. Cancer epigenetics. *Hum Mol Genet.* 2005;14 Spec No 1:R65–R76.
12. Verma M, Dunn BK, Ross S, et al. Early detection and risk assessment: proceedings and recommendations from the Workshop on Epigenetics in Cancer Prevention. *Ann N Y Acad Sci.* 2003;983:298–319.
13. Kaneda A, Wang CJ, Cheong R, et al. Enhanced sensitivity to IGF-II signaling links loss of imprinting of IGF2 to increased cell proliferation and tumor risk. *Proc Natl Acad Sci USA.* 2007;104:20926–20931.
14. Luedi PP, Dietrich FS, Weidman JR, Bosko JM, Jirtle RL, Hartemink AJ. Computational and experimental identification of novel human imprinted genes. *Genome Res.* 2007;17:1723–1730.
15. Bjornsson HT, Brown LJ, Fallin MD, et al. Epigenetic specificity of loss of imprinting of the IGF2 gene in Wilms tumors. *J Natl Cancer Inst.* 2007;99:1270–1273.
16. Byun HM, Wong HL, Birnstein EA, Wolff EM, Liang G, Yang AS. Examination of IGF2 and H19 loss of imprinting in bladder cancer. *Cancer Res.* 2007;67:10753–10758.
17. Hede K. Imprinting may provide cancer prevention tools. *J Natl Cancer Inst.* 2007;99:424–426.
18. Hunter P. The silence of genes. Is genomic imprinting the software of evolution or just a battleground for gender conflict? *EMBO Rep.* 2007;8:441–443.
19. Szyf M. The dynamic epigenome and its implications in toxicology. *Toxicol Sci.* 2007;100:7–23.
20. Takeuchi S, Hofmann WK, Tsukasaki K, et al. Loss of H19 imprinting in adult T-cell leukaemia/lymphoma. *Br J Haematol.* 2007;137:380–381.

21. Watanabe N, Haruta M, Soejima H, et al. Duplication of the paternal IGF2 allele in trisomy 11 and elevated expression levels of IGF2 mRNA in congenital mesoblastic nephroma of the cellular or mixed type. *Genes Chromosomes Cancer.* 2007;46:929–935.

22. Waterland RA, Michels KB. Epigenetic epidemiology of the developmental origins hypothesis. *Annu Rev Nutr.* 2007;27:363–388.

23. Estecio MR, Yan PS, Ibrahim AE, et al. High-throughput methylation profiling by MCA coupled to CpG island microarray. *Genome Res.* 2007;17:1529–1536.

24. Minamoto T, Mai M, Ronai Z. K-ras mutation: early detection in molecular diagnosis and risk assessment of colorectal, pancreas, and lung cancers—a review. *Cancer Detect Prev.* 2000;24:1–12.

25. Muller HM, Oberwalder M, Fiegl H, et al. Methylation changes in faecal DNA: a marker for colorectal cancer screening? *Lancet.* 2004;363:1283–1285.

26. Ng CS, Zhang J, Wan S, et al. Tumor p16M is a possible marker of advanced stage in non-small cell lung cancer. *J Surg Oncol.* 2002;79:101–106.

27. Tascilar M, Caspers E, Sturm PD, Goggins M, Hruban RH, Offerhaus GJ. Role of tumor markers and mutations in cells and pancreatic juice in the diagnosis of pancreatic cancer. *Ann Oncol.* 1999;10(Suppl 4):107–110.

28. O'Brien MJ, Yang S, Mack C, et al. Comparison of microsatellite instability, CpG island methylation phenotype, BRAF and KRAS status in serrated polyps and traditional adenomas indicates separate pathways to distinct colorectal carcinoma end points. *Am J Surg Pathol.* 2006;30:1491–1501.

29. Hoque MO, Kim MS, Ostrow KL, et al. Genome-wide promoter analysis uncovers portions of the cancer methylome. *Cancer Res.* 2008;68:2661–2670.

30. Chilukamarri L, Hancock AL, Malik S, et al. Hypomethylation and aberrant expression of the glioma pathogenesis-related 1 gene in Wilms tumors. *Neoplasia.* 2007;9:970–978.

31. Ladd-Acosta C, Pevsner J, Sabunciyan S, et al. DNA methylation signatures within the human brain. *Am J Hum Genet.* 2007;81:1304–1315.

32. Klump B, Hsieh CJ, Nehls O, et al. Methylation status of p14ARF and p16INK4a as detected in pancreatic secretions. *Br J Cancer.* 2003;88:217–222.

33. Marsit CJ, Houseman EA, Christensen BC, et al. Examination of a CpG island methylator phenotype and implications of methylation profiles in solid tumors. *Cancer Res.* 2006;66:10621–10629.

34. Marsit CJ, Houseman EA, Schned AR, Karagas MR, Kelsey KT. Promoter hypermethylation is associated with current smoking, age, gender and survival in bladder cancer. *Carcinogenesis.* 2007;28:1745–1751.

35. Marsit CJ, Karagas MR, Schned A, Kelsey KT. Carcinogen exposure and epigenetic silencing in bladder cancer. *Ann N Y Acad Sci.* 2006;1076:810–821.

36. Robertson KD, Keyomarsi K, Gonzales FA, Velicescu M, Jones PA. Differential mRNA expression of the human DNA methyltransferases (DNMTs) 1, 3a and 3b during the G(0)/G(1) to S phase transition in normal and tumor cells. *Nucleic Acids Res.* 2000;28:2108–2113.

37. Jair KW, Bachman KE, Suzuki H, et al. De novo CpG island methylation in human cancer cells. *Cancer Res.* 2006;66:682–692.

38. Kerr KM, Galler JS, Hagen JA, Laird PW, Laird-Offringa IA. The role of DNA methylation in the development and progression of lung adenocarcinoma. *Dis Markers.* 2007;23:5–30.

39. Laird PW. The power and the promise of DNA methylation markers. *Nat Rev Cancer.* 2003;3:253–266.

40. Ogino S, Cantor M, Kawasaki T, et al. CpG island methylator phenotype (CIMP) of colorectal cancer is best characterised by quantitative DNA methylation analysis and prospective cohort studies. *Gut.* 2006;55:1000–1006.

41. Wei SH, Brown R, Huang TH. Aberrant DNA methylation in ovarian cancer: is there an epigenetic predisposition to drug response? *Ann N Y Acad Sci.* 2003;983:243–250.
42. Nephew KP, Huang TH. Epigenetic gene silencing in cancer initiation and progression. *Cancer Lett.* 2003;190:125–133.
43. Esteller M. Aberrant DNA methylation as a cancer-inducing mechanism. *Annu Rev Pharmacol Toxicol.* 2005;45:629–656.
44. Jeronimo C, Usadel H, Henrique R, et al. Quantitation of GSTP1 methylation in non-neoplastic prostatic tissue and organ-confined prostate adenocarcinoma. *J Natl Cancer Inst.* 2001;93:1747–1752.
45. Hanaoka M, Shimizu K, Shigemura M, et al. Cloning of the hamster p16 gene 5' upstream region and its aberrant methylation patterns in pancreatic cancer. *Biochem Biophys Res Commun.* 2005;333:1249–1253.
46. House MG, Herman JG, Guo MZ, et al. Aberrant hypermethylation of tumor suppressor genes in pancreatic endocrine neoplasms. *Ann Surg.* 2003;238:423–431; discussion 431–422.
47. Tan SH, Ida H, Lau QC, et al. Detection of promoter hypermethylation in serum samples of cancer patients by methylation-specific polymerase chain reaction for tumour suppressor genes including RUNX3. *Oncol Rep.* 2007;18:1225–1230.
48. Cairns P, Esteller M, Herman JG, et al. Molecular detection of prostate cancer in urine by GSTP1 hypermethylation. *Clin Cancer Res.* 2001;7:2727–2730.
49. Sova P, Feng Q Geiss G, et al. Discovery of novel methylation biomarkers in cervical carcinoma by global demethylation and microarray analysis. *Cancer Epidemiol Biomarkers Prev.* 2006;15:114–123.
50. Feng Q, Hawes SE, Stern JE, et al. Promoter hypermethylation of tumor suppressor genes in urine from patients with cervical neoplasia. *Cancer Epidemiol Biomarkers Prev.* 2007;16:1178–1184.
51. Shames DS, Girard L, Gao B, et al. A genome-wide screen for promoter methylation in lung cancer identifies novel methylation markers for multiple malignancies. *PLoS Med.* 2006;3:e486.
52. Shames DS, Minna JD, Gazdar AF. DNA methylation in health, disease, and cancer. *Curr Mol Med.* 2007;7:85–102.
53. Ogino S, Odze RD, Kawasaki T, et al. Correlation of pathologic features with CpG island methylator phenotype (CIMP) by quantitative DNA methylation analysis in colorectal carcinoma. *Am J Surg Pathol.* 2006;30:1175–1183.
54. Weisenberger DJ, Siegmund KD, Campan M, et al. CpG island methylator phenotype underlies sporadic microsatellite instability and is tightly associated with BRAF mutation in colorectal cancer. *Nat Genet.* 2006;38:787–793.
55. Brock MV, Hooker CM, Ota-Machida E, et al. DNA methylation markers and early recurrence in stage I lung cancer. *N Engl J Med.* 2008;358:1118–1128.
56. Yan Q, Zhang ZF, Chen XP, et al. Reduced T-cadherin expression and promoter methylation are associated with the development and progression of hepatocellular carcinoma. *Int J Oncol.* 2008;32:1057–1063.
57. Henrique R, Jeronimo C. Molecular detection of prostate cancer: a role for GSTP1 hypermethylation. *Eur Urol.* 2004;46:660–669; discussion 669.
58. Kawakami K, Brabender J, Lord RV, et al. Hypermethylated APC DNA in plasma and prognosis of patients with esophageal adenocarcinoma. *J Natl Cancer Inst.* 2000;92:1805–1811.
59. Pullarkat ST, Stoehlmacher J, Ghaderi V, et al. Thymidylate synthase gene polymorphism determines response and toxicity of 5-FU chemotherapy. *Pharmacogenomics J.* 2001;1:65–70.

60. Rodriguez FJ, Thibodeau SN, Jenkins RB, et al. MGMT immunohistochemical expression and promoter methylation in human glioblastoma. *Appl Immunohistochem Mol Morphol.* 2008;16:59–65.
61. Moore LE, Huang WY, Chung J, Hayes RB. Epidemiologic considerations to assess altered DNA methylation from environmental exposures in cancer. *Ann N Y Acad Sci.* 2003;983:181–196.
62. Foddis R, Vivaldi A, Filiberti R, et al. Serum mesothelin dosages in follow-up of previously exposed workers. *Giornale italiano di medicina del lavoro ed ergonomia.* 2007;29:342–345.
63. Guglielmi G, Ciberti A, Foddis R, et al. Medical surveillance of previously asbestos-exposed workers: report of a case of lung cancer with high level of serum mesothelin. *Giornale italiano di medicina del lavoro ed ergonomia.* 2007;29:345–346.
64. Hirao T, Bueno R, Chen CJ, Gordon GJ, Heilig E, Kelsey KT. Alterations of the p16(INK4) locus in human malignant mesothelial tumors. *Carcinogenesis.* 2002;23:1127–1130.
65. Dolinoy DC, Jirtle RL. Environmental epigenomics in human health and disease. *Environ Mol Mutagen.* 2008;49:4–8.
66. Belinsky SA, Liechty KC, Gentry FD, et al. Promoter hypermethylation of multiple genes in sputum precedes lung cancer incidence in a high-risk cohort. *Cancer Res.* 2006;66:3338–3344.
67. Kalantari M, Calleja-Macias IE, Tewari D, et al. Conserved methylation patterns of human papillomavirus type 16 DNA in asymptomatic infection and cervical neoplasia. *J Virol.* 2004;78:12762–12772.
68. Kim K, Garner-Hamrick PA, Fisher C, Lee D, Lambert PF. Methylation patterns of papillomavirus DNA, its influence on E2 function, and implications in viral infection. *J Virol.* 2003;77:12450–12459.
69. Widschwendter A, Gattringer C, Ivarsson L, et al. Analysis of aberrant DNA methylation and human papillomavirus DNA in cervicovaginal specimens to detect invasive cervical cancer and its precursors. *Clin Cancer Res.* 2004;10:3396–3400.
70. Ushiku T, Chong JM, Uozaki H, et al. p73 gene promoter methylation in Epstein-Barr virus-associated gastric carcinoma. *Int J Cancer.* 2007;120:60–66.
71. Minarovits J. Epigenotypes of latent herpesvirus genomes. *Curr Top Microbiol Immunol.* 2006;310:61–80.
72. Nardone G, Compare D, De Colibus P, de Nucci G, Rocco A. Helicobacter pylori and epigenetic mechanisms underlying gastric carcinogenesis. *Dig Dis.* 2007;25:225–229.
73. Di Bartolo DL, Cannon M, Liu YF, et al. KSHV LANA inhibits TGF-{beta} signaling through epigenetic silencing of the TGF-{beta} type II receptor. *Blood.* 2008;111:4731–4740.
74. Carrillo-Infante C, Abbadessa G, Bagella L, Giordano A. Viral infections as a cause of cancer (review). *Int J Oncol.* 2007;30:1521–1528.
75. Verma M. Viral genes and methylation. *Ann N Y Acad Sci.* 2003;983:170–180.
76. Rao SP, Rechsteiner MP, Berger C, Sigrist JA, Nadal D, Bernasconi M. Zebularine reactivates silenced E-cadherin but unlike 5-Azacytidine does not induce switching from latent to lytic Epstein-Barr virus infection in Burkitt's lymphoma Akata cells. *Mol Cancer.* 2007;6:3.
77. Maekita T, Nakazawa K, Mihara M, et al. High levels of aberrant DNA methylation in Helicobacter pylori-infected gastric mucosae and its possible association with gastric cancer risk. *Clin Cancer Res.* 2006;12:989–995.
78. Perri F, Cotugno R, Piepoli A, et al. Aberrant DNA methylation in non-neoplastic gastric mucosa of H. Pylori infected patients and effect of eradication. *Am J Gastroenterol.* 2007;102:1361–1371.

79. Vale FF, Vitor JM. Genomic methylation: a tool for typing Helicobacter pylori isolates. *Appl Environ Microbiol.* 2007;73:4243–4249.

80. Huang Q, Su X, Ai L, Li M, Fan CY, Weiss LM. Promoter hypermethylation of multiple genes in gastric lymphoma. *Leuk Lymphoma.* 2007;48:1988–1996.

81. Waterland RA, Lin JR, Smith CA, Jirtle RL. Post-weaning diet affects genomic imprinting at the insulin-like growth factor 2 (Igf2) locus. *Hum Mol Genet.* 2006;15:705–716.

82. Chang HS, Anway MD, Rekow SS, Skinner MK. Transgenerational epigenetic imprinting of the male germline by endocrine disruptor exposure during gonadal sex determination. *Endocrinology.* 2006;147:5524–5541.

83. Crews D, Gore AC, Hsu TS, et al. Transgenerational epigenetic imprints on mate preference. *Proc Natl Acad Sci USA.* 2007;104:5942–5946.

84. Skinner MK, Anway MD. Seminiferous cord formation and germ-cell programming: epigenetic transgenerational actions of endocrine disruptors. *Ann N Y Acad Sci* 2005;1061:18–32.

85. Zoeller RT. Endocrine disruptors: do family lines carry an epigenetic record of previous generations' exposures? *Endocrinology.* 2006;147:5513–5514.

86. Barciszewska AM, Murawa D, Gawronska I, Murawa P, Nowak S, Barciszewska MZ. Analysis of 5-methylcytosine in DNA of breast and colon cancer tissues. *IUBMB Life.* 2007;59:765–770.

87. Melnikov AA, Scholtens DM, Wiley EL, Khan SA, Levenson VV. Array-based multiplex analysis of DNA methylation in breast cancer tissues. *J Mol Diagn.* 2008;10:93–101.

88. Nakano H, Nakamura Y, Soda H, et al. Methylation status of breast cancer resistance protein detected by methylation-specific polymerase chain reaction analysis is correlated inversely with its expression in drug-resistant lung cancer cells. *Cancer.* 2008;112(5):1122–1130.

89. Ordway JM, Budiman MA, Korshunova Y, et al. Identification of novel high-frequency DNA methylation changes in breast cancer. *PLoS ONE.* 2007;2:e1314.

90. Shukla S, Mirza S, Sharma G, Parshad R, Gupta SD, Ralhan R. Detection of RASSF1A and RARbeta hypermethylation in serum DNA from breast cancer patients. *Epigenetics.* 2006;1:88–93.

91. Stearns V, Zhou Q, Davidson NE. Epigenetic regulation as a new target for breast cancer therapy. *Cancer Invest.* 2007;25:659–665.

92. Monje L, Varayoud J, Luque EH, Ramos JG. Neonatal exposure to bisphenol A modifies the abundance of estrogen receptor alpha transcripts with alternative 5'-untranslated regions in the female rat preoptic area. *J Endocrinol.* 2007;194:201–212.

93. Li S, Hansman R, Newbold R, Davis B, McLachlan JA, Barrett JC. Neonatal diethylstilbestrol exposure induces persistent elevation of c-fos expression and hypomethylation in its exon-4 in mouse uterus. *Mol Carcinog.* 2003;38:78–84.

94. Sinclair KD, Lea RG, Rees WD, Young LE. The developmental origins of health and disease: current theories and epigenetic mechanisms. *Soc Reprod Fertil Suppl.* 2007;64:425–443.

95. Poulsen P, Esteller M, Vaag A, Fraga MF. The epigenetic basis of twin discordance in age-related diseases. *Pediatr Res.* 2007;61:38R–42R.

96. Fraga MF, Ballestar E, Paz MF, et al. Epigenetic differences arise during the lifetime of monozygotic twins. *Proc Natl Acad Sci USA.* 2005;102:10604–10609.

97. Weidman JR, Dolinoy DC, Murphy SK, Jirtle RL. Cancer susceptibility: epigenetic manifestation of environmental exposures. *Cancer J.* 2007;13:9–16.

98. Bakalova R. RNA interference—about the reality to be exploited in cancer therapy. *Methods Find Exp Clin Pharmacol.* 2007;29:417–421.

99. Dong-Dong L. Small interfering RNA (siRNA) inhibited human liver cancer cell line SMMC7721 proliferation and tumorigenesis. *Hepatogastroenterology.* 2007;54:1731–1735.

100. Navakanit R, Graidist P, Leeanansaksiri W, Dechsukum C. Growth inhibition of breast cancer cell line MCF-7 by siRNA silencing of Wilms tumor 1 gene. *J Med Assoc Thai*. 2007;90:2416–2421.

101. Sampson VB, Rong NH, Han J, et al. MicroRNA let-7a down-regulates MYC and reverts MYC-induced growth in Burkitt lymphoma cells. *Cancer Res*. 2007;67:9762–9770.

102. Jones PA, Martienssen R. A blueprint for a Human Epigenome Project: the AACR Human Epigenome Workshop. *Cancer Res*. 2005;65:11241–11246.

103. An W. Histone acetylation and methylation: combinatorial players for transcriptional regulation. *Subcell Biochem*. 2007;41:351–369.

104. Marks PA, Breslow R. Dimethyl sulfoxide to vorinostat: development of this histone deacetylase inhibitor as an anticancer drug. *Nat Biotechnol*. 2007;25:84–90.

105. Shankar S, Srivastava RK. Histone deacetylase inhibitors: mechanisms and clinical significance in cancer: HDAC inhibitor-induced apoptosis. *Adv Exp Med Biol*. 2008;615:261–298.

106. Korkmaz A, Reiter RJ. Epigenetic regulation: a new research area for melatonin? *J Pineal Res*. 2008;44:41–44.

107. Dokmanovic M, Clarke C, Marks PA. Histone deacetylase inhibitors: overview and perspectives. *Mol Cancer Res*. 2007;5:981–989.

108. Kim TY, Bang YJ, Robertson KD. Histone deacetylase inhibitors for cancer therapy. *Epigenetics*. 2006;1:14–23.

109. Arce C, Perez-Plasencia C, Gonzalez-Fierro A, et al. A proof-of-principle study of epigenetic therapy added to neoadjuvant doxorubicin cyclophosphamide for locally advanced breast cancer. *PLoS ONE*. 2006;1:e98.

110. Mazieres J, Tovar D, He B, et al. Epigenetic regulation of RhoB loss of expression in lung cancer. *BMC Cancer*. 2007;7:220.

111. Gore SD. Combination therapy with DNA methyltransferase inhibitors in hematologic malignancies. *Nat Clin Pract*. 2005;2(Suppl 1):S30–S35.

112. Kelly WK, Marks PA. Drug insight: Histone deacetylase inhibitors—development of the new targeted anticancer agent suberoylanilide hydroxamic acid. *Nat Clin Pract*. 2005;2:150–157.

113. Piekarz R, Bates S. A review of depsipeptide and other histone deacetylase inhibitors in clinical trials. *Curr Pharm Des*. 2004;10:2289–2298.

114. Piekarz RL, Sackett DL, Bates SE. Histone deacetylase inhibitors and demethylating agents: clinical development of histone deacetylase inhibitors for cancer therapy. *Cancer J*. 2007;13:30–39.

115. Bruserud O, Stapnes C, Tronstad KJ, Ryningen A, Anensen N, Gjertsen BT. Protein lysine acetylation in normal and leukaemic haematopoiesis: HDACs as possible therapeutic targets in adult AML. *Expert Opin Ther Targets*. 2006;10:51–68.

116. Karagiannis TC, El-Osta A. Will broad-spectrum histone deacetylase inhibitors be superseded by more specific compounds? *Leukemia*. 2007;21:61–65.

117. Sanchez-Gonzalez B, Yang H, Bueso-Ramos C, et al. Antileukemia activity of the combination of an anthracycline with a histone deacetylase inhibitor. *Blood*. 2006;108:1174–1182.

118. Kano Y, Akutsu M, Tsunoda S, et al. Cytotoxic effects of histone deacetylase inhibitor FK228 (depsipeptide, formally named FR901228) in combination with conventional anti-leukemia/lymphoma agents against human leukemia/lymphoma cell lines. *Invest New Drugs*. 2007;25:31–40.

119. Lundqvist A, Abrams SI, Schrump DS, et al. Bortezomib and depsipeptide sensitize tumors to tumor necrosis factor-related apoptosis-inducing ligand: a novel method to potentiate natural killer cell tumor cytotoxicity. *Cancer Res*. 2006;66:7317–7325.

120. Butler LM, Liapis V, Bouralexis S, et al. The histone deacetylase inhibitor, suberoyla-nilide hydroxamic acid, overcomes resistance of human breast cancer cells to Apo2L/TRAIL. *Int J Cancer.* 2006;119:944–954.

121. Qi H, Ratnam M. Synergistic induction of folate receptor beta by all-trans retinoic acid and histone deacetylase inhibitors in acute myelogenous leukemia cells: mecha-nism and utility in enhancing selective growth inhibition by antifolates. *Cancer Res.* 2006;66:5875–5882.

122. Garber K. Purchase of Aton spotlights HDAC inhibitors. *Nat Biotechnol.* 2004; 22:364–365.

123. Richards DA, Boehm KA, Waterhouse DM, et al. Gemcitabine plus CI-994 offers no advantage over gemcitabine alone in the treatment of patients with advanced pancreatic cancer: results of a phase II randomized, double-blind, placebo-controlled, multicenter study. *Ann Oncol.* 2006;17:1096–1102.

124. Loprevite M, Tiseo M, Grossi F, et al. In vitro study of CI-994, a histone deacetylase inhibitor, in non-small cell lung cancer cell lines. *Oncol Res.* 2005;15:39–48.

125. Bug G, Ritter M, Wassmann B, et al. Clinical trial of valproic acid and all-trans retinoic acid in patients with poor-risk acute myeloid leukemia. *Cancer.* 2005; 104:2717–2725.

126. Bug G, Schwarz K, Schoch C, et al. Effect of histone deacetylase inhibitor valproic acid on progenitor cells of acute myeloid leukemia. *Haematologica.* 2007;92:542–545.

127. Cheng JC, Matsen CB, Gonzales FA, et al. Inhibition of DNA methylation and reactiva-tion of silenced genes by zebularine. *J Natl Cancer Inst.* 2003;95:399–409.

128. Kawasaki H, Taira K. Induction of DNA methylation and gene silencing by short inter-fering RNAs in human cells. *Nature.* 2004;431:211–217.

129. Veerla S, Panagopoulos I, Jin Y, Lindgren D, Hoglund M. Promoter analysis of epigeneti-cally controlled genes in bladder cancer. *Genes Chromosomes Cancer.* 2008;47:368–378.

130. Martinez R, Schackert G. Epigenetic aberrations in malignant gliomas: an open door leading to better understanding and treatment. *Epigenetics.* 2007;2:147–150.

131. Everhard S, Kaloshi G, Criniere E, et al. MGMT methylation: a marker of response to temozolomide in low-grade gliomas. *Ann Neurol.* 2006;60:740–743.

132. Snell C, Krypuy M, Wong EM, Loughrey MB, Dobrovic A. BRCA1 promoter methyla-tion in peripheral blood DNA of mutation negative familial breast cancer patients with a BRCA1 tumour phenotype. *Breast Cancer Res.* 2008;10:R12.

133. Hwang KT, Han W, Bae JY, et al. Downregulation of the RUNX3 gene by promoter hypermethylation and hemizygous deletion in breast cancer. *J Korean Med Sci.* 2007;22(Suppl):S24–S31.

134. Wendt MK, Cooper AN, Dwinell MB. Epigenetic silencing of CXCL12 increases the metastatic potential of mammary carcinoma cells. *Oncogene.* 2008;27:1461–1471.

135. Mirza S, Sharma G, Prasad CP, et al. Promoter hypermethylation of TMS1, BRCA1, ERalpha and PRB in serum and tumor DNA of invasive ductal breast carcinoma patients. *Life Sci.* 2007;81:280–287.

136. Versmold B, Felsberg J, Mikeska T, et al. Epigenetic silencing of the candidate tumor suppressor gene PROX1 in sporadic breast cancer. *Int J Cancer.* 2007;121:547–554.

137. Sharma G, Mirza S, Prasad CP, Srivastava A, Gupta SD, Ralhan R. Promoter hyperm-ethylation of p16INK4A, p14ARF, CyclinD2 and Slit2 in serum and tumor DNA from breast cancer patients. *Life Sci.* 2007;80:1873–1881.

138. Coyle YM, Xie XJ, Lewis CM, Bu D, Milchgrub S, Euhus DM. Role of physical activity in modulating breast cancer risk as defined by APC and RASSF1A promoter hypermethylation in nonmalignant breast tissue. *Cancer Epidemiol Biomarkers Prev.* 2007;16:192–196.

139. Caldeira JR, Prando EC, Quevedo FC, Neto FA, RainhoCA, Rogatto SR. CDH1 promoter hypermethylation and E-cadherin protein expression in infiltrating breast cancer. *BMC Cancer.* 2006;6:48.
140. Airoldi I, Cocco C, Di Carlo E, et al. Methylation of the IL-12Rbeta2 gene as novel tumor escape mechanism for pediatric B-acute lymphoblastic leukemia cells. *Cancer Res.* 2006;66:3978–3980.
141. Iacopetta B, Grieu F, Li W, et al. APC gene methylation is inversely correlated with features of the CpG island methylator phenotype in colorectal cancer. *Int J Cancer.* 2006;119:2272–2278.
142. Miyakura Y, Sugano K, Akasu T, et al. Extensive but hemiallelic methylation of the hMLH1 promoter region in early-onset sporadic colon cancers with microsatellite instability. *Clin Gastroenterol Hepatol.* 2004;2:147–156.
143. Zighelboim I, Goodfellow PJ, Schmidt AP, et al. Differential methylation hybridization array of endometrial cancers reveals two novel cancer-specific methylation markers. *Clin Cancer Res.* 2007;13:2882–2889.
144. Huang Y, Peters CJ, Fitzgerald RC, Gjerset RA. Progressive silencing of p14ARF in oesophageal adenocarcinoma. *J Cell Mol Med.* February 2008;13(2):398–409.
145. Chan AO, Chu KM, Huang C, et al. Association between Helicobacter pylori infection and interleukin 1beta polymorphism predispose to CpG island methylation in gastric cancer. *Gut.* 2007;56:595–597.
146. Miyamoto K, Ushijima T. Diagnostic and therapeutic applications of epigenetics. *Jpn J Clin Oncol.* 2005;35:293–301.
147. Su PF, Lee TC, Lin PJ, et al. Differential DNA methylation associated with hepatitis B virus infection in hepatocellular carcinoma. *Int J Cancer.* 2007;121:1257–1264.
148. Feng Q, Hawes SE, Stern JE, et al. DNA methylation in tumor and matched normal tissues from non-small cell lung cancer patients. *Cancer Epidemiol Biomarkers Prev.* 2008;17:645–654.
149. Lo KW, Huang DP. Genetic and epigenetic changes in nasopharyngeal carcinoma. *Semin Cancer Biol.* 2002;12:451–462.
150. Shi H, Guo J, Duff DJ, et al. Discovery of novel epigenetic markers in non-Hodgkin's lymphoma. *Carcinogenesis.* 2007;28:60–70.
151. Lim SL, Smith P, Syed N, et al. Promoter hypermethylation of FANCF and outcome in advanced ovarian cancer. *Br J Cancer.* 2008;98:1452–1456.
152. Wiley A, Katsaros D, Chen H, et al. Aberrant promoter methylation of multiple genes in malignant ovarian tumors and in ovarian tumors with low malignant potential. *Cancer.* 2006;107:299–308.
153. Tokita T, Maesawa C, Kimura T, et al. Methylation status of the SOCS3 gene in human malignant melanomas. *Int J Oncol.* 2007;30:689–694.
154. Murao K, Kubo Y, Ohtani N, Hara E, Arase S. Epigenetic abnormalities in cutaneous squamous cell carcinomas: frequent inactivation of the RB1/p16 and p53 pathways. *Br J Dermatol.* 2006;155:999–1005.
155. van Doorn R, Zoutman WH, Dijkman R, et al. Epigenetic profiling of cutaneous T-cell lymphoma: promoter hypermethylation of multiple tumor suppressor genes including BCL7a, PTPRG, and p73. *J Clin Oncol.* 2005;23:3886–3896.
156. Hoon DS, Spugnardi M, Kuo C, Huang SK, Morton DL, Taback B. Profiling epigenetic inactivation of tumor suppressor genes in tumors and plasma from cutaneous melanoma patients. *Oncogene.* 2004;23:4014–4022.
157. Pfeifer GP, Dammann R. Methylation of the tumor suppressor gene RASSF1A in human tumors. *Biochemistry (Mosc).* 2005;70:576–583.
158. Shin JY, Kim HS, Park J, Park JB, Lee JY. Mechanism for inactivation of the KIP family cyclin-dependent kinase inhibitor genes in gastric cancer cells. *Cancer Res.* 2000;60:262–265.

159. Cheng JC, Weisenberger DJ, Gonzales FA, et al. Continuous zebularine treatment effectively sustains demethylation in human bladder cancer cells. *Mol Cell Biol.* 2004;24:1270–1278.

160. Marquez VE, Barchi JJ, Jr, Kelley JA, et al. Zebularine: a unique molecule for an epigenetically based strategy in cancer chemotherapy. The magic of its chemistry and biology. *Nucleosides Nucleotides Nucleic Acids.* 2005;24:305–318.

161. Bolden JE, Peart MJ, Johnstone RW. Anticancer activities of histone deacetylase inhibitors. *Nature Rev.* 2006;5:769–784.

162. Dai Z, Liu S, Marcucci G, Sadee W. 5-Aza-2'-deoxycytidine and depsipeptide synergistically induce expression of BIK (BCL2-interacting killer). *Biochem Biophys Res Commun.* 2006;351:455–461.

163. Ahrendt SA, Chow JT, Xu LH, et al. Molecular detection of tumor cells in bronchoalveolar lavage fluid from patients with early stage lung cancer. *J Natl Cancer Inst.* 1999;91:332–339.

164. Rohatgi N, Kaur J, Srivastava A, Ralhan R. Smokeless tobacco (khaini) extracts modulate gene expression in epithelial cell culture from an oral hyperplasia. *Oral Oncol.* 2005;41:806–820.

165. Virmani A, Rathi A, Heda S, et al. Aberrant methylation of the cyclin D2 promoter in primary small cell, nonsmall cell lung and breast cancers. *Int J Cancer.* 2003;107:341–345.

166. Tanaka H, Sato H, Sato N, et al. Adding HPV16 testing to abnormal cervical smear detection is useful for predicting CIN3: a prospective study. *Acta Obstet Gynecol Scand.* 2004;83:497–500.

167. Palmisano ME, Gaffga AM, Daigle J, et al. Detection of human papillomavirus DNA in self-administered vaginal swabs as compared to cervical swabs. *International journal of STD & AIDS.* 2003;14:560–567.

168. Sathyanarayana UG, Maruyama R, Padar A, et al. Molecular detection of noninvasive and invasive bladder tumor tissues and exfoliated cells by aberrant promoter methylation of laminin-5 encoding genes. *Cancer Res.* 2004;64:1425–1430.

169. Wang SS, Smiraglia DJ, Wu YZ, et al. Identification of novel methylation markers in cervical cancer using restriction landmark genomic scanning. *Cancer Res.* 2008;68:2489–2497.

170. Muretto P, Ruzzo A, Pizzagalli F, et al. Endogastric capsule for E-cadherin gene (CDH1) promoter hypermethylation assessment in DNA from gastric juice of diffuse gastric cancer patients. *Ann Oncol.* 2008;19:516–519.

171. Rosas SL, Koch W, da Costa Carvalho MG, et al. Promoter hypermethylation patterns of p16, O6-methylguanine-DNA-methyltransferase, and death-associated protein kinase in tumors and saliva of head and neck cancer patients. *Cancer Res.* 2001;61:939–942.

172. Leng S, Stidley CA, Willink R, et al. Double-strand break damage and associated DNA repair genes predispose smokers to gene methylation. *Cancer Res.* 2008;68:3049–3056.

173. Palmisano WA, Divine KK, Saccomanno G, et al. Predicting lung cancer by detecting aberrant promoter methylation in sputum. *Cancer Res.* 2000;60:5954–5958.

174. Ahmed FE, Vos P, iJames S, et al. Transcriptomic molecular markers for screening human colon cancer in stool and tissue. *Cancer Genomics Proteomics.* 2007;4:1–20.

175. Goessl C, Krause H, Muller M, et al. Fluorescent methylation-specific polymerase chain reaction for DNA-based detection of prostate cancer in bodily fluids. *Cancer Res.* 2000;60:5941–5945.

176. Hoque MO, Begum S, Topaloglu O, et al. Quantitative detection of promoter hypermethylation of multiple genes in the tumor, urine, and serum DNA of patients with renal cancer. *Cancer Res.* 2004;64:5511–5517.

177. Verma M, Seminara D, Arena FJ, John C, Iwamoto K, Hartmuller V. Genetic and epigenetic biomarkers in cancer: improving diagnosis, risk assessment, and disease stratification. *Mol Diagn Ther.* 2006;10:1–15.

178. Verma M. Pancreatic cancer epidemiology. *Technol Cancer Res Treat.* 2005;4:295–301.
179. Ward EM, Sabbioni G, DeBord DG, et al. Monitoring of aromatic amine exposures in workers at a chemical plant with a known bladder cancer excess. *J Natl Cancer Inst.* 1996;88:1046–1052.
180. Kampa M, Castanas E. Human health effects of air pollution. *Environ Pollut.* January 2008;151(2):362–367.
181. Chien JW, Au DH, Barnett MJ, Goodman GE. Spirometry, rapid FEV1 decline, and lung cancer among asbestos exposed heavy smokers. *Copd.* 2007;4:339–346.
182. Gamble J. Risk of gastrointestinal cancers from inhalation and ingestion of asbestos. *Regul Toxicol Pharmacol.* October 2008;52(1 Suppl):S124–S153.
183. Darbre PD. Environmental oestrogens, cosmetics and breast cancer. *Best Pract Res.* 2006;20:121–143.
184. Salnikow K, Zhitkovich A. Genetic and epigenetic mechanisms in metal carcinogenesis and cocarcinogenesis: nickel, arsenic, and chromium. *Chem Res Toxicol.* 2008;21:28–44.
185. Edwards TM, Myers JP. Environmental exposures and gene regulation in disease etiology. *Environ Health Perspect.* 2007;115:1264–1270.
186. Carpenter DO. Polychlorinated biphenyls (PCBs): routes of exposure and effects on human health. *Rev Environ Health.* 2006;21:1–23.
187. Dolinoy DC, Huang D, Jirtle RL. Maternal nutrient supplementation counteracts bisphenol A-induced DNA hypomethylation in early development. *Proc Natl Acad Sci USA.* 2007;104:13056–13061.
188. Golka K, Weistenhofer W. Fire fighters, combustion products, and urothelial cancer. *J Toxicol Environ Health.* 2008;11:32–44.
189. Lock EA, Reed CJ. Trichloroethylene: mechanisms of renal toxicity and renal cancer and relevance to risk assessment. *Toxicol Sci.* 2006;91:313–331.

29

The use of family history in public health practice: the epidemiologic view

Rodolfo Valdez, Muin J. Khoury, and Paula W. Yoon

Introduction

With the advent of molecular genetics, the accelerated mapping of human genes to specific chromosome locations was made possible without the use of detailed pedigrees. Moreover, following the sequencing of the human genome, new techniques now allow for the scanning of entire genomes in search of genes or gene markers associated with a given trait, regardless of the pattern of inheritance. Among these major advances, however, it is not likely that an instrument as useful as family history will be rendered obsolete as a genomic tool. In this chapter we will argue not only that the use of family history will continue to be valid in clinical settings, but also that family history is poised to become a tool of widespread use in public health settings. Since our emphasis will be on the latter argument, we will address the clinical aspects of family history briefly.

Family History in the Clinical Setting

A well-documented family history for a suspected genetic condition should include a standard pedigree with three generations of relatives, age and sex of each relative, age at onset of the condition for the affected relatives, and age at death and cause of death for the deceased relatives. Complementary information could include ethnic background, adoption, consanguinity, and reproductive history. Such information is rich in clinical applications (1). For example, it could help

- establish the genetic nature of a condition and its pattern of inheritance
- identify healthy family members at risk and to estimate their risk for a condition
- diagnose some conditions
- decide on type and frequency of screening and diagnostic tests
- anticipate the development and decide on the management of a condition
- assess the probability that future family members will inherit a condition
- educate patients and their relatives about the probabilistic nature of genetic inheritance and the influence of environmental factors on inherited conditions.

These applications of family history in the clinical setting will gain even more importance as the discovery of new genes and phenotypes accumulates at a rapid pace. For example, the pattern of inheritance of all these new genes and phenotypes will surely need clarification and family history is a great tool for this task. Genes spread through families and their expression is ultimately affected by the environment shared by family members. The timely collection, interpretation, and translation of family history information into routine health care practice will be the domain of clinical genetics for the foreseeable future.

Family History in the Public Health Setting

Family History Captures the Joint Effect of Genes and Environment on Phenotypes

Several diseases of great public health importance for their high prevalence in the general population are thought to have a genetic component; however, they do not seem to follow Mendelian patterns of inheritance. And even if they did, the number of genetic loci involved would make it extremely difficult to discern these patterns. Moreover, additional genetic and nongenetic factors (i.e., gene–gene and gene–environment interactions) may compound the difficulty of unveiling these already intricate patterns. The high level of difficulty, however, has not deterred efforts to bring to light the genetic component of major diseases such as cancer, heart disease, diabetes, and many other chronic diseases. Almost daily there are scientific reports of genes or genetic markers found associated with a major disease. Furthermore, meta-analyses and systematic reviews begin to show some consistency among a few gene–disease associations that have been replicated. But for major chronic diseases like diabetes, the effect sizes of these associations remain small, and therefore of uncertain utility in public health (2).

Family health history can be the tool of choice as a first step toward examining the role that genes and environment play in the emergence of complex conditions in populations. Complex conditions that result from the interaction of genes and environment are more likely to concur among close relatives for several reasons: first, close relatives share a substantial proportion of their genes; second, close relatives might have been exposed to the same environment for prolonged periods of their lives; third, shared family life and culture bring the opportunity to acquire and practice long-lasting habits and behaviors that ultimately may affect health.

The observation that the risk for a condition is elevated among the close relatives of a person already affected with that condition has broad practical applications in public health. For example, the collection of family history from index cases became a very important tool to track and control infectious disease outbreaks early in the past century (3). Hence, the knowledge of the familial aggregation of a condition may help to control it, even when the mechanism of transmission is unknown.

Family History as a Risk Assessment Tool

A large and growing body of evidence indicates that family history can in fact be counted as a risk factor that is significantly and independently associated with several diseases of public health importance (specific examples will be discussed later in this chapter). However, the widespread use of family history in preventive medicine has been hindered by several factors, which include difficulty in allocating time to collect the information during visits to health care providers, inadequate systems for data collection and decision support, limited knowledge and skill among health care personnel for interpreting family histories and for counseling patients according to their familial risk, and unclear reimbursement policies (4).

In our opinion, a major obstacle for the widespread use of family history in public health is the lack of a standard approach to define familial risk. A good definition should convey properly the health risks associated with having relatives affected with a condition. More often than not, family history is casually defined in epidemiologic studies as a dichotomous variable (positive/negative) depending on the presence or absence of one or more affected individuals among the close (first- or second-degree) relatives of a healthy patient or proband. To fully realize the potential of family history as a public health tool, a more systematic approach to risk assessment is necessary. At a minimum, a family history collected to assess familial risk for a condition should include the following (5)

- the type and degree of relationship among family members (pedigree)
- age and sex of each relative
- age at diagnosis for each family member affected with the condition
- age, cause, and date of death if the relative has died
- ethnicity and ancestry may be important in some cases
- chronic habits and behaviors that might influence health among relatives.

There are tools designed to assess familial risk based on this type of information. The next step, their implementation in public health settings, should be subjected to the same standards required for genetic tests and other well-established risk assessment tools. The current standards are known as the ACCE framework, first designed to assess the benefits and risks of genetic tests (6). This framework includes four elements to be evaluated: (i) analytical validity (ability to identify the true health status); (ii) clinical validity (ability to accurately predict disease status); (iii) clinical utility (capability of motivating positive changes in health care systems and personal behaviors); and (iv) ethical, legal, and social issues (see Chapter 24).

Family History as a Risk Factor

In the next section we will present ample, current evidence supporting the association between family history and the risk of several major chronic diseases. Even though this evidence is highly suggestive of a distinct genetic influence on these diseases, it is virtually impossible to distinguish the genetic from the environmental contributions to the development of these diseases. In any case, most studies were not designed to test the independence of these contributions.

In addition, family history has been used to detect preclinical signs of some diseases. Table 29.1 presents examples of studies that report physiological alterations, which may lead to chronic disease, among healthy individuals with diseased relatives. Despite differences in the definitions of family history, the implication that family history can detect early signs of disease is clear. And the public health implications of such detection are promising, as early detection is a desirable goal in disease prevention.

Recent Epidemiologic Findings Using Family History

Family history, alone or in combination with other risk factors, can identify individuals and families who are at increased risk for chronic diseases. Ultimately, we believe, family history can play a role in the prevention and management of common chronic diseases through risk assessment in populations and interventions in high-risk groups. The assessment of familial risk can be the basis for recommendations that may include lifestyle changes, screening, chemoprevention, and genetic testing (16). For example, the United States Preventive Services Task Force (USPSTF) has issued recommendations based on relevant family history. These recommendations include screening and the adoption of certain behaviors to prevent breast cancer, colorectal cancer, dyslipidemias, cardiovascular disease, and abdominal aortic aneurysm (17).

Cardiovascular Disease

Epidemiologic evidence indicates that family history is a significant and prevalent risk factor for many common diseases such as cardiovascular disease (CVD), type 2 diabetes, and cancer. One of the first population-based studies to examine the association between family medical history and cardiovascular disease was the Health Family Tree Study in Utah (18). This study showed not only that family history of coronary heart disease (CHD) and the occurrence of the disease were strongly related but, perhaps more importantly, that the disease and associated risk factors were clustered in a small proportion of families (high risk). Data from 122,155 families showed that 72% of early onset cases of CHD (aged < 55 years) in the population was concentrated in just 14% of all families. Likewise, 86% of cases of early onset stroke was concentrated in just 11% of families. In the 20 years since findings from the Utah study were first reported, hundreds of papers have been published on the association between family history and CVD and the use of family history for predicting disease (19). Recent studies have focused on determining which characteristics of family history contribute most to the risk increase (e.g., number of affected relatives, lineage, age of onset, type of relative). Many studies have shown that the association gains strength as the number of affected first-degree relatives increases (20–22) and the age at onset of the disease decreases (22–25). Interestingly, several studies have shown that having a sibling with CVD may confer

Table 29.1 Sample of studies reporting the effect of family history on a trait that precedes a condition or disease

Condition	Precursor Trait	Definition of Family History	Effect Attributed to Family History
Alzheimer disease	Rate of glucose metabolism in the brain	Only mother or father diagnosed with the disease at age 65–80 years	Healthy adults (age: 48–80 years) with a maternal family history had a lower cerebral metabolic rate of glucose than comparable subjects with just paternal or no family history (7).
Cardiovascular disease	Endothelium-dependent vasodilation (EDV)	Both parents with type 2 diabetes	Normal adults (average age around 38 years) with a family history had a significantly lower EDV than comparable subjects with no family history (8).
Cardiovascular disease	Intimal-medial thickness of the common carotid artery (IMT CCA)	Diabetes family history score that includes only first-degree relatives older than the participant (parents, siblings)	IMT CCA was increased among adult (average age around 40 years) Mexican Americans without diabetes but with a higher burden of the disease among their older first-degree relatives (9).
Colorectal cancer	Colorectal polyps	One or more first-degree relatives reported to have had cancer of the colon, rectum, or large bowel	The risk of colon cancer among subjects who reported at least one first-degree relative with colorectal polyps was approximately double the risk of those who did not (10).
Diabetes	Insulin action	Both parents with type 2 diabetes	Normoglycemic adults (average age around 30 years) with a family history had significantly reduced indicators of glucose disposal at baseline and developed diabetes, two decades later, at a rate 10–20 times the rate of comparable subjects with no family history (11).

(Continued)

Table 29.1 Continued

Condition	Precursor Trait	Definition of Family History	Effect Attributed to Family History
Diabetes	Beta cell function and insulin sensitivity	First- or second-degree relative with diabetes, confirmed by treatment or by interview with other relatives if deceased	Healthy children (aged 12–15 years), mostly of Hispanic background, with a family history were more likely to have a lower insulin secretory capacity and a lower rate of glucose disposal than comparable children with no family history (12).
Diabetes	Impaired glucose tolerance (IGT)	Type 2 diabetes in at least one parent, a sibling, or a grandparent	About one in three overweight Hispanic children (average age: 11 years) with a family history has IGT. The association is independent of the severity of overweight (13).
Diabetes	Insulin sensitivity	Presence of known family members with type 2 diabetes in any of three generations (siblings, parents, or grandparents)	Healthy white children (average age around 12 years) with a family history showed lower insulin sensitivity and insulin clearance capability than comparable children with no family history (14).
Obesity, diabetes	Expression of adiponectin receptor genes and the concentration of adiponectin in plasma	At least two known first-degree relatives with diabetes	Healthy adult Mexican Americans (aged 30–40 years) with a family history showed a significantly lower gene expression and lower plasma concentrations of adiponectin than comparable subjects with no family history (15).

a greater risk for the disease than having an affected parent (20,26,27). For example, data from the Framingham Offspring Study, a prospective study with validated CVD events, indicate that having a sibling with CVD resulted in greater risk for the disease (OR = 2.0) than having an affected parent (OR = 1.5), even after adjusting for age and traditional risk factors (26).

Less is known about stroke and family history, although several studies have shown increased risk for stroke associated with having parents and other first-degree relatives with the disease (28–35). It has been reported that having a first-degree relative diagnosed with any vascular event before age 65 years was associated with a two-fold increased risk of ischemic stroke (35). In a case-control study of women aged 18–44 years, the risk of hemorrhagic or ischemic stroke was double for the cases with parental or sibling history of stroke (32). Another study, using a three-tiered familial risk stratification method, found that people in the high familial risk stratum were about four times more likely to report having had a stroke compared to people in the moderate and average risk strata, independently of demographic factors and other health conditions (36). Among patients who suffered a transient ischemic attack, family history of stroke and family history of myocardial infarction were associated with hypertension (37). Hypertension is one of the strongest risk factors for stroke and has been found to aggregate in families (38–40). Despite the epidemiologic evidence that family history of stroke is an independent risk factor for stroke, its use for risk assessment, alone or in combination with other risk factors such as hypertension, has been limited.

Recent research on the association of family history of CHD and the risk for the disease supports the use of family history in the detection of intermediate phenotypes or subclinical signs of disease. The Johns Hopkins Sibling study identified asymptomatic women aged 30–59 years who were the sisters of women hospitalized with premature CHD (41). Framingham global coronary risk scores were then calculated for the asymptomatic sisters. Ninety-eight percent of these women were classified as low risk, but one out of three of them had significant coronary atherosclerosis based on their coronary artery calcification (CAC) scores. Similarly, among asymptomatic individuals enrolled in the Multi-Ethnic Study of Atherosclerosis, a significant association, which varied by type of relative, was found between family history and CAC (42). The association was strongest in participants reporting a family history in both a parent and a sibling (OR = 2.7), followed by a sibling only (OR = 2.1), and a parent only (OR = 1.5). This type of evidence has led to the modification of existing risk algorithms to add family history and other novel risk factors (43,44). For example, a modified version of the Framingham Risk Score, the Reynolds Risk Score, includes the usual risk factors plus parental history of early myocardial infarction (age < 60 years) and C-reactive protein, an inflammatory marker. When applied to a cohort of healthy women aged 45 years and older who had been followed up for 10 years, the Reynolds score greatly improved the accuracy of the risk estimation compared to the current ATP-III prediction scores. Nearly 50% of the women classified at intermediate risk by the ATP-III scores were more accurately reclassified into the higher and lower risk categories by the Reynolds score. Obviously, more validation needs to be done for risk algorithms that include family history of CHD, but the evidence clearly suggests that individuals with a family history may benefit from strategies to screen and treat early several risk factors for CHD.

Diabetes

It has been well established that the risk of diabetes among those with a family history of the disease is greater than the risk in the general population. Most studies report a two- to six-fold increased risk independent of other risk factors (45). And there seems to be a dose response effect: the risk is higher when both parents are affected than when only one parent is affected (46–49). A few studies have also suggested that a maternal history may be associated with greater risk than paternal history (50,51). Studies employing a familial risk stratification methodology have shown that the association between familial risk and diabetes is graded and independent of other major risk factors (49,52,53). Data from the 2004 HealthStyles national survey evaluated a three-tiered familial risk stratification algorithm (52). For the stratification, the algorithm considered the number of relatives with diabetes, their degree of relationship, the lineage or side of the family with cases of diabetes, and age at diagnosis. Diabetes was assessed by self-report. Compared to respondents with a weak familial risk for diabetes, moderate and strong familial risk categories were associated respectively with 3.6-fold (95% CI: 2.8, 4.7) and 7.6-fold (95% CI: 5.9, 9.8) increase in diabetes after adjusting for common demographic factors. A more recent analysis (53), with 6-year data from the National Health and Nutrition Examination Survey (NHANES, 1999–2004, $n = 16,388$ adults), included three risk categories: (i) *high*: at least two first-degree relatives, or one first-degree and at least two second-degree relatives with diabetes from the same lineage; (ii) *moderate*: just one first-degree and one second-degree relative with diabetes, or only one first-degree relative with diabetes, or at least two second-degree relatives with diabetes from the same maternal or paternal line; (iii) *average*: no family history of diabetes or, at most, one second-degree relative with diabetes. Diabetes was assessed by self-report or a fasting plasma glucose measurement. Overall, 70% of the U.S. adults were in the average, 23% in the moderate, and 7% in the high familial risk category for diabetes. After accounting for sex, race/ethnicity, age, body mass index, hypertension, income, and education, the odds of having diabetes for people in the moderate and high familial risk categories, when compared to the average, were 2.3 and 5.5 times higher, respectively. Another study (49), using NHANES data from 1999 to 2002, showed a significant association between high familial risk and the presence of diabetes among people who did not know they had the disease. Undiagnosed cases of diabetes were detected by fasting plasma glucose. Since, nationally, nearly one-third of people with diabetes are not aware they have the disease (54), family history is a potential screening tool to not only identify people with an intermediate phenotype of the disease (prediabetes), but to find those who already have diabetes but have not been diagnosed.

Many screening tools have been developed for early detection of type 2 diabetes. These tools include noninvasive measurements like age, gender, body mass index, and family history to facilitate their use in a primary care setting and even outside of a clinical setting (55–61). These tools may be of great value as a first step in serial diagnostic strategies and for raising awareness of diabetes risk factors in community settings. However, studies have repeatedly shown that screening tools developed in one population rarely apply to others. Sensitivities, specificities, and predictive values are usually higher for the population where the tool was developed (62,63). This may be due to differences in population characteristics and in the distribution of risk factors. Risk assessment tools for diabetes may have to be adapted or recalibrated to the populations where they are being used.

Even the recommendations to screen for diabetes with glucose measurements are not uniform. The USPSTF recommends screening for type 2 diabetes in adults with hypertension or dyslipidemias (64). The USPSTF does not recommend universal diabetes screening for adults. The American Diabetes Association recommends screening every 3 years for adults beginning at age 45. But adults with a family history of diabetes, obesity, or other characteristics should be screened at younger ages and more frequently, every 1–2 years (65). Although screening criteria differ, there is evidence that family history influences screening practices in the primary care setting. It has been reported that having a family history of diabetes is strongly associated with providers ordering a plasma glucose test even after adjusting for the patient's age, weight, and blood pressure (OR =2.9; 95% CI: 1.3, 6.7). However, having a first-degree relative with diabetes did not influence the providers recommending diet or exercise counseling (66). A few population-based studies have found that family history of diabetes was associated with greater awareness of risk and higher reporting of risk-reducing behaviors (67,68). The prevention of type 2 diabetes in high-risk individuals involves the adoption of lifestyle behaviors that have proven difficult to change and maintain. It remains to be seen whether using family history to personalize risk might empower people at above average risk to seek medical advice and practice healthy behaviors.

Cancer

Based on substantial epidemiologic evidence, family history is already a key component of risk assessment for many cancers. It is estimated that 5–10% of cancers have a strong hereditary basis. Examples of these include hereditary nonpolyposis colorectal cancer (HNPCC) (69) and breast and ovarian cancers associated with the *BRCA1* and *BRCA2* genes (70). Approximately 10–30% of cancers are considered familial. These cancers cluster in families but the genetic mutations that may cause them are not known. Familial cancers may be due to shared susceptibility genes and common environments and behaviors. Much work has been done on developing cancer risk assessment tools based on family history. Clinicians and genetic counselors have been using self-administered questionnaires for many years to gather detailed information about cancer among first- and second-degree relatives. A more recent trend is the use of computerized assessment tools that include sophisticated algorithms that assign risk categories, and in some cases recommend strategies for disease prevention, early detection, and genetic testing (71,72). Automating the risk assessment process has highlighted the need to validate and standardize the risk assessment algorithms being used in these tools. Recently the USPSTF issued a clinical guideline defining family history criteria that could be used to identify women who should be referred for genetic risk assessment and testing for breast and ovarian cancer susceptibility (73). Much of the evidence for creating risk algorithms based on family history, including the USPSTF guidelines, comes from clinical data sets and case-control studies that have used registries of cancer patients. Population-based studies are needed to evaluate the effectiveness of these algorithms in other settings. The need for the evaluation of the clinical validity of these algorithms is exemplified by a recent study in which six different cancer family history screening protocols were applied to the same cohort of women aged 21–55 years. The proportion of women who met the criteria for genetic testing ranged from 4.4% to 7.8%, depending on the protocol used. Based on the Kappa statistic, the protocols had only low to fair agreement (74).

From a public health perspective, it is hoped that awareness of family history of cancer might motivate people to adhere to screening guidelines. In 2004, only 51.8% of U.S. adults aged 50 years or older had recently undergone a sigmoidoscopy or colonoscopy or a fecal occult blood test (FOBT). This figure varied by state: from 42.5% in Mississippi to 64.6% in Rhode Island (75). Barriers are numerous, but any strategy that could improve participation in colorectal cancer screening would likely have an impact on morbidity and mortality from this disease. As with CVD and diabetes, there are few data describing the impact of familial risk assessment for cancer on the adoption of health-related behaviors (76). As an alternative, decision analysis methods have been used to estimate the impact of family-based screening (77,78). The clinical and economic impact of using family history to identify persons for colorectal cancer screening younger than age 50 years has been estimated: for the year 2004 approximately one million people would have been eligible for early colonoscopy, resulting in 2,800 invasive cancers detected and 29,300 life years gained, at a total cost of $900 million. This works out to a discounted cost per life year gained of about $58,000. While results from these simulation studies are promising, further data are needed to determine the effectiveness of this strategy for disease prevention and the social burden of the disease.

Summary and Conclusion

The use of family history and pedigrees has a venerable history in genetics. This use long precedes the discoveries that firmly established the rules of inheritance; however, those discoveries and more recent advances in genetics and genomics have not weakened and actually may have strengthened the role that this simple but informative tool can play in medicine and public health. On the one hand, the fast pace of current gene discoveries has created new and exciting challenges for clinical geneticists who must rely on family histories for many aspects of their work. On the other hand, family history appears to act as a good proxy for the genetic component of some diseases of major public health importance. This is not to deny that family history also reflects the actions of environments that family members have shared totally or partially—genes don't operate in a vacuum, after all. It is rather to affirm that, at least for some diseases, family history can be interpreted as a risk exposure that starts at birth. It is then expected that individuals with a family history for these diseases will show intermediate phenotypes or preclinical signs of the disease earlier in life than individuals without such family history. This interpretation has obvious implications for public health. Indeed, many guidelines consider family history of a disease as a relevant criterion for early screening and as a trigger of more aggressive approaches to prevention.

Despite its importance, family history still faces many barriers to becoming fully established as a clinical and public health tool. The initial barrier is the lack of a systematic approach to collecting and interpreting family history as a risk factor. Fortunately, in the past few years there has been a renewed interest in doing research aimed at overcoming this barrier. As a result of this renewed interest, we should expect in the near future great improvements in the following areas: (i) the collection, storage, and retrieval of family history information through the use of computers; (ii) the interpretation of the health risks associated with family history for major diseases; (iii) the development of algorithms to capture the distribution of familial risk in populations; (iv) the incorporation of familial risk into electronic medical records; (v) the organization and delivery of evidence-based advice for the prevention of major diseases where familial risk is elevated; (vi) the performance of cost-effectiveness studies to evaluate the use of family history in the clinical and the public health settings.

References

1. Bennett RL. *The Practical Guide to the Genetic Family History.* New York: Wiley-Liss Inc.; 1999.
2. Zeggini E, Scott LJ, Saxena R, Voight BF. Meta-analysis of genome-wide association data and large-scale replication identifies additional susceptibility loci for type 2 diabetes. *Nat Genet.* 2008;40:638–645.
3. Frost WH. The familial aggregation of infectious diseases. *Am J Public Health.* 1938;28:7–13.
4. Suther S, Goodson P. Barriers to the provision of genetic services by primary care physicians: a systematic review of the literature. *Genet Med.* 2003;5:70–76.
5. Bennett RL. The family medical history. *Prim Care Clin Office Pract.* 2004;31:479–495.
6. Yoon PW, Scheuner MT, Khoury MJ. Research priorities for evaluating family history in the prevention of common chronic diseases. *Am J Prev Med.* 2003;24:128–135.
7. Mosconi L, Brys M, Switalski R, et al. Maternal family history of Alzheimer's disease predisposes to reduced brain glucose metabolism. *Proc Natl Acad Sci USA.* 2007;104:19067–19072.

8. Goldfine AB, Beckman JA, Betensky RA, et al. Family history of diabetes is a major determinant of endothelial function. *J Am Coll Cardiol.* 2006;47:2456–2461.

9. Kao WHL, Hsueh WC, Rainwater DL, et al. Family history of type 2 diabetes is associated with increased carotid artery intimal-medial thickness in Mexican Americans. *Diabetes Care.* 2005;28:1882–1889.

10. Kerber RA, Slattery ML, Potter JD, Caan BJ, Edwards SL. Risk of colon cancer associated with a family history of cancer or colorectal polyps: the Diet, Activity, and Reproduction in Colon Cancer Study. *Int J Cancer.* 1998;78:157–160.

11. Goldfine AB, Bouche C, Parker RA, et al. Insulin resistance is a poor predictor of type 2 diabetes in individuals with no family history of disease. *Proc Natl Acad Sci USA.* 2003;100:2724–2729.

12. Rosenbaum M, Nonas C, Horlick M, et al. β-cell function and insulin sensitivity in early adolescence: association with body fatness and family history of type 2 diabetes mellitus. *J Clin Endocrinol Metab.* 2004;89:5469–5476.

13. Goran MI, Bergman RN, Avila Q, et al. Impaired glucose tolerance and reduced β-cell function in overweight latino children with a positive family history for type 2 diabetes. *J Clin Endocrinol Metab.* 2004;89:207–212.

14. Arslanian SA, Bacha F, Saad R, Gungor N. Family history of type 2 diabetes is associated with decreased insulin sensitivity and an impaired balance between insulin sensitivity and insulin secretion in white youth. *Diabetes Care.* 2005;28:127–131.

15. Civitarese AE, Jenkinson CP, Richardson D, et al. Adiponectin receptors gene expression and insulin sensitivity in non-diabetic Mexican Americans with or without a family history of Type 2 diabetes. *Diabetologia.* 2004;47:816–820.

16. Scheuner MT, Yoon PW, Khoury MJ. Contribution of Mendelian disorders to common chronic disease: opportunities for recognition, intervention, and prevention. *Am J Med Genet C Semin Med Genet.* 2004;125C:50–65.

17. Wattendorf DJ, Hadley DW. Family history: the three-generation pedigree. *Am Fam Physician.* 2005;72:441–448.

18. Hunt SC, Williams RR, Barlow GK. A comparison of positive family history definitions for defining risk of future disease. *J Chronic Dis.* 1986;39:809–821.

19. Kardia SL, Modell SM, Peyser PA. Family-centered approaches to understanding and preventing coronary heart disease. *Am J Prev Med.* 2003;24:143–151.

20. Silberberg JS, Wlodarczyk J, Fryer J, Robertson R, Hensley MJ. Risk associated with various definitions of family history of coronary heart disease. The Newcastle Family History Study II. *Am J Epidemiol.* 1998;147:1133–1139.

21. Bertuzzi M, Negri E, Tavani A, La Vecchia C. Family history of ischemic heart disease and risk of acute myocardial infarction. *Prev Med.* 2003;37:183–187.

22. Scheuner MT, Whitworth WC, McGruder H, Yoon PW, Khoury MJ. Expanding the definition of a positive family history for early-onset coronary heart disease. *Genet Med.* 2006;8:491–501.

23. Brown DW, Giles WH, Burke W, Greenlund KJ, Croft JB. Familial aggregation of early-onset myocardial infarction. *Community Genet.* 2002;5:232–238.

24. Sesso HD, Lee IM, Gaziano JM, Rexrode KM, Glynn RJ, Buring JE. Maternal and paternal history of myocardial infarction and risk of cardiovascular disease in men and women. *Circulation.* 2001;104:393–398.

25. Vaidya D, Yanek LR, Moy TF, Pearson TA, Becker LC, Becker DM. Incidence of coronary artery disease in siblings of patients with premature coronary artery disease: 10 years of follow-up. *Am J Cardiol.* 2007;100:1410–1415.

26. Murabito JM, Pencina MJ, Nam BH, et al. Sibling cardiovascular disease as a risk factor for cardiovascular disease in middle-aged adults. *JAMA.* 2005;294:3117–3123.

27. Friedlander Y, Arbogast P, Schwartz SM, et al. Family history as a risk factor for early onset myocardial infarction in young women. *Atherosclerosis*. 2001;156:201–207.

28. Liao D, Myers R, Hunt S, et al. Familial history of stroke and stroke risk. The Family Heart Study. *Stroke*. 1997;28:1908–1912.

29. Tentschert S, Greisenegger S, Wimmer R, Lang W, Lalouschek W. Association of parental history of stroke with clinical parameters in patients with ischemic stroke or transient ischemic attack. *Stroke*. 2003;34:2114–2119.

30. Jousilahti P, Rastenyte D, Tuomilehto J, Sarti C, Vartiainen E. Parental history of cardiovascular disease and risk of stroke. A prospective follow-up of 14371 middle-aged men and women in Finland. *Stroke*. 1997;28:1361–1366.

31. Khaw KT, Barrett-Connor E. Family history of stroke as an independent predictor of ischemic heart disease in men and stroke in women. *Am J Epidemiol*. 1986;123:59–66.

32. Kim H, Friedlander Y, Longstreth WT, Jr, Edwards KL, Schwartz SM, Siscovick DS. Family history as a risk factor for stroke in young women. *Am J Prev Med*. 2004;27:391–396.

33. Wannamethee SG, Shaper AG, Ebrahim S. History of parental death from stroke or heart trouble and the risk of stroke in middle-aged men. *Stroke*. 1996;27:1492–1498.

34. Jood K, Ladenvall C, Rosengren A, Blomstrand C, Jern C. Family history in ischemic stroke before 70 years of age: the Sahlgrenska Academy Study on Ischemic Stroke. *Stroke*. 2005;36:1383–1387.

35. Jerrard-Dunne P, Cloud G, Hassan A, Markus HS. Evaluating the genetic component of ischemic stroke subtypes: a family history study. *Stroke*. 2003;34:1364–1369.

36. Mvundura M, McGruder H, Khoury MJ, Valdez R, Yoon PW. Family history as a risk factor for early-onset stroke/transient ischemic attack among U.S. Adults. *Public Health Genomics* (DOI:10.1159/000209879) Published Online: March 23, 2009.

37. Flossmann E, Rothwell PM. Family history of stroke in patients with transient ischemic attack in relation to hypertension and other intermediate phenotypes. *Stroke*. 2005;36:830–835.

38. Feinberg WM, Albers GW, Barnett HJM, et al. Guidelines for the management of transient ischemic attacks. *Stroke*. 1994;25:1320–1335.

39. Arnett DK. Heritability of hypertension and target organ damage (Chapter A78). In: Izzo JL, Black HR, Goodfriend TL, eds. *Hypertension Primer: The Essentials of High Blood Pressure*. Lippincott: Williams & Wilkins; 2003:227.

40. Seidlerová J, Bochud M, Staessen JA, et al. Heritability and intrafamilial aggregation of arterial characteristics. *J Hypertens*. 2008;26:721–728.

41. Michos ED, Vasamreddy CR, Becker DM, et al. Women with a low Framingham risk score and a family history of premature coronary heart disease have a high prevalence of subclinical coronary atherosclerosis. *Am Heart J*. 2005;150:1276–1281.

42. Nasir K, Budoff MJ, Wong ND, et al. Family history of premature coronary heart disease and coronary artery calcification: Multi-Ethnic Study of Atherosclerosis (MESA). *Circulation*. 2007;116:619–626.

43. Ridker PM, Buring JE, Rifai N, Cook NR. Development and validation of improved algorithms for the assessment of global cardiovascular risk in women: the Reynolds Risk Score. *JAMA*. 2007;297:611–619.

44. Hippisley-Cox J, Coupland C, Vinogradova Y, Robson J, May M, Brindle P. Derivation and validation of QRISK, a new cardiovascular disease risk score for the United Kingdom: prospective open cohort study. *BMJ*. 2007;335(7611):136.

45. Harrison TA, Hindorff LA, Kim H, et al. Family history of diabetes as a potential public health tool. *Am J Prev Med*. 2003;24:152–159.

46. Knowler WC, Pettitt DJ, Savage PJ, Bennett PH. Diabetes incidence in Pima Indians: contributions of obesity and parental diabetes. *Am J Epidemiol*. 1981;113:144–156.

47. Bjørnholt JV, Erikssen G, Liestøl K, Jervell J, Thaulow E, Erikssen J. Type 2 diabetes and maternal family history: an impact beyond slow glucose removal rate and fasting hyperglycemia in low-risk individuals? Results from 22.5 years of follow-up of healthy nondiabetic men. *Diabetes Care.* 2000;23:1255–1259.

48. Meigs JB, Cupples LA, Wilson PW. Parental transmission of type 2 diabetes: the Framingham Offspring Study. *Diabetes.* 2000;49:2201–2207.

49. Annis AM, Caulder MS, Cook ML, Duquette D. Family history, diabetes, and other demographic and risk factors among participants of the National Health and Nutrition Examination Survey 1999–2002. *Prev Chronic Dis.* 2005;2(2):A19.

50. Mitchell BD, Valdez R, Hazuda HP, Haffner SM, Monterrosa A, Stern MP. Differences in the prevalence of diabetes and impaired glucose tolerance according to maternal or paternal history of diabetes. *Diabetes Care.* 1993;16:1262–1267.

51. Lin RS, Lee WC, Lee YT, Chou P, Fu CC. Maternal role in type 2 diabetes mellitus: indirect evidence for a mitochondrial inheritance. *Int J Epidemiol.* 1994;23:886–890.

52. Hariri S, Yoon PW, Qureshi N, Valdez R, Scheuner MT, Khoury MJ. Family history of type 2 diabetes: a population-based screening tool for prevention? *Genet Med.* 2006;8:102–108.

53. Valdez R, Yoon PW, Liu T, Khoury MJ. Family history and prevalence of diabetes in the U.S. population: the 6-year results from the National Health and Nutrition Examination Survey (1999–2004). *Diabetes Care.* 2007;10:2517–2522.

54. Centers for Disease Control and Prevention. National diabetes fact sheet: general information and national estimates on diabetes in the United States, 2007. Atlanta, GA: U.S. Department of Health and Human Services, Centers for Disease Control and Prevention, 2008. Available at http://www.cdc.gov/diabetes/pubs/pdf/ndfs_2007.pdf. Accessed October 15, 2008.

55. Ramachandran A, Snehalatha C, Vijay V, Wareham NJ, Colagiuri S. Derivation and validation of diabetes risk score for urban Asian Indians. *Diabetes Res Clin Pract.* 2005;70:63–70.

56. Aekplakorn W, Bunnag P, Woodward M, et al. A risk score for predicting incident diabetes in the Thai population. *Diabetes Care.* 2006;29:1872–1877.

57. Al-Lawati JA, Tuomilehto J. Diabetes risk score in Oman: a tool to identify prevalent type 2 diabetes among Arabs of the Middle East. *Diabetes Res Clin Pract.* 2007;77:438–444.

58. Glümer C, Carstensen B, Sandbæk A, Lauritzen T, Jørgensen T, Borch-Johnsen K. A Danish diabetes risk score for targeted screening: the Inter99 study. *Diabetes Care.* 2004;27:727–733.

59. Schmidt MI, Duncan BB, Bang H, et al. Identifying individuals at high risk for diabetes: the atherosclerosis risk in communities study. *Diabetes Care.* 2005;28:2013–2018.

60. Ruige JB, de Neeling JN, Kostense PJ, Bouter LM, Heine RJ. Performance of an NIDDM screening questionnaire based on symptoms and risk factors. *Diabetes Care.* 1997;20:491–496.

61. American Diabetes Association. Diabetes Risk Calculator. Available at http://www.diabetes.org/risk-test.jsp. Accessed October 15, 2008.

62. Rathmann W, Martin S, Haastert B, et al. Performance of screening questionnaires and risk scores for undiagnosed diabetes: the KORA Survey 2000. *Arch Intern Med.* 2005;165:436–441.

63. Glümer C, Vistisen D, Borch-Johnsen K, Colagiuri S. Risk scores for type 2 diabetes can be applied in some populations but not all. *Diabetes Care.* 2006;29:410–414.

64. Norris SL, Kansagara D, Bougatsos C, Fu R. Screening adults for type 2 diabetes: a review of the evidence for the U.S. Preventive Services Task Force. *Ann Intern Med.* 2008;148:855–868.

65. American Diabetes Association. Screening for type 2 diabetes. *Diabetes Care.* 2004; 27:S11–S14.

66. Murff HJ, Rothman RL, Byrne DW, Syngal S. The impact of family history of diabetes on glucose testing and counseling behavior in primary care. *Diabetes Care.* 2004;27:2247–2248.

67. Baptiste-Roberts K, Gary TL, Beckles GL, et al. Family history of diabetes, awareness of risk factors, and health behaviors among African Americans. *Am J Public Health.* 2007;97:907–912.

68. Qureshi N, Kai J. Informing patients of familial diabetes mellitus risk: How do they respond? A cross-sectional survey. *BMC Health Serv Res.* 2008;8:37.

69. Lynch HT, de la Chapelle A. Hereditary colorectal cancer. *N Engl J Med.* 2003; 348:919–932.

70. Peto J, Collins N, Barfoot R, et al. Prevalence of BRCA1 and BRCA2 gene mutations in patients with early-onset breast cancer. *J Natl Cancer Inst.* 1999;91:943–949.

71. Acheson LS, Zyzanski SJ, Stange KC, Deptowicz A, Wiesner GL. Validation of a self-administered, computerized tool for collecting and displaying the family history of cancer. *J Clin Oncol.* 2006;24:5395–5402.

72. Sweet KM, Bradley TL, Westman JA. Identification and referral of families at high risk for cancer susceptibility. *J Clin Oncol.* 2002;20:528–537.

73. Nelson HD, Huffman LH, Fu R, Harris EL. Genetic risk assessment and BRCA mutation testing for breast and ovarian cancer susceptibility: systematic evidence review for the U.S. Preventive Services Task Force. *Ann Intern Med.* 2005;143:362–379.

74. Palomaki GE, McClain MR, Steinort K, Sifri R, LoPresti L, Haddow JE. Screen-positive rates and agreement among six family history screening protocols for breast/ovarian cancer in a population-based cohort of 21- to 55-year-old women. *Genet Med.* 2006;8:161–168.

75. American Cancer Society. *Cancer Prevention & Early Detection Facts & Figures 2007.* Atlanta: American Cancer Society; 2007.

76. Audrain-McGovern J, Hughes C, Patterson F. Effecting behavior change: awareness of family history. *Am J Prev Med.* 2003;24:183–189.

77. Tyagi A, Morris J. Using decision analytic methods to assess the utility of family history tools. *Am J Prev Med.* 2003;24:199–207.

78. Ramsey SD, Burke W, Pinsky L, Clarke L, Newcomb P, Khoury MJ. Family history assessment to detect increased risk for colorectal cancer: conceptual considerations and a preliminary economic analysis. *Cancer Epidemiol Biomarkers Prev.* 2005;14:2494–2500.

V

CASE STUDIES: ASSESSING THE USE OF GENETIC INFORMATION IN PRACTICE FOR SPECIFIC DISEASES

30

Cytochrome P450 testing in the treatment of depression

Iris Grossman, Mugdha Thakur, and David B. Matchar

Objective

Personalized medicine has been the leading concept in the evolution and maturation of "pharmacogenetics"—a scientific discipline first conceived over half a decade ago (1) and centered around genetic variation and its impact on pharmacology and toxicology. The notion of "individually tailoring" treatment to patients according to their genetic makeup is particularly sought after in disease models that lack clear drug prescription guidelines and thus default into "trial-and-error" treatment paradigms. Psychiatry has been one of the leading fields to employ pharmacogenetic research to assist in the management of chronic, common, suboptimally managed conditions, the most publicly relevant of which is depression (only about 60% of patients respond favorably (2)). In the years 2006–2007 alone several comprehensive review papers were published on the pharmacogenetics of antidepressants, suggesting an imminent application in daily practice (3–6). Furthermore, Roche announced in January 2005 that the microarray-based AmpliChip® CYP450 Test was cleared by the U.S. Food and Drug Administration (FDA) for diagnostic use in the United States, with direct indication for antidepressant treatment in the diagnostic test insert: "The enzyme encoded by *CYP2D6* metabolizes many antidepressants..." "The impact of these polymorphisms upon the pharmacokinetics of antidepressants..." also was exemplified on their website at the time by a case study of a patient treated with selective serotonin reuptake inhibitors (SSRIs) to support the use of *CYP450* testing to guide SSRI prescriptions. While the latter milestone recognizes the potential significance of genetics in drug response and safety modification, critical review of the available evidence supporting these statements was clearly required, and motivated the Evaluation of Genomic Applications in Practice and Prevention (EGAPP) Working Group to request an evidence review, which was funded by the Office of Public Health Genomics at the Centers for Disease Control and Prevention (CDC), and commissioned to us through the Agency for Healthcare Research and Quality (AHRQ). We composed an evidence report entitled "Testing for cytochrome P450 polymorphisms in adults with nonpsychotic depression treated with selective serotonin reuptake inhibitors (SSRIs)" (7). The overarching question identified by EGAPP was focused on the clinical utility of *CYP450* genotyping, and the usefulness of genetic predictors in this therapeutic area relating to medical, personal, and/or public health decision making.

Background

Major Depressive Disorder and Selective Serotonin Reuptake Inhibitors

Major depressive disorder (MDD) is widely distributed in the population and is usually associated with substantial symptom severity and role impairment (7). It is estimated to be the second leading cause of death and disability by the year 2020 worldwide (8). Despite available therapies, this burden remains enormous, mainly due to high rates of nonresponse and resistance to available treatments (9). In the recently completed landmark STAR*D trial, the response rate (rate of improvement in symptoms) was 47% and the remission rate (rate of substantial improvement, with only minimal residual symptoms) only 33% after 14 weeks of treatment with a selective serotonin reuptake inhibitor (SSRI) (10).

First-line treatment for MDD is currently composed of agents in the SSRI class. These have quickly dominated the antidepressant market, offering improved tolerability and relative safety in overdose in comparison with the older generation tricyclic antidepressants (TCAs). However, treatment of MDD with SSRIs is not without challenges. The suggested dosing schedules for individual SSRIs may lead to adverse effects in some patients, and longer time to response in others. Thus a trial and error approach is often required when prescribing SSRIs to patients.

Cytochrome P450 Enzyme Family and Its Potential Impact on Clinical Practice

The cytochrome P450 (CYP) enzyme system is responsible for the phase I metabolism of most drugs, including both antidepressants and antipsychotics. *CYP2D6* is the enzyme for which genetic variation has been best characterized and investigated in relation to subsequent phenotypic and clinical association in various therapeutic areas and for a multitude of pharmaceutical agents. Sixty-seven genetic variants of the *CYP2D6* gene and over 100 total subvariants have been characterized thus far (11). *In vitro* and *in vivo* studies indicate the translation of diploid combinations of these alleles into one of four phenotypic classes: (i) Poor Metabolizers (PM, comprising ~2–8% of most ethnic groups) exhibit complete deficiency of enzyme activity and demonstrate the most clinically significant phenotype; (ii) Intermediate Metabolizers (IM, comprising ~10–15% of most ethnic groups) display reduced enzyme activity; (iii) Extensive Metabolizers (EM, comprising ~70–80% of most ethnic groups) exhibit normal enzyme activity; and (iv) Ultra-rapid Metabolizers (UM, comprising ~2–5% of most ethnic groups) demonstrate extremely high enzymatic activity. The *CYP2C* family comprises *CYP2C8, CYP2C9, CYP2C18,* and

CYP2C19. The variant allele *CYP2C9*2* includes a genetic sequence polymorphism that leads to an amino acid change in position 144 of the protein, where Cysteine in *CYP2C9*2* replaces Arginine in the wild-type (normal activity) CYP2C9 enzyme (also referred to as *CYP2C9*1*). This Arg144Cys alteration leads to various degrees of impaired CYP2C9 catalytic activity, while the *CYP2C9*3* allele exhibits reduced catalytic activity across the majority of tested substrates (12). The markedly decreased activity alleles *CYP2C19*2* and *CYP2C19*3* lead to various degrees of impaired enzymatic activity, depending on the ethnic background of carriers: in Japanese, three distinct levels of activity have been reported (13) (i.e., PM, IM, and EM), while in Caucasians only two levels of activity have been reported (i.e., EM and PM). The *CYP2C19*17* allele translates into ultrarapid enzymatic activity, depending on substrate (14).

Of note, there are racial differences in the frequency of function-altering polymorphisms. Table 30.1 registers the frequency of the major alleles in select world populations. It should be mentioned that the PM, IM, EM, and UM phenotypes of enzymatic activity comprise two-allele combinations (i.e., genotypes) that each individual carries. These genotypes may include homozygous combinations (i.e., carriage of identical alleles, such as *CYP2D6*1/CYP2D6*1*) or heterozygous (i.e., carriage of nonidentical alleles, such as *CYP2D6*1/CYP2D6*4*). Additionally, the same enzyme variant may have different activity levels toward different drugs. For example, the enzyme product of the *CYP2D6*17* allele, which demonstrates "reduced" activity toward dextromethorphan, bufuralol, and debrisoquine, relative to the reference normal activity homozygous *CYP2D6*1* genotype, has been

Table 30.1 Allele frequencies of *CYP2D6* variants in select populations

CYP2D6 variant	Predicted enzymatic function*	Caucasian (Europe) (15)	Caucasian (U.S.) (15)	African-American (15)	Swedish (16)
*1	Normal	33–36%	27–40%	29–35%	36.7%
2 (35)	Normal	22–33%	26–34%	18–27%	32.4%
*3	Deficient	1–4%	1–1.4%	<1%	1.4%
*4	Deficient	12–23%	18–23%	6–9%	24.4%
*5	Deficient	2–7%	2–4%	6–7%	4.3%
*6	Deficient	1–1.4%	1%	<1%	0.9%
*9	Decreased activity	0–2.6%	2–3%	<1%	—
*10	Decreased activity	1.4–2%	2–8%	3–8%	—
*17	Decreased activity	<1%	<1%	15–26%	—
*41	Decreased activity	20%	—	—	—
*1×N	Increased activity	<1%	<1%	1.3%	—
*2×N	Increased activity	1.5%	<1%	1.3%	—
*4×N	Deficient	<1%	<1%	2.3%	—

Source: Adopted from Matchar et al. (7).
*Predicted enzymatic activity is listed as demonstrated toward most relevant substrates in most ethnic groups.

reported to have increased metabolic activity with other medications, such as halo-peridol (17) and risperidone (18) in specific populations.

CYP450 enzymes—primarily CYP2D6, CYP2C19, and CYP2C9—are involved in the metabolism of all of the SSRIs (19), and for a given SSRI, more than one CYP450 enzyme may be involved in its metabolism (20,21). It is important to note that enzymes other than CYP450 enzymes are also involved in SSRI metabolism (22,23). Additionally, it is noteworthy that CYP2D6 with identical pharmaco-logic and molecular properties to those of the hepatic CYP2D6 enzyme has been identified in microsomal fractions in the brain. Hence, CYP2D6 may potentially contribute to local clearance of psychotropics at the site of action. Differences in personality traits between CYP2D6 EMs and PMs were noted in both Swedish and Spanish healthy white subjects, also suggesting that there may be an endogenous substrate for CYP2D6 in the brain (24).

Genetic Testing for Key CYP450 Polymorphisms in MDD

Currently there are no proven methods to ensure selection of a clinically effective SSRI agent for the individual patient, resulting in low response rates, subsequent low compliance, and an increased risk of side effects. Genetic *CYP450* polymorphisms, if proven to directly affect clinical outcomes, could potentially aid the selection of an effective SSRI and/or guide decisions about appropriate dosing to optimize effi-cacy and tolerability for each patient. Numerous laboratories offer genetic testing for *CYP450* polymorphisms, mainly supporting clinical trials and a growing market of patient management and direct-to-consumer selling. A significant recent devel-opment was the approval by the U.S. Food and Drug Administration (FDA) of the Roche AmpliChip CYP450 Test for this purpose (25,26). However, whether such testing produces any real benefits at all, is controversial at best. We carried out a systematic review of the available literature using standard methods of evidence-based medicine to inform the future use of genetic testing in the treatment of MDD with SSRIs, as well as to guide research priorities in service of optimal patient care. While several broad reviews have been published on this topic in the years 2006–2007 (3–6), none has analytically applied a systematic survey of all available evidence to address the usefulness and benefit of this diagnostic tool, weighing all relevant analytical, laboratory, and medical aspects of its application. In order to inform the establishment of treatment guidelines, the principles of evidence-based medicine (EBM) guided us through: (i) establishing key questions relevant to clin-ical management (such as whether patients with specific characteristics are likely to benefit from testing in terms of time to improvement or avoidance of adverse effects); (ii) constructing an analytic framework for examining the questions, here linking the use of a test to establishment of genotype, to prediction of phenotype, to therapeutic decision making, to clinical outcome (i.e., analytic validity, clinical validity, and clinical utility); (iii) identifying and synthesizing soundly designed published studies; and (iv) interpreting the evidence. We applied this approach to evaluating *CYP2D6* diagnostic testing as a potential clinical aid supporting a safer or/and more efficient SSRI prescription for MDD management in routine clinical practice.

Materials and Methods

Full details on the literature search, methodology, and strategy have been presented elsewhere (7,27,28). Briefly, the primary source of literature was MEDLINE (1966–May 2006). In addition, data from the FDA website describing the operating characteristics of the Roche AmpliChip CYP450 Test (25,26) were included. Paired researchers independently reviewed all abstracts. The methodological approach adopted was designed to address each component relevant to future formulation of evidence-based recommendations by the EGAPP Working Group for the use of genetic testing in depression treatment decision making. To this end an analytic framework was developed and is presented in Figure 30.1.

Overall, each fully reviewed article was evaluated for methodological quality. For the question regarding analytic validity, we assessed quality of studies based on questions in the "Analytic validity, Clinical validity, Clinical utility and associated Ethical, legal and social implications" (ACCE) model for evaluation of genetic testing (29). For all other questions for which we could identify data that was not covered by the ACCE framework, we elected to use criteria developed by the Oxford Centre for Evidence-based Medicine (30). These included evaluations of individual studies based on type of study (therapy versus prognosis versus prevalence) and strength of study design.

It is notable that the definitions of sensitivity and specificity in their classical sense are most directly applicable to tests with dichotomous results (mutation present or absent). Because there are multiple *CYP450* polymorphisms that can be assessed, and each study may provide information on only a subset of polymorphisms, analytic sensitivity was defined operationally as the proportion of known genotype challenge samples that are correctly identified by the test under evaluation. Similarly, analytic specificity was defined operationally as the proportion of known wild-type challenge samples that are correctly identified by the test under evaluation.

An additional search was performed at the end of 2007 using the exact same criteria reported above. None of the newly identified articles contributed substantially to the body of evidence pertaining to the current investigation, and the conclusions thus remain unchanged.

Results

Literature Search

A total of 1,200 abstracts were identified, of which 140 met criteria for full-text evaluation. Thirty-seven articles met the final inclusion criteria and addressed the relationship between *CYP450* polymorphisms and SSRI metabolism, safety, efficacy,

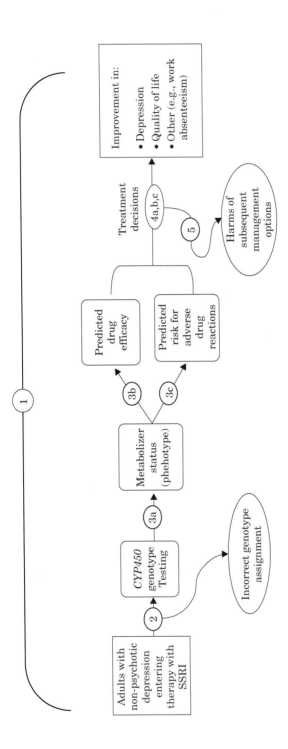

Figure 30.1 Analytic framework guiding evidence review on CYP450 genotyping in SSRI treatment of major depression.

Within the domain of testing and depression management, the analytic framework depicted in Figure 30.1 provides an explicit link between the use of the test and the various health outcomes of importance to decision makers. Such a framework also clarifies the relevant key questions posed by the EGAPP:

*   *Question 1 (overarching question): Does testing for cytochrome P450 (CYP450) polymorphisms in adults entering SSRI treatment for nonpsychotic depression lead to improvement in outcomes, or are testing results useful in medical, personal, or public health decision making?*
*   *Question 2: What is the analytic validity of tests that identify key CYP450 polymorphisms?*

- *Question 3a: How well do particular CYP450 genotypes predict metabolism of particular SSRIs? Do factors such as race/ethnicity, diet, or other medications, affect this association?*
- *Question 3b: How well does CYP450 testing predict drug efficacy? Do factors such as race/ethnicity, diet, or other medications, affect this association?*
- *Question 3c: How well does CYP450 testing predict adverse drug reactions? Do factors such as race/ethnicity, diet, or other medications, affect this association?*
- *Question 4a: Does CYP450 testing influence depression management decisions by patients and providers in ways that could improve or worsen outcomes?*
- *Question 4b: Does the identification of the CYP450 genotypes in adults entering SSRI treatment for nonpsychotic depression lead to improved clinical outcomes compared to not testing?*
- *Question 4c: Are the testing results useful in medical, personal, or public health decision making?*
- *Question 5: What are the harms associated with testing for CYP450 polymorphisms and subsequent management options?*

and clinical outcomes. The interrater agreement for inclusion of abstracts (kappa statistic) ranged from -0.037 to 0.613.

The sections ahead include our findings regarding analytic validity, clinical validity, and clinical utility.

Analytic Validity

Analytic validity assessment refers to analytic sensitivity, specificity, laboratory quality control, and assay robustness (i.e., how resistant is the assay to changes in pre-analytic and analytic variables?). We calculated these parameters for CYP2D6 and CYP2C19 and other relevant CYP450 enzymes.

CYP2D6. We identified nine reports that compared clinical methods for genotyping *CYP2D6* polymorphisms to a reference standard. Of these, only two (26,31) provided a comparison to the gold standard, DNA sequencing.

Combining all studies, the analytic sensitivity and specificity results for each tested genotype were 100% and ≥94.12%, respectively (with the exception of Schaffeler et al. (32) reporting a sensitivity of 91.67% to detect the genotype combination of a duplication allele with a single copy allele). However, only 26 of about 100 known *CYP2D6* polymorphisms (http://www.cypalleles.ki.se/) were evaluated in the included studies (detailed tables are provided elsewhere (7)).

Quality control methods were utilized, but there was no standard procedure followed, no consistent testing of assay robustness, and little investigation of pre-analytic and analytic bias. New studies published in 2007 add virtually no new data to the established analytic properties of *CYP2D6* genotyping. Unfortunately, even recent studies lack basic details on this component: for example, Crescenti et al. (33) evaluated only a small subset of the polymorphisms (*3, *4, *5, and *6) in a Spanish population of 290 individuals recruited in trauma centers. They did not employ comparison to the gold standard.

Gene deletion and duplication studies had lower sensitivity and specificity, further compounded by the limitation that there is no accepted gold standard for such tests (33).

CYP2C19. We identified three reports that compared clinical methods for genotyping *CYP2C19* polymorphisms to a reference standard. Only one study provided a comparison to the gold standard, DNA sequencing (25).

All three studies reported a high sensitivity and specificity (96.43–100%). However, each study focused on detection of two out of the three common *CYP2C19* alleles (*2, *3, and *4). Quality control procedures varied across studies.

Other CYPs. We identified one report that compared clinical methods for genotyping *CYP2C9* polymorphisms to a reference standard (34). We identified two studies that compared methods for *CYP2C8* polymorphisms (35,36), and one for *CYP1A1* polymorphisms (37), to a reference standard. All of these studies had very high sensitivity (100%) and specificity (100%).

Melis et al. (38) recently reported employing the Tag-IT technology (FDA-approved (2005) currently only for *CFTR* genotyping as a diagnostic for cystic fibrosis) in determination of *CYP2D6, CYP2C9,* and *CYP2C19* genotyping. One strength of their paper was the fact that assay calibration utilized DNA samples from the Coriell Institute for Medical Research (NJ, U.S.A.) on an array of ethnicities: Caucasian, Japanese, Chinese, Southeast Asian, African American, and Middle Eastern ancestry. The report concludes that the *CYP2C9* and *CYP2C19* assays were particularly robust and were easily implemented in the clinical laboratory. The *CYP2D6* assay was "somewhat less robust" due to challenges with interpretation of the genotypes, including the nucleotide variation from C to T in position 2850 of the genetic sequence, as well as the inability to characterize the number and the allele type involved when gene duplication occurs. The greatest methodological flaw of this paper is the fact that no comparator methods were employed, nor were the samples cross identified by independent investigators.

Clinical Validity

Clinical validity defines how well do particular *CYP* genotypes detect or predict the associated phenotype(s) of interest: metabolism (serving as an intermediate endophenotype), efficacy (positive response), and induced adverse effects of particular SSRIs.

(i)   *Evidence pertaining to the relationship between CYP450 polymorphisms and SSRI metabolism*: Data extracted from prolonged drug exposure studies in clinical populations was reviewed and calculations of confidence intervals for differences in mean SSRI levels between homozygous EM and comparator groups (PM, heterozygous EM, etc.) were performed when available. Comparison across studies showed little consistency (7), including a total of 11 studies, which were conducted in clinical populations who had achieved steady state after multiple doses, and which were cross-sectional in design. It should be mentioned, however, that a trend toward significant differences in the level of total active metabolites in fluoxetine treated patients were seen between *CYP2C9* EMs and PMs (39,40). Overall, these were based on small population sizes (ranging from 11 to 124 subjects) (7) and are thus underpowered to draw any definitive conclusions.

Since the original evidence report, several additional studies were identified that tested the relationship between *CYP* polymorphisms and SSRI metabolism. Three of these enhance the body of evidence associating *CYP450* genotypes with metabolic effects. In a study by Shams et al. (41), serum concentrations of venlafaxine and its metabolites were investigated in 100 patients and genotyping was performed if the ratios were abnormal. Extremely low metabolite/parent drug ratios were 100% correlated with *CYP2D6* PM genotypes ($n = 4$), extremely high ratios were 100% correlated with UM ($n = 6$), and IM correlated with carriers of a single functional allele ($n = 5$). In a different study *CYP2C19* PM genotypes were reported as associated with significantly reduced oral clearance of citalopram in 53 Chinese adult patients (42).

Of interest, Zourkova et al. (43) reported a shift in the actual metabolic phenotype in 55 *CYP2D6* genotyped Czech anxiety and/or depressive disorder patients treated with paroxetine 10–40 mg daily for long periods of time (2–16 months). Transition from extensive to slower phenotype was detected in about 60% of patients.

(ii) *Evidence pertaining to the relationship between CYP450 polymorphisms and SSRI treatment efficacy:* Overall, only eight studies were identified that examined the association between CYP450 genotypes and SSRI efficacy. Efficacy was largely defined as response rate based on the improvement in depression measures, which varied across studies. The most commonly used measures were Montgomery-Asberg Depression Rating Scale (MADRS), Hamilton depression scale (HAM-D), and Clinical Global Impression (CGI) scale. Six of the studies investigated *CYP2D6* polymorphisms alone, one study also tested *2C9* and *2C19* polymorphisms, and the most comprehensive analysis of drug metabolizing enzyme variants examined *2D6, 2C19, 3A4, 3A5* as well as the gene encoding the Pgp transporter (*ABCB1* or *MDR1*) in the Sequenced Treatment Alternatives to Relieve Depression (STAR*D) cohort (44). On the whole, the studies did not show a consistent relationship between CYP450 genotype and antidepressant efficacy (7). Results from studies employing comparison groups ($n = 5$) are provided in Table 30.2.

Recently, Peters et al. (44) tested 15 functional polymorphisms in 5 pharmacokinetic genes relevant to the metabolism and elimination of the SSRI citalopram in the largest study yet evaluated in this field. MDD patients enrolled in the STAR*D trial were analyzed in a discovery set ($n = 831$) and a validation set ($n = 1,046$). Results showed no association of SSRI metabolic enzyme polymorphisms with either efficacy or tolerability, illustrating lack of clinical validity and further suggesting little likelihood of clinical utility of genetic testing for the management of depression with citalopram.

(iii) *Evidence pertaining to the relationship between CYP450 polymorphisms and SSRI treatment tolerability:* Adverse SSRI reactions were the most commonly included and most extensively analyzed endpoint in *CYP* genetic studies, yet limited number of subjects, substantial heterogeneity in study design, measurements, reported parameters, and patients' characteristics limit the extent of conclusions that can be drawn regarding *CYP* polymorphisms and SSRI treatment tolerability. A summary of results is given in Table 30.3 for studies employing comparison groups.

The most comprehensive evidence reported thus far of genetic variants associated with SSRI tolerability was recently published based on the STAR*D trial and employed a sizable tested marker list that did not include *CYP* variants (45) (see below).

Clinical Utility

Evidence pertaining to the use of *CYP450* polymorphism testing to select SSRI drug and/or dose and its subsequent treatment outcomes

Table 30.2 CYP450 predicted phenotypes and efficacy of SSRIs in MDD patients

Study	Patient characteristics	SSRI(s)	Alleles of interest	Predicted phenotypes	Results
Shams et al., 2006 (41)	25 depressive patients (selected out of 100 based on metabolic rate)	Venlafaxine	2D6 *1, *3, *4, *5, *6 and *9, as well as duplications	PM: 16%; IM: 20%; EM: 36% UM: 28%	No association was detected with efficacy defined as improvement in CGI scale score.
Peters et al., 2008 (44)	831 depressive patients in the discovery set, ~300 Caucasians and ~60 African-American (dependent on response definition)	Citalopram	2D6 *1, *3, *4, *5, *6, *7, *8, *9; 3A4 *1B; 3A5 *3C; 2C19 *2, *3, *17; ABCB1 C1236T, G2677T, C3435T	2D6 PM = 5% (Caucasian), 2% (African-American); 2C19 PM = 2% (Caucasians and African-American)	No association was detected and replicated between metabolizer status or genotype of any of the tested variants and response to treatment defined as at least 50% reduction in QIDS-SR score, dosage or length of treatment period in trial.
Gerstenberg et al., 2003 (46)	49 depressive Japanese patients	Fluvoxamine	2D6 *1, *3, *4, *5, *10	EMs = 25%; IMs = 55%; PMs = 20%	Final MADRS score, and proportion of responders defined as MADRS score < 10 was not significantly different in the three metabolic status groups.
Grasmader et al., 2004 (47)	70 depressive patients (refers to Caucasians in conclusion)	Fluvoxamine, paroxetine, sertraline, citalopram	CYP2C9 *1, *2, *3, CYP2C19*1 and *2, 2D6 *1 to *9 and gene duplication	NR	Plasma concentration above or below lower limit of presumed therapeutic levels did not predict improvement in CGI scores.
Murphy et al., 2003 (48)	246 depressive patients	Paroxetine (and mirtazapine)	2D6: 16 alleles, deletion, duplication, and *41 allele	PMs = 6.5%; IMs = 10.5%; UMs = 4%; EMs = 79%	No differences between PM + IM vs. EM + UM groups in depression outcomes defined by improvement in CGI scores.

Abbreviations: CGI = Clinical Global Impressions Scale; EM(s) = extensive metabolizer(s); HAM-D = Hamilton Rating Scale for Depression; IM(s) = intermediate metabolizer(s); MADRS = Montgomery-Åsberg Depression Rating Scale; NR = not reported; PMs = poor metabolizer(s); SSRI(s) = selective serotonin reuptake inhibitor(s); UM(s) = ultrarapid metabolizer(s); QIDS-SR = Quick Inventory of Depressive Symptomatology (Self-Report version).

Table 30.3 CYP450 predicted phenotypes and adverse effects associated with SSRIs in MDD patients

Study/ design	Patient characteristics	SSRI(s)	Alleles of interest	Predicted phenotypes	Results
Chen et al., 1996 (49)	74 patients	Paroxetine, fluoxetine, sertraline, fluvoxamine, (also TCAs)	2D6–A, B, D, E, and T alleles	NR	PM phenotype was significantly more frequent in depressed patients ($n = 18$; 44%) reporting adverse effects to substrate of 2D6 compared to a random group ($n = 56$; 21%) of depressed patients ($p < 0.05$), or compared to the general population.
Rau et al., 2004 (50)	28 patients with adverse effects to SSRIs (9 patients), SNRIs	Various SSRIs	2D6 *1, *3, *4, *6, *2, *8, *10, *14, *41, *5	PM: 29% IM: 7% EM: 64% UM: 0	29% PMs compared to 7% in the German population ($p < 0.0001$). There were no differences across groups in frequency of dose reduction, stopping treatment, reducing or terminating antidepressant, or number of adverse effects.
Gerstenberg et al., 2003 (46)	49 depressive Japanese patients	Fluvoxamine	2D6 *1, *3, *4, *5, *10	PM: 20% EM: 25% IM: 55%	Incidence of adverse effects (nausea) was not significantly different across the three groups.
Murphy et al., 2003 (48)	246 depressive patients	Paroxetine	2D6: 16 alleles, deletion, duplication, and *41 allele	PM: 6.5% IM: 10.5% UM: 4% EM: 79%	No differences between PM + IM vs EM + UM groups in severity of adverse effects or frequency of discontinuation.
Roberts et al., 2004 (51)	65 depressive patients	Fluoxetine	2D6 *1-*16, *19, *20	PM: 9% EM: 91%	PMs were no more likely to experience adverse effects than EMs and were no more likely to drop out of the study than EMs.
Suzuki et al., 2006 (52)	97 depressive Japanese patients	Fluvoxamine	2D6 *1, *5, *10	PM: 22.7% EM: 77.3%	Greater prevalence of GI side effects in PMs compared to EMs ($p = 0.043$; CI 1.019–3.254). Discontinuation rates similar between PMs and EMs.
McAlpine et al., 2007 (53)	38 patients identified out of 199 study patients with no therapeutic response	Venlafaxine	2D6 *1, *2A, *3, *4, *5, *6, *7, *8, *9, *10, *11, *12, *17, and *41	EM+IM: 87%; PM: 13%	A difference in dosage level between patients with no fully active allele (<75 mg) and those with at least 1 fully active allele (>150 mg) was statistically significant ($p < .002$).

Study	Patients	Drug	Genotype variants	Metabolizer status	Findings
Peters et al., 2008 (44)	831 depressive patients in the discovery set, 565 Caucasians and 98 African-Americans, validation set: 679 Caucasians and 99 African-Americans	Citalopram	2D6 *1, *3, *4, *5, *6, *7, *8, *9; 3A4 *1B; 3A5 *3C; 2C19 *2, *3, *17; ABCB1 C1236T, G2677T, C3435T	2D6 PM: 5% (Caucasian), 2% (African-American); 2C19 PM: 2% (Caucasians and African-American)	No association was detected and replicated between metabolizer status or genotype of any of the tested variants and treatment tolerance.
Zourkova et al., 2007 (43)	55 Czech anxiety and depressive patients	Paroxetine	2D6 *1, *3, *4, *5, *6	EM: 65%; IM/PM: 35%	It is unclear whether the results reported relate to genotype-derived metabolic status or actual measures. Several sexual dysfunction items in ASEX were nominally significant when contrasted between EM and PM in female alone.
Shams et al., 2006 (41)	25 depressive patients (selected out of 100 based on metabolic rate)	Venlafaxine	2D6 *1, *3, *4, *5, *6, and *9, as well as duplications	PM: 16%; IM: 20%; EM: 36% UM: 28%	PMs had significantly more side effects ($p < 0.005$) as compared with EMs.
Yin et al., 2006 (42)	53 Chinese mood and anxiety patients	Citalopram	2C19 *1, *2, *3	EM_{IM}: 40%; EM_{III}: 47%; PM: 13%	No statistically significant association was found between genotype groups and TSES, despite significant association between oral clearance and both genotype and TSES.
Kropp et al., 2006 (54)	229 depressive and schizophrenic patients		2C19 *2; 2D6 *1, *3, *4, *5, and *6		HT and HM patients for the defective alleles required longer hospitalization (median 57.5 vs 40 days).

Abbreviations: CI = confidence interval; DSM-IV = *Diagnostic and Statistical Manual for Mental Disorders, 4th edition*; EM(s) = extensive metabolizer(s); GI = gastrointestinal; HAM-D = Hamilton Rating Scale for Depression; IM(s) = intermediate metabolizer(s); MADRS = Montgomery-Åsberg Depression Rating Scale; NR = not reported; PMs = poor metabolizer(s); SNRI(s) = serotonin/norepinephrine reuptake inhibitors; SSRI(s) = selective serotonin reuptake inhibitor(s); TCAs = tricyclic antidepressants; UM(s) = ultrarapid metabolizer(s); HT = heterozygous; HM = Homozygous; TSES = Toronto Side Effects Scale; SNPs = single nucleotide polymorphisms; ASEX = Arizona Sexual Experience Scale.

No studies were identified that examined the clinical utility and cost-effectiveness of *CYP450* testing for the management of SSRI treatment in the clinic.

Other Plausible Candidates for Improving Clinical Management of SSRI Treatment

Publications in very recent years overwhelmingly suggest that genetic variation related to various aspects of the SSRI mode-of-action and the underlying pathophysiology of depression are plausible candidates for use in improving clinical management of depression. Binder and Holsboer determine in their 2006 review (4) that "it is clear, that non-*CYP450* candidate systems have to be considered in the pharmacogenetics of antidepressant drugs, such as neuropeptidergic systems, the hypothalamus-pituitary adrenal (HPA) axis and neurotrophic systems." While a detailed evaluation is outside of the scope of the current chapter, a brief review of recent developments pertaining to pharmacogenetic non-*CYP* markers is provided below.

Other drug metabolizing enzymes and transporters (DMETs) interacting with SSRIs may display genetic variability that is predictive of clinically relevant endpoints. A striking example was published recently in *Neuron* (55). In this study, antidepressants were first tested and screened for transport across the blood-brain-barrier (BBB) through the active efflux pump p-glycoprotein (P-gp) in knockout mice. Thereafter, polymorphic sites across the entire ABCB1 gene region (encoding P-gp) were genotyped in an MDD patient population and tested for association with remission after 4–6 weeks of treatment. Several single nucleotide polymorphisms (SNPs) were identified and confirmed in a follow-up case-control study. However, the small sample sizes and conflicting findings by others (e.g., the STAR*D cohort (44)) indicate that further investigation will be crucial before such testing can be advocated clinically.

The most comprehensive pharmacogenetic study yet performed in MDD patients was the STAR*D trial (10). Four major discoveries have been made, replicated, and published based on the careful analysis of this sizable cohort, which increase our understanding of MDD pathophysiology and PGx substantially. First, McMahon et al. (56) identified a marker in *HTR2A*, which was robustly and consistently associated with both response and remission phenotypes after 3–6 weeks of therapy. This association was significant in Caucasian and overall populations but not in the African-American subpopulation (n= 170–261, depending on phenotype). In a follow-up report, Paddock et al. (57) used the full set of 1,816 genotyped individuals in STAR*D (33% increase in sample size) with 634 psychiatrically healthy controls. Two SNPs passed the significance threshold in both the discovery and replication groups: the previously identified *HTR2A* polymorphism and a SNP in *GRIK4*. However, no clinical specificity or sensitivity calculation was reported, and appropriately designed studies would need to be conducted to assess the predictive value of these variants as response markers.

The third STAR*D publication reported an association between genetic variants in *KCNK2 (TREK1)* and resistance to antidepressant treatment, regardless of class (58). In rodents, *TREK1* is inhibited by therapeutic doses of SSRIs, and in its absence mice express a depression-resistant phenotype, insensitive to SSRI treatment (59). However, this has not yet been independently validated.

In the STAR*D analysis of citalopram-induced suicide ideation (45), case-control analysis was performed between 120 treatment emergent suicidal ideation patients and 1,742 patients without this adverse event, both ascertained by self-reported questionnaire responses. A logistic regression stepwise selection model including two markers (in *GRIK2* and *GRIA3*), remission and race was highly and consistently associated with treatment emergent suicidal ideation both in women (likelihood ratio $\chi^2 = 20.7$, $p = 0.0009$) and in men (likelihood ratio $\chi^2 = 34.8$, $p < 0.0001$). Shortly after this publication, **NeuroMark** designed the Mark-C genetic test for suicidal ideation in patients treated with citalopram. The product is intended first for investigational use only, pending results from two confirmatory trials, appropriately powered to assess specificity, sensitivity, and predictive value.

It can be argued that the combined effects of multiple genes, encoding molecules that function in various aspects of a drug's mode-of-action and downstream pathways, would serve as better markers for drug response and safety. Several examples in the field of psychiatry already suggest **synergistic** effect of *CYP2D6* and *5-HT2A* SNPs on fluvoxamine-induced side effects in Japanese depressed patients (52); or an increased predisposition to citalopram-induced suicidal ideation by markers in **both** *GRIA3* and *GRIK2* (45). Moreover, the biological roles that drug-metabolizing enzymes play in physiology and pathophysiology may further confound investigations focused on pharmacogenetic endpoints. To this end it may be important to take into consideration the reported increased susceptibility for MDD by carriers of *CYP2C9*3* and *5-HTTLPR-S* (60), as well as the fact that *CYP2D6* may contribute to regeneration of serotonin from 5-methoxytryptamine in the brain. These associations, if confirmed and shown to convey large effects, could introduce bias into retrospective pharmacogenetic studies.

Lastly, Binder and Holsboer (4) indicate that studies of *5-HTTLPR* genotype and response to antidepressant drugs provide promising evidence for the potential utility of pharmacogenetics in MDD (61). Further research is warranted, however, in order to reconcile discrepancies in findings across different ethnic groups (4), a potential involvement of this gene in the placebo response (62), potential bias of publication, allelic heterogeneity in this gene (63), as well as combined effects with other relevant variants (60). To this end, a Dutch study published in 2007 employed a decision-analytical model to assess whether pretreatment genetic testing for *5-HTTLPR* could be an efficient tool in the treatment of depression (64). The study compared empirical SSRI treatment assignment to a genetic testing approach prior to drug class prescription. Predicted nonresponders to SSRI could be assigned to receive serotonin-norepinephrine reuptake inhibitors (SNRIs) or TCAs. The simulated allele frequencies and response rates were based on previously published reports. The results suggested a potential benefit in clinical outcomes, as predicted by remission rates in each of the treatment arms after 6 weeks, and more so during 12 weeks of follow-up. While these are encouraging findings, they were based on a theoretical model and did not take into account cost assessments and the reimbursement and clinical guidelines employed in each country specifically.

Discussion

There is a paucity of evidence regarding the use of *CYP450* genotyping as a guide to the management of SSRIs for patients with depression. While studies of the technical characteristics of tests are generally adequate (albeit incomplete), very few reliable and meaningful clinical studies address the key questions related to clinical utility.

Comparison of the results of available tests for *CYP450* genotype with a reference standard suggests that the analytic sensitivity and specificity of available tests are generally high, although some serious concerns remain. In the evaluation of gene deletions and duplications, assessing the magnitude of the potential error in these analytic parameters is limited by the lack of an established gold standard for gene copy number. Another concern is that few *CYP450* variants were interrogated by the studies we identified, which focused particularly on the more common variants in Caucasians. Only a few studies reported performance relative to the gold standard of DNA sequencing; all were applied to a limited number of samples (resulting in wide confidence intervals for analytic sensitivity and specificity); and there was no standard assessment report scheme for evaluation of quality control or assay robustness, preventing an objective performance evaluation of each method, as well as comparison between reports.

In depressed patients who have reached a steady-state concentration of an SSRI, the limited existing data do not demonstrate a clear correlation between CYP450 metabolizer status and (i) SSRI concentrations (an intermediate outcome), (ii) efficacy of SSRIs, or (iii) tolerability of SSRIs. There were several limitations to the studies addressing these questions. In addition to having small sample sizes, many reports did not take into account concurrent medications that may inhibit or induce certain CYP450 enzymes thus affecting metabolism of CYP450 metabolized drugs. Additionally, we did not identify any studies that examined effects of CYP450 inhibition/induction together with genetic polymorphisms of *CYP450* enzymes (e.g., is there an additive effect of a CYP2D6 inhibitor medication in a CYP2D6 poor metabolizer [PM] subject such that SSRI levels are higher than the levels without such an inhibitor medication in a CYP2D6 PM subject?). Several studies looked at limited genotypes and did not account for the fact that more than one CYP450 enzyme may be involved in the metabolism of a specific SSRI. Most studies examining the clinical outcomes of efficacy or adverse effects did not comment on blinding between treating clinicians and those responsible for interpreting results of genetic testing, or patient blinding. Many studies grouped together multiple SSRIs, or SSRIs and other antidepressants. This approach can potentially confound results because of variability in contribution of different CYP450 enzymes to metabolism of different SSRIs and other antidepressants, and variability in CYP450 inhibition by different SSRIs.

We did not identify any studies that addressed whether testing for *CYP450* polymorphisms in adults entering SSRI treatment of depression leads to improved clinical outcomes compared to not testing. An alternative to clinical trials of testing versus no-testing strategies is the use of decision modeling. This approach has been used in order to model some of the decisions that may be involved in genetic testing and the actions required based on the genetic information. The inferences of such models may illustrate some of the problems that may be faced by randomized clinical trials in these areas, including their utility in specific populations. While these would require strong assumptions—in particular that the association between genotype and response to treatment reflects cause and effect—decision analytic models such as the one published by Smits et al. (64) could provide a useful guide to the selection and design of further clinical studies.

Future Research

We propose the following types of studies to fill in the gaps in existing knowledge regarding *CYP450* genotyping in the treatment of depression with SSRIs:

1. Studies of *CYP450* genotyping in a large variety of populations to ascertain analytic sensitivity and specificity of genotyping in real-world settings:

   It is essential that such studies explore a large range of the known possible polymorphisms functionally affecting each enzyme, refraining from focusing solely on the detection of the major alleles relevant to Caucasians and African-Americans. In order to reliably assess the performance of these tests, the sample sizes employed must demonstrate sufficient statistical power to report results within narrow margins of confidence intervals, repeatedly and consistently concluding identical genotype calls.

2. Studies that better describe the *CYP450* polymorphism-associated differences in the rate of metabolism of each individual SSRI in different ethnic groups:

   These should overcome the limitations of current literature addressing this issue, such that they are adequately powered, address individual SSRIs, and account for diet and comedications, particularly *CYP450* inhibiting or inducing drugs.

3. Multigenic pathway analysis studies that provide guidance regarding extent of variation in depression treatment response attributable to CYP450 enzymes and other pharmacokinetic and pharmacodynamic molecules of relevance:

   These studies will be challenging due to the number of potential inter actions and the large samples needed to unravel the gene–gene interactions, as well as gene–environment interactions. As our technological and analytical abilities improve, whole genome scans will be useful tools in further elucidating relevant mechanisms and guiding hypothesis-free exploratory analyses in a standardized fashion (65).

4. Studies that ascertain the predictive value of *CYP450* genotyping in depression treatment outcomes, and its impact on medical or personal decision making:

The ideal study would be a large randomized trial of prospective *CYP450* genotyping-guided treatment versus treatment as usual (66). Such a trial should be in keeping with design standards aimed at minimizing bias (e.g., using intent-to-treat analysis, blinding of physicians and patients), maximizing generalizability (e.g., representative of individuals with severe depression), and including meaningful outcomes (e.g., short-term treatment success, satisfaction, resource utilization). Such a study would provide answers about rates of dropouts/nonresponse in individuals who were genotyped versus those who were not. It would also provide data about treatment decisions by providers and patients, based on genotyping, and the outcome of such genotyping-guided treatment (e.g., different SSRI choices, higher starting doses in ultrarapid metabolizers or lower doses in poor metabolizers) in comparison to the current practice of "trial and error." It may also provide valuable information about harms (such as inaccurate testing, poor or incorrect interpretation of test results, inappropriate employment by healthcare providers, privacy and confidentiality liabilities, etc.).

5. Studies that examine the importance to patients of potential outcomes, such as time to response or quality of life during the early treatment of depression:

Appropriate measures in such a study would be utility measures, including "willingness-to-pay."

6. Studies that address how genotyping affects actual decision making and clinical outcomes. Possible designs would be cohort studies that monitor how specific genotypes relate to treatment choices and subsequent resource utilization.

Summary

In summary, although there is evidence demonstrating high analytic sensitivity and specificity of *CYP450* genotyping for common variants, the available data fail to support a clear correlation between *CYP* polymorphisms and SSRI levels, SSRI efficacy, or tolerability. There are no data regarding whether testing leads to improved outcomes as against not testing in the treatment of depression. There is a critical need to design research studies to fill these knowledge gaps. If shown to be useful, *CYP450* genotyping will make the most impact by reducing the trial and error currently inherent in SSRI treatment, thereby decreasing morbidity and improving quality of life in patients with depression. The results of our comprehensive review were submitted to CDC and the EGAPP Working Group in January 2007. A recommendation statement (28) from the independent EGAPP Working Group, based on the findings of our review as well as complementary and confirmatory analyses, reinforced the authors' recommendations. Moreover, the NIH's Secretary's Advisory Committee on Genetics, Health and Society (SACGHS) published their final draft report on the overall usefulness of genetic tests in the USA in 2008 (67). The 15-member expert panel concluded that federal regulation and oversight of genetic tests is inadequate and a growing number of the tests are being marketed with unproven, ambiguous, false or misleading claims (68). The panel noted that "there is currently no requirement that test providers disclose information to support claims about the accuracy and validity of testing", and physicians and patients cannot be sure a test will provide the promised results in daily clinical practice settings." Thus the overarching question addressed in this report may be broadly applied to other pharmaceuticals: "what is the clinical utility of genetic tests, and what is the usefulness of genetic predictors relating to medical, personal and/or public health decision-making". The answer is, in most cases, a resounding "not yet" (with a small but growing list of genetic biomarkers approved by the FDA for personalized medicine application (69).

Considering the high prevalence of depressive disorders and the length of time required to determine whether a given antidepressant is successful or not, there may be a valuable benefit at the population level if even a small benefit can be demonstrated at the individual level. As a whole, the herein proposed translational study designs are required to indisputably proof the utility, cost effectiveness, robustness and predictive value in daily health care settings (warfarin (70), abacavir (71)).

Note: This chapter is largely based on the evidence report published by the authors (see Reference 7).

References

1. Gurwitz D, Motulsky AG. "Drug reactions, enzymes, and biochemical genetics": 50 years later. *Pharmacogenomics.* 2007;8:1479–1484.
2. Steimer W, Muller B, Leucht S, Kissling W. Pharmacogenetics: a new diagnostic tool in the management of antidepressive drug therapy. *Clin Chim Acta.* 2001;308:33–41.
3. Black JL, III, O'Kane DJ, Mrazek DA. The impact of CYP allelic variation on antidepressant metabolism: a review. *Expert Opin Drug Metab Toxicol.* 2007;3:21–31.
4. Binder EB, Holsboer F. Pharmacogenomics and antidepressant drugs. *Ann Med.* 2006;38:82–94.
5. de Leon J, Armstrong SC, Cozza KL. Clinical guidelines for psychiatrists for the use of pharmacogenetic testing for CYP450 2D6 and CYP450 2C19. *Psychosomatics.* 2006;47:75–85.
6. Perlis RH. Pharmacogenetic studies of antidepressant response: how far from the clinic? *Psychiatr Clin North Am.* 2007;30:125–138.
7. Matchar DB, Thakur ME, Grossman I, et al. Testing for cytochrome P450 polymorphisms in adults with non-psychotic depression treated with selective serotonin reuptake inhibitors (SSRIs). *Evid Rep Technol Assess (Full Rep).* 2007;146:1–77.
8. Murray CJ, Lopez AD. Alternative projections of mortality and disability by cause 1990–2020: Global Burden of Disease Study. *Lancet.* 1997;349:1498–1504.
9. Kirsch I, Deacon BJ, Huedo-Medina TB, Scoboria A, Moore TJ, Johnson BT. Initial severity and antidepressant benefits: a meta-analysis of data submitted to the Food and Drug Administration. *Plos Med.* 2008;5:260–268.

10. Trivedi MH, Rush AJ, Wisniewski SR, et al. Evaluation of outcomes with citalopram for depression using measurement-based care in STAR*D: implications for clinical practice. *Am J Psychiatry.* 2006;163:28–40.

11. Home Page of the Human Cytochrome P450 (CYP) Allele Nomenclature Committee. Available at http://www.cypalleles.ki.se/. Last accessed January 1, 2004.

12. Xie HG, Prasad HC, Kim RB, Stein CM. CYP2C9 allelic variants: ethnic distribution and functional significance. *Adv Drug Deliv Rev.* 2002;54:1257–1270.

13. Furuta T, Sugimoto M, Shirai N, Ishizaki T. CYP2C19 pharmacogenomics associated with therapy of Helicobacter pylori infection and gastro-esophageal reflux diseases with a proton pump inhibitor. *Pharmacogenomics.* 2007;8:1199–1210.

14. Sim SC, Risinger C, Dahl ML, et al. A common novel CYP2C19 gene variant causes ultrarapid drug metabolism relevant for the drug response to proton pump inhibitors and antidepressants. *Clin Pharmacol Ther.* 2006;79:103–113.

15. Bradford LD. CYP2D6 allele frequency in European Caucasians, Asians, Africans and their descendants. *Pharmacogenomics.* 2002;3(2):229–243.

16. Zackrisson AL, Holmgren P, Gladh AB, et al. Fatal intoxication cases: cytochrome P450 2D6 and 2C19 genotype distributions. *Eur J Clin Pharmacol.* 2004;60(8):547–552.

17. Bogni A, Monshouwer M, Moscone A, et al. Substrate specific metabolism by polymorphic cytochrome P450 2D6 alleles. *Toxicol In Vitro.* 2005;19:621–629.

18. Cai WM, Nikoloff DM, Pan RM, et al. CYP2D6 genetic variation in healthy adults and psychiatric African-American subjects: implications for clinical practice and genetic testing. *Pharmacogenomics J.* 2006;6:343–350.

19. Brosen K. Some aspects of genetic polymorphism in the biotransformation of antidepressants. *Therapie.* 2004;59:5–12.

20. Margolis JM, O'Donnell JP, Mankowski DC, Ekins S, Obach RS. (R)-, (S)-, and racemic fluoxetine N-demethylation by human cytochrome P450 enzymes. *Drug Metab Dispos.* 2000;28:1187–1191.

21. Olesen OV, Linnet K. Studies on the stereoselective metabolism of citalopram by human liver microsomes and cDNA-expressed cytochrome P450 enzymes. *Pharmacology.* 1999;59:298–309.

22. Mandrioli R, Forti GC, Raggi MA. Fluoxetine metabolism and pharmacological interactions: the role of cytochrome p450. *Curr Drug Metab.* 2006;7:127–133.

23. Obach RS, Cox LM, Tremaine LM. Sertraline is metabolized by multiple cytochrome P450 enzymes, monoamine oxidases, and glucuronyl transferases in human: an in vitro study. *Drug Metab Dispos.* 2005;33:262–270.

24. Llerena A, Edman G, Cobaleda J, Benitez J, Schalling D, Bertilsson L. Relationship between personality and debrisoquine hydroxylation capacity. Suggestion of an endogenous neuroactive substrate or product of the cytochrome P4502D6. *Acta Psychiatr Scand.* 1993;87:23–28.

25. Roche Molecular Systems I. U.S. Food and Drug Administration 510(k) Substantial Equivalence Determination Decision Summary for Roche AmpliChip CYP450 microarray for identifying CYP2C19 genotype (510(k) Number k043576). Available at http://www.accessdata.fda.gov/cdrh_docs/pdf4/K043576.pdf. Last accessed June 11, 2009.

26. Roche Molecular Systems I. U.S. Food and Drug Administration 510(k) Substantial Equivalence Determination Decision Summary for Roche AmpliChip CYP450 microarray for identifying CYP2D6 genotype (510(k) Number k042259). Available at http://www.accessdata.fda.gov/cdrh_docs/reviews/K042259.pdf. Last accessed June 11, 2009.

27. Thakur M, Grossman I, McCrory DC, et al. Review of evidence for genetic testing for CYP450 polymorphisms in management of patients with nonpsychotic depression with selective serotonin reuptake inhibitors. *Genet Med.* 2007;9:826–835.

28. Recommendations from the EGAPP Working Group: testing for cytochrome P450 polymorphisms in adults with nonpsychotic depression treated with selective serotonin reuptake inhibitors. *Genet Med.* 2007;9:819–825.

29. Centers for Disease Control and Prevention. ACCE Model for Evaluation of Genetic Testing. Available at www.cdc.gov/genomics/gtesting/ACCE.htm. Last accessed June 11, 2009.

30. Phillips B, Ball C, Sackett D. Oxford Centre for Evidence-based Medicine Levels of Evidence. Available at www.cebm.net/levels_of_evidence.asp#levels. Accessed January 1, 2001.

31. Hersberger M, Marti-Jaun J, Rentsch K, et al. Rapid detection of the CYP2D6*3, CYP2D6*4, and CYP2D6*6 alleles by tetra-primer PCR and of the CYP2D6*5 allele by multiplex long PCR. *Clin Chem* 2000;46(8 Pt 1):1072–1077.

32. Schaeffeler E, Schwab M, Eichelbaum M, et al. CYP2D6 genotyping strategy based on gene copy number determination by TaqMan real-time PCR. *Hum Mutat* 2003;22(6):476–485.

33. Crescenti A, Mas S, Gasso P, Baiget M, Bernardo M, Lafuente A. Simultaneous genotyping of CYP2D6*3, *4, *5 and *6 polymorphisms in a Spanish population through multiplex long polymerase chain reaction and minisequencing multiplex single base extension analysis. *Clin Exp Pharmacol Physiol.* 2007;34:992–997.

34. Eriksson S, Berg LM, Wadelius M, et al. Cytochrome p450 genotyping by multiplexed real-time DNA sequencing with pyrosequencing technology. *Assay Drug Dev Technol* 2002;1(1Pt 1):49–59.

35. Muthiah YD, Lee WL, Teh LK, et al. A simple multiplex PCR method for the concurrent detection of three CYP2C8 variants. *Clin Chim Acta* 2004;349(1–2):191–198.

36. Weise A, Grundler S, Zaumsegel D, et al. Development and evaluation of a rapid and reliable method for cytochrome P450 2C8 genotyping. *Clin Lab* 2004;50(3–4):141–148.

37. Wu X, Zhou Y, Xu S. Detection of CYP I A1 polymorphisms with a colorimetric method based on mismatch hybridization. *Clin Chim Acta* 2002;323(1–2):103–109.

38. Melis R, Lyon E, McMillin GA. Determination of CYP2D6, CYP2C9 and CYP2C19 genotypes with Tag-It mutation detection assays. *Expert Rev Mol Diagn.* 2006;6:811–820.

39. Scordo MG, Spina E, Dahl ML, Gatti G, Perucca E. Influence of CYP2C9, 2C19 and 2D6 genetic polymorphisms on the steady-state plasma concentrations of the enantiomers of fluoxetine and norfluoxetine. *Basic Clin Pharmacol Toxicol.* 2005;97:296–301.

40. Llerena A, Dorado P, Berecz R, Gonzalez AP, Penas-Lledo EM. Effect of CYP2D6 and CYP2C9 genotypes on fluoxetine and norfluoxetine plasma concentrations during steady-state conditions. *Eur J Clin Pharmacol.* 2004;59:869–873.

41. Shams ME, Arneth B, Hiemke C, et al. CYP2D6 polymorphism and clinical effect of the antidepressant venlafaxine. *J Clin Pharm Ther.* 2006;31:493–502.

42. Yin OQ, Wing YK, Cheung Y, et al. Phenotype-genotype relationship and clinical effects of citalopram in Chinese patients. *J Clin Psychopharmacol.* 2006;26:367–372.

43. Zourkova A, Ceskova E, Hadasova E, Ravcukova B. Links among paroxetine-induced sexual dysfunctions, gender, and CYP2D6 activity. *J Sex Marital Ther.* 2007;33:343–355.

44. Peters EJ, Slager SL, Kraft JB, et al. Pharmacokinetic genes do not influence response or tolerance to citalopram in the STAR*D sample. *PLoS One.* 2008;3(4):e1872.

45. Laje G, Paddock S, Manji H, et al. Genetic markers of suicidal ideation emerging during citalopram treatment of major depression. *Am J Psychiatry.* 2007;164:1530–1538.

46. Gerstenberg G, Aoshima T, Fukasawa T, et al. Relationship between clinical effects of fluvoxamine and the steady-state plasma concentrations of fluvoxamine and its major metabolite fluvoxamino acid in Japanese depressed patients. *Psychopharmacology (Berl).* 2003;167:443–448.

47. Grasmader K, Verwohlt PL, Rietschel M, et al. Impact of polymorphisms of cytochrome-P450 isoenzymes 2C9, 2C19 and 2D6 on plasma concentrations and

clinical effects of antidepressants in a naturalistic clinical setting. *Eur J Clin Pharmacol.* 2004;60:329–336.

48. Murphy GM, Jr, Kremer C, Rodrigues HE, Schatzberg AF. Pharmacogenetics of antidepressant medication intolerance. *Am J Psychiatry.* 2003;160:1830–1835.

49. Chen S, Chou WH, Blouin RA, et al. The cytochrome P450 2D6 (CYP2D6) enzyme polymorphism: screening costs and influence on clinical outcomes in psychiatry. *Clin Pharmacol Ther.* 1996;60:522–534.

50. Rau T, Wohlleben G, Wuttke H, et al. CYP2D6 genotype: impact on adverse effects and nonresponse during treatment with antidepressants-a pilot study. *Clin Pharmacol Ther.* 2004;75:386–393.

51. Roberts RL, Mulder RT, Joyce PR, Luty SE, Kennedy MA. No evidence of increased adverse drug reactions in cytochrome P450 CYP2D6 poor metabolizers treated with fluoxetine or nortriptyline. *Hum Psychopharmacol.* 2004;19:17–23.

52. Suzuki Y, Sawamura K, Someya T. Polymorphisms in the 5-hydroxytryptamine 2A receptor and CytochromeP4502D6 genes synergistically predict fluvoxamine-induced side effects in japanese depressed patients. *Neuropsychopharmacology.* 2006;31:825–831.

53. McAlpine DE, O'Kane DJ, Black JL, Mrazek DA. Cytochrome P450 2D6 genotype variation and venlafaxine dosage. *Mayo Clin Proc.* 2007;82:1065–1068.

54. Kropp S, Lichtinghagen R, Winterstein K, Schlimme J, Schneider U. Cytochrome P-450 2D6 and 2C19 polymorphisms and length of hospitalization in psychiatry. *Clin Lab.* 2006;52:237–240.

55. Uhr M, Tontsch A, Namendorf C, et al. Polymorphisms in the drug transporter gene ABCB1 predict antidepressant treatment response in depression. *Neuron.* 2008;57:203–209.

56. McMahon FJ, Buervenich S, Charney D, et al. Variation in the gene encoding the serotonin 2A receptor is associated with outcome of antidepressant treatment. *Am J Hum Genet.* 2006;78:804–814.

57. Paddock S, Laje G, Charney D, et al. Association of GRIK4 with outcome of antidepressant treatment in he STAR*D cohort. *Am J Psychiatry.* 2007;164:1181–1188.

58. Perlis RH, Moorjani P, Fagerness J, et al. Pharmacogenetic Analysis of Genes Implicated in Rodent Models of Antidepressant Response: Association of TREK1 and Treatment Resistance in the STAR(*)D Study. *Neuropsychopharmacology.* 2008;33(12):2810–2819.

59. Honore E. The neuronal background K2P channels: focus on TREK1. *Nat Rev Neurosci.* 2007;8:251–261.

60. Dorado P, Penas-Lledo EM, Gonzalez AP, Caceres MC, Cobaleda J, Llerena A. Increased risk for major depression associated with the short allele of the serotonin transporter promoter region (5-HTTLPR-S) and the CYP2C9*3 allele. *Fundam Clin Pharmacol.* 2007;21:451–453.

61. Serretti A, Kato M, De Ronchi D, Kinoshita T. Meta-analysis of serotonin transporter gene promoter polymorphism (5-HTTLPR) association with selective serotonin reuptake inhibitor efficacy in depressed patients. *Mol Psychiatry.* 2007;12:247–257.

62. Durham LK, Webb SM, Milos PM, Clary CM, Seymour AB. The serotonin transporter polymorphism, 5HTTLPR, is associated with a faster response time to sertraline in an elderly population with major depressive disorder. *Psychopharmacology (Berl).* 2004;174:525–529.

63. Hu XZ, Rush AJ, Charney D, et al. Association between a functional serotonin transporter promoter polymorphism and citalopram treatment in adult outpatients with major depression. *Arch Gen Psychiatry.* 2007;64:783–792.

64. Smits KM, Smits LJ, Schouten JS, Peeters FP, Prins MH. Does pretreatment testing for serotonin transporter polymorphisms lead to earlier effects of drug treatment in patients with major depression? A decision-analytic model. *Clin Ther.* 2007;29:691–702.
65. Kingsmore SF, Lindquist IE, Mudge J, Gessler DD, Beavis WD. Genome-wide association studies: progress and potential for drug discovery and development. *Nat Rev Drug Discov.* 2008;7(3):221–230.
66. Grossman I. Routine pharmacogenetic testing in clinical practice: dream or reality? *Pharmacogenomics.* 2007;8:1449–1459.
67. Peer R. Growth of genetic tests concerns federal panel. *New York Times.* January 18, 2008:A12.
68. Report of the Secretary's Advisory Committeeon Genetics, Health, and Society. U.S. System of Oversight of Genetic Testing: A Response to the Charge of the Secretary of Health and Human Services. Available at http://oba.od.nih.gov/oba/SACGHS/reports/SACGHS_oversight_report.pdf. Accessed June 11, 2009.
69. U.S. FDA, Table of Valid Genomic Biomarkers in the Context of Approved Drug Labels. Available at http://www.fda.gov/Drugs/ScienceResearch/ResearchAreas/Pharmacogenetics/ucm083378.htm. Accessed June 11, 2009.
70. Schelleman H, Chen Z, Kealey C, et al. Warfarin response and vitamin K epoxide reductase complex 1 in African Americans and Caucasians. *Clin Pharmacol Ther.* 2007;81:742–747.
71. Mallal S, Phillips E, Carosi G, et al. HLA-B*5701 screening for hypersensitivity to abacavir. *N Engl J Med.* 2008;358:568–579.

31

A Rapid-ACCE review of *CYP2C9* and *VKORC1* allele testing to inform warfarin dosing in adults at elevated risk for thrombotic events to avoid serious bleeding

Monica R. McClain, Glenn E. Palomaki, Margaret Piper, and James E. Haddow

Introduction

This chapter describes the results from a Rapid-ACCE review (**A**nalytic validity, **C**linical validity, **C**linical utility, and **E**thical, legal, and social implications), designed to facilitate the transition of genetic tests from investigational settings to clinical and public health practice (1,2). The ACCE model is composed of a standard set of 44 questions, and builds on the methodologies and terminology introduced by the Secretary's Advisory Committee on Genetic Testing (3). A Rapid-ACCE review will usually address all 44 questions, but may be used when the literature base is limited, resources (e.g., time, funds) are limited, and/or a specific limited application is being considered for evaluation. Rapid-ACCE reviews are discussed in more detail in Chapter 24. Prior to evaluating the components of ACCE, the genetic test, clinical disorder, clinical scenario/intended use must be defined.

In this review, the genetic test is *CYP2C9* and *VKORC1* genotyping, the disorder is serious bleeding, and the clinical scenario is adults at elevated risk for thrombotic events who are candidates for warfarin. These two genes are responsible for much of the observed differences in drug metabolism between individuals. The full Rapid-ACCE review is available online (www.acmg.net) and a summary has been published (4). This chapter has been updated with recently published studies. Understanding the extent of benefit to be gained by testing is important, because: (i) up to 2 million new warfarin patients per year might have genetic tests performed, (ii) a yearly average of 870 adverse drug events due to warfarin were reported to the Food and Drug Administration (FDA) between 1998 and 2005 (5), and over 30,000 admissions to emergency rooms associated with anticoagulant usage per year occur in the United States (6), (iii) the FDA has recently revised the Coumadin label (and will revise the generic warfarin label) to include genomic test information without mandating genetic testing, and (iv) *CYP2C9/VKORC1* testing services are readily available.

Warfarin (Coumadin) is a widely used oral anticoagulant that acts by inhibiting vitamin K-dependent coagulation factors. Indications include prophylaxis and/or treatment of atrial fibrillation, myocardial infarction, cardiac valve replacement, venous thrombosis, and pulmonary embolism. Hemorrhagic events are a complication of warfarin drug treatment due to the narrow therapeutic range. Thrombotic events are also a consequence of the narrow therapeutic range, but this chapter is limited to the hemorrhagic events. The target range for monitoring warfarin therapy is defined by the International Normalized Ratio (INR) value being between 2.0 and 3.0 (slightly lower or higher for some conditions). The INR is a standardized measure of the patient's prothrombin time (PT). This allows for results to be compared across laboratories and test reagents (7). INR monitoring usually begins 2–3 days after the initial dosing (8). In a hospital setting, patients may be monitored daily, while in an outpatient setting, monitoring may be reduced to two or three times each week. If the INR is stable, the interval between testing can be gradually increased up to every 4 weeks. The risk for serious bleeding increases when INR values reach 4.0 or higher. Such elevations are more likely to occur within the first few weeks, before a stable INR is achieved. The goal of long-term anticoagulation monitoring is to maintain the patient in the INR target range; success is measured as percent time in the therapeutic range and avoidance of adverse events. The stability of therapy over time may be influenced by changes in other medications (including over-the-counter medications and nutraceuticals), health status changes that affect warfarin metabolism or vitamin K-dependent coagulation factors, dietary or gastrointestinal factors affecting vitamin K (e.g., alcohol use, irregular ingestion of vitamin K-rich foods, changes in intestinal absorption capacity). The health care provider should monitor, at appropriate intervals, any changes in status, and make necessary and appropriate dose adjustments to maintain the target INR. In addition, patient communication, education, and compliance are important determinants of success. Finally, active intervention may be required when the INR is excessively prolonged and the patient has active bleeding or is at high risk for bleeding.

The recently FDA-approved change in the warfarin label provides information on how people with certain genetic differences may respond to warfarin. This use of genetic information to inform the prescribing of drugs is known as pharmacogenetics or pharmacogenomics. Variations in two genes are known to be associated with the warfarin dose that results in a patient maintaining a stable INR. These genes are *CYP2C9* and *VKORC1*. It is likely that maintenance doses of warfarin will continue to be primarily based on INR measurements, but genotyping may be of help with initial dosing and obtaining stable INR more quickly. The intended use of *CYP2C9* and *VKORC1* genotyping is to predict an individual's maintenance warfarin dose by incorporating demographic, clinical, and gene variant data (both *CYP2C9* and *VKORC1*). This can be used as the initial dose to limit high INR values (overanticoagulation) that are associated with serious bleeding events, and to decrease the time required to reach the target INR. There are limited data on whether this intervention can reduce the incidence of high INR values, the time to stable INR, or the occurrence of serious bleeding events.

Analytic Validity

Analytic validity refers to the ability of a test to measure the genotype of interest both accurately and reliably.

The cytochrome P450 complex is a group of hepatic microsomal enzymes responsible for the oxidative metabolism of various substrates (pharmacokinetics). Thirty-seven *CYP2C9* haplotypes containing over 100 sequence variants have been identified. However, the literature tends to focus on only two of these, which are designated as *2 (R144C, 3608C>T) and *3 (I359L, 42614A>C). The *1 designation is reserved for the wild-type allele. In the European Caucasian population, the frequencies of the *2 and *3 variants are approximately 12.2% and 7.9%, respectively (9). Using these allele frequencies, we calculated the genotype frequencies found in Table 31.1. Individuals with the wild genotype reach a warfarin steady state in 3–5 days. Heterozygotes for *2 and *3 require 6–8 days and 12–15 days, respectively (10). Three additional variants (*4 [I359T, 42615T>C]; *5 [D360E, 42619C>G]; and *6 [10601delA, 818delA]) are sometimes mentioned for inclusion in a testing panel for African-Americans or Asian-Americans. However, even in these populations, the allele frequencies for *4, *5, and *6 are less than 1% (11). Table 31.2 shows the most common *CYP2C9* genotypes, their associated warfarin metabolic rates and associated nomenclature.

Variants in the gene encoding *VKORC1* also influence the response to warfarin via reduced enzyme activity (pharmacodynamics). The clinically relevant variants (-1639G>A, 1173C>T, 1542G>C, 2255T>C, 3730G>A) in non-Hispanic Caucasians are in strong linkage disequilibrium. The literature uses conflicting nomenclatures

Table 31.1 *CYP2C9* and *VKORC1* common allele designations and associated single nucleotide polymorphisms (SNPs) in European Caucasians

Genotype *CYP2C9* (9)	Nucleotide Position (2 alleles)	Prevalence (%)[1]
*1/*1 (no variant)	wild + wild	63.8
*1/*2	wild + 3608C>T	19.5
*1/*3	wild + 42614A>C	12.6
*2/*2	3608C>T + 3608C>T	1.9
*2/*3	3608C>T + 42614A>C	1.5
*3/*3	42614A>C + 42614A>C	0.6
VKORC1 (12–15)		
BB (no variant)	wild + wild	35
AB	wild + (−1639G>A, 1173C>T, 1542G>C, 2255T>C, 3730G>A[2])	47
AA	2 * (−1639G>A, 1173C>T, 1542G>C, 2255T>C, 3730G>A)	18

[1] In non-Hispanic Caucasians when testing is restricted to the *2 and *3 variants
[2] These five SNPs are in strong linkage disequilibrium. Therefore, we have combined them.

Table 31.2 *CYP2C9* variants and their relationship to warfarin metabolism and a *VKORC1* variant and its relationship to gene expression

CYP2C9		
Genotype	Metabolism	Nomenclature
*1/*1	Extensive, rapid, ultrametabolizer	Normal, wild
*1/*2	Intermediate	Heterozygote
*1/*3	Poor, slow	Heterozygote
*2/*3	Poor, slow	Compound heterozygote
*2/*2	Poor, slow	Homozygote
*3/*3	Poor, slow, extremely slow	Homozygote
VKORC1		
Genotype	Enzyme production	Nomenclature
BB	Low (patient needs higher warfarin dose)	Normal, Wild
AB	Medium	Heterozygote
AA	High (patient needs lower warfarin dose)	Homozygote

to refer to these variants. We have chosen that used by Rieder et al. (16). Table 31.2 shows the relationship between *VKORC1* genotype and warfarin dose. The frequencies of these genotypes have been estimated from data reported by several studies, using a random effects model (12–15). Among non-Hispanic Caucasians, these frequencies are 35%, 47%, and 18% for the BB, AB, and AA genotypes, respectively (Table 31.1). The frequencies of these genotypes vary by race/ethnicity (17–23). While *VKORC1* variants are considerably more common than those of *CYP2C9*, there are fewer data available that characterize their analytic validity and clinical validity.

Nearly all available data for analytic validity refer to the detection of two variants in the *CYP2C9* gene; few data are available on detecting the variants in the *VKORC1* gene. Based on seven studies reporting performance in the analytic phase of testing (Table 31.3), assays for the common *CYP2C9* genotypes (*1/*2 and *1/*3) have an analytic sensitivity of 100% (95% CI 96.7–100%) (24). The analytic specificity is also 100% (95% CI 98.2–100%). Based on sparse data for the less common *CYP2C9* genotypes (*2/*2, *2/*3, and *3/*3) the analytic sensitivity of selected assay systems is still 100%, but the confidence interval is wider (95% CI 75–100%) (17). The bottom of Table 31.3 also contains information from the gray literature regarding both *CYP2C9* and *VKORC1* testing. There is one publication that reported the analytic sensitivity of a *VKORC1* variant (-1639) by three genotyping platforms (25); however, there were insufficient data given to include this information in Table 31.3. The analytic sensitivity was reported to be 99% (95% CI 96–100%), 99% (95% CI 96–100%), and 100% (95% CI 97–100%), for the INFINITI analyzer, Invader assay, and Tag-It assay, respectively. No published information is available from which pre- or postanalytic errors can be estimated. Depending on the methodology, sample type, and sample condition, 1–5% of samples may experience repeated assay failures

Table 31.3 Analytic validity of CYP2C9 (restricted to the *2 and *3 variants) and VKORC1 testing

Reference	Year	Assay Method	Referent Method	CYP2C9 ANALYTIC SENSITIVITY (TEST RESULT/REFERENT RESULT)					ANALYTIC SPECIFICITY
				(*1/*2)	(*2/*2)	(*1/*3)	(*3/*3)	(*2/*3)	(*1/*1)
Hillman M. et al.	2004	LightCycler	Sequencing	2/2	1/1	—	1/1	1/1	4/4
Pickering J, et al.	2004	Luminex, eSensor	Sequencing	15/15	1/1	13/13	—	2/2	70/70
Wen S, et al.	2003	Microarray	Sequencing	—	—	7/7	—	—	13/13
Zainuddin A, et al.	2003	Nested PCR	Sequencing	3/3	—	5/5	2/2	2/2	28/28
Eriksson S, et al.	2002	Pyrosequencing	PCR-RFLP	9/9	—	5/5	—	—	9/9
Aquilante C, et al.	2004	Pyrosequencing	PCR-RFLP	—	—	—	—	—	—
Burian M, et al.	2002	LightCycler	PCR-RFLP	27/27	1/1	10/10	1/1	1/1	79/79
			Total	**56/56**	**3/3**	**40/40**	**4/4**	**6/6**	**203/203**
Third Wave Tech	2006	Invader, Tag-It, Pyro	Sequencing	9/9	3/3	6/6	2/2	6/6	9/9
ARUP Laboratory	2006	Invader, Tag-It	Sequencing	9/9	—	1/1	—	—	21/21
LabCorp	2006	Invader, Tag-It	PCR-RFLP	6/6	1/1	5/5	1/1	4/4	5/5
VKORC1				**(AB)**	**(AA)**				**(BB)**
Third Wave Tech	2006	Invader, Pyro	Sequencing	16/16	12/12				7/7
ARUP	2006	Invader	Sequencing	10/10	4/4				17/17
LabCorp	2006	Invader	PCR-RFLP, Sequencing	10/10	5/5				7/7

ARUP, Associated Regional and University Pathologists.

resulting in inconclusive test results (26) (see Question 16 in the full review for personal communications containing additional data). These failures can be viewed as reducing the analytic sensitivity and specificity.

Based on other molecular tests that have been studied in more detail (*CFTR* (27,28) and *HFE* (29)), working estimates of overall analytic sensitivity and specificity for the common *CYP2C9* genotypes are 98–99% and 99.5–99.75%, respectively. Too few data exist to estimate these rates for *VKORC1* genotyping. Nearly all available data are based on DNA extracted from whole blood samples. Other sample types (e.g., mouthwash) have been mentioned (30), but data are sparse. Using these estimates for *CYP2C9*, incorrect genotype assignments would be expected to be relatively rare (1 in 50 to 1 in 200) among any genotype group. At least 12 laboratories in the United States now offer *CYP2C9* and/or *VKORC1* genotyping for clinical use (see full review, Table 31.4). Several manufacturers offer reagents to test for variants in both genes.

It appears that the methodologies used to identify *CYP2C9* and *VKORC1* variants can easily be completed in a day. Thus, turnaround time greater than 2 or 3 days will be because of slow transport of samples, because laboratory does not run the assay every day. Neither of these issues would be expected to impact analytic validity (other than to perhaps improve the quality of samples by shortening transport time). On at least one website offering testing, the laboratory turnaround time is stated to be 1 day (http://www.kimballgenetics.com/tests.html).

The Genetic Testing Quality Control Materials Program at the CDC assists genetic testing laboratories in obtaining validated quality control materials. As part of this program, 96 samples from Coriell Cell Repositories (Camden, NJ) were genotyped for *CYP2C9* and *VKORC1* variants (http://wwwn.cdc.gov/dls/genetics/rmmaterials/MaterialsAvailability.aspx). Two laboratories used the Tag-It (TM Bioscience) methodology to analyze the *CYP2C9* gene, and both identified the same genotypes in all samples. Two other laboratories sequenced the *VKORC1* gene, and both identified the same genotypes in all samples. Laboratories validating new assays can purchase these samples with known genotypes.

The College of American Pathologists (CAP) has established a working group consisting of members from the CAP/ACMG Biochemical and Molecular Genetics, Special Chemistry, Toxicology and Coagulation Committees, to develop a Pharmacogenetics (PGx) Survey. This PGx Survey began in 2008, with two shipments (April and September). Each shipment will contain two different vials of 25 μg each of extracted DNA, which participants will be able to test for genetic variations in the *CYP2C19, CYP2C9, CYP2D6, UGT1A1*, and *VKORC1* genes.

Missing or incomplete data in the literature are identified as gaps in knowledge in the Rapid-ACCE review. Missing or incomplete data pertaining to analytic validity include:

- which *CYP2C9/VKORC1* variants should be part of a clinical panel
- poorly defined analytic validity for the less common *CYP2C9* genotype (e.g., *3/*3)

- lack of published data on analytic validity for *VKORC1* against a "gold standard"
- whether clinical laboratories are able to offer an appropriately validated test (e.g., variants included, turnaround time, costs, sample types, internal analytic validity studies)
- limited information on long-term performance/consistency of methods (within-laboratory variability)
- data showing between-laboratory consistency
- overall estimate of analytic performance including pre- and postanalytic error rates
- method-specific and sample-specific failure rates
- data from the external proficiency testing program.

Clinical Validity

Clinical validity refers to the ability of a test to detect or predict the disorder/phenotype of interest.

CYP2C9 Genotypes and INR Values

Clinical validity was examined using one intermediate outcome (elevated International Normalized Ratios, INRs), as well as the health outcome of severe bleeding. INR values above 3.0 are twice as likely among *CYP2C9* heterozygotes (relative risk of 2.0 or higher), and are more likely to occur in the first and second week (induction phase) after warfarin initiation than in the third week or later (Table 31.4). This information is based on only two studies that were designed and analyzed differently (31). A third study found a weak correlation between the rate of

Table 31.4 Relative risk of INR values above 3.0 during warfarin induction, stratified by *CYP2C9* genotype

	Week After Induction	Lindh et al., 2005	Peyvandi et al., 2004	All
Relative risk (*2 versus *1/*1)	1	2.8 (1.2–6.7)*		
	2	2.1 (1.2–3.7)	1.9 (1.3–2.9)	1.8 (1.3–2.3)
	3	1.0 (0.5–1.8)		
Relative risk (*3 versus *1/*1)	1	5.4 (2.5–12)		
	2	3.5 (2.1–5.8)	2.0 (1.3–3.1)	2.5 (1.3–4.5)
	3	1.1 (0.6–2.0)		

*95% confidence interval.
*2 includes *1/*2 and *2/*2.
*3 includes *1/*3, *3/*3, and *2/*3.

change in the INR values (slope) and *CYP2C9* genotype (nonwild genotypes had a higher slope, $p = 0.05$) (32).

CYP2C9 Genotypes and Severe Bleeding

Clinical sensitivity is defined as the proportion of individuals with the outcome of interest (severe bleeding) that has a genotype other than wild (i.e., *1/*2, *2/*2, *2/*3, *1/*3, *3/*3). This is synonymous with the detection rate. With nonwild *CYP2C9* genotypes grouped together from three studies, the clinical sensitivity of *CYP2C9* to identify serious bleeding events is 45% (95% CI 34–55%) (33), indicating that about half of all serious bleeding events occur among *CYP2C9* wild-type individuals (Table 31.5). Clinical specificity is defined as the proportion of individuals with no severe bleeding that has the wild (*1/*1) genotype. One minus the clinical specificity is the false-positive rate. The false-positive rate indicates the proportion of individuals without a bleeding event that has a nonwild genotype. Overall, the clinical specificity of *CYP2C9* is 68% (95% CI 57–77%). The correspondingly high false-positive rate (32%) is because nonwild *CYP2C9* genotypes are relatively common and most will not experience serious bleeding. The relative risk for serious bleeding in nonwild versus *1/*1 individuals is 1.4 (95% CI 0.9–3.1%, not significant). The attributable risk is estimated to be 3.1%.

Figure 31.1 shows the relationship between these parameters in a population with a serious bleeding rate of 5%. The prevalence of serious bleeding among populations varies widely (<1–17%) depending on many factors (11,12,14,15) (e.g., indication for warfarin, age, comorbidities, definition of serious bleeding and other drug use). The positive predictive value (PPV) is estimated to be 7% (95% CI 0.2–33.9%) (i.e., 1 of every 15 patients with a nonwild *CYP2C9* genotype will suffer a bleeding event). Because nonwild *CYP2C9* genotypes are relatively common and the prevalence of serious bleeding is low, most will not experience serious bleeding. When

Table 31.5 Clinical sensitivity, clinical specificity, relative risk, and attributable risk for severe bleeding events (wild versus nonwild *CYP2C9* genotype)

Study	Clinical Sensitivity (%)	Clinical Specificity (%)	Relative Risk (%)	Attributable Risk (%)
Ogg et al. (33)[*]	23	87	1.85	7
Margaglione et al. (10)[†]	67	53	1.91	12
Higashi et al. (12–16,34)	50	78	2.19	15
Wadelius et al. (20)	33	66	0.96	0
Limdi et al. (12–16,34)	43	60	1.12	0
Summary (Higashi, Wadelius, and Limdi) (95% CI)	**45** (34–55)	**68** (57–77)	**1.4** (0.9–2.4)	**3.1** (0–10)

[*]Considered only *3 genotypes (these estimates are not included in the summary line).
[†]Wild *CYP2C9* genotype frequency in Italy is low (these estimates are not included in the summary line).

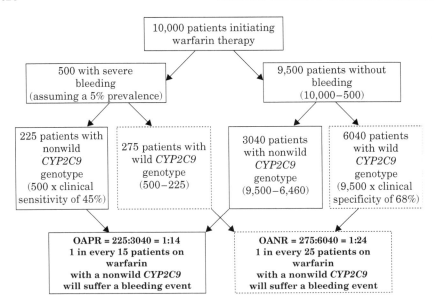

Figure 31.1 Flow diagram showing episodes of severe bleeding in a hypothetical cohort of 10,000 individuals initiating warfarin treatment, stratified by CYP2C9 genotype. The estimates used in this figure were derived from published literature summarized in this evidence-based review. The solid bordered boxes are used to calculate the odds of being affected, given a positive result (nonwild genotype), while the dotted bordered boxes are used to calculate the odds of being affected given a negative result (wild genotype).
OAPR = odds of being affected given a positive result (nonwild genotypes)
OANR = odds of being affected given a negative result (wild genotype)

the prevalence of serious bleeding is allowed to range from 1% to 17%, the PPV ranges from 1.4% to 33.3%, respectively. Figure 31.1 also shows that the negative predictive value (NPV) is estimated to be 96% (95% CI 79.6–99.9%) (i.e., 24 of every 25 patients with a wild *CYP2C9* genotype will not suffer a bleeding event). Again, allowing the prevalence of serious bleeding to range from 1% to 17%, the NPV ranges from 99.2% (95% CI 95.5–100.0%) to 83.3% (95% CI 35.9–99.6%), respectively.

VKORC1 Genotypes and Severe Bleeding

One study has reported the association of *VKORC1* genotype and risk of hemorrhagic complications among African-Americans and European-Americans on warfarin therapy (35,36). The incident rate for minor or major hemorrhage was not significantly different for patients with a *VKORC1* variant compared to the wild-type genotype (sensitivity [95% CI] = 43% [39–44]; specificity [95% CI] = 60% [58–61]; relative risk [95% CI] = 1.1 [0.6–2.0]; attributable risk = <1%).

CYP2C9 Genotype and Steady State Warfarin Modeling

In addition to warfarin dose requirements, *CYP2C9* genotyping also provides information concerning time to steady state of warfarin plasma levels. The results of modeling time to steady state warfarin in three genotypes (*1/*1, *1/*2, and *1/*3) have been reported (35). Each genotype is provided with a targeted dose (5, 3, and 1.6 mg, respectively). Wild-type individuals reach steady state within 3–5 days. This is much faster than the 6–8 days for those with a *1/*2 genotype or the 12–15 days for a *1/*3 genotype (35). This delay may have long-term INR monitoring implications when warfarin doses are being modified.

CYP2C9 and VKORC1 Genotype and
Warfarin Steady State Dose

Although not considered a direct measure of clinical validity, *CYP2C9* genotypes are strongly related to warfarin dose, once the INR has stabilized. Compared with the wild genotype (*1/*1), warfarin dose is reduced by 22%, 36%, 43%, 53%, and 76% among individuals with the *1/*2, *1/*3, *2/*2, *2/*3, and *3/*3 genotypes, respectively (Figure 31.2) (37). Compared with the heterozygote *VKORC1* genotype (indicated by AB), warfarin dose is increased by 35% among individuals with the BB genotype and reduced by 32% among those with the AA genotype (38). Figure 31.3 displays modeled distributions of stable warfarin dose for the three most common *CYP2C9* genotypes, derived using data from one study (39). Although there are clear reductions in the average levels, there is considerable overlap among these three groups. The three *VKORC1* genotypes also have considerable overlap of stable warfarin dose (data not shown). *CYP2C9* and *VKORC1* genotypes contribute

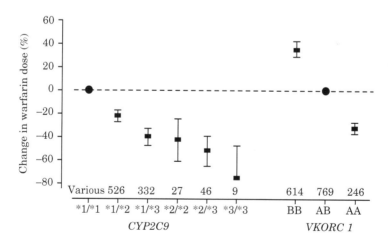

*Figure 31.2 Change in warfarin dose at stable INR by CYP2C9 or VKORC1 genotype. This meta-analysis includes ten data sets for CYP2C9 genotyping and seven data sets for VKORC1 genotyping. The referent categories (horizontal dotted line) were chosen because they included the largest proportion of the population for each gene. The numbers above each genotype indicate the number of samples included in the analysis. For the CYP2C9 reference category, the number varied from a high of 1,757 for the comparison with the *1/*3 genotype to a low of 476 for the *3/*3 genotype comparison.*

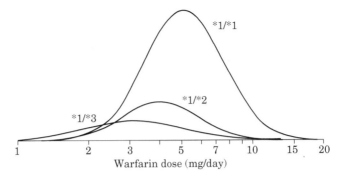

Figure 31.3 Overlapping distributions of warfarin dose at stable INR for three CYP2C9 genotypes. The modeled distributions of oral warfarin dose are shown on a logarithmic horizontal axis. The areas of the three distributions are in direct relation to their prevalence (*1/*1 being the most common). Although the reduction in stable warfarin dose is clearly visible for the *1/*2 and *1/*3 genotype, there is considerable overlap of the three distributions.

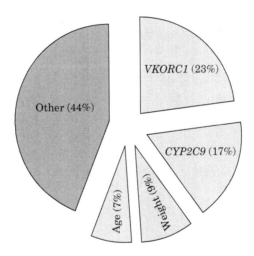

Figure 31.4 Pie chart showing the known sources of variability in warfarin dose needed for a stable INR. Each estimate is based on a summary analysis of partial r^2 values from multivariate regression analysis reported in six studies that included genotyping on both CYP2C9 and VKORC1.

relatively independent information about stable warfarin dose (Figure 31.4) (40–42). Based on six studies that involved testing for both genes in a population with a steady state INR, *VKORC1* genotyping explains a slightly higher proportion of overall variability in warfarin dose (23%) than *CYP2C9* genotyping (17%) (42). This is because the *VKORC1* genotypes associated with changes in dosage are more common in the Caucasian population. Other important factors in predicting warfarin dose are body weight (9% of variability) and age (7% of variability).

Table 31.6 Estimates of warfarin dose (mg) at stable INR, stratified by *CYP2C9* and *VKORC1* genotype

| | cyp2c9 Genotype | | | | | |
| | Rapid | Inter | | Poor | | |
VKORC1 Genotype	*1/*1	*1/*2	*1/*3	*2/*2	*2/*3	*3/*3
High (BB)	6.7	5.4	4.5	4.4	3.6	3.0
Medium (AB)	4.8	3.9	3.2	3.2	2.6	2.2
Low (AA)	3.5	2.8	2.3	2.3	1.9	1.6

Source: From www.WarfarinDosing.org, for a 65-year-old Caucasian non-Hispanic male with a body surface area of 1.96 m² (weight = 180 lbs, height = 5′ 8″) with an initial INR of 0.75 and a target INR of 2.75. He is a non-smoker with no liver disease and is taking no relevant drugs (e.g., amiodarone, statin). The indication for warfarin is atrial fibrillation.

Two recent studies have been published that provide warfarin-dosing models incorporating both *CYP2C9* and *VKORC1* variants (35,36). Both of these models include logarithmic transformation for warfarin dose and both *CYP2C9* *2 and *3 genotypes. In addition, one of these models includes prior warfarin doses and INR values (35). Table 31.6 shows the variations in warfarin dose that were computed by a comprehensive (but unpublished) warfarin-dosing model (www.WarfarinDosing.org) that accounts for both *CYP2C9* and *VKORC1* genotyping, as well as several other known covariates. Table 31.7 shows warfarin doses relative to the most common subgroup (*CYP2C9* = *1/*1, and *VKORC1* = AB) comprising 30% of the Caucasian population. The display highlights that individuals with certain genotypes will actually receive a higher warfarin dose (e.g., 40% higher dose in *1/*1, BB), compared to those with the most common genotype. Four dosing models have been published that do not include both an appropriate transformation for warfarin dose (e.g., logarithmic) and allow for observed difference in warfarin doses for the *1/*2 versus *1/*3 genotypes (11,12,14,15). Missing or incomplete data pertaining to clinical validity include:

- the clinical sensitivity, clinical specificity, relative risk, and attributable risk of severe bleeding in the *VKORC1* genotypes and in *CYP2C9* and *VKORC1* genotypes combined
- the contribution of genetic versus other influences toward bleeding in various racial/ethnic populations
- the positive and negative predictive values (PPV and NPV) for severe bleeding in the *VKORC1* genotypes, and *CYP2C9* and *VKORC1* genotypes combined
- how the difference in dosage would be best presented to clinicians who are initiating treatment in warfarin-naïve individuals to ensure that a targeted dose will account for all known important sources of variation
- the roles of other genes in the pharmacokinetics and pharmacodynamics of warfarin and their impact on warfarin dosage requirements

Table 31.7 Relative adjustments to warfarin dose at stable INR, stratified
by *CYP2C9* and *VKORC1* genotype and estimated frequency per 1000

	cyp2c9 Genotype						
	Rapid	*Inter*	*Poor*				*Frequency*
VKORCI Genotype	*1/*1	*1/*2	*1/*3	*2/*2	*2/*3	*3/*3	**/ 1000**
High (BB)	140% (223)	113% (68)	94% (44)	92% (5)	75% (7)	63% (2)	(350)
Medium (AB)	100% (300)	81% (92)	67% (59)	67% (7)	54% (9)	46% (3)	(470)
Low (AA)	73% (115)	58% (35)	48% (23)	48% (3)	40% (3)	33% (1)	(180)
Frequency/1,000	(638)	(195)	(126)	(15)	(19)	(6)	(1,000)

The boxed entry (*1/*1; AB) is the most common combination of *CYP2C9/VKORC1* genotypes (300 per 1,000) and is considered the referent group (100% dose). Other entries are represented as a percentage of this dose (e.g., 140% indicates a 40% increase in predicted dose to achieve a stable INR).

Frequencies are derived from the allele frequencies for *CYP2C9* of 12.2% and 7.9% for *2 and *3, respectively, and for the BB, AB, and AA genotype frequencies of 35%, 47%, and 18%, respectively. The two sets of allele frequencies are considered to be independent.

Source: From www.warfarindosing.org, for a 65-year old Caucasian with a body surface area of 1.96 m² (weight = 180 lbs, height = 5' 8") with a target INR of 2.75, who is a nonsmoker and is taking no other relevant drugs.

Clinical Utility

Clinical utility is defined as the benefits and risks associated with the introduction of a test into clinical practice, and includes economic analyses to determine the financial impact of such testing. One small pilot randomized trial enrolled 38 patients and found six serious bleeding events among the 20 patients with standard warfarin dosing versus two bleeding events among the 18 receiving model-based dosing using *CYP2C9* genotyping (37). These results are not statistically significant, but show acceptability of the randomized design.

A recent prospective randomized controlled study in Israel reported that patients who received *CYP2C9* genotype-guided warfarin dosing ($n = 93$) reached their first therapeutic INR 2.7 days earlier than those patients who received standard warfarin dosing ($n = 93$) (HR 2.89, 95% CI 2.1–4.0, $p < 0.001$) (38). The *2 and *3 variants were included in the dosing model. The time spent in the therapeutic range during the induction phase was 45% versus 24% for the genotype-guided dose group and the standard dose group, respectively ($p < 0.001$). The time required to reach stable anticoagulation phase was 14 days for the genotype-guided dose group compared with 32 days for the standard dose group (HR 4.23, 95% CI 2.9–6.1, $p < 0.001$). The time spent in the therapeutic range from induction to stable anticoagulation phase was 80% versus 63% for the genotype-guided dose group and the standard dose group, respectively ($p < 0.001$). A single serious bleeding event occurred in a control group patient, whose INR was within target range.

A second randomized trial in Utah also compared outcomes between patients who received genotype-guided warfarin dosing ($n = 101$) and those who received standard dosing ($n = 99$) (39). The genotype-guided warfarin dosing took into account the *2 and *3 variants in the *CYP2C9* gene and the 1173C>T variant in the *VKORC1* gene. This study found no significant difference between the groups in time within therapeutic range (69.7% versus 68.6%, for genotype-guided dosing and standard dosing, respectively, $p = 0.74$). The number of serious adverse events was nearly equal for the genotype-guided group ($n = 4$) and the standard dose group ($n = 5$) (OR 0.78, 95% CI 0.2–2.98, $p = 0.71$), and were unrelated to out-of-range INRs.

Additional randomized trials are underway to provide further information regarding the clinical effectiveness of *CYP2C9* and *VKORC1* genotyping to inform warfarin dosing. Some of these trials are using severe bleeding as the outcome, while others are targeting intermediate measures such as reducing the time to achieve stable INR, and the percentage of time in range during dose stabilization.

Using estimates of clinical validity described earlier (Figure 31.1), along with several assumptions of clinical utility (e.g., cost of testing and the effectiveness of targeted warfarin dose to avoid serious bleeding), the number of individuals that must be tested to avoid one serious bleeding event ranges from 48 to 385. The cost per serious bleeding event averted ranges from $14,500 to $95,900. Key assumptions that strongly influence this cost estimate are the effectiveness of targeted warfarin dose (range 80–20% in a sensitivity analysis) and the cost of genetic testing (range $300–$500).

Economic outcomes and decision analysis studies on genetic and pharmacogenetic testing have been published (40–42). One recently released analysis suggests that genetic testing prior to warfarin dosing will avoid many severe bleeding events and result in large cost savings (42). However, close examination of this study reveals that the authors made several assumptions that may not be valid. These assumptions include: targeted dosing by genotype will be 100% effective in reducing bleeding events to the level of that in individuals with the wild genotype; more effective dosing will reduce the rate of strokes; the rate of bleeding events is higher than expected; and the estimate of new warfarin users per year is high. Missing or incomplete data pertaining to clinical utility include:

- the clinical utility of genotyping prior to warfarin dosing (e.g., is there a reduction in time to stable INR, is there a reduction in severe bleeding events?)
- cost-effectiveness of *VKORC1* testing alone, or in combination with *CYP2C9*
- the impact of the timing of genotyping (e.g., prior to initial dose or 2–3 days after initial warfarin treatment)
- validated educational materials for patients and providers
- long-term monitoring plans
- guidelines for evaluating program performance.

Ethical, Legal, and Social Implications (ELSI)

Pharmacogenetic testing might be perceived as carrying less serious ELSI than other types of genetic testing. For example, a variant that alters response to a drug (e.g., a *CYP2C9* or *VKORC1* genotype) might carry less potential for discrimination, privacy/confidentiality, and stigmatization than a mutation that is predictive of a debilitating and/or fatal disease (e.g., Huntington disease). However, a premise does exist that pharmacogenetic tests may be used to classify groups that face discrimination in health care, resulting in prejudice and stigmatization. Furthermore, stratifying the population into genetic subgroups could mean that the costs of developing new drugs tailored to the needs of a given small subgroup might be prohibitively expensive and might not be developed. Even if this premise should be validated, an individual will still avoid harm, if found to be in a genetic subgroup for which an existing therapy is known to be harmful, in that inappropriate treatment will be avoided.

The Nuffield Council on Bioethics Report suggests that "the likelihood that pharmacogenomic data will be of relevance to family members is low" (43). However, since single nucleotide polymorphism (SNP) testing has not been widely studied and SNPs are heritable, it may be too early to decide definitively if this statement will be upheld.

Pharmacogenetic testing for *CYP2D6*, in the context of tamoxifen use, is already being marketed directly to consumers (www.DNAdirect.com). Standalone *CYP2D6* testing for generalized drug metabolism is advertised, but not yet available. The issues of direct-to-consumer marketing of genetic tests have been discussed elsewhere. It is likely that *CYP2C9* and *VKORC1* testing will also be offered directly to consumers in the near future.

It has been recommended that, if information about unrelated medicines or diseases is likely to be obtained from pharmacogenetic testing, or if the results of the test will have a significant impact on the health or lifestyle of the patient, written consent may be appropriate. Even if it is decided that consent is not required, written information (e.g., education materials) should be supplied.

Legal implications may arise as pharmacogenetic testing becomes widespread. For instance, will providers and drug companies be held liable for not considering genetic information? Should pharmacies store genotype information obtained for one application and use it when dispensing other drugs utilizing the same metabolic pathway? Finally, the new FDA-revised warfarin label may make conducting randomized controlled trials more difficult.

The issues discussed in this section are all considered gaps in knowledge and will require further monitoring and documentation to further describe the ethical, legal, and social implications of pharmacogenetic testing.

Summary

There exists compelling evidence for the association between *CYP2C9* and *VKORC1* genotypes and stable warfarin dose. Based on the recommendation by the Clinical

Pharmacology Subcommittee of the Advisory Committee for Pharmaceutical Sciences, the FDA updated the warfarin label to include information on how people with certain genetic differences may respond to warfarin. Specifically, people with *CYP2C9* and *VKORC1* variants may need lower warfarin doses than those without variants. However, due to the absence of evidence from a randomized trial showing that genotype-based warfarin dosing improves clinical outcomes (e.g., severe bleeding), the updated label does not recommend or require pharmacogenetic testing.

Few data are available to evaluate the association between *CYP2C9* genotype and stable INR during the induction phase, when the risk of severe bleeding is highest. There are limited data on the clinical validity of *CYP2C9* genotyping to predict severe bleeding events, and even fewer data for *VKORC1* genotypes. The clinical utility of DNA testing in this clinical scenario is to "personalize" an individual's initial warfarin dose by incorporating demographic, clinical, and genotype data (*CYP2C9* and *VKORC1*) as a way to limit high INR values (overanticoagulation) that are associated with an increased risk of serious bleeding events. No large study has yet shown this to be acceptable or effective. Several randomized trials are underway addressing various components related to clinical effectiveness of *CYP2C9* and *VKORC1* genotyping to inform warfarin dosing as a way to reduce serious bleeding. It is possible that the trial setting may influence study outcomes. For example, in the setting of a warfarin clinic that is highly focused on achieving and maintaining appropriate target INR levels, the introduction of genotyping might not result in any real benefit. Alternatively, if the setting were less structured, without stringent monitoring of INR levels, genotyping might result in a large net benefit. This highlights the need for genotyping to be put into the context of existing efforts to "personalize" warfarin dosage based on demographic and clinical factors.

In the meantime, there may be selected circumstances in which *CYP2C9* and *VKORC1* genotyping might be warranted. The American College of Medical Genetics has issued a policy statement regarding the use of *CYP2C9* and *VKORC1* testing to inform warfarin dosing (44). Routine testing in a population of warfarin-naïve patients would, of course, be necessary in the context of any organized clinical trial. Outside of this setting, selective testing might be useful as part of individual patient care in the relatively uncommon situations when stabilizing the INR is found to be particularly difficult and/or time consuming or when the warfarin dose is surprisingly high, or low. Several ethical, legal, and social implications were identified as part of this evidence review that would need to be monitored if testing were to become widespread, in order to help ensure equitable, nondiscriminatory, and confidential *CYP2C9* and *VKORC1* testing.

Acknowledgment

Funding was provided by the American College of Medical Genetics Foundation (ACMGF). Tm Bioscience (Toronto, Canada, acquired in 2006 by Luminex, Austin, TX) provided the ACMGF with partial funding for this study.

We thank David Flockhart, MD, PhD, Indiana University School of Medicine, Indianapolis, Indiana; Dennis O'Kane, PhD, Mayo Clinic, Rochester, Minnesota; Michael Watson, PhD, American College of Medical Genetics, Washington, DC; Marc S. Williams, MD, Clinical Genetics Institute, LDS Hospital, Salt Lake City, Utah for their oversight and comments.

We also thank Amy Brower, PhD, Third Wave Technologies, Madison, Wisconsin; LabCorp, Burlington, NC; Brian Gage, MD, Washington University School of Medicine, St. Louis, Missouri; Roy Gandolfi, MD, Intermountain Healthcare, West Valley City, Utah; Elaine Lyon, PhD, ARUP, Salt Lake City, Utah; David Veenstra, PharmD, University of Washington, Seattle, Washington; Ann Wittkowsky, PharmD, University of Washington Medical Center, Seattle, Washington for their submission of unpublished data, discussions and/or comments.

References

1. Haddow JE, Palomaki GE. ACCE: a model process for evaluating data on emerging genetic tests. In: Khoury MJ, Little J, Burke W, eds. *Human Genome Epidemiology: A Scientific Foundation for Using Genetic Information to Improve Health and Prevent Disease.* Oxford: Oxford University Press; 2003:217–233.

2. Gudgeon JM, McClain MR, Palomaki GE, Williams MS. Rapid ACCE: experience with a rapid and structured approach for evaluating gene-based testing. *Genet Med.* July 2007;9(7):473–478.

3. Enhancing the oversight of genetic tests: Recommendations of the SACGT. http://www4. od.nih.gov/oba/sacgt/reports/oversight_report.pdf. Accessed 7/1/08.

4. McClain MR, Palomaki GE, Piper M, Haddow JE. A rapid-ACCE review of CYP2C9 and VKORC1 alleles testing to inform warfarin dosing in adults at elevated risk for thrombotic events to avoid serious bleeding. *Genet Med.* February 2008;10(2):89–98.

5. Moore TJ, Cohen MR, Furberg CD. Serious adverse drug events reported to the Food and Drug Administration, 1998–2005. *Arch Intern Med.* September 10, 2007;167(16):1752–1759.

6. Budnitz DS, Pollock DA, Weidenbach KN, Mendelsohn AB, Schroeder TJ, Annest JL. National surveillance of emergency department visits for outpatient adverse drug events. *JAMA.* October 18, 2006;296(15):1858–1866.

7. Johnston M, Harrison L, Moffat K, Willan A, Hirsh J. Reliability of the international normalized ratio for monitoring the induction phase of warfarin: comparison with the prothrombin time ratio. *J Lab Clin Med.* August 1996;128(2):214–217.

8. Hirsh J, Guyatt GH, Albers GW, Schunemann HJ. The seventh ACCP conference on antithrombotic and thrombolytic therapy: evidence-based guidelines. *Chest.* 2004;126:172S–173S.

9. Sanderson S, Emery J, Higgins J. CYP2C9 gene variants, drug dose, and bleeding risk in warfarin-treated patients: a HuGEnet systematic review and meta-analysis. *Genet Med.* February 2005;7(2):97–104.

10. Linder MW, Looney S, Adams JE, 3rd, et al. Warfarin dose adjustments based on CYP2C9 genetic polymorphisms. *J Thromb Thrombolysis.* December 2002;14(3):227–232.

11. Takahashi H, Wilkinson GR, Nutescu EA, et al. Different contributions of polymorphisms in VKORC1 and CYP2C9 to intra- and inter-population differences in maintenance dose of warfarin in Japanese, Caucasians and African-Americans. *Pharmacogenet Genomics.* February 2006;16(2):101–110.

12. Aquilante CL, Langaee TY, Lopez LM, et al. Influence of coagulation factor, vitamin K epoxide reductase complex subunit 1, and cytochrome P450 2C9 gene polymorphisms on warfarin dose requirements. *Clin Pharmacol Ther.* April 2006;79(4):291–302.

13. D'Andrea G, D'Ambrosio RL, Di Perna P, et al. A polymorphism in the VKORC1 gene is associated with an interindividual variability in the dose-anticoagulant effect of warfarin. *Blood.* January 15, 2005;105(2):645–649.

14. Sconce EA, Khan TI, Wynne HA, et al. The impact of CYP2C9 and VKORC1 genetic polymorphism and patient characteristics upon warfarin dose requirements: proposal for a new dosing regimen. *Blood.* October 1, 2005;106(7):2329–2333.

15. Vecsler M, Loebstein R, Almog S, et al. Combined genetic profiles of components and regulators of the vitamin K-dependent gamma-carboxylation system affect individual sensitivity to warfarin. *Thromb Haemost.* February 2006;95(2):205–211.

16. Rieder MJ, Reiner AP, Gage BF, et al. Effect of VKORC1 haplotypes on transcriptional regulation and warfarin dose. *N Engl J Med.* June 2, 2005;352(22):2285–2293.

17. Aquilante CL, Lobmeyer MT, Langaee TY, Johnson JA. Comparison of cytochrome P450 2C9 genotyping methods and implications for the clinical laboratory. *Pharmacotherapy.* June 2004;24(6):720–726.

18. Burian M, Grosch S, Tegeder I, Geisslinger G. Validation of a new fluorogenic real-time PCR assay for detection of CYP2C9 allelic variants and CYP2C9 allelic distribution in a German population. *Br J Clin Pharmacol.* November 2002;54(5):518–521.

19. Eriksson S, Berg LM, Wadelius M, Alderborn A. Cytochrome p450 genotyping by multiplexed real-time dna sequencing with pyrosequencing technology. *Assay Drug Dev Technol.* November 2002;1(1 Pt 1):49–59.

20. Hillman MA, Wilke RA, Caldwell MD, Berg RL, Glurich I, Burmester JK. Relative impact of covariates in prescribing warfarin according to CYP2C9 genotype. *Pharmacogenetics.* August 2004;14(8):539–547.

21. Pickering JW, McMillin GA, Gedge F, Hill HR, Lyon E. Flow cytometric assay for genotyping cytochrome p450 2C9 and 2C19: comparison with a microelectronic DNA array. *Am J Pharmacogenomics.* 2004;4(3):199–207.

22. Wen SY, Wang H, Sun OJ, Wang SQ. Rapid detection of the known SNPs of CYP2C9 using oligonucleotide microarray. *World J Gastroenterol.* June 2003;9(6):1342–1346.

23. Zainuddin Z, Teh LK, Suhaimi AW, Salleh MZ, Ismail R. A simple method for the detection of CYP2C9 polymorphisms: nested allele-specific multiplex polymerase chain reaction. *Clin Chim Acta.* October 2003;336(1–2):97–102.

24. Eby CS, King C, Gage B. Evaluation of commercial platforms for rapid genotyping of polymorphisms affecting therapeutic warfarin dose. *J Thromb Thrombolysis.* November 14, 2007;25(1):99.

25. Palomaki GE, Bradley LA, Richards CS, Haddow JE. Analytic validity of cystic fibrosis testing: a preliminary estimate. *Genet Med.* January–February 2003;5(1):15–20.

26. Hruska MW, Frye RF, Langaee TY. Pyrosequencing method for genotyping cytochrome P450 CYP2C8 and CYP2C9 enzymes. *Clin Chem.* December 2004;50(12):2392–2395.

27. Lindh JD, Lundgren S, Holm L, Alfredsson L, Rane A. Several-fold increase in risk of overanticoagulation by CYP2C9 mutations. *Clin Pharmacol Ther.* November 2005;78(5):540–550.

28. Peyvandi F, Spreafico M, Siboni SM, Moia M, Mannucci PM. CYP2C9 genotypes and dose requirements during the induction phase of oral anticoagulant therapy. *Clin Pharmacol Ther.* March 2004;75(3):198–203.

29. Wilke RA, Berg RL, Vidaillet HJ, Caldwell MD, Burmester JK, Hillman MA. Impact of age, CYP2C9 genotype and concomitant medication on the rate of rise for prothrombin time during the first 30 days of warfarin therapy. *Clin Med Res.* November 2005;3(4):207–213.

30. Ogg MS, Brennan P, Meade T, Humphries SE. CYP2C9*3 allelic variant and bleeding complications. *Lancet.* September 25, 1999;354(9184):1124.

31. Margaglione M, Colaizzo D, D'Andrea G, et al. Genetic modulation of oral anticoagulation with warfarin. *Thromb Haemost.* November 2000;84(5):775–778.

32. Wadelius M, Sorlin K, Wallerman O, et al. Warfarin sensitivity related to CYP2C9, CYP3A5, ABCB1 (MDR1) and other factors. *Pharmacogenomics J.* 2004;4(1):40–48.

33. Limdi NA, McGwin G, Goldstein JA, et al. Influence of CYP2C9 and VKORC1 1173C/T Genotype on the Risk of Hemorrhagic Complications in African-American and European-American Patients on Warfarin. *Clin Pharmacol Ther.* February 2008;83(2):312–321. Epub July 25, 2007.

34. Wadelius M, Chen LY, Downes K, et al. Common VKORC1 and GGCX polymorphisms associated with warfarin dose. *Pharmacogenomics J.* 2005;5(4):262–270.

35. Millican E, Jacobsen-Lenzini PA, Milligan PE, et al. Genetic-based dosing in orthopaedic patients beginning warfarin therapy. *Blood.* March 26, 2007(110):1511–1515.

36. Zhu Y, Shennan M, Reynolds KK, et al. Estimation of Warfarin Maintenance Dose Based on VKORC1 (-1639 G>A) and CYP2C9 Genotypes. *Clin Chem.* July 2007;53(7):1199–1205.

37. Hillman MA, Wilke RA, Yale SH, et al. A prospective, randomized pilot trial of model-based warfarin dose initiation using CYP2C9 genotype and clinical data. *Clin Med Res.* August 2005;3(3):137–145.

38. Caraco Y, Blotnick S, Muszkat M. CYP2C9 genotype-guided warfarin prescribing enhances the efficacy and safety of anticoagulation: a prospective randomized controlled study. *Clin Pharmacol Ther.* March 2008;83(3):460–470. Epub September 12, 2007.

39. Anderson JL, Horne BD, Stevens SM, et al. Randomized trial of genotype-guided versus standard warfarin dosing in patients initiating oral anticoagulation. *Circulation.* November 7, 2007;116(22):2563–2570. Epub November 7, 2007.

40. Higashi MK, Veenstra DL. Managed care in the genomics era: assessing the cost effectiveness of genetic tests. *Am J Manag Care.* July 2003;9(7):493–500.

41. You JH, Chan FW, Wong RS, Cheng G. The potential clinical and economic outcomes of pharmacogenetics-oriented management of warfarin therapy—a decision analysis. *Thromb Haemost.* September 2004;92(3):590–597.

42. McWilliam A, Lutter R, Nardinelli C. Health care savings from personalizing medicine using genetic testing: the case of warfarin. 2006, AEI-Brookings Joint Center for Regulatory Studies.

43. *Pharmacogenetics: Ethical Issues.* London, UK: Nuffield Council on Bioethics; 2003.

44. Flockhart DA, O'Kane D, Williams MS, et al. Pharmacogenetic testing of CYP2C9 and VKORC1 alleles for warfarin. *Genet Med.* February 2008;10(2):139–150.

32

Hereditary hemochromatosis: population screening for gene mutations

Diana B. Petitti

Introduction

A summary of the state of knowledge about hereditary hemochromatosis written 15 years ago would read thus:

> Hemochromatosis, characterized by cirrhosis, diabetes, and bronzing of the skin, is an autosomal recessive condition due to mutation of the gene that regulates intestinal iron absorption. The genetic mutation, when present in the homozygous state, leads to the progressive deposition of excess iron in the liver, pancreas, heart, pituitary gland, and joints. Iron overload ultimately causes organ failure, principally liver failure, and death. The gene mutation causing hemochromatosis is highly prevalent in the United States, enough to warrant a program of universal screening of adults in primary care settings.

Today's scenario is much more complex for hereditary hemochromatosis. More importantly, experience with hereditary hemochromatosis shows that screening for genetic mutations requires evidence that permits certainty about three things: (i) the prevalence of the mutation(s) of the gene in diverse populations; (ii) the likelihood of development of disease in those with the mutation(s); and (iii) the ability of interventions to alter favorably the natural history of the disease in those with the mutation(s). Early anticipation of the need for research to address these issues could reduce the time between the discovery of a gene–disease association and the beneficial application of this knowledge to population health.

History

Trousseau, a French physician, is credited with the first published description, in 1865, of cases of a syndrome characterized by the triad of diabetes, cirrhosis, and a generalized darkening to "bronze" in skin color (1). In 1889, von Recklinghausen established that the discoloration of the skin and tissues in patients with this syndrome was accompanied by the deposition of iron (2). He named the iron-storage pigment in patients with the syndrome "hemosiderin" from the Greek *síderos* for iron and *haima* for blood because he thought the pigment came from blood. The clinical condition was named "hemochromatosis" from the Greek *haima* for blood and *chrôma* for color.

Over the next five decades, numerous case reports and case series were published describing this syndrome. It was variously considered to be a complication of diabetes, a complication of cirrhosis or, because of the similarity of its liver pathology to that in Wilson's disease, a result of chronic copper poisoning. There was, however, no consensus about the cause.

In 1935, in a "meta-series," Sheldon summarized information on more than 300 cases of hemochromatosis reported in the world literature (3). He concluded that the hallmark of hemochromatosis was deposition of iron in tissues throughout the body. He was the first to suggest that hemochromatosis was a familial disorder.

By the mid-1960s, clinical cases of the triad of diabetes, cirrhosis, and skin discoloration with increased tissue iron were virtually universally called "hemochromatosis," or "idiopathic hemochromatosis." Its familial nature was recognized, but controversy about whether it was a genetic disease persisted.

In the 1960s, MacDonald and colleagues provided epidemiologic evidence to support a genetic basis for idiopathic hemochromatosis (4). In 1976, French researchers showed an association of idiopathic hemochromatosis with HLA-A3 and HLA-B4 (5). In 1996, Feder et al. (6) identified two specific mutations of a single gene, the *HFE* gene, in more than 90% of patients with the clinical features of idiopathic hemochromatosis. Beutler et al. (7) reported virtually identical findings in an independent analysis of 147 clinically diagnosed cases. The contribution of mutations in a specific gene to the clinical condition originally described by Trousseau was established.

Terminology

Confusion

In the period from Sheldon's publication until the late 1970s, the term "hemochromatosis" denoted the clinical disease characterized by diabetes, cirrhosis, and skin discoloration due to tissue iron deposition. The term "hemosiderosis" was used to describe the presence of an increase in iron stores with or without tissue damage.

Starting in the late 1970s, the term "hemochromatosis" began to be used in different ways by different people. Most importantly, it began to be used not only to describe clinical cases of classical hemochromatosis, but also to describe an increase in iron stores whether or not accompanied by tissue damage. That is, what was previously called hemosiderosis became hemochromatosis!

In 1996, after identification of specific gene mutations in patients with the triad of features seen in the cases originally reported by Trousseau (6,7), the term "hemochromatosis" began to be used often to describe having a genotype that could *potentially* lead to disease with these features. It also was sometimes used to refer to any genotype that could *potentially* lead to increased iron stores.

Different authors, and even the same authors writing at different times, have used the term "hemochromatosis" in different ways. Understandably, the lack of clarity of terms causes confusion and makes it somewhat difficult to read the literature.

Terminology and Scope

This chapter uses the term "hemochromatosis" to describe both (i) the presence of increased iron stores from any cause, and (ii) the presence of any gene mutation that has been found to lead or potentially lead to an increase in iron stores. This terminology is the same as that used by Beutler in his chapter on Disorders of Iron Metabolism in the 2006 edition of the textbook, *Williams Hematology* (8). "Iron overload" is used to describe increases in iron stores measured in either serum or tissue.

Hemochromatosis is usually divided into primary and secondary hemochromatosis (8). Secondary hemochromatosis is defined as iron overload from extrinsic causes such as exposure to red cell blood products from, for example, repeated red cell transfusions to treat anemia. All other hemochromatoses are primary (nonsecondary). This chapter is limited to primary hemochromatoses. More specifically, the chapter deals only with "hereditary hemochromatosis" (HHC), which is defined as primary iron overload associated with (known) gene mutations.

Primary Hemochromatosis Classification

Overview

Table 32.1 summarizes the classification of hemochromatosis and iron overload syndrome and what is known (February 2008) about the genes and mutations that have been found in people with clinical disease due to iron overload (8,9).

It is now known that there is more than one gene whose mutation(s) can cause iron overload and widespread tissue damage as a consequence of iron overload. That is, there is not a single condition of HHC. Rather, there are multiple HHCs.

Hereditary Hemochromatosis Type 1

The clinical disease consisting of the triad of diabetes, cirrhosis, and skin discoloration with widespread tissue iron deposition described by Trousseau is now called HHC type 1 or "classical" hemochromatosis. Two single-base substitutions (C282Y and H63D) in a single gene—the *HFE* gene—were found in 90% of clinically diagnosed HHC type 1 cases in the first two reports about the gene mutation (6,7). In both of these series, C282Y homozygosity was found in 83% of clinical cases.

Later research confirmed that about 80–90% of white patients with clinical HHC are homozygous for the C282Y mutation of the *HFE* gene; an additional 3–6% are compound C282Y/H63D heterozygotes (8,9). A third mutation of the *HFE* gene, the S65C mutation, is also associated with clinically manifest HHC type 1 in whites, accounting for about 1% of clinical cases in patients without either a C182Y or H63D

Table 32.1 Primary hemochromatosis

Name of Condition or Syndrome	Type Designation	Clinical Features	Pathophysiology	Chromosome OMIM Number	Encoded Protein (Gene)	Detection
Classical hemochromatosis	HHC Type 1	Accumulation of iron in tissues with organ damage leading to diabetes, cirrhosis, bronze skin color in middle age; M > F	Increased intestinal iron absorption	6p3 235200	??? (HFE)	Gene mutation C282Y/C282Y C282Y/H63D Elevated transferrin Elevated ferritin
Juvenile hemochromatosis	HHC Type 2 Subtype A	Rapid accumulation of iron in tissues starting from birth with types of organ damage as in HHC type 1 but organ failure is observed at ages less than 30 years; hypogonadism is common at presentation; M = F	Increased intestinal iron absorption	1q21 602390	hemojuvelin (HJV)	Elevated transferrin Elevated ferritin
	HHC Type 2 Subtype B		Increased intestinal iron absorption	19q13.1 606464	Hepcidin antimicrobial peptide (HAMP)	Elevated transferrin Elevated ferritin
TfR2 hemochromatosis	HHC Type 3	Same as HHC Type 1	Increased intestinal iron absorption	7q 604250	transferrin receptor-2 (TFR2)	Elevated transferrin Elevated ferritin
Ferroportin-related iron overload	HHC Type 4		Abnormal retention of iron	2q32 606069	ferroportin (SLC11A3)	Low or normal transferrin Elevated ferritin

Other Genetic

Aceruloplasminemia	None	Accumulation of iron prominently in the brain but also in liver and in pancreas	Reduced iron transport due to ferrioxidase deficiency	604290	ceruloplasmin	Elevated ferritin Anemia
Neonatal hemochromatosis	None			231100	Unknown	None
OTHER						
African iron overload syndrome	None	Hepatomegaly, cirrhosis, impotence, diabetes; anemia	Increased iron absorption in response to dietary exposure	601105	?ferroportin? (SCL40A1)?	Elevated transferrin Elevated ferritin Mild anemia

Modified from Beutler (8) and Pietrangelo (9).

mutation (10). Other variations of the *HFE* gene have been reported in clinical cases of HHC type 1 (11) and the general population.

In HHC type 1, iron absorption from the gastrointestinal tract is increased, causing higher than average levels of serum iron and increased iron storage. A consequence is deposition of iron in the liver, pancreas, heart, joints, and the pituitary gland, leading to organ failure in middle age in some people.

Men are more likely to be observed in clinical series of HHC type 1. In one large series of clinical HC cases in Brittany ($n = 711$, all presumably whites), the ratio of men to women was 3:1 in clinical HC cases that were C282Y homozygotes and 7:1 in clinical cases that were non-C282Y homozygotes (10). The interaction of mutations of the *HFE* gene was suggested as an explanation for the difference in the sex ratio between C282Y homozygotes and nonhomozygotes. Emerging data indicates that HHC is determined by complex mutation–mutation, gene–gene, and gene–environment interactions.

Hereditary Hemochromatosis Type 2A, Type 2B, Type 3, and Type 4

Juvenile hemochromatosis, now called HHC type 2, is a rare autosomal recessive condition that results in rapid accumulation of iron beginning in early life (8,9). The clinical features of the condition are the same as in HHC type 1 except that organ failure occurs before age 30, hypogonadism is a common clinical presentation, and males and females are equally affected. HHC type 2 is subdivided into HHC type 2A and HHC type 2B. HHC type 2A is associated with mutations in the JVC gene that encodes hemojuvelin and maps to chromosome 1 (12). HHC type 2B is associated with mutations in the HAMP gene that encodes hepcidin and maps to chromosome 19 (13).

Hepcidin is believed to affect the intestinal absorption; hemojuvelin modulates hepcidin expression (9). Increased iron absorption is observed in both HHC type 2A and type 2B.

The clinical condition observed in HHC type 3 is indistinguishable from that in HHC type 1. It is also characterized by increased intestinal iron absorption (8,9). It is inherited as an autosomal recessive condition. HHC type 3 is associated with mutations in the transferrin receptor-2 gene (14).

HHC type 4 differs from the other HHCs in that it is inherited in an autosomal dominant pattern (8). Iron accumulates in the reticuloendothelial space. The clinical condition in patients with HHC type 4 is the same as in patients with HHC type 1, but milder. The condition is associated with a mutation in the *SLC40A1* gene (15), which encodes ferroportin, a main iron export protein.

Other Hemochromatoses with a Known Genetic Contribution

Iron overload occurs in a number of hereditary conditions including atransferrinemia, aceruloplasminemia, X-linked hereditary sideroblastic anemia, thalassemia major, congenital dyserythropoietic anemia, various red cell deficiencies, Friederich's ataxia, and Hallervorden–Spatz syndrome (16,17). In some of these, iron deposition may lead to a clinical condition that is like hereditary hemochromatosis, although subtle differences may be found on closer examination. Aceruloplasminemia, for example, is a rare autosomal recessive disorder that results from deficiency in ceruloplasmin ferrioxidase activity due to a mutation in the ceruloplasmin gene (18). Accumulation of iron in the central nervous system is a prominent feature.

Neonatal hemochromatosis is a rare gestational condition in which iron accumulates in fetal tissues in a distribution similar to that seen in HHC type 1 (8). Although the condition is suspected to have a genetic basis, neither HHC type 1 nor other iron storage diseases have been identified in siblings or parents of probands (19), and no pathologic mutations have been found in genes implicated in iron metabolism (beta-2-microglobulin, *HFE*, and haem oxygenases 1 and 2 (20)). Maternal factors may be important in at least some cases (21).

African Iron Overload

African iron overload was first observed in Africans in South Africa. The condition was considered to be due solely to high dietary intake of iron due to consumption of homemade beer brewed in iron barrels (22). Once considered benign, it is now known that iron overload in Africans can lead to cirrhosis, diabetes, and widespread deposition of iron in tissues and cause a clinical condition that is indistinguishable from HHC type 1 (23). Iron overload unexplained by diet, supplements, or transfusion is also found in black African Americans (24,25).

As early as 1992, it was considered that African iron overload might be due to an interaction of one or more genes with dietary iron intake (26). The C282Y mutation in the *HFE* gene does not explain iron overload in Africans (27).

Two reports have linked higher ferritin levels in both Africans and African Americans with a mutation (G248H) in the *ferroportin 1* gene (28,29). However, in one study, only 2 of 13 African American patients with severe clinical disease due to iron overload were heterozygous for this mutation (30). In another study in African Americans (31), the Q248H-associated risk of iron overload in African Americans was 1.57 (95% CI 0.52, 4.72), which was not statistically significant.

The contributions of genes, environment, and their interactions to iron absorption, transport, and the development of hemochromatosis in African Americans are not well understood and are being actively investigated.

Population Screening for Mutations That Cause Hereditary Hemochromatosis

Overview

Population screening for hemochromatosis has been discussed many times over the past 20 years (32–38). The possibility of screening for the gene mutation that is associated with most clinical cases of HHC type 1 became a reality after identification of the *HFE* gene and development of a test. Treatment with periodic phlebotomy reduces iron stores and probably prevents progression to clinical disease in those with iron overload. Importantly, the gene mutation associated with HHC type 1 has a high prevalence in some populations.

In 2005, the United States Preventive Services Task Force (USPSTF) recommended against population screening for *HFE* gene mutations that cause HHC (39). This organization recommended against population screening for gene mutation because of the low prevalence of unexplained liver disease in the general population and uncertainty about how often clinically important disease develops in people homozygous for the C282Y mutation. Uncertainty about the ability of phlebotomy treatment to prevent the consequences of iron overload in people homozygous for the mutation was also a consideration.

In 2006, the Clinical Molecular Genetics Society published a guideline that stated that "population screening is not currently recommended primarily due to the penetrance issue surrounding the C282Y mutation" (40). In 2008, the Swedish Council on Technology Assessment in Health Care joined the USPSTF in recommending against screening for hemochromatosis in Sweden using genetic testing (41).

Prevalence of Mutations Associated with Clinical Disease

The prevalence of homozygosity for the C282Y and H63D mutation of the *HFE* gene varies by race and, within whites, by geography. Table 32.2 shows data from the Hemochromatosis and Iron Overload Study (HEIRS (42)), which was conducted in the United States and Canada and involved more than 100,000 participants. In HEIRS, the prevalence of C282Y homozygosity was very low in blacks and Native Americans (<1 per 1,000). In Asians in the United States (42) and elsewhere (43), the mutation is almost nonexistent. The prevalence of C282Y homozygosity in non-Hispanic whites in HEIRS was 4.4 per 1,000. However, the best estimate of prevalence of C282Y homozygosity in whites in the United States—3.3 per 1,000— comes from Steinberg et al. (44), who assessed a representative population of whites in the United States. The prevalence of the C282Y homozygosity varies from 2 to 8 per 1,000 in white European populations and whites of European origin living in Australia and New Zealand (43).

In populations where the prevalence of the C282Y mutation is negligible or zero, the value of screening to identify C282Y heterozygotes is also negligible or zero. Thus, mutation screening in Asians, Africans, African Americans, Native Americans, Pacific Islanders, and Hispanics would have no value.

Natural History of C282Y Homozygosity

The natural history of C282Y homozygosity remains uncertain. It is a critical issue in deciding whether and whom to screen. The best evidence to address the question of disease development in C282Y homozygotes derives from population-based cohort studies with long follow-up and systematic examination of individuals who

Table 32.2 Prevalence per 1,000 of C282Y and H63D homozygosity and C282Y/H63D compound heterozygosity by ethnicity in the United States

Place	Number	c282y/c282y		c282y/h63d		h63d/h63d	
		Prevalence / 1,000	(95% CI)	Prevalence / 1,000	(95% CI)	Prevalence / 1,000	(95% CI)
United States							
White	44,082	4.4	(4.2, 4.7)	20	(20, 21)	24	(23, 24)
Native American	648	1.1	(0.61, 2.0)	7.7	(0.6, 1.1)	13	(10, 18)
Hispanic	12,459	0.27	(0.22, 0.32)	3.3	(0.3, −0.4)	11	(10, 11)
Black	21,124	0.14	(0.12, 0.17)	0.71	(0.1, 0.1)	0.89	(0.81, 0.97)
Pacific Islander	698	0.12	(0.043, 0.32)	0.96	(0.55,1.7)	2	(1.2, 3.2)
Asian	12,772	0.00039	(0.00015, 0.0010)	0.055	(0.029, 0.093)	2	(1.7, 2.2)

Table data are adapted from the Hemochromatosis and Iron-Overload Screening (HEIRS) study (Adams et al.) (42)

are C282Y homozygotes. Ascertainment of liver disease is important because it is the most serious documented consequence of iron overload due to the C282Y mutation.

In their systematic evidence review conducted for the USPSTF, Whitlock et al. (45) identified two population-based cohort studies that assessed the risk of clinical hemochromatosis (46,47). Both studies were rated as fair to good in quality. A third population-based cohort study published in 2008 (48) provides evidence on this issue. It would likely be rated fair to good. Table 32.3 summarizes these three studies and their findings.

All three studies were done either in almost exclusively white and European populations (e.g., Australia and Copenhagen before the 1990s) or enrolled only white people of European lineage. All of them assessed C282Y mutations in participants and attempted to determine whether the C282Y homozygotes developed serious clinical disease putatively related to iron overload, including but not limited to liver disease and diabetes. Two of the studies (47,48) assessed iron overload using transferrin saturation and ferritin in C282Y homozygotes and/or evaluated the trajectory of serum iron parameters in the C282Y homozygotes.

The prevalence of C282Y homozygosity was 5.2 per 1,000 in one Australian study (46) and 6.8 per 1,000 in the other (48). The prevalence of C282Y homozygosity was 2.5 per 1,000 in the Copenhagen study (46). In the two studies with serum iron measures (46,47), C282Y homozygous men were much more likely to have or to develop possible iron overload based on serum tests.

Serious clinical disease developed in 14% of C282Y male homozygotes (1 in 7) men in the Copenhagen study followed for 25 years (46), 50% of men (2 in 6) in the Brusselton study followed for 17 years (47), and 28.4% of the men (21 in 74) in the Melbourne study followed for 12 years (48). Aggregating across the three studies, only 1% of women (1 in 106) who were C282Y homozygotes developed serious clinical disease.

In all three studies, follow-up was incomplete and information on clinically manifest disease in C282Y homozygotes was poor or missing. People with a clinical diagnosis of hemochromatosis at the time of entry into the study were sometimes not counted as having serious clinical disease unless they were examined in the study. The results of the Melbourne study (48) were affected by the use of phlebotomy to treat people identified as C282Y homozygotes because of participation in the study. Finally, the age of subjects at entry and their attained ages at the end of follow-up varied. In none of the studies was there more than 70% of subjects 65+ years of age at the end of published follow-up. Because the development of clinical liver disease increases with age, none of the studies has yet to provide a complete picture of serious morbidity developing over the entire lifespan in people who are C282Y homozygotes.

Using data from the two studies published at the time of the review (46,47), Whitlock et al. (45) estimated that 25–60% of C282Y homozygotes would develop clinical disease. The upper bound of this estimate was based on an assumption that

Table 32.3 Population-based follow-up studies of C282Y homozygosity

Author and Reference Place Duration of Follow-up	Number Tested	% White/Northern European	Number C282Y Homozygotes	Prevalence of C282Y Homozygosity	Elevated Iron Parameters in C282Y Homozygotes	Serious Clinical Disease* in C282Y Homozygotes with Follow-up
Andersen et al. (46) Copenhagen, Denmark 25 years	9,174	>95%	n=23	2.5/1,000	No data	Female 0/16 0% Male 1/7 14%
Olynyk et al. (47) Brusselton, Australia 17 years	3,011	100%	n=16	5.3/1,000	Both transferrin and ferritin elevated Female 2/6 33% Male 4/4 100%	Female 0/6 0% Male 3/6 50%
Allen et al. (48) Melbourne, Australia 12 years	29,676	100%	n=203	6.8/1,000	Ferritin >1000 µg/L Female 7/84 8.3% Male 33/74 44.6%	Female 1/84 1.2% Male 21/74 28.4%

* Clinical diagnosis of hemochromatosis; liver fibrosis or cirrhosis at examination; diabetes mellitus attributed to hemochromatosis; liver fibrosis or cirrhosis at examination; diabetes mellitus attributed to hemochromatosis in Andersen et al. (46) and Olynyk et al. (47). Allen et al. (48) also considered joint disease and elevated liver enzymes as serious clinical conditions attributed to hemochromatosis.

all 3 of the 23 participants in the Copenhagen study known to be C282Y homozygotes who died before examination and all 25 of the nonparticipants in the genetic screening component of the study who were expected to be C282Y homozygotes would have developed clinical disease. Sixty percent is thus the extreme upper bound for development of clinical disease in C282Y homozygotes. The estimate applies only to men even as an extreme upper bound. This conclusion is not altered by findings in the Allen et al. study (48).

The low likelihood of development of clinical disease in European and American white women with C282Y homozygosity argues strongly against mutation screening of women of any race/ethnicity.

Alteration of Progression to Disease in C282Y Homozygotes

There is no point in finding people who have mutations associated with disease unless the progression to disease in people with the mutation can be favorably altered. Phlebotomy reduces iron stores. It is a clinically accepted approach for the treatment of hemochromatosis and is widely believed to improve outcomes in people with documented iron overload and/or clinical disease. Phlebotomy is also used to decrease iron stores in people who are identified as C282Y/C282Y homozygotes to prevent progression to clinical disease.

The 2004 American College of Physicians systematic review of hemochromatosis screening (49) identified 409 potentially relevant publications about the effect of phlebotomy on outcomes in clinical hemochromatosis. After screening the 409 studies and judging them against explicit quality standards, only two—Milman et al. (50) and Niederau et al. (51)—met the American College of Physicians standards. A third study published in 2006 (52) provides outcome information based on liver biopsies and is discussed here.

The first study (50) involved patients with clinical HC who were not genotyped but who probably had HHC type 1 based on clinical signs and the geography and timeframe (Denmark from 1951 to 1975). It compared survival after an average of 8.5 years in the 128 patients who were adequately phlebotomized with survival in those who were inadequately phlebotomized. At 5 years, the estimated survival of adequately phlebotomized patients ($n = 66$) was 93% compared with 48% for inadequately phlebotomized patients ($n = 62$). At 10 years, estimated survival was 78% for adequately phlebotomized patients compared with 32% for inadequately phlebotomized patients.

The second study (51) involved 185 patients with clinical HC who were not genotyped but who probably had HHC type 1 based on clinical signs and symptoms and geography and time (Dusseldorf, Germany 1982–1991). It assessed the results of baseline and repeat biopsies before and after the use of phlebotomy treatment that lasted an average of 14 years. Forty-two patients (23%) had improved liver histology, two (1%) had liver pathology that deteriorated, and 141 (76%) had liver histology that did not change. The findings are interpreted as evidence of an effect of phlebotomy in halting progression of liver damage.

The third study (52) evaluated longitudinal changes in hepatic fibrosis in 20 patients (of 25 who had two biopsies) who were C282Y homozygotes. It showed decreases in hepatic fibrosis after phlebotomy in C282Y homozygotes.

The evidence on the effectiveness of phlebotomy for treatment of clinical HC has limitations. No study involved randomization, but randomization might not be possible because of the strongly held belief in treatment efficacy. On the other hand, the studies are consistent in finding a beneficial effect of phlebotomy; harms have not been identified; cost and inconvenience are unmeasured. The beginning age for phlebotomy in people with mutations, the best phlebotomy regimen, and the precise risks remain undefined.

Gene–Environment Interactions in HHC Type 1

The suggested explanation for the lower rate of serious clinical disease in female C282Y homozygotes is menstrual blood loss. Anecdotal reports and some data from longitudinal studies of C282Y homozygotes and clinical studies link C282Y homozygosity with drinking alcohol. In both of the longitudinal Australian studies that followed C282Y homozygotes, men drank more alcohol than women (47,48). The possibility that differences in alcohol consumption contribute to the higher risk of developing clinical disease in male compared with female C282Y homozygotes should be studied.

Data from the Brusselton study suggest that the trajectory of serum iron parameters is highly variable between individuals over time (47). Factors other than blood loss and alcohol use, both genetic and environmental, could affect the development of clinical disease in C282Y homozygotes. Dietary iron intake and exposure to iron through ingestion of supplements and in water may modify the development of disease in C282Y homozygotes. This is another important avenue for further research.

Selective Screening of High-Risk Groups

Early enthusiasm for universal population-based screening for genetic mutations in the *HFE* gene has waned. Targeted screening of high-risk groups (e.g., white men of Celtic origin) remains an option. Targeted screening for most diseases is an efficient way to make screening programs less costly and to minimize screening harms due to false positives.

Iron overload defined as high serum ferritin and/or cirrhosis has been found in a high proportion of C282Y homozygotes identified through family screening of probands—patients who are C282Y homozygotes and have clinical disease (53). The prevalence of C282Y homozygosity among family members of probands is higher than in the general population (54).

Screening family members of probands has been recommended by some experts (55,56). The USPSTF made no specific recommendation against screening the family member of probands (40).

There is a strong case for screening the brothers of male and female probands (clinical cases of HHC type 1) for iron overload based on serum tests of iron overload at age 35–40 years. The likelihood of the proband being a C282Y homozygote is at least 80%, and 40% of brothers are likely to be C282Y homozygotes. Even if only 20% of homozygotes develop clinically manifest disease, as many as 8% of the brothers of probands might have a poor clinical course. The consequences of failure to detect iron overload in a male relative of a documented case of clinically manifest HHC type 1 are potentially large.

Screening for the C282Y mutation in other groups that have been suggested as being at high risk of clinical disease that can be caused by the mutation—for example, people with diabetes, arthritis, cirrhosis—is discussed in detail by Whitlock et al. (45). The evidence provides no support for screening for the C282Y mutation in any population group except male relatives of HHC type 1 probands.

Summary and Conclusion

Hemochromatosis continues to fascinate and puzzle. It encompasses issues of importance to basic scientists, clinical researchers, clinicians, epidemiologists, public health professionals, and policy makers. Understanding its history, the evolution of our knowledge about it, and the current state of knowledge provides rich insights into the genetics of disease and the complexity of the genetic determinants of disease and health in humans. This chapter touches only briefly on the many lessons that can be learned by considering hemochromatosis in historical context.

References

1. Trousseau A. Glycosurie, diabète sucré. In: Baillière et fils, editor. *Clinique Médicale de l'Hôtel-Dieu de Paris,* 2nd ed, Vol. 2. Paris: 1865:663–698.
2. von Recklinghausen FD. Ueber Haemachromatose. *Tageblatt Versammlung Dtsche Naturforscheer Arzte Heidelberg.* 1889;62:324–325.
3. Sheldon JH. *Haemochromatosis.* London: Oxford University Press; 1935.
4. MacDonald RA. Idiopathic hemochromatosis. Genetic or acquired? *Prog Hematol.* 1966;5:324–353.
5. Simon M, Bourel M, Fauchet R, Genetet B. Association of HLA-A3 and HLA-B14 antigens with idiopathic hemochromatosis. *Gut.* 1976;17:332–334.
6. Feder JN, Gnirke A, Thomas W, et al. A novel MHC class I-like gene is mutated in patients with hereditary haemochromatosis. *Nat Genet.* 1996;13:399–408.
7. Beutler E, Gelbart T, West C, et al. Mutation analysis in hereditary hemochromatosis. *Blood Cells Mol Dis.* 1996;22:187–194.
8. Beutler E. Disorders of iron metabolism. In: Lichtman MA, Beutler E, Kipps TJ, Seligsohn U, Koushansky K, Pachal JT, eds. *Willams Hematology.* New York: McGraw-Hill; 2006:511–553.
9. Pietrangelo A. Hereditary hemochromatosis—a new look at an old disease. *N Engl J Med.* 2004;350:2383–2397.
10. Mura C, Raguenes O, Férec C. HFE mutations analysis in 711 hemochromatosis probands: evidence for S65C implication in mild form of hemochromatosis. *Blood.* 1999;93:2502–2505.

11. Wallace DF, Dooley JS, Walker AP. A novel mutation of HFE explains the classical phenotype of genetic hemochromatosis in a C282Y heterozygote. *Gastroenterology.* 1999;116:1409–1412.

12. Papanikolaou G, Samuels ME, Ludwig EH, et al. Genetic abnormalities and juvenile hemochromatosis: mutations of the HJV gene encoding hemojuvelin. *Blood.* 2004;103:4669–4671.

13. Majore S, Binni F, Pennese A, De Santis A, Crisi A, Grammatico P. HAMP gene mutation c.208T>C (p.C70R) identified in an Italian patient with severe hereditary hemochromatosis. *Hum Mutat.* 2004;23:400.

14. Camaschella C, Roetto A, Cali A, et al. The gene TFR2 is mutated in a new type of haemochromatosis mapping to 7q22. *Nat Genet.* 2000;25:14–15.

15. Montosi G, Donovan A, Totaro A, et al. Autosomal-dominant hemochromatosis is associated with a mutation in the ferroportin (SLC11A3) gene. *J Clin Invest.* 2001;108:619–623.

16. Beutler E, Felitti V, Gelbart T, Ho N. Genetics of iron storage and hemochromatosis. *Drug Metab Dispos.* 2001;29:494–499.

17. Ponka P. Rare causes of hereditary iron overload. *Semin Hematol.* 2002;39:249–262.

18. Loreal O, Turlin B, Pgeon C, et al. Aceruloplasminemia: new clinical, pathophysiological and therapeutic insights. *J Hepatol.* 2002;36:851–856.

19. Dalhoj J, Klaer H, Wiggers P, Grandy RW, Jones RL, Knisely AS. Iron storage disease in parents and sibs of infants with hemochromatosis: 30-year follow-up. *Am J Med Genet.* 1990;37:342–345.

20. Kelly AL, Lunt PW, Rodrigues F, et al. Classification and genetic feature of neonatal hemochromatosis: a study of 27 affected pedigrees and molecular analysis of genes implicated in iron metabolism. *J Med Genet.* 2001;38:599–610.

21. Knisely AS, Mieli-Vergani G, Whitington PF. Neonatal hemochromatosis. *Gastroenterol Clin North Am.* 2003;32:877–889, vi–vii.

22. Bothwell TH, Seftel H, Jacob P, Torrance JD, Baumslag N. Iron overload in Bantu subjects. Studies on the availability of iron in Bantu beer. *Am J Clin Nutr.* 1964;14:47–51.

23. MacPhail AP, Mandishona EM, Bloom PD, Paterson AC, Rouault TA, Gordeuk VR. Measurements of iron status and survival in African iron overload. *S Afr Med J.* 1999;89:966–972.

24. Barton JC, Edwards CQ, Bertoli LF, Shroyer TW, Hudson SL. Iron overload in African Americans. *Am J Med.* 1995;99:616–623.

25. Wurapa RK, Gordeuk VR, Brittenham, GM, Khiyami A, Schechter GP, Edwards CQ. Primary iron overload in African Americans. *Am J Med.* 1996;101:9–18.

26. Gordeuk V, Mukiibi J, Hasstedt SJ, et al. Iron overload in Africa. Interaction between a gene and dietary iron content. *N Engl J Med.* 1992;326:95–100.

27. McNamara L, MacPhail AP, Gordeuk VR, Hasstedt SJ, Rouault T. Is there a link between African iron overload and the described mutations of the hereditary haemochromatosis gene? *Br J Haematol.* 1998;102:1176–1178.

28. Gordeuk VR, Caleffi A, Corradini E, et al. Iron overload in Africans and African-Americans and a common mutation in the SCL40A1 (ferroportin 1) gene. *Blood Cells Mol Dis.* 2003;31:299–304.

29. Beutler E, Barton JC, Felitti VJ, et al. Ferroportin 1 (SCL40A1) variant associated with iron overload in African-Americans. *Blood Cells Mol Dis.* 2003;31:305–309.

30. Barton JC, Acton RT, Rivers CA, et al. Genotypic and phenotypic heterogeneity of African Americans with primary iron overload. *Blood Cells Mol Dis.* November–December 2003;31(3):310–319.

31. Barton JC, Acton RT, Lee PL, West C. SLC40A1 Q248H allele frequency and Q248H-associated risk of non-HFE iron overload in person of sub-Saharan African descent. *Blood Cells Mol Dis.* 2007;39:206–211.

32. Edwards CQ, Kushner JP. Screening for hemochromatosis. *N Engl J Med.* 1993;328:1616–1620.
33. Bradley LA, Haddow JE, Palomaki GE. Population screening for haemochromatosis: a unifying analysis of published intervention trials. *J Med Screen.* 1996;3:178–187.
34. Witte DL, Crosby WH, Edwards CQ, Fairbanks VF, Mitros FA. Practice guideline development task force of the College of American Pathologists. Hereditary hemochromatosis. *Clinica Chimica Acta.* 1996;245:139–200.
35. Cogswell ME, McDonnell SM, Khoury MJ, Franks AL, Burke W, Brittenham G. Iron overload, public health, and genetics: evaluating the evidence for hemochromatosis screening. *Ann Intern Med.* 1998;129:971–979.
36. Cogswell ME, Burke W, McDonnell SM, Franks AL. Screening for hemochromatosis. A public health perspective. *Am J Prev Med.* 1999;16:134–140.
37. Njajou OT, Alizadeh BZ, van Duijn CM. Is genetic screening for hemochromatosis worthwhile? *Eur J Epidemiol.* 2004;19:101–108.
38. Allen K, Williamson R. Screening for hereditary hemochromatosis should be implemented now. *BMJ.* 2000;320:183–184.
39. U.S. Preventive Services Task Force. Screening for hemochromatosis: recommendation statement. *Ann Intern Med.* 2006;145:204–208.
40. Screening for hemochromatosis by genetic testing. Available at http://www.sbu.se/en/Medical-Science-and-practice/Vetenskap-och-praxis/2259/. Accessed June 18, 2009.
41. King C, Barton DE. Best practice guidelines for the molecular genetic diagnosis of Type 1 (HFE-related) hereditary haemochromatosis. *BMC Med Genet.* 2006;7:81.
42. Adams PC, Reboussin DM, Barton JC, et al. Hemochromatosis and iron-overload screening in a racially diverse population. *N Engl J Med.* 2005;352:1769–1778.
43. Merryweather-Clarke AT, Pointon JJ, Shearman JD, Robson KJ. Global prevalence of the putative haemochromatosis mutation. *J Med Genet.* 1997;34:275–278.
44. Steinberg KK, Cogswell ME, Chang JC, et al. Prevalence of C282Y and H63D mutations in the hemochromatosis (HFE) gene in the United States. *JAMA.* 2001;285:2216–2222.
45. Whitlock EP, Garlitz BA, Harris EL, Beil TL, Smith PR. Screening for hereditary hemochromatosis: a systematic review for the U.S. Preventive Services Task Force. *Ann Intern Med.* 2006;145:209–223.
46. Andersen RV, Tybjaerg-Hansen A, Appleyard M, Birgens H, Nordestgaard BG. Hemochromatosis mutations in the general population: iron overload progression rate. *Blood.* 2004;103:2914–2919.
47. Olynyk JK, Cullen DJ, Aquilia S, Rossi E, Summerville L, Powell LW. A population-based study of the clinical expression of the hemochromatosis gene. *N Engl J Med.* 1999;341:718–724.
48. Allen KJ, Gurrin LC, Constantine CC, et al. Iron-overload-related disease in HFE hereditary hemochromatosis. *N Engl J Med.* 2008;358:221–230.
49. Schmitt B, Golub RM, Green R. Screening primary care patients for hereditary hemochromatosis with transferring saturation and serum ferritin: systematic review for the American College of Physicians. *Ann Intern Med.* 2005;43:522–526.
50. Milman N, Pedersen P, A Steig T, Byg KE, Graudal N, Fenger K. Clinically overt hereditary hemochromotosis in Denmark 1948–1985: epidemiology, risk factors of significance for long-term survival, and causes of death in 179 patients. *Ann Hematol.* 2001;80:737–744.
51. Niederau C, Fischer R, Purschel A, Stremmel W, Haussinger D, Strohmeyer G. Long-term survival in patients with hereditary hemochromatosis. *Gastroenterology.* 1996;110:1107–1119.
52. Powell LW, Dixon JL, Ramm GA, et al. Hemochromatosis in asymptomatic subjects with or without a family history. *Arch Intern Med.* 2006;166:294–301.

53. Barton JC, Rothenberg BE, Bertoli LF, Acton RT. Diagnosis of hemochromatosis in family members of probands: a comparison of phenotyping and HFE genotyping. *Genet Med.* 1999;1:89–93.

54. McCune CA, Ravine D, Worwood M, Jackson HA, Evans HM, Hutton D. Screening for hereditary haemochromatosis within families and beyond. *Lancet.* 2003;362:1897–1898.

55. Imperatore G, Pinsky LE, Motulsky A, Reyes M, Bradley LA, Burke W. Hereditary hemochromatosis: perspectives of public health, medical genetics, and primary care. *Genet Med.* 2003;5:1–8.

56. Harrison H, Adams PC. Hemochromatosis. Common genes, uncommon illness? *Can Fam Physician.* 2002;48:1326–1333.

Index

Note: Page numbers in *italics* denote figures and tables.

Printed in the USA/Agawam, MA
May 16, 2013

575354.059